LANGUAGE DISORDERS

A Functional Approach to Assessment and Intervention in Children

SEVENTH EDITION

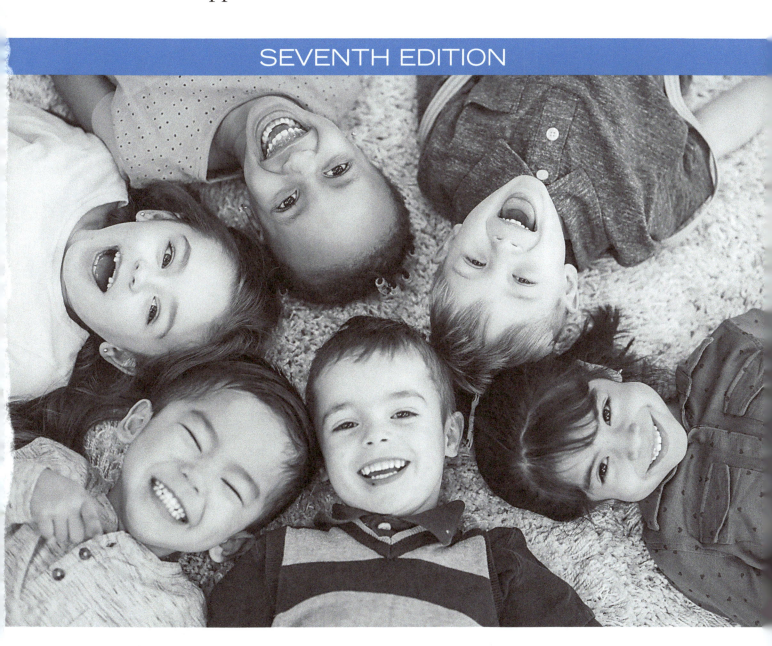

LANGUAGE DISORDERS

A Functional Approach to Assessment and Intervention in Children

SEVENTH EDITION

Robert E. Owens, Jr., PhD, CCC-SLP

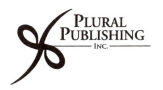

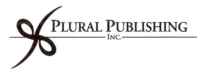

5521 Ruffin Road
San Diego, CA 92123

e-mail: information@pluralpublishing.com
Website: https://www.pluralpublishing.com

Copyright © 2024 by Plural Publishing, Inc.

Typeset in 10.5/14 Stone Serif by Flanagan's Publishing Services, Inc.
Printed in the United States of America by Integrated Books International

All rights, including that of translation, reserved. No part of this publication may be reproduced, stored in a retrieval system, or transmitted in any form or by any means, electronic, mechanical, recording, or otherwise, including photocopying, recording, taping, Web distribution, or information storage and retrieval systems without the prior written consent of the publisher.

This book was previously published by Pearson Education, Inc.

For permission to use material from this text, contact us by
Telephone: (866) 758-7251
Fax: (888) 758-7255
e-mail: permissions@pluralpublishing.com

Every attempt has been made to contact the copyright holders for material originally printed in another source. If any have been inadvertently overlooked, the publisher will gladly make the necessary arrangements at the first opportunity.

Library of Congress Cataloging-in-Publication Data

Names: Owens, Robert E., Jr., 1944- author.
Title: Language disorders : a functional approach to assessment and
  intervention in children / Robert E. Owens, Jr.
Description: Seventh edition. | San Diego, CA : Plural Publishing, Inc.,
  [2024] | Includes bibliographical references and index.
Identifiers: LCCN 2022034971 (print) | LCCN 2022034972 (ebook) | ISBN
  9781635504132 (paperback) | ISBN 1635504139 (paperback) | ISBN
  9781635504149 (ebook)
Subjects: MESH: Language Disorders | Language Therapy | Child | Infant
Classification: LCC RJ496.L35 (print) | LCC RJ496.L35 (ebook) | NLM WL
  340.2 | DDC 618.92/855--dc23/eng/20220826
LC record available at https://lccn.loc.gov/2022034971
LC ebook record available at https://lccn.loc.gov/2022034972

Contents

Preface .... *xiii*

Acknowledgments .... *xv*

CHAPTER 1. A FUNCTIONAL LANGUAGE APPROACH — 1

Language and Language Disorders 2
Traditional and Functional Models 4
    Traditional Intervention Approaches 4
    The Functional Approach 5
Role of Pragmatics in Intervention 6
    Dimensions of Communication Context 9
    Summary 9
Role of Generalization in Intervention 10
    Variables That Affect Generalization 11
Evidence-Based Practice 17
Getting "It" 19
Conclusion 20

CHAPTER 2. LANGUAGE DISORDERS — 23

Developmental and Educational Outcomes 24
Possible Risk and Related Factors 26
    Neurological Basis 27
    Aspects of Language Affected 28
Information Processing 29
    Attention 29
    Discrimination 30
    Organization 30
    Memory 30
    Processes 30
    Summary 31
Diagnostic Categories 32
    Continuum of Function 33
    Broad Groupings 34

Developmental Language Disorders... 34
Social Communication Disorder 49
Conclusion.. 52

CHAPTER 3. LANGUAGE DISORDERS ASSOCIATED WITH OTHER DISORDERS   55

Language Disorders Associated With Autism Spectrum Disorder................... 56
Development 57
Characteristics... 58
Risk Factors 59
Language Characteristics 59
Possible Causal Factors 64
Summary 66
Language Disorders Associated With Learning Disability/Specific 66
Learning Disorder
Description 67
Language Characteristics 68
Possible Causal Factors 70
Dyslexia/Specific Learning Disorder With Impairment in Reading 72
and Writing
Similar Disorders: Attention-Deficit/Hyperactivity Disorder 72
Seemingly Similar Disorders: Prenatal Drug and Alcohol Exposure 74
Summary 76
Language Disorders Associated With Intellectual Developmental Disorder 76
Language Characteristics 79
Possible Causal Factors 82
Language Disorders Associated With Neurocognitive Disorders................... 86
Traumatic Brain Injury 86
Cerebrovascular Accident... 90
Summary 91
Language Disorders Associated With Maltreatment: Neglect and Abuse 91
Language Characteristics 92
Possible Causal Factors 93
Summary 94
Language Disorders Associated With Less Frequent Disorders.................... 94
Late Language Emergence 95
Childhood Schizophrenia 96
Selective Mutism... 97
Otitis Media... 97
Deafness 97
Implications.. 98
Conclusion... 98

CHAPTER 4. EARLY COMMUNICATION INTERVENTION — 101

Legal Basis for Early Intervention	102
The Early Intervention Model	103
Children Served in ECI Programs	108
Established Risk	108
At-Risk Children	113
ECI Assessment	118
Transdisciplinary Model of Assessment	119
Family Concerns, Priorities, and Resources	120
Informal Communication Assessment	120
Formal Assessment	128
Organizing an Early Language and Communication Assessment	128
Considerations for Infants With Culturally/Linguistically Diverse Backgrounds	133
ECI Intervention	133
Use of Daily Routines	134
Telehealth	134
Record Keeping	134
Intervention Strategies	135
Natural Settings and Partners	135
Culturally Responsive Intervention	138
A Hybrid Model	139
Intervention for Children With Autism Spectrum Disorder	140
Augmentative and Alternative Communication	144
Types of AAC	145
Evidence-Based Practice	145
Assessment	146
AAC Intervention	148
Summary	154
Conclusion	155

CHAPTER 5. ASSESSMENT OF PRESCHOOL AND SCHOOL-AGE CHILDREN WITH LANGUAGE DISORDERS — 157

Psychometric Versus Descriptive Procedures	160
Normalist Assessment Measures	161
Descriptive Assessment Approaches	168
An Integrated Functional Assessment Strategy	174
Referral, Screening, Questionnaire, and Interview	175
Observation	177
Formal Language Testing	180

Assessment of Related Cognitive Factors 188
Dynamic Assessment 192
Sampling 192
Conclusion 193

CHAPTER 6. LANGUAGE SAMPLING — 195

Extent of Language Sampling Use 196
Planning a Language Sample 196
Representativeness 196
Language Sampling Contexts 198
Collecting a Language Sample 207
Conversational Samples 207
Narrative Samples 218
Recording the Sample 224
Collecting Samples of Written Language 224
Transcribing the Oral Sample 224
Utterances 226
Conclusion 228

CHAPTER 7. LANGUAGE SAMPLE ANALYSIS — 231

Levels of Language Sample Analysis 232
Communication Event 232
Across Utterances and Partners 251
Within Utterances 256
Narrative Analysis 284
Macrostructure Analysis 285
Microstructure Analysis 293
Reliability and Validity 300
Summary 301
Computer-Assisted Language Sample Analysis (CLSA) 301
Conclusion 303

CHAPTER 8. ASSESSMENT OF CHILDREN FROM CULTURALLY AND LINGUISTICALLY DIVERSE BACKGROUNDS — 305

Difference or Disorder? 306
State of Service Delivery 307
Lack of Academic Preparation 308
Unfamiliarity With Different Languages and Cultures 308

viii

Lack of Appropriate Assessment Tools 315
Summary 316
Language Assessment of a Child Who Is an ELL 316
Who Are ELLs? 317
Importance of Accurate Assessment 319
Overcoming Bias in Assessment of ELLs 319
An Integrated Model for Assessment for ELLs 322
Components 322
Language Assessment of Children Speaking NMAE 342
Careful Use of Standardized Tests 342
Alternative Assessment Approaches 344
Model of Language Assessment of a Child Who Speaks NMAE 346
Components 346
Conclusion 351

CHAPTER 9. A FUNCTIONAL INTERVENTION MODEL — 355

Guidelines 357
Be a Reinforcer 358
Closely Approximate Natural Learning 359
Follow Developmental Guidelines 359
Follow the Child's Lead 360
Actively Involve the Child 362
Remember the Influence of Context on Language 362
Use the Scripts Found in Familiar Events 362
Design a Generalization Plan First 363
Generalization Variables 363
Teaching Targets 364
Teaching Items 365
Method of Teaching 367
Language Teachers 370
Teaching Cues 379
Contingencies 380
Location 381
Conclusion 382

CHAPTER 10. MANIPULATING CONTEXT — 385

Nonlinguistic Contexts 386
Linguistic Contexts 389
Exposure to Grammatical Targets 389
Explicit Instruction 391

Conversational Milieu 393
Conversations: Top-Down Teaching 411
Conclusion 412

CHAPTER 11. SPECIFIC INTERVENTION TECHNIQUES   417

Cognitive Considerations 418
    Information Processing 419
Pragmatics 421
    Social Skills and Autism Spectrum Disorder 421
    Intentions 422
    Conversational Abilities 427
    Narration 436
Semantics 444
    Vocabulary and Word Meaning 444
    Semantic Categories and Relational Webs 454
    Word Retrieval and Categorization 461
    Comprehension 466
    Figurative Language 467
    Verbal Working Memory 469
Syntax and Morphology 472
    Morphology 472
    Word Order and Sentence Types 482
Children With CLD Backgrounds 488
Use of Microcomputers 491
Conclusion 492

CHAPTER 12. CLASSROOM FUNCTIONAL INTERVENTION   495

Background and Rationale: Recent Educational Changes 497
    Common Core State Standards 497
    Response to Intervention 498
    Inclusion 500
    Collaborative Teaching 501
    Summary 503
Role of the Speech-Language Pathologist 503
    Relating to Others 503
Language Intervention and Language Arts 505
Elements of a Classroom Model 506
    Identification of Children at Risk 506
Curriculum-Based Intervention 513
    CBLI Model 513

Classroom Demands.. 515
Instructional Approaches.. 517
Linguistic Awareness Intervention Within the Classroom........................ 518
Preschool 518
School-Age and Adolescent.. 524
Summary 526
Language Facilitation 527
Classroom Language Requirements 527
Talking With Children 537
Classroom Support for Children With Working Memory Deficits 539
Instituting a Classroom Model... 543
Conclusion 547

CHAPTER 13. LITERACY IMPAIRMENTS: LANGUAGE IN A VISUAL MODE — 549

Reading.. 551
Reading Comprehension and Inferencing 552
Reading Problems 553
Children With Culturally Linguistically Diverse Backgrounds.................. 557
Reading and Language Disorders 558
Contribution of Linguistic Awareness.................................... 559
Deficits in Comprehension... 560
Deficits in Inferencing... 561
Dyslexia 562
Assessment of Reading 564
Data Collection.. 564
Data Analysis 568
Assessment of Phonological Awareness 569
Assessment of Morphological Awareness................................. 569
Assessment of Comprehension... 570
Early Assessment of Dyslexia 570
Reading Assessment for Children With ASD 572
Language-Based Reading Intervention...................................... 573
Early Literacy Intervention 573
Preschool Emerging Literacy 574
School-Age Intervention 581
Writing.. 595
Writing Problems... 596
Assessment of Writing 598
Data Collection.. 598
Data Analysis 600
Spelling Assessment 603
Language-Based Writing Intervention 605

Extended Writing... 605
Spelling 609
Sentence Construction and Composition 612
Conclusion 613

Afterword *615*
Appendices
   A. Formal Language Measures 617
   B. SUGAR (Sampling Utterances and Grammatical Analysis Revised) 621
       Procedures
   C. Comparison of Computer-Based Language Sample Analysis Methods 629
   D. Selected English Morphological Prefixes and Suffixes 633
   E. Non-Majority American English Dialects and English Influenced by 635
       Other Languages
   F. Indirect Elicitation Techniques 641
   G. Intervention Activities and Language Targets............................... 643
   H. Use of Children's Literature in Preschool Classrooms 649
Glossary.. *657*
References *663*
Index.. *735*

Preface

The seventh edition of *Language Disorders: A Functional Approach to Assessment and Intervention in Children* is a special treat for me because I have joined a new publisher, Plural Publishing. I must admit that I was cautious but have found Plural to be welcoming and supportive. It already feels like home.

As with previous editions, this one is an exhaustive compilation of hundreds of professional studies conducted by my colleagues in the field. To this, I've added my own scholarly and clinical work in speech-language pathology with both presymbolic and symbolic children with language disorders.

When I was a student, my academic department was called Speech and Hearing Disorders. There was no language. I'm thankful for the pioneers and for my contemporaries who have brought the field of language disorders into its maturity.

The subtitle for the text is "a functional approach." This approach goes by other names, such as environmental or conversational, and includes elements of several other models. Where I have borrowed someone's model, ideas, or techniques, full credit is given to that person. I find assessment and intervention to be an adaptation of a little of this and a little of that within an overall theoretical framework.

Readers should read this text with my biases in mind. I do not approach language intervention as I might teaching arithmetic. One plus one may always be two, regardless of the context, but "May I have a cookie, please" only works when we consider the context. And that's my point, teaching language is different.

Context is essential to assessment and intervention with language. Now you can stop reading this book. You've got it all.

I've made some content decisions that should be explained. I group all children with language problems, both delays and disorders, under the general rubric of *language disorders*. This expedient decision was made recognizing that this text would not be addressing specific disorder populations except where applicable. In general, we address the generic child with a language disorder.

I hope you'll be pleased with this edition. Professors who've used previous editions will notice some new additions and changes in emphasis. These are based on professional feedback, reviewers' comments, student input, and the changing nature of speech and language services. Here is a partial list of updates and modifications:

- The text is thoroughly updated with the addition of several hundred new sources. This is the result of many hours of reading or perusing journal articles. In all honesty, I also looked at some other texts on this topic to see how the authors organized and explained language disorders.

- You'll find greater emphasis on autism spectrum disorder (ASD) in view of the increasing numbers of children being diagnosed with this disorder.

- I've added a whole new section on developmental language disorders (DLD), a new and more inclusive term than those used before. These children have always been with us but under a variety of different names.

- Chapter 2 of the previous edition has been divided into two chapters to accommodate the new information we have on language disorders. In this volume, Chapter 2 focuses solely on language disorders, such as DLD, and Chapter 3 focuses on language disorders associated with other disorders, such as ASD.

- I've gathered together the various discussions of assessment with children with culturally linguistically diverse backgrounds into a beefier chapter, giving this discussion its rightful place. I'm thrilled by the increasingly diverse nature of U.S. society and believe it's essential that we serve those children who need our services to the best of our ability.

- Fortunately, the number of meta-analyses focusing on the best evidence-based practices continues to increase, enabling us to say more on evidence-based practice. Wherever I've been able to find these professional articles, I have incorporated their results, even when they don't conform to what I might believe. That's how we learn and grow, isn't it?

- The chapters on language and narrative analysis have been strengthened and consolidated into one. Since the last edition, I've devoted myself, with the expert help of Stacey Pavelko, PhD, to development of SUGAR (Sampling Utterances and Grammatical Analysis Revised), an easy, valid, diagnostically accurate, and totally cost-free language sample analysis tool. This development enabled me to discuss SUGAR in a text for the first time. As much as possible, I've attempted to give other methods their due and to tone down my enthusiasm for my own work. Still, I invite you to visit sugarlanguage.org and see for yourself. We keep updating our development and research, so check back often.

I hope you are pleased with the results and will find this text useful.

Those who use the methods found within these pages tell me that they and their clients find them to be useful, effective, adaptable, and fun. Time will tell if you agree.

Acknowledgments

No text is written without the aid of other people. First, I thank the reviewers of this edition; I have tried to heed their sound advice.

No text is undertaken by the author alone, and I have been fortunate to have the support of some wonderful people. First, I acknowledge my colleagues at The College of Saint Rose. My department of Communication Sciences and Disorders co-chairs, Drs. Dave DeBonis and Jack Pickering, are a perfect example of leading with a light touch. It's a special treat to co-teach Counseling in Communication Disorders with Jack. Other amazing colleagues include, in alphabetic order, Katelynn Carroll, Sarah Coons, Lottie Dunbar, Jessica Evans, Kelly Fagan, Julie Hart, Nathan Holt, Wendy Kolakowski, Zhaleh Lavasani, Dr. Deirdre Muldoon, Grace Paster, Director of Clinical Education Melissa Spring, Lynn Stephens, Dr. Julia Unger, and Victoria Vestal. Somehow, through COVID, working together, we managed to fulfill our teaching and supervising mission. What a truly wonderful group of dedicated professionals and all-around warm, welcoming people! Our program is exciting, innovative, and dynamic.

My family and extended family also deserve thanks for their understanding and support. This includes my three children, Jason, Todd, and Jessica, and my grandchildren, The Divine Ms. Cassidy, Dakota, and Zavier.

Over the past several years, I've had the great joy to work closely with Dr. Stacey Pavelko in the development of SUGAR (Sampling Utterances and Grammatical Analysis Revised). Stacey is extremely intelligent and creative and a great researcher, making my job that much easier.

I would be remiss if I didn't acknowledge the inspiration of my dearest friend, Addie Haas, PhD, a former department chair in Communication Disorders at SUNY New Paltz. Although we've both aged and our adventures have matured along with us, she remains my kind, generous, loving friend.

In addition, special thanks and much love to my partner at O and M Education, Moon Byungchoon, for his patience, support, and perseverance. He was of great help with this text, doing work I did not have time to accomplish.

*To my grandson Dakota
whose developmental challenges as a child and young teen
can teach us all about the power of the human spirit*

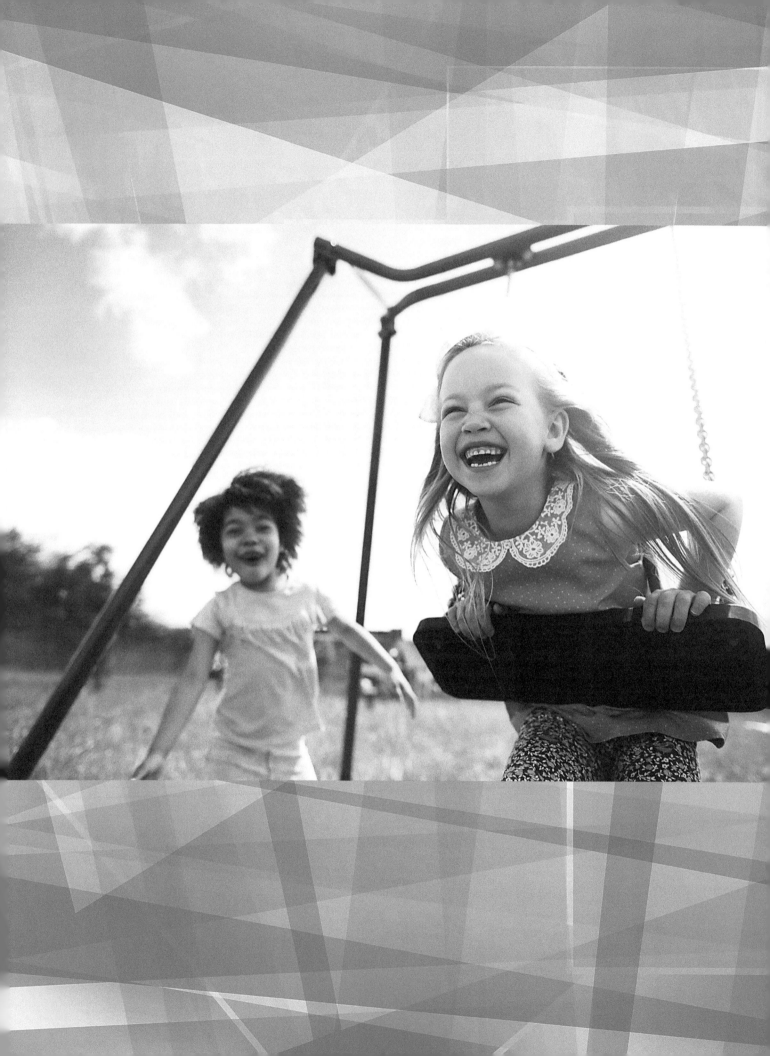

CHAPTER 1
A FUNCTIONAL LANGUAGE APPROACH

*A*ustin is a preschooler who struggles with language. He didn't begin to use words until age 2 years, and although he's progressed with the help of his parents, preschool teacher, and speech-language pathologist (SLP), progress has been slow. In all honesty, his spoken language sounds more like a typical 2-year-old than a child about to begin kindergarten. He did poorly on his school district's kindergarten readiness exam, and his preschool teacher has recommended that he remain in preschool for an additional year.

Although Austin is a sociable child and is well-liked by his teacher, the other children have begun to shun him because of his language. He often plays alone despite his good social skills. He rarely speaks in complete sentences, and words are often lacking their morphological endings, tense markers, and articles, as in "Mommy go store." Shorter words are often omitted. Although he's a bright child, his SLP, preschool teacher, and parents are concerned that he'll do poorly in school, especially with reading and writing.

Austin is a child with a language disorder who's having difficulty figuring out and learning the language code of his family and community. He's just one of the many children with a language disorder that you'll meet as a school-based SLP. It's my hope that this book and the excellent instruction your professor provides will give you some of the tools to address the challenges children like Austin face daily.

I've been an SLP and college professor for well over 40 years, but I began my career just as you are, sitting in classes, taking notes, reading texts, and eager for but fearful of my first clinical experience. This book is my attempt to give you as much information about language disorders as possible in the shortest space possible. The text is thick and filled with information because this topic is complicated.

Remember your language development course and how complicated that was. Now we'll be exploring how that process can go wrong, and how you as an SLP assess a child's language and plan and carry out intervention.

Even after we've spent all these words in discussing the topic, we'll have only skimmed the surface. You will spend your professional career continually updating this knowledge. And yet, each new child with a language disorder that you meet will challenge your knowledge, your skill, and your creativity. It's what makes the field of language disorder so challenging and rewarding.

So, let's proceed together. If you have concerns as we go, if I've made a mistake or confused you, or if I've been insensitive about a topic at some point, please let me know. I value your input.

Throughout this book, to the best of my ability, I have used evidence-based practice (EBP) as the basis for this text. I have attempted to research each topic, weigh the data, and make informed decisions prior to passing the knowledge on to you. If you are unfamiliar with EBP, I'll explain it at the end of the chapter. For now, let's begin with the basic concepts of **language disorder** and **functional language intervention**.

> ***Food for Thought:*** **Stop and think for a moment about language development. Pick one area that might have challenged you. Now imagine that you are 3 or 4 years old. Where might you go astray or struggle. That's what children with language disorders face.**

Language and Language Disorders

Communication and language skills are essential to a child's ability to engage in social relationships and access learning experiences. As you'll recall, language is a vehicle for communication and is primarily used in conversations. As such, *language is the social tool* that we use to accomplish our goals when we communicate. In other words, language can be viewed as a dynamic process. If we take this view, it changes our approach to language intervention. We become interested in the *how* more than in the *what*. It is that aspect of language intervention that I wish for us to explore through this book.

In the field of communication disorders, the study and remediation of language disorders are relatively new. Until the mid-1970s, around the time I was a graduate student, there was little emphasis on language disorders in children outside of childhood speech disorders. My academic department's name was "Speech and Hearing Disorders," and I was bluntly told by the chair that my PhD was not in language disorders. That didn't exist. So, I and others, with the help of a few innovative professors, had to teach ourselves.

In the late 1990s, two large studies came out of the University of Iowa demonstrating that language disorders were independent of speech disorders (Shriberg et al., 1999; Tomblin et al., 1997). Co-occurrence of speech and language disorders, adjusting for age expectations, was estimated at less than 2%. Nor are the two conditions likely to share a common cause.

Furthermore, children with language disorders, in the absence of any other disorders, were least likely to receive intervention despite the Iowa study's documentation that around 7% of monolingual American English-speaking kindergarten-age children like Austin, who were without other diagnosed developmental disorders, had language disorders despite having normal or above-normal range nonverbal IQs. An additional 3% of children were in the borderline range of low nonverbal IQs and also had language disorders. Similar estimates have been reported in other population-based studies (Frazier Norbury et al., 2016).

CHAPTER 1 A FUNCTIONAL LANGUAGE APPROACH

Think of it. Seven to ten or more percent of children had a disorder that only recently had not even been recognized as such.

The wheel turned slowly. Our primary professional organization became the American Speech-Language-Hearing Association (ASHA) in 1978 but left the "L" for language out of the acronym. Two decades later, in 1997, the *Journal of Speech and Hearing Research* became the *Journal of Speech, Language, and Hearing Research*, the premier professional journal in our field. Now there's a special interest group within ASHA devoted solely to language disorders in children. And the caseloads of school-based SLPs are bursting with these children.

ASHA defines *language disorder* as follows:

> A language disorder is impaired comprehension and/or use of spoken, written and/or other symbol systems. This disorder may involve (1) the form of language (phonology, morphology, syntax), (2) the content of language (semantics), and/or (3) the function of language in communication (pragmatics) in any combination. (Ad Hoc Committee on Service Delivery in the Schools, 1993, p. 40)

An international consortium (CATALISE) using a consensus method reached an agreed upon definition (Bishop et al., 2017) in which language disorders refers to difficulties that occur alone or co-occur with other disorders. These disorders cause impairment in daily functioning within the child's environment.

The term *language disorder* does not apply to children with language difference, such as a child who speaks a non-mainstream dialect of American English or is learning English subsequent to using another language.

For our purposes, we'll consider the term *language disorder* to refer to a heterogeneous group of developmental disorders, acquired disorders, delays, or any combination of these principally characterized by deficits and/or immaturities in the use of spoken and/or written language for comprehension and/or production purposes that may involve the form, content, or function of language in any combination. Language disorder may persist across the lifetime of the individual and may vary in symptoms, manifestations, effects, and severity over time and as a consequence of context, content, and learning task. As noted previously, language differences, found in some individuals who are English language learners (ELLs) and those using different dialects, do not in themselves constitute language disorders.

In attempting to clarify the definition of language disorder, we have, no doubt, raised more questions than we have answered. For example, causal factors, such as prematurity, although important, are omitted from the definition because of their diverse nature and the lack of clear causal links in many children with language disorders, such as Austin. In general, causal categories are not directly related to many language behaviors. Likewise, diagnostic categories, such as traumatic brain injury, are not included in my definition for many of the same reasons. The definition also states that language differences are not disorders, even though the general public and some professionals often confuse the two.

We'll explore all of these issues in Chapter 2 and the chapters that follow. For now, relax a little and let's discuss functional language intervention, the subtitle to this text.

Let's begin with a more traditional model of language intervention and compare it to a functional model.

> ***Food for Thought:*** **Might a child who is learning English as a second language also have a language disorder? How would you determine that fact?**

Traditional and Functional Models

The professional with primary responsibility for assessment and intervention with children with language disorders is the SLP. SLPs, you'll find, wear many hats—team members, team teachers, teachers and parent trainers, collaborators, advocates, and language facilitators, to name a few.

These many roles reflect a growing recognition that viewing a child and their communication as the sole source of the disorder is an outmoded concept. Increasingly, language intervention is becoming family and/or classroom centered and environmentally based. Professional concern is shifting from strictly language targets, such as individual morphological endings or vocabulary words, to a more functional, holistic approach focusing on the child's overall communication effectiveness. Read that last sentence again because it is the essence of this text.

Traditional Intervention Approaches

The traditional approach to teaching language is a highly structured, behavioral one, emphasizing the teaching of specific language features within a stimulus-response-reinforcement model. This approach is presented in Figure 1–1. In practice, this means that the SLP controls the situation and cues the child to respond, after which the adult reinforces correct responses or provides corrective feedback and progresses to the next cue. Thus, language is not seen as a process but a product or response elicited by a stimulus or produced in anticipation of reinforcement. There is a certain logic here.

Stimulus-response-reinforcement models of intervention such as this have often taken the form of questions by an SLP and answers by a child or directives by an SLP for a child to respond. Typical stimulus utterances by an SLP might include "Did you say that correctly?" or "Tell me the whole thing." The SLP's responses are based on the correctness of production and might include "Good talking!" or "Repeat it again correctly three times."

Many SLPs prefer a traditional structured approach because they can predict accurately the response of the child to the teaching stimuli. In addition, structured behavioral approaches increase the probability that the child will make the appropriate, desired response. Language lessons usually are scripted as drills and, therefore, are repetitive and predictable for the SLP.

In a structured behavioral approach, the child can become a passive learner. The SLP's overall style is highly directive. In other words, the clinical procedure is unidirectional

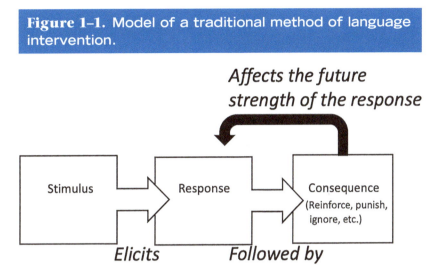

Figure 1–1. Model of a traditional method of language intervention.

and adult-oriented. Unfortunately, used alone, these approaches are inadequate for developing meaningful uses for the newly acquired language feature. Something's missing.

Although structured behavioral approaches that exhibit intensity, consistency, and organization have been successful in teaching some language skills, they exhibit a major weakness—generalization. For example, the failure of language-teaching targets to generalize to other uses is one of the major criticisms of intervention with children with autism spectrum disorders. Could that failing rest with the highly behavioral methods used with these children?

The Functional Approach

In contrast to traditional models, functional approaches give more control to the child and decrease the amount of structure in intervention activities. Measures of improvement are increased successful communication rather than simply the number of correct responses. Procedures used by the SLP and the child's communication partners more closely resemble those in the language-learning environment of children. In addition, the everyday environment of the child is included in the training.

A functional language approach to assessment and intervention, as described in this text, targets language used as a vehicle for communication. It's a communication-first approach. The focus is the overall communication of the child with a language disorder and of those who communicate with the child. As stated, the goal is better communication that works in the child's natural communicative environment.

In a functional language approach, conversation between a child and their communication partners becomes the vehicle for change. By manipulating the linguistic and nonlinguistic contexts within which a child's utterances occur, the partner facilitates the use of certain structures and provides evaluative feedback while maintaining the conversational flow. That last sentence is another one worth rereading. From the early data collection stages through the intervention process, the SLP and other communication partners are concerned with the enhancement of the child's overall communication.

Functional language approaches have been shown in clinical research to increase mean length of utterance and multiword utterance production, the overall quantity of spontaneous communication, pragmatic skills, vocabulary growth, language complexity, receptive labeling, and intelligibility and the use of learned forms in novel utterances in children with a variety of language disorders and causes. Even minimally symbolic children—those using no words or just a few—can benefit from a more conversational milieu.

Interestingly, functional interactive approaches improve generalization even when the immediate results differ little from those of more directive methods. And as an additional benefit, a functional conversational approach can yield more positive behaviors from the child, such as smiling, laughing, and engagement in activities, with significantly more verbal initiation, than does a strictly imitation approach. In contrast, the child learning through a structured traditional approach is more likely to be quiet and passive.

Naturally, the effectiveness of any language-teaching strategy will vary with the characteristics of the child with a language disorder and the content being taught. For example, children with learning disabilities may benefit more from specific language teaching than do other children with language disorders. Similarly, children with more severe language disorders initially benefit more from a structured imitative approach. That doesn't mean that you as an SLP need to stop there. Although imitation is a quick method for getting a desired response, learning doesn't hold and generalization is weak.

I've probably raised more issues than answered your questions. Don't worry. We have a whole book to examine a functional approach and to address your doubts and concerns. My goal in this chapter was simply to pique your interest. To help you digest all this information so far, Table 1–1 offers a simplified comparison of the traditional and functional models.

> **Food for Thought:** Even though I've been vague, can you imagine what the outline of a functional method of language intervention might entail in comparison to a more traditional model. Try to do this without peeking at Table 1–1.

In the remainder of this chapter, we'll further define a functional language approach and explore a rationale for it. This rationale is based on the primacy of pragmatics in language and language intervention and on the generalization of language intervention to everyday contexts. Then, we'll wrap up the chapter with a brief discussion of EBP, which is the basis of this text and what we practice as a profession.

Role of Pragmatics in Intervention

As you'll recall, pragmatics consists of the intentions or communication goals of each speaker and of the linguistic adjustments made by each speaker for the listener in order

Table 1–1. Comparison of Traditional and Functional Intervention Approaches

Traditional Model	Functional Model
Individual or small group	Individual, small group, large group, or an entire class
Clinical situation	Actual communication situation
Isolated language targets	Relationship of linguistic units stressed as target is used in conversation
Begin with small units of language and build up to conversation	Target conversation as "fixing" the child's language as needed with minimal prompts
Stress on modeling, imitation, practice, and drill	Conversational techniques stressing successful communication
Use in conversations stressed in final stages of intervention	Use is optimized as a vehicle for intervention
Child's behavior and language constrained by adult	Increased opportunity to use the new language feature in a wide variety of contexts
Little real conversation and use	Premised on real conversation and use
Little involvement of significant others	Parents and teachers used as agents of change

to accomplish these goals. Most features of language are affected by pragmatic aspects of the conversational context. For example, a speaker's selection of pronouns involves more than syntactic and semantic considerations. The conversational partners must be aware of the preceding linguistic information and of each other's point of reference. For example, a noun reference is used before the speaker can refer to it with a pronoun. In addition, pronouns such as *I* and *you* depend on who's speaking.

In an earlier era, interest by SLPs in psycholinguistics led to a therapeutic emphasis on increasing syntactic complexity. With a therapeutic shift in interest to semantics or meaning in the early 1970s came a new recognition of the importance of cognitive or intellectual readiness. The influence of sociolinguistics and pragmatics in the late 1970s and 1980s has led to interest in conversational rules and contextual factors. Everyday contexts provide a backdrop for linguistic performance.

Likewise, among those working with individuals with communication disorders, the focus has shifted to the communication process itself. Previously, for example, children's behaviors were considered either appropriate or inappropriate to the stimulus-reinforcement situation. When emphasis shifts to pragmatics and to the processes that underlie language use, however, the child's language can be considered on its own terms. For example, does it serve a purpose for the child within their communication context?

Older approaches have tended to emphasize children's deficits with the goal of fixing what's wrong. In contrast, a functional approach stresses what a child needs in order to accomplish their communication goals. It follows that intervention should provide contexts for actively engaging children in communication. In shifting the focus away from the disorder, the goal of intervention becomes increasing opportunities for supporting a child's participation in everyday communication situations. It's a new recognition that a language disorder is not a thing residing in a child but a dynamic process reflecting the child and the communication context in which the communication occurs.

Increasingly, SLPs are recognizing that the structure and content of language are heavily influenced by the conversational constraints of the communication context. This view of language necessitates a very different approach to language intervention. In effect, functional intervention moves from an entity approach, which targets discrete isolated bits of language, to a systems or holistic approach, which targets language within the overall communication process. The major implication is a change in both the targets and the methods of teaching. If pragmatics is just one of five equal aspects of language, as seen on the left in Figure 1–2, then it offers yet another set of rules to teach and the methodology need not change much. The teaching still can emphasize the *what* with little change in the *how*, which can continue in a structured behavioral paradigm that I've called a traditional method.

In contrast, an approach in which pragmatics is seen as the overall organizing aspect of language, shown on the right in Figure 1–2, necessitates a more interactive conversational teaching approach, one that mirrors the environment in which the language will be used. Therapy becomes child-oriented rather than error-oriented, and conversation is viewed as both the teaching and transfer environment. I'm calling this a functional approach.

Figure 1–2. Models of how aspects of language are related.

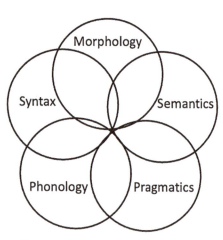

Pragmatics is one of five equal and interrelated aspects of language

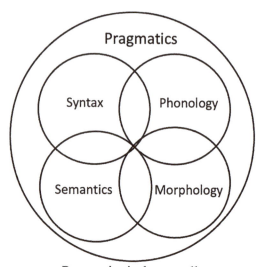

Pragmatics is the overall organizing aspect of language

Dimensions of Communication Context

Language is purposeful and takes place within a dynamic context that affects form and content and may, in turn, be affected by them. Context consists of a complex interaction of many factors:

- *Purpose*, which affects what to say and how to say it. Here's pragmatics again.
- *Content* or topic, which affects the form and the style.
- *Type of discourse* or characteristic type of structure related to the purpose. An argument differs from a bedtime story in many ways.
- *Participant characteristics*, such as background knowledge, roles, life experiences, moods, group identity and shared rules, willingness to take risks, relative age, status, familiarity, and relationship in time and space, affect the context.
- *Setting and activity*, including circumstances of the communication situation, can affect language, especially the choice of vocabulary.
- *Mode of discourse*, such as speech, signing, and writing, require very different types of interaction from the participants.

Within a conversation, participants continually must assess these factors and their changing relationships. Now, it should be easier to see why consideration of the pragmatic context is an essential feature of effective language intervention.

> ***Food for Thought:*** Imagine telling a narrative to a friend. Now imagine the same story being told to a group of seniors whom you've never met and who will not understand some of the words you used. Do these factors affect the story being told?

An SLP must be a master of the conversational context. Unfortunately, it is too easy to rely on overworked verbal cues that keep the adult in control, such as "Tell me about this picture" or "What do you want?" to elicit certain language structures. There are better, more creative ways to elicit the same structures, but the SLP must be willing to relinquish some of that control and use more creative brain power. If an SLP knows the dimensions of a communication context and understands how these dimensions are likely to affect communication, the SLP can manipulate them more efficiently. I'll explain how later in the text.

Summary

In the clinical setting, SLPs need to be aware of the effects of context on communication. How well children with language disorders regulate their relationships with other people depends on their ability to monitor aspects of the context. Given the dynamic nature of conversational contexts, it is essential that intervention also address generalization to the child's everyday communication contexts.

Role of Generalization in Intervention

One of the most challenging aspects of language intervention is generalization, or carryover, to nonteaching situations. Time and again, we SLPs bemoan the fact that although Johnny performed correctly during intervention, he could not transfer this performance to the playground, classroom, or home. When language features taught in one setting are not generalized to other content and contexts, the child's goal of communicative competence is not realized. Consideration of generalization shapes many aspects of a functional intervention approach.

Lack of generalization can be a function of several factors, including the material selected for teaching, the learning characteristics of a child, and the design of the teaching. Stimuli present in the clinical setting that directly or indirectly affect learning may not be found in other settings. Some of these stimuli, such as teaching cues, have intended effects, whereas others, such as an SLP's presence, may have quite unintended ones. In addition, clinical cues and consequences used for teaching, such as reinforcement, may be very different from those encountered in everyday situations, thus removing the motivation to use the behavior elsewhere.

For our purposes, let's consider generalization to be the ongoing interactive process of clients and their newly acquired language feature with the communication environment (Figure 1–3). For example, if we are trying to teach a child the new word *doggie*, we

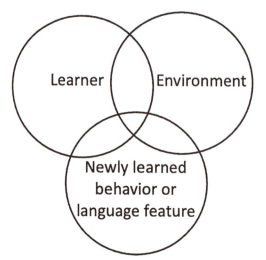

Figure 1–3. Generalization schematic.

Generalization is the interaction of the individual, the newly learned behavior or language feature, and the environment. All three must be present for generalization to occur.

might repeat the word several times in the presence of the family dog and then cue the child with "Say doggie." If the child repeats the word only in this situation, she has not learned to use the word. If she says the word spontaneously and in the presence of other dogs, however, then we can reasonably assume that the child has learned the word and its use. In other words, the content taught has generalized.

The factors that affect generalization lie within the content being taught, the learner, and the teaching context but will vary as particular aspects of the teaching situation change. If a response is to occur in a nonteaching situation, such as a classroom, then some aspects of that situation should be present in the teaching situation to signal that the response should occur. In other words, an SLP must consider the effects of the teaching context on generalization to everyday contexts.

Language intervention may not generalize for myriad reasons, such as being taught out of context, representing neither a child's communicative functions nor linguistic knowledge or experiences, or presenting few authentic communicative opportunities. To some extent, generalization is also a result of the procedures used and of the variables manipulated in language intervention.

With each client, an SLP needs to ask: Will this procedure (or target) work in the child's everyday environment? Is there a need within the everyday communication of the child for the feature that is being targeted, and do the methods used in its teaching reflect that everyday context of the child? In a meeting with a student SLP, the answer to these questions was no. As a result, we decided to forgo other morphological targets and focus on past tense *-ed* because his class was working on "storytelling." In other words, we opted for a more functional approach that targeted useful skills in the everyday environment of the client rather than choosing another language target.

Variables That Affect Generalization

Generalization is an essential part of learning. Even the young child using their first word must learn to generalize its use to novel content and contexts. At first, the word *doggie* may be used with other four-legged animals. From feedback—"No, honey, that's a kitty"—the child abstracts those cases in which the word *doggie* is correct and those in which it is not. The child is learning those contexts that obligate the use of *doggie* and those that preclude its use. In other words, while refining the definition of the word, the child learns which contexts regulate application of the language rules.

Likewise, a young child who can say, "May I have a cookie, please?" has not truly learned this new utterance until it is used in the appropriate contexts just as you haven't learned to ski until you go out into the snow. Likewise, the child learns the appropriate contextual cues, such as the presence of cookies, that govern use of the utterance. Now the utterance "works" for the child. It's functional.

The contexts in which intervention takes place influence what a child actually learns. In fact, correctness is not inherent in a child's response itself but is found in the response in context. Saying "May I have a cookie, please?" when you're in line at the bank is inappropriate.

The relationship of context to learning is not a simple one, and the stimuli controlling a response may be multiple. Likewise, learning to ask questions without comprehending when you need to do so is also inappropriate. Part of this is recognizing what you know and what you don't.

In a similar way, generalization is an integral part of the language intervention process. Thoughts on generalization should not be left until after intervention has finalized. Generalization is not a single-line entry at the end of the lesson plan, nor is it homework. It's an integral part of intervention.

To facilitate the acquisition of truly functional language—language that works for the child—it is essential that you as an SLP learn to manipulate the variables related to generalization throughout the therapeutic process. In a functional model, generalization is an essential element at every step. Table 1–2 includes a list of the major generalization variables. As we consider each variable, we're roughing in the outline of a functional approach.

Broad Categories of Generalization Variables

Generalization variables are of two broad types: content generalization and context generalization. Let's briefly describe each before discussing the variables included in each type.

Content Generalization. Content is the *what* of teaching. Content generalization occurs when the child induces a language rule from examples and from actual use. Thus, the new feature (e.g., plural *-s*) may be used with content not previously taught, such as words not used in the therapy situation. Content generalization is affected by the targets chosen and by the specific choice of teaching items.

Context Generalization. If content is the *what*, context is the *how*. Context generalization occurs when the client uses the newly learned language feature within everyday communication, such as in the classroom, at home, or in play. In each of these contexts, there are differences in persons present and different linguistic and nonlinguistic events that precede and follow the newly learned behavior. Generalization can be facilitated

Table 1–2. Variables That Affect Generalization	
Content generalization	Training targets
	Training items
Context generalization	Method of training
	Language facilitators
	Training cues
	Consequences
	Location of training

Variables

Let's briefly look at each variable. We'll come back to them later when we begin to design an intervention approach in Chapter 9.

Teaching Targets. The very complexity of language makes it impossible for an SLP to teach everything that a child needs to become a competent communicator. Target selection, therefore, is a conscious process with far-reaching implications.

Functional target selection is based as much as possible on the actual needs and interests of each child within their communication environments. The focus of instruction is on increasing the effectiveness of child-initiated communication.

Although there is a tendency for beginning SLPs to target specific language deficits, such as plural -*s*, as an end in themselves, intervention goals can focus on stimulating the language acquisition process beyond the immediate target (Fey et al., 2003). We can best serve a child with a language disorder if we enhance their existing resources for learning language more effectively within the intervention context and beyond.

Not all language features occur with equal frequency. It may be necessary, therefore, to create more frequent opportunities for a feature to occur. An SLP can create activities and modify the environment to increase the need for the target.

Generalization is also a function of the scope of the teaching target and of the child's characteristics and linguistic experience with the target. In general, language rules with broad scope generalize more easily than those with more restricted scope.

The scope of rule application can be a function of the way it is taught. Narrow, restricted teaching reduces teaching targets to easily identifiable and observable units that may not be found in everyday use environments. For example, plural nouns rarely occur in isolation devoid of a purpose or intention.

In conclusion, teaching targets should be selected on the basis of each child's actual communication needs and abilities. The targets selected for teaching should be functional or useful in a client's everyday communication environment.

Teaching Items. The items selected for intervention, such as the specific verbs to be used in teaching the past tense -*ed* or the sentences to be used in teaching negation, and the linguistic complexity of these intervention items also can influence generalization. In general, it is best if these items come from the natural communication environment of the child. Structured observation of this environment can aid intervention programming. For example, an active child may use the verbs *walk*, *jump*, and *hop* frequently. It is more likely that use of the past tense -*ed* will generalize if these frequently occurring words are used in intervention.

Individualization is important because of the many potentially different use environments. A child in a classroom may have very different content to discuss than does a child at home.

Targeted linguistic forms can be taught across several contexts. For example, negatives used with auxiliary verbs can occur in declaratives ("That won't fit"), imperatives ("Don't touch that"), interrogatives ("Don't you want to go?"), and intentions, such as denying ("I wouldn't do it") or requesting information ("Why can't you go?").

For optimum generalization, then, it is necessary to select teaching items from a child's everyday environment. In addition, these items should be taught across different linguistic forms and/or functions and across both linguistic and nonlinguistic contexts.

Method of Teaching. Teaching discrete bits of language devoid of the communication context fragments learning, allowing minute analysis units to eclipse intentionality and synergy. In other words, language use is overlooked. Intervention that focuses on these specific, discrete, structural entities fosters drills and didactic (*cue-respond-reinforce*) teaching. These, in turn, adversely affect the flow, intentionality, and meaningfulness of language.

If language is viewed holistically, then the teaching of language involves much more than just teaching words and structures. Clients learn strategies for comprehending language directed to them and for generating novel utterances within several conversational contexts.

To optimize generalization, teaching could occur within actual use in a conversational context. It makes sense to use conversations to teach for where we use language most, in conversations. Teaching in the use context makes good common sense.

Another way of saying this is that our intervention methodology should flow logically from our concept of language. If *language is a social tool* and if the goal is to teach for generalized use, then it follows that language should be taught in conditions similar to the ultimate use environment. It is important, therefore, to view context not as a backdrop for but as the ongoing process of intervention.

It would be foolish to assume that conversational methods alone will guarantee successful learning and generalization for every child with a language disorder. A successful SLP will blend methods together as required by the child.

Language Facilitators. Let's begin this discussion topic by focusing on children with typically developing language (TDL). Factors that can contribute to poor language outcomes for children with TDL are reduced language input within caregiver–child interactions, less than optimal adult strategies such as use of directives ("Get your coat"), low maternal education, and low socioeconomic status (Sultana et al., 2019). Notice the prominence of caregivers.

Good language partners are facilitators who increase a child's potential for communication success. Parents and caregivers, teachers, aides, and others, in addition to the SLP, can act as language facilitators because of their relationship with and the amount of time each spends with the child.

Interactional pairs, such as a caregiver and a child, form a unique communication context, and it is essential that the child experience newly learned language in a number of these contexts. Language will differ within the context created by a child with each communication partner. Thus, generalization depends on the number of communication partners we can involve in the intervention process. Austin, mentioned at the beginning of the chapter, would most likely benefit if I involve his parents and teachers in the intervention process.

Programs that involve a child's communication partners, especially parents and caregivers, produce greater gains for children than do programs that do not. Parents and other caregivers offer a channel for generalizing to the natural environment of the home. The key in working with families, especially in early intervention with infants and toddlers, is mutual respect and individualization of services based on each family's priorities and concerns (Sandall et al., 2001).

Some cultural beliefs may be at variance with the use of parents or caregivers as language facilitators. For example, some Mexican American mothers believe that schools have the main responsibility for educating children and that parents should not be actively involved (Rodriguez & Olswang, 2003). Still, these mothers can be enticed into taking a more active role in language intervention if an SLP builds positive rapport and collaboration and is respectful of culturally held beliefs.

Intervention need not be limited to just families. When daycare staff are trained to respond to children's initiations, to engage children, to model simplified language, and to encourage peer interactions, it has a significant effect on the language production of preschool children (Girolametto et al., 2003). The same is true for school-age children.

With the involvement of others, the traditional role of an SLP changes. In essence, the SLP becomes a programmer of a child's environment, manipulating the variables to ensure successful communication and generalization. The SLP acts as a consultant, helping each child–partner dyad finely tune its conversational behaviors.

Teaching Cues. Goals for the child should include both initiating and responding behaviors in the situations in which each is appropriate. Therefore, an SLP considers teaching language through a great variety of both linguistic and nonlinguistic cues. The adult encourages child utterances by subtle manipulation of the context and responds to the child in an appropriate manner. A functional language approach adapts these techniques as naturally as possible to intervention.

Contingencies or Consequences. The nature of the reinforcement used in teaching is also a strong determiner of generalization. Said simply, everyday natural consequences are best. If the child requests a paintbrush, she should be given one, unless, of course, there is a good reason not to give it. If that is the case, then the child should not have been required to learn that request.

Most of the time, we're reinforced in conversation by the other person's reply. As an SLP, you can use verbal reinforcers found in the natural communication environment. Verbal or social consequences such as "Good talking," encountered only rarely if at all in the course of everyday conversations, should be discontinued in favor of more natural responses, such as attention or a simple conversational reply.

Verbal responses that combine feedback about correctness/incorrectness with additional information can be both a language-learning opportunity and a communicative turn that maintains the conversational flow. "Good talking" ends social interaction by commenting on the correctness of the child's utterance only and leaving little that the child can say in return.

Not every utterance is reinforced in the natural environment. In the course of everyday conversations, many utterances elicit no response. In traditional language intervention, however, every utterance by the child may be reinforced. Interestingly, intermittent reinforcement, which more closely resembles the real world, is stronger and more resistant to loss of the behavior.

Location. The location of teaching involves not only places but also events. For maximum generalization, language should be taught in various locations, such as the home, clinic, school, or unit, and in the activities in which it is used, such as play or household chores. For young children like Austin, mentioned previously, play is a very natural setting for intervention.

As much as possible, language should be taught within the daily activities of the child. Daily routines can provide a familiar framework within which language can occur. The familiar situation provides a frame that allows for a degree of automatization important in the acquisition of language. Often called *incidental teaching*, this approach attempts to ensure that a child learns and has ample opportunity to use language within naturally occurring activities. Generalization increases with the similarity of the learning situation to the transfer situation.

The ideal teaching situation is one in which a child with a language disorder is engaged in some meaningful activity with a conversational partner who models appropriate language forms and functions. In this way, a child learns language in the conversational context in which it is likely to occur. It is within these everyday events that language is acquired naturally and to these events that the newly learned language is to generalize.

Within these daily events are naturally occurring communication sequences. Daily events, such as phone calls, friendly meetings, dinner preparation, and play, can provide a framework for language and for incidental language teaching. The frame provides a guide to help the participants organize their language and their language learning. Routines and familiar situations provide support. As an SLP, you can plan conversational roles and language teaching through the use of such daily events.

Summary

A basic goal of intervention should be to help a child achieve greater flexibility in the learning and use of language in written and oral modalities of comprehension and production. Such language intervention can be a dynamic process of exchange that occurs during natural events in different environments and with different conversational partners. The variables relative to content and context can, if manipulated carefully, facilitate generalization of newly learned language features and make intervention seem more natural.

> *Food for Thought:* Does is make intuitive sense to you that the similarity of the teaching and generalization contexts fosters carryover? Why? Why not? What questions does it raise for you?

Evidence-Based Practice

As SLPs, we should be concerned with providing the best, most well-grounded intervention for our clients that is humanly possible. In other words, we should do what works or is most effective. Discerning efficacy and providing the most efficacious intervention is a portion of something called **evidence-based practice**. In EBP, decision making is informed by a combination of

- scientific evidence,
- clinical experience, and
- client needs.

Research is combined with reason when making decisions about treatment approaches. Evidence-based practice is based on two assumptions (Bernstein Ratner, 2006):

- Clinical skills grow from the current available data, not simply from experience.
- The expert SLP continually seeks new therapeutic information to improve efficacy.

Note that it is up to each of us, as professionals, to use the best clinical methods available.

Not all clinical evidence is created equal. Professional journals, called peer-reviewed journals, in which each submitted manuscript is critiqued by other experts in the field and accepted or rejected on the basis of the quality of the research, are the best source of information. Once research has been located, you as an SLP are left to decide how much information is enough, how to resolve seemingly conflicting results, and how to adapt the information to individual clients.

Some assistance comes in the form of meta-analyses. In **meta-analysis**, professional researchers compile all relevant research, rank it in terms of strength of the findings, and select their overall finding(s) from the strongest research. In general, the best research compares the efficacy of an intervention method with similar groups to which children have been randomly assigned so as not to bias the results. It is best if data collectors do not know to which group children are assigned and use valid and reliable measures of performance. Other studies in the form of single-subject findings, clinical notes, or anecdotal reports are used in meta-analysis to support the stronger ones.

It is important as an SLP to recognize that efficacy is never an all-or-nothing proposition (Law, 2004; Rescorla, 2005). We cannot, for example, promise a "cure." As an old-timer, I've had both knees and both shoulders rebuilt, and although these joints now function better than they did prior to surgery and physical therapy, they are not the joints I had when I was 20 years old. I have regained a portion of my former strength and agility, but it is not perfect. It was not a "cure." Neither is our intervention in speech-language pathology, especially given the many variables that can affect intervention outcomes. This fact makes careful understanding and application of recommended intervention techniques critical.

The decision-making process in EBP is systematic and includes the following several steps (S. Gillam & Gillam, 2006; Porzsolt et al., 2003):

- Determine the information needed and ask the correct clinical question. Questions should include information on the client's performance, the environment, the intervention approach, and the desired outcomes.

- Find studies that address the clinical question. The ASHA website is a valuable resource for articles published in ASHA journals and hundreds of other affiliated journals. Effective use of the Internet is addressed later.

- Determine the level of evidence and critically evaluate the studies. The quality of information differs and should be prioritized by an SLP. This has already been accomplished if a meta-analysis exists. As an SLP, you must also determine that the participants in the study compare well with the specific child in question.

- Evaluate the information for the specific case in question. Issues include the associated costs of intervention in time and money, cultural variables of the child and family, student–caregiver involvement and opinions, child's interests, and agency policies and philosophy.

- Integrate the information and make a decision.

- Evaluate treatment outcomes to measure efficacy. Of special significance is the use of the targeted language features in everyday natural speaking situations.

These steps alone will not guarantee the best outcome, but they do provide a systematic method for decision making.

Although the Internet may be filled with ideas, as an SLP, you should be cautious. Because of the potential for misinformation when researching on the Internet, it is important that an SLP use the most appropriate methods for investigating and retrieving information. Search engines such as Google search the entire open Internet and often provide information from secondary or tertiary sources or information that is not based on peer-reviewed research at all. It's important to know who authored the information and/or sponsors the site, the purpose and nature of the site, and the currency of the information (Nail-Chiwetula & Bernstein Ratner, 2006). For example, a site sponsored by an intervention materials company may try to promote intervention methods using its materials. Even academic (.edu) or government (.gov) sites may present non-peer-reviewed information. For example, educational sites may present student papers submitted for specific courses. Useful professional sites include the following:

- The American Speech-Language-Hearing Association (https://www.asha.org/publications/) offers full text of all articles in its journals for ASHA or National Student Speech-Language-Hearing Association members. Your college library most likely subscribes to these publications which gives you access.

- PubMed (http://www.ncbi.nlm.nih.gov/entrez/query.fcgi) is a free database offered by the National Library of Medicine. Full-text articles are unavailable.

Many university libraries offer several databases relevant to speech-language pathology, including CINAHL, ERIC, Language and Language Behavior Abstracts (LLBA), MEDLINE, and PsycINFO. Many offer full-text access. Article abstracts do not provide sufficient information for evaluating the quality of research reported.

As you can imagine, combing journals for clinical results to guide EBP practices can be time-consuming. Half the SLPs polled in one study stated that they didn't have sufficient professional time to devote to the process of EBP (Zipoli & Kennedy, 2005). A first step, of course, is to critically evaluate one's own clinical practices for their efficiency and effectiveness. In centers with more than one SLP or in local professional organizations, SLPs can form EBP research groups that will benefit from the input and the data-keeping and possible research efforts of each member. Another source of pooled knowledge is ASHA's Special Interest Group 1 of SIG1, which is devoted to language disorders. Together, you can explore the best practices to use with children with language impairment.

I've only skimmed the surface. All graduate programs offer a course in research, which will be the best place to receive in-depth information on EBP.

Finally, I have to the best of my ability provided evidence-based information throughout this text. It's an almost overwhelming task when faced with a book with the scope of this one. I leave it to others to decide if I succeeded.

> **Food for Thought:** Does this all seem a bit overwhelming? I'm sure it does. As we proceed, try to become more comfortable with the information. Make it part of your professional persona. Imagine yourself providing assessment and intervention for a child with a language disorder.

Getting "It"

Before we wrap this chapter up, let me make a few comments on application of a functional model of language intervention. A colleague who uses a functional approach related to me that she is questioned by other SLPs in her school district who wonder how she learned to make therapy look so natural and to engage children so well while genuinely seeming to enjoy herself. I can't promise all that, but I'll try to open your eyes to a model of assessment and intervention that, although unique, does not preclude using other approaches.

After I had presented an all-day workshop, an older SLP approached me to tell me she used many functional methods she had read in this book and found them to be very effective. Somewhat humbled, I thanked her, but as I turned to continue packing up, she took my arm firmly and said, "You don't understand. I get it. I get it." As I turned back to her, she explained that functional intervention is not the same as using someone's published language intervention program; it's a philosophy of intervention that influences everything she does with children and adults with language disorders.

In this book, we are going to explore that "it," a functional philosophy of language intervention. I want you to get "it" too. There are many pieces to this model but, fortunately, an inability to use one portion, such as working with a parent or caregiver, does not preclude using others, such as teaching through conversation. Nor does use of functional methods negate the need for more traditional methods with some clients and at some times during intervention.

Conclusion

Language is an essential part of life, and you as an SLPs will be the link between a child and their environment. Functional language intervention focuses on the child with a language disorder and brings the environment into intervention to the maximum extent possible.

A functional approach emphasizes both nurturant and naturalistic methods. The nurturant aspect requires an SLP or other language facilitator to relinquish control to the child and to respond to the child's communication initiations. The naturalistic aspect emphasizes everyday events and contexts because language makes sense only when used within a communication context. The SLP becomes a master in the manipulation of that context in order to facilitate communication and generalization.

As much as possible, language is taught while and where it is actually being used in everyday contexts. As a result, the language learning generalizes.

Learning and generalization are the result of good planning based on a knowledge of the variables that affect generalization and the individual needs of each child. The content selected for teaching and the context within which this teaching takes place are both important aspects of the learning and generalization process. The SLP helps the child determine the best response to fulfill their initiations within contexts that facilitate their intervention targets. Although the role of an SLP within the functional language paradigm changes from primary direct service provider to a language facilitator and consultant, the SLP still has primary responsibility for planning and implementing intervention.

Some professionals cast a wary eye on implementation of such conversational and communication-based approaches to language intervention. The fear is that intervention will deteriorate into a "Hey, man, what's happenin'?" approach, too open-ended to be effective in changing client behavior. Although this danger does exist, it is not inherent in functional approaches. As this text progresses, we'll discuss assessment and intervention procedures that enable SLPs to maintain a teaching momentum within the more natural context of conversation. It's productive, fun, and, where data exist, evidence based.

In the following chapters, we'll explore language disorders, assessment, and intervention. After a discussion of children with language disorders, such as Austin, we'll discuss the assessment process and the collection and analysis of conversational and narrative data. In the following chapters, an intervention paradigm and various techniques are presented, along with discussion of special applications to the classroom environment and to literacy.

That's where were going. So, buckle in, we're about to begin.

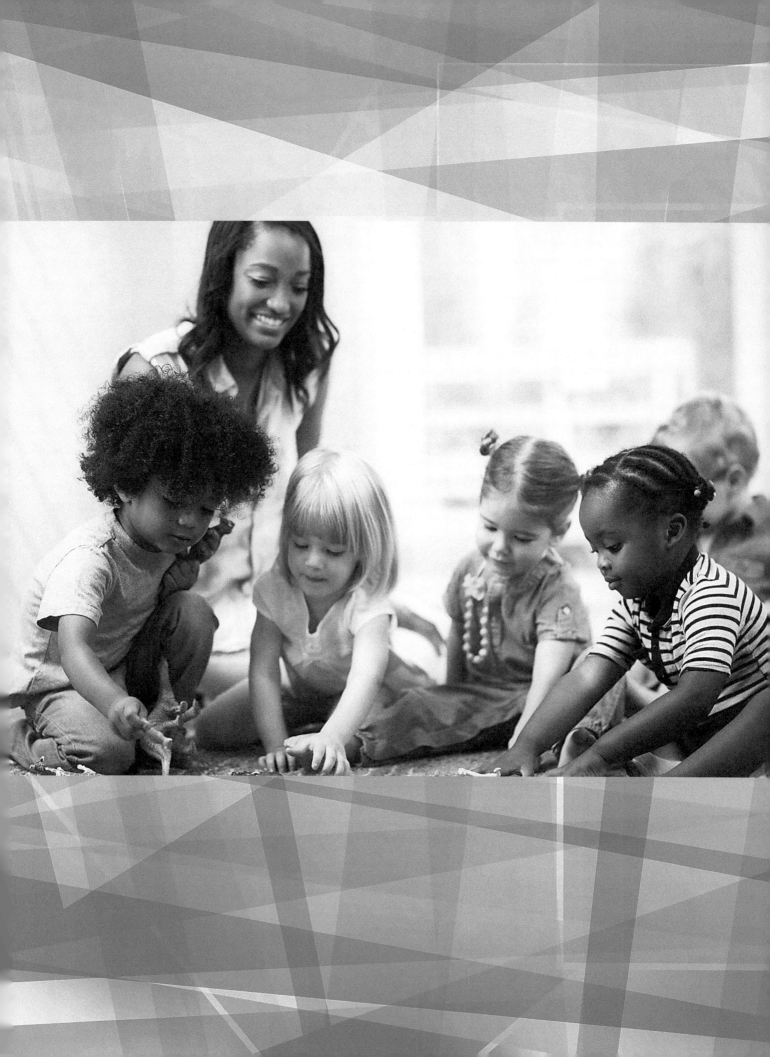

CHAPTER 2
LANGUAGE DISORDERS

Juan is a bright second grader who struggles with language. He has difficulty following directions and often misunderstands his teacher's directives. Reading is especially difficult, and in addition to poor decoding skills or sounding out written words, he doesn't seem to comprehend what he's read.

He speaks in short sentences and seems easily confused while producing longer, more complicated ones. The result is frequent stops and starts, half-finished thoughts, and reattempts. Similarly, his words are often truncated and short words are confused, such as saying, "Hims got some relax." This all gives his language a choppy, disconnected character. In addition, he has consistent speech sound error.

His vocabulary is limited, and he tends to repeat words rather than finding other word choices. In interactions with peers, he seems shy and is teased for not being more actively involved. When teased, he sometimes responds aggressively or simply withdraws.

Juan, like many of the children described in this chapter, may have impairments in other areas of development as well. For example, children with intellectual disability are going to experience slower maturity in all developmental areas, not just language. It is reported that some children with language disorder have nonverbal deficits, as well, in memory and in motor tasks. This and other reported differences may reflect actual deficits or may be confounded by the linguistic aspects of the tasks used to assess a child's behavior. We still have much to learn from these children.

In this and the next chapter, we'll discuss the most common diagnostic categories of children with language disorder. Please remember that we are describing groups of children, not individuals. No child with a learning disability may exhibit all of the characteristics ascribed to these children in this text. I'll try to explain commonalities and differences across various disorders and to explore the most common language problems seen by speech-language pathologists (SLPs).

Although at least one exhaustive study failed to establish reliable rates of incidence, prevalence, and outcomes for speech and language disorders in the general population (Raghavan et al., 2018), it is estimated that at the time of school entry, approximately two or three pupils in every class of 30 or approximately 10% will have severe enough language disorders to hinder academic progress. Another study reported that from preschool into elementary school, approximately 3% of children display persistent language disorder, 5% transient language disorder, and 6.5% late-onset language disorder (Zambrana et al., 2014).

In a population of more than 12,000 children, a third study found the prevalence of language disorders to be 9.92% (Frazier Norbury et al., 2016). The prevalence of language disorders of unknown origin was 7.58%, and that of language disorders associated with intellectual disability and/or existing medical diagnosis was 2.34%. The second value seems low and to some extent may reflect some school districts and states underreporting in an effort to save money. According to their logic, if a child's language is within the normal range for that disorder population, such as those with intellectual disability, which we'll explore later, then the child does not have a language disorder and thus the school district does not have to provide services even though the child's language is well below that of children with typically developing language (TDL). Call it budgetary restraint if you like; I call it unethical. We have consigned that child to a lower standard and lower expectations.

The prevalence of communication disorders is higher for children from low socioeconomic status (SES) backgrounds. According to a recent national report by the U.S. Social Security Administration's Supplemental Security Income Program, children in low-income families are more likely than the general population to exhibit disabilities (McNeilly, 2016). Although approximately 21% of children in the United States live in low-income households, 26% of children with speech and language disorders live in these same households.

Developmental and Educational Outcomes

A child with a language disorder often displays elevated symptoms of social, emotional, and behavioral problems relative to peers with TDL and lags in expected academic progress. A child with a language disorder associated with known medical diagnosis and/or intellectual disability may display even more severe deficits.

Although there is individual variation across children with language disorders, prelinguistic development is a relatively stable measure and a predictor of later language development. A longitudinal study of monolingual Finnish-speaking children found continuity from prelinguistic development to later early school-age language ability, meaning that those children who lag behind in early communication development are likely to have language disorders later (Määttä et al., 2016).

Preschool children with late-emerging language are relatively common but may be difficult to detect during the preschool years, although we must continue to try. Children who are identified as late talkers at 24 to 31 months still have a weakness in language-related skills in late adolescence (Rescorla, 2009). Although most perform in the average range on all language and reading tasks at age 17 years, they do significantly more poorly in vocabulary/grammar and verbal memory than SES-matched peers with TDL.

We can roughly characterize children as having three developmental trajectories from preschool into elementary school. These can be described as resolving, persisting, and emerging (Snowling et al., 2016):

- *Resolving.* Language and literacy outcomes are relatively good for those with resolving language disorder. Unfortunately, as high as 35% of those who appear to have resolved their language disorder by age 5½ years may relapse in adolescence as language demands increase.

- *Persisting.* Children whose language disorders persist frequently experience reading and writing (literacy) difficulties.
- *Emerging.* A significant proportion of children with average language abilities in preschool have language disorders that emerged later in elementary school. A high proportion of these children have a family risk of dyslexia and persistent reading difficulties.

Children with a language disorder and those with TDL have similar but divergent developmental paths. Both groups of children have more rapid language growth in preschool. In school age, however, the slowing of development appears to occur at age 7 years for children with TDL and at age 5 years for those with a language disorder. Even with language intervention, language growth appears to slow at an earlier age for children with a language disorder than for children with TDL (Schmitt et al., 2017).

> ***Food for Thought:*** Do these data suggest the importance of beginning language intervention early? Is elementary school too late to intervene for some? Are we missing opportunities to change children's chances of school success?

Compared with their peers with TDL, 4- to 6-year-old children with language disorders show little relative change in their language skills without intervention (Klem et al., 2015). These and other data suggest that a child with a language disorder at age 5 years may experience persistent language difficulties. In addition, the poorer school readiness of a child with a language disorder may mean that they don't fully benefit from the more advanced language of the classroom (Rimm-Kaufman et al., 2000; Spaulding, 2010).

The long-term effects of language disorder for many children are not good, especially without intervention. An Australian longitudinal study found that children identified with communication impairment (CI) at age 4 to 5 years performed significantly more poorly at age 7 to 9 years than their peers with TDL on both teacher and parent assessments and on language testing (McCormack et al., 2011). Parents and teachers reported slower progression in reading, writing, and overall school achievement. The children with CI reported more bullying, poorer peer relationships, and less enjoyment of school than did their peers. These differences were found across age, gender, ethnicity, and SES.

Young adults with language disorder, even those in higher education, may experience persistent deficits in the lexical–semantic system. This can be seen in semantic fluency or the ability to name members of categories quickly and efficiently (Hall et al., 2017). This ability affects categorization and writing flexibility. In addition, there can be a co-occurrence of language disorder with reading disorder or dyslexia (McArthur et al., 2000) and with other disorders, such as autism spectrum disorder (ASD). Looking at other aspects of life, compared to peers, children with language disorders had poorer outcomes in literacy, but also in mental health, and even employment at age 34 years (Law et al., 2009).

Children with language disorders are at greater risk for difficulties with behavior regulation. In general, children with lower behavior regulation gain less over the academic year than do peers with higher behavior regulation (Schmitt et al., 2014).

We're safe in saying that children with language disorders have poorer academic attainment (Schoon et al., 2010), fewer social relationships (Durkin & Conti-Ramsden, 2007), less independence (Conti-Ramsden & Durkin, 2008; Howlin et al., 2000); experience more peer neglect and bullying—chronic stressors that can lead to socioemotional problems (Barkley, 2006; Tomblin, 2014), and poorer employment (Clegg et al., 2005; Howlin et al., 2000) than their peers with TDL. As an SLP, you'll have the responsibility of identifying and intervening with these children.

> *Food for Thought:* Did the possible outcomes relative to language disorders surprise you? Are the scope and seriousness of language disorders becoming more apparent?

Possible Risk and Related Factors

The biggest risk factors for language disorders include (Brignell et al., 2018; Harrison & McLeod, 2010; McNeilly, 2016; Zambrana et al., 2014)

- being male;
- having ongoing hearing problems;
- having a more reactive temperament;
- coming from a low SES background;
- exhibiting poor early communicative skills;
- having a family history suggesting a genetic and/or environmental link in some cases; and
- having a low IQ.

In contrast, protective factors are

- having a more persistent and sociable temperament; and
- higher levels of maternal well-being.

Familial risk for writing and reading difficulties greatly increases the odds for late-onset and persistent language disorder (Zambrana et al., 2014).

Prenatal and/or early postnatal exposure to certain chemicals may also be associated with language delays or disorders. Several studies of polychlorinated biphenyls, lead, and mercury have reported exposure-related reductions in overall IQ and/or verbal skills that persist into middle or late childhood (Dzwilewski & Schantz, 2015).

CHAPTER 2 LANGUAGE DISORDERS

In addition, mothers of preschool children diagnosed with language disorders are less sensitive and exhibit more depression than mothers of children whose language disorder has been resolved (La Paro et al., 2004). Measures of maternal sensitivity include to what degree a mother is a supportive presence and respects her child's autonomy. This is not to suggest that mothers or other caregivers are a causal factor. The differences we see may be a contributing factor, an accompaniment, or a reaction to a child's disorder.

Neurological Basis

Although childhood language disorders are common, researchers have yet to identify a singular neurological source. These efforts are complicated by the nature of the disorder and also by the co-occurrence of other disorders. We are at a point, however, at which we can say that limited evidence exists for regional brain anomalies in the primary language processing centers.

Neuroimaging has so far not identified a specific area that is the neural basis of language disorders. Cortical and subcortical anomalies have been reported in a widespread area in the brain (Liégeois et al., 2014). One area, the superior temporal gyri, has emerged (Figure 2–1). Increasing accuracy in processing complex sentences is correlated with the blood-oxygen-level-dependent activation in both Broca's area and the posterior portion of the superior temporal gyrus, a critical switching area where Wernicke's area intersects with the angular and supramarginal gyri.

Figure 2–1. Neurological areas associated with language disorder.

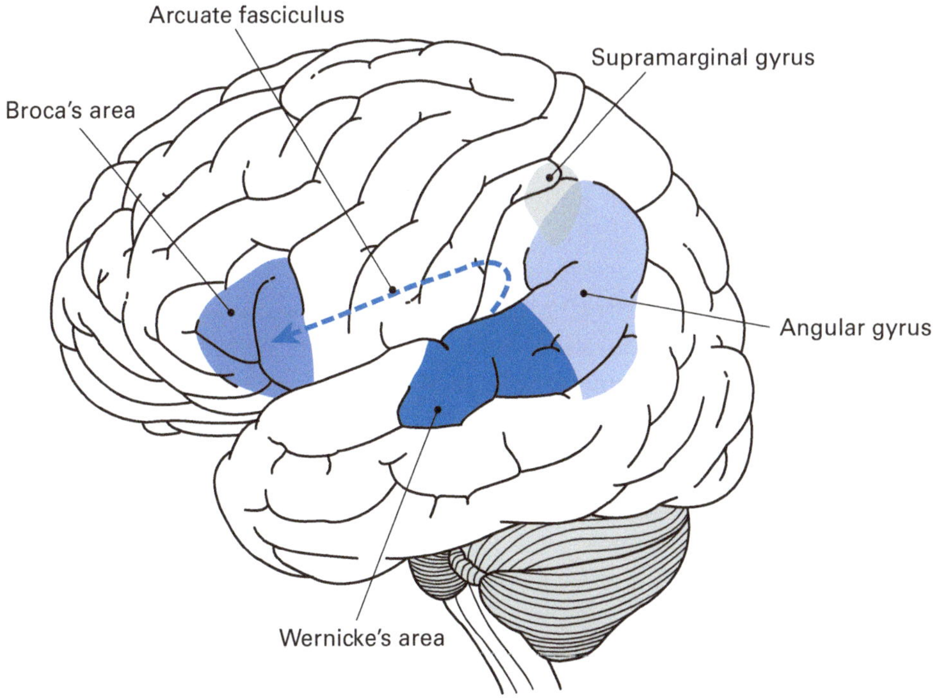

Both accuracy and speed of processing are correlated with maturation of the arcuate fasciculus, the white matter fiber connecting Broca's and the temporal areas mentioned. You may recall from language development that the arcuate fasciculus travels below the brain surface and is especially important for language production. Neuroimaging has found abnormalities in the arcuate fasciculus, although several other areas, primarily in the left hemisphere, have been implicated in language disorders as well (A. Morgan et al., 2016).

Aspects of Language Affected

Language disorders can also affect other aspects of communication. For example, although young preschool children with language disorders gesture more frequently than children with TDL (Iverson & Braddock, 2011), deficits in gestural accuracy occur alongside difficulties with spoken communication (Wray et al., 2017).

In addition, language disorders may not be as confined to specific areas of language as once thought. For example, it may seem at first glance that children have difficulty with only one aspect of language, such as syntax, but in reality they often have deficits across the different aspects of language and the processes of communication in general. Many children with pragmatic difficulties also demonstrate poor receptive vocabulary and poor picture-naming abilities. In addition, many of these children also make more semantic errors, nonrelated errors, and omissions and circumlocutions than their peers with TDL (Ketelaars et al., 2011).

It's easy to assume from these data that children with language disorders perform like younger children with similar receptive language skills. That would be incorrect and would overlook the struggles children with language disorders have with both comprehension and comprehension monitoring, two distinct but related processes.

When we comprehend, we construct meaning, and when we don't, comprehension monitoring helps us detect that a problem has occurred and attempt to correct it and thus improve the accuracy of our representation of the meaning. These judgments of communication breakdown and repair are part of a preschooler's emerging metacognitive and metalinguistic abilities. Comprehension monitoring may lie at the intersection of linguistic and cognitive processing. As such, comprehension monitoring calls into play a child's understanding of diverse areas of language, such as pertinent vocabulary, basic grammatical forms, and a rudimentary story representation, as well as skills of detecting errors, evaluation, and regulations of one's own behavior, which are executive functions (Skarakis-Doyle et al., 2005).

Typical language learning occurs naturally through interaction and conversation with others. This requires that a child be able to

- perceive sequenced acoustic events of short duration;
- attend actively, to be responsive, and to anticipate stimuli;
- use symbols; and
- invent syntax from the language of the environment.

In addition, the child must have enough mental energy to do all of these simultaneously. To accomplish this requires the child to efficiently and effectively monitor and manipulate language information. This takes us to a brief review of information processing.

Information Processing

Prior to discussing specific disorders, it may be helpful to quickly review the information processing system that serves both thought and language. New research is indicating the importance of this system and of the processing of information for both language development and language disorder. It is hoped that this information is a review from language development.

Each individual processes information in a somewhat different manner. These differences can be explained by structural differences in individual brains and by learned differences, such as the way in which each of us approaches problem-solving. These learned differences influence, among other things, decisions about attending, schemes for organization, and rules and strategies for handling information.

Information processing can be divided into four steps: attention, discrimination, organization, and memory or retrieval. These are presented in Figure 2–2.

Attention

Attention includes automatic activation of the brain, orientation that focuses awareness, and focus. When the brain focuses on a stimulus, a neural or mental "model" is formed

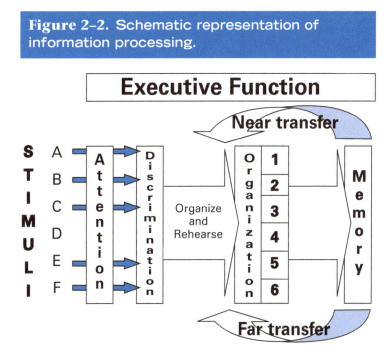

Figure 2–2. Schematic representation of information processing.

in working memory that allows further processing to occur. A child with poor attending skills may not pay attention to important stimuli, with the result that the child will have poor discrimination.

Discrimination

Discrimination is the ability to identify stimuli from a field of competing stimuli. We might also call this process *perception*. Decisions are made on the similarity or dissimilarity of stimuli within working memory. Information is compared to similar information held in long-term memory.

Incoming linguistic information undergoes two types of synthesis: simultaneous and successive. In simultaneous coding, the overall meaning of the message is coded. In contrast, successive coding occurs in linear fashion, one at a time. Language is processed at the unit level rather than holistically. Both processes are used for decoding and encoding of linguistic and nonlinguistic information.

Organization

Organization is the categorization of information for storage and later retrieval. Information that is organized is more easily retrievable. Material that is unorganized or poorly organized will hinder later recall and quickly overload memory capacity. Information is stored in networks that relate to all aspects of stored information. The more associations formed, the better memory and retrieval function.

Memory

Memory is the retrieval of stored information. The capacity for storage and the speed and accuracy of retrieval increase with maturity. Retrieval is limited and dependent on environmental cues, the frequency of previous retrieval, competition from other memory items, and the age of learned information. It is easiest to retrieve information that has been frequently retrieved, has few competing memory items, has distinct environmental cues, and was learned recently and well.

Processes

The simplicity of this discussion doesn't do justice to this complex process. Let's consider transfer, levels of processing, working memory, and central executive function.

Transfer

Although not one of the four steps, transfer or generalization—the application of learned material to previously unlearned information or to new contexts—is important for learning. Transfer exists along a continuum of near to far. Near transfer involves only minimal difference between stored and new information. In contrast, far transfer involves substantial difference. As you might assume, near transfer is easier.

Levels of Processing

Processing occurs on many levels simultaneously (Snyder et al., 2002). At bottom levels, processing is shallow and involves primarily perceptual analysis. In contrast, top levels of processing are more elaborate and associate the new information with knowledge already stored in the brain. As you might surmise, top processing results in better memory because of the associations formed.

Less complex stimuli are initially processed via perceptual analysis at bottom levels and then forwarded to working memory for more elaborate encoding—a process called bottom-up processing—and storage in long-term memory. For more elaborate stimuli, such as language, the brain activates higher, or top-level, processes, such as linguistic and word knowledge. Through these processes, the brain formulates "guesses" of what's coming next, and the low-level processes analyze incoming information perceptually to determine how it fits. In other words, language is "heard" in accordance with the guesses that are based on stored linguistic information and the message so far (Samuel, 2001).

The processes may operate either automatically or in a controlled fashion based on the amount and type of information incoming, the demands of the task, and the capacity of the individual. In contrast to automatic processes, controlled ones are performed consciously and intentionally and make considerable demands on the resources of the brain.

Working Memory

Working memory (WM), which is discussed in more detail later, is the "place" where information, such as an incoming or outgoing sentence, is held while it is processed (R. Gillam & Bedore, 2000). While encoding and decoding, WM must have enough capacity to handle complex information but be flexible to keep up with changing input.

Executive Function

The brain's central executive function (CEF) determines the cognitive resources needed and monitors and evaluates their application while controlling the flow of information. Thus, the CEF is responsible for selective attention and for the coordination and inhibition of stimuli and concepts. Children with language disorder may exhibit difficulty with executive function (EF) in the ways in which they attend to and perceive information and the ways in which concepts are represented (R. Gillam et al., 2002).

If a child with language disorder uses too much energy in bottom-level analyses, they may be limiting the amount of language processed. Too much energy expended in bottom-level analysis—because of poor attending, poor working memory, poor discrimination, or poor organization and/or retrieval—limits the child's ability to process language automatically at higher levels of functioning.

EF is also important for WM. We'll discuss both in more detail in our consideration of developmental language disorders.

Summary

As we proceed, you'll see that information processing can break down at any step. For example, attention abilities of children are associated with their language performance in school (Mahurin-Smith et al., 2017). Children with language disorders have been found to have attention deficits in both visual and auditory modalities, although, as you might expect, the auditory–linguistic deficits are more pronounced (Danahy Ebert & Kohnert, 2011).

Successful participation in conversational give and take requires active monitoring of one's own comprehension. In narratives, preschool children with language disorders demonstrate poorer comprehension monitoring, including error detection, evaluation, and correction, than their peers with TDL (Skarakis-Doyle & Dempsey, 2008).

Many of the children described in the following section have problems in more than one of these areas. As we discuss each language disorder, try to keep these typical abilities in mind.

> ***Food for Thought:*** **How might information processing cause or be related to a language disorder?**

Diagnostic Categories

I hate to put people into boxes and maybe you do too. For the sake of ease of understanding, our discussions throughout this text will focus on clusters of children based on their type of language disorder. It's important to remember, however, that on a daily basis, you as an SLP will be working with individual children and not with categories. A label doesn't relieve us as SLPs of the responsibility to individualize our assessment and intervention efforts.

There is a danger in describing categories of children and then assigning children to these categories. Although categories are helpful for discussion, they can become self-fulfilling. It is important to remember that the child is not learning disabled but, rather, is a child with a learning disability. The distinction is important.

Some educators and parents see labeling as irrelevant. A few reject labels outright. They would argue that among other things, labels

- focus on what's wrong with a child while ignoring environmental limitations;
- stigmatize a child and become self-fulfilling;
- substitute for a thorough description of a child's many facets;
- obscure individual differences;
- can confuse discussions unless strictly defined; and
- give the false impression that they explain a child's difficulties.

All of these are valid concerns, and to these, we might add that the dividing line between typical and disordered is arbitrary, which further clouds any distinctions we make.

CHAPTER 2 LANGUAGE DISORDERS

As a counterpoint, a lack of labels and definitions could minimize children's language difficulties because we would then be left with no clear criteria for deciding who requires professional help. Although there are both advantages and disadvantages in classifying children who exhibit language difficulties, labels are necessary in order to ensure that children receive the services they require and deserve. In addition, labels and categories of disorder can increase our knowledge of the nature and causes of language disorders. In some ways, a lack of agreement about language disorders can impede clinical and research considerations as well as impact access to services.

In addition, consistent accurate nomenclature can facilitate communication with families and clients, professionals, policymakers, the media, and across the research community. In other words, agreed-upon category names allow us to communicate effectively with one another, such as in a textbook.

Continuum of Function

Recently, we've begun to think of disorders in terms of function. From this perspective, neurodevelopmental language deficits are continuous across the entire population, varying only in degree. This perspective is revolutionary for the entire field of disability.

A child with a disability isn't categorically different from a typical child but represents a position along a continuum or spectrum of function. Thus, diagnosis highlights the severity of the functional impact rather than an arbitrary cut-off based on test scores. From this perspective, a child would be considered to have a language disorder if the child's language abilities prevent adequate functioning in life settings, such as family, school, and community.

Using me as an example, I have a slight learning disability. Maybe you do too. It's evident when I write and place words in the wrong order and when I confuse words that sound the same. Sometimes it's funny and at other times downright embarrassing. In addition, I'm easily distracted. But, and here's the important difference, I can still *function* in the world without any accommodations, so I am not considered to have a disorder. I compensate by being extremely organized and that keeps me on track. Another compensation, so as not to be distracted, I try not to sit facing a video or TV screen in a restaurant or play music when I'm writing or reading. The notion of functionality is consistent with the requirement outlined in the Individuals with Disabilities Education Act (2004) and the goals of the Every Student Succeeds Act (2015), in which a child should receive special education supports when their disabilities adversely affect academic performance.

I know this discussion may seem picky, but it's worth our time to stay with it, if for no other reason than to help you understand that our categories and terms are not set in stone. On the contrary, terminology in the field of communication disorders and in special education seems to be constantly in flux. For example, during the past 80 years or so, we have moved thankfully from the horrific terms "idiot" and "moron" through "retarded person" to "mentally retarded person" to "individual with mental retardation" and on to our current "individual with intellectual developmental disorder" (IDD). In part, the changes represent our attempts to clarify and better label, describe, and understand the disorders we encounter.

> *Food for Thought:* Does the notion of disordered behavior on the same continuum as typical behavior challenge your thinking of disorders? At the very least, you might begin to wonder where the dividing line, if it exists, is located.

Broad Groupings

We can roughly divide children with language disorders into two broad groups: those children with seemingly unexplained language problems and those who have other co-occurring or comorbid conditions, such as IDD, that affect their language development and use.

The following discussion begins with children who seem to exhibit only a language disorder with no associated disorders. Then, in Chapter 3 we turn to language disorders co-occurring with other disorders, such as ASD. I promise you that we'll thoroughly explore each disorder category in detail and distinguish one from another.

Discussing of language disorder categories can cause us to overlook the similarities that exist between children classified within different categories. In addition, many children with language disorders cannot be easily described by any of the categories discussed in these chapters. For example, there is a higher prevalence rate of ASD in children with Down syndrome, which is approximately 20%, than in the general population, in which it is approximately 2% (DiGuiseppi et al., 2010; Warner et al., 2014; Wester Oxelgren et al., 2017). Each child represents a unique set of circumstances, so language assessment and intervention must be individualized.

Unfortunately, we are unable to discuss all possible language disorders associated with other disorders. Table 2–1 presents the language disorders we discuss.

Some identifiable disorders have been omitted because of the small numbers of children or the paucity of research data. Others—for example, Tourette syndrome, a neurological movement disorder that affects up to 3% of children and consists of uncontrolled motor and phonic tics (Jankovic, 2001)—have been omitted because concomitant behaviors place the disorder in a somewhat specialized category and also because language disorder is tangential to the primary disorder. In addition, language disorders resulting from low birth weight, prolonged hospitalization, or multiple births are not discussed separately and may be found within other categories described in this chapter (Hemphill et al., 2002). Finally, deafness has also been omitted because of the very broad range of issues relative to hearing, speech, and language. Issues of deafness deserve their own text.

After you complete each category, stop and review what you know so far. Otherwise, as we keep adding to your pile, the different language disorders will all begin to look alike.

Developmental Language Disorders

In many ways, as you'll soon see, developmental language disorders (DLD) are defined by what they are not. Developmental language disorders have no obvious cause and seem

Table 2–1. Primary Categories of Language Disorders	
Language disorders	Development language disorder (DLD)
	Social communication disorder (SCD)
Language disorders associated with another disorder	Autism spectrum disorder (ASD)
	Learning disability/specific learning disorder (LD)
	Intellectual developmental disorder (IDD)
	Neurological disorders
	Traumatic brain injury (TBI)
	Cardiovascular accident (CVA)
	Maltreatment and neglect
	Other
	Late language emergence (LLE)
	Childhood schizophrenia
	Selective mutism
	Otitis media
	Deafness

not to affect or be affected by anatomical, physical, or intellectual problems. Children with DLD may appear to be delayed, although the language problem is not the result of early language delay or other co-occurring disorders. In fact, children with DLD are unlike children with TDL at every stage of development.

There is a mismatch between the percentage of children with DLD who are considered eligible for clinical services and estimates based on the prevalence of DLD from community samples (McGregor, 2019). There is more need than there are services, which are underfunded, in part, because of the perception that fewer children are affected. It's a circular conundrum.

This mismatch may reflect a lack of awareness of DLD; the less obvious nature of DLD compared with other disorders; and potential conflict with parents, caregivers, and administrators when a child is diagnosed within the schools. Most families and staff do not understand that it is within an SLP's scope of practice to diagnose DLD.

These children are underidentified, identified late, or not identified at all, especially if they are not male, White, or wealthy, or from well-educated families (Catts et al., 2012; Frazier Norbury et al., 2016; P. Morgan et al., 2016; Wittke & Spaulding, 2018). A general lack of awareness of DLD results in inadequate service delivery (McGregor et al., 2020). However, children with DLD will be the bulk of your caseload as a school-based SLP.

Although professional organizations and publications, plus school districts are retiring an older term *specific language impairment* (SLI) in favor of DLD, the lion's share of the research is with children with SLI. It is hoped that you can see how that poses a bit of a dilemma as I attempt to describe DLD. So, here's my thought. I will not use the term SLI unless absolutely necessary and instead I'll speak of "the majority of children with DLD," which would be correct.

Description

Like Juan, described previously, children with DLD seem typical in other ways except language. Unfortunately, without intervention, most will not catch up to other children their age. Children with DLD have a seemingly unexplained deficit in language abilities despite appropriate environmental stimulation and cognitive abilities and no neurological disorders (Bishop et al., 2017; Leonard, 2014; National Institute of Deafness and Other Communication Disorders, 2017).

The presence of DLD in preschool and later is a strong predictor of the disorder in the future. The longer it persists, the higher the chance or probability—as high as 90% in one study—that it will continue (Miniscalco et al., 2018; Snowling et al., 2000).

Although we will characterize children with DLD as having typical intelligence, the range of "typical" is wide. One meta-analysis of 131 studies reported that as a group, children with SLI were in the low normal range for nonverbal or nonlanguage intelligence (Gallinat & Spaulding, 2014). Children with DLD exhibit deficits in a variety of nonverbal tasks, such as manipulating images and hypothesis testing, suggesting impaired or delayed cognitive functioning (Mainela-Arnold et al., 2006).

Language skills are significant predictors of performance in all school subject areas for children with DLD. As might be expected, these children have greater difficulty with curriculum that's more heavily reliant on language abilities, such as English and language arts. Science and mathematics are affected to lesser degrees, especially on nonlanguage-based tasks (Durkin et al., 2015).

A meta-analysis of case history factors and SLI, the bulk of those with DLD, identified the following five factors that are predictive for the majority of children with DLD (Rudolph, 2017):

- Late language emergence
- Maternal education level
- 5-min Apgar score (a health measure used with newborns and explained more in Chapter 4)
- Birth order
- Biological sex

The ability gap between children with DLD and those without doesn't close with age, but children with higher nonverbal IQs and/or mothers with higher education seem not to lag behind their peers with TDL as much. These factors are risk factors, not causes.

> *Food for Thought:* Were you surprised to find that a language disorder could exist seemingly on its own? We often only envision language disorders associated with other disorders, such as traumatic brain injury.

Psychosocial Adjustment

A majority of children with DLD are likely to have the following:

- A high risk for reading disorders (Catts, 2004; Catts et al., 2014)
- Low academic achievement and increased risk for stopping education at the high school level (Tomblin, 2014)
- Peer relationship difficulties (Durkin & Conti-Ramsden, 2007)
- Heightened risk for peer victimization and bullying (Redmond, 2011)
- Increased risk for being identified as having attention-deficit/hyperactive disorder
- Increased social anxiety in early childhood (Brownlie et al., 2016)

In general, the majority of children with DLD are perceived more negatively by both teachers and peers (Segebert DeThorne & Watkins, 2001).

Young children with DLD may have behavior problems that decrease with age (Redmond & Rice, 2002). In elementary school, children with DLD take minor roles in cooperative learning, contribute little, and have fewer high-level negotiating strategies than their language-matched peers developing typically. By late elementary school or middle school, language problems take their toll on self-esteem, and these children perceive themselves negatively in scholastic competence, social acceptance, and behavior conduct (Jerome et al., 2002).

Given that communication is fundamental to the initiation and maintenance of successful peer relationships (Ladd et al., 2012; Rubin et al., 2012), it's not surprising that children with DLD often have peer problems. One longitudinal study found that for these children, peer relations is the most developmentally vulnerable area of functioning (St Clair et al., 2011). As might be expected, risk of poor peer relations is greatest for children with pragmatic difficulties. In establishing peer relationships, prosocial behavior is the strongest factor, consisting of behaviors such as being considerate of others' feeling, sharing, helping those in distress, being kind to younger children, and volunteering to help others.

Children at risk for DLD demonstrate increased emotional difficulties that are likely a function of early language difficulties and emotional self-regulation abilities (St Clair et al., 2019). Overall, children who are more social, possess better pragmatic language skills, and have lower levels of emotional problems have fewer problems in developing peer relations.

The majority of school-age children with DLD often experience difficulties in socioemotional functioning related to language and to social cognition, the ability to process, store, and apply information about other people and social situations. These children often have difficulties with emotional competence, which puts them at risk for victimization and bullying. Forty percent of 7- and 8-year-old children with SLI report physical bullying in school compared with 10% of children with TDL (Redmond, 2011). These findings suggest that bullying may be a major negative factor in the psychosocial health of children with DLD. Children who are victimized report higher levels of sadness and fear.

Poor pragmatic skills are related to poor social outcomes. As a result, by the time they get to junior high, many adolescents with DLD perceive themselves negatively in scholastic competence, social acceptance, and behavioral conduct, characterized by choosing to act in the accepted manner (Jerome et al., 2002).

Compared to school-age children with TDL, the majority of those with DLD, especially those with expressive language deficits, are less successful at initiating play interactions. These children withdraw and engage in more individual play and onlooking behaviors (Hart et al., 2004; Liiva & Cleave, 2005). Their reticence is characterized by staring at other children but not reacting, doing nothing even when there are many opportunities, and demonstrating fear of approaching other children. We saw this with Juan at the beginning of this chapter. Reticence and extreme aloneness may lead to rejection by others in middle and high school (Rubin et al., 2002).

In addition, those with DLD tend to have more aggressive behavior (Winstanley et al., 2018). Fortunately, young adults with a history of DLD who received intervention during their school years report less contact with their local police than age-matched peers with DLD who lack intervention.

Language and literacy play an increasingly larger role in adolescent independent functioning. Adolescents with DLD are less independent than their peers with TDL (Conti-Ramsden & Durkin, 2008). As these teens transition into adulthood, parents and caregivers express concern about their level of independence, quality of peer relations, their social behavior, and the presence of behavioral issues (Conti-Ramsden et al., 2008).

Research demonstrates that there is a correlation between language ability in adolescence and self-esteem in young adulthood. Young adults with a history of language disorders enter adulthood less socially confident than their peers with TDL (Durkin et al., 2017; Wadman et al., 2008). Those with language disorders have poorer self-esteem and social self-efficacy and are more shy than peers with TDL. Women with DLD have almost three times the risk for sexual assault in adulthood as adults with typical language (Brownlie et al., 2007, 2017).

Language Characteristics

Developmental language disorder is a persistent language disorder that is evident early in development. It's likely that a child with DLD will become an adult with poor language skills, especially in language form, which is the primary aspect of language affected.

Children with DLD begin to use single words and to combine words at a later age than children with TDL. The trajectory of their subsequent language growth is similar to but less advanced than that of children with TDL. Growth begins to slow in preadolescence, prior to reaching a par with their peers (Rice, 2012, 2017).

Among school-age children and adolescents with DLD, there is a deficit in the ability to detect regularities in language, such as verb endings and sentence structure. These are, you'll recall, related to the frequency of occurrence of these language structures (Lammertink et al., 2017). In development, children with TDL use these regularities to determine the underlying rules. Specific language problems found in many children with DLD are presented in Table 2–2.

The use of frequency information (how often something occurs) to identify underlying rules and meaning is called statistical learning. A simplistic explanation of the importance of statistical learning is that words and grammar that are heard more

CHAPTER 2 LANGUAGE DISORDERS

Table 2–2. Language Characteristics of Children With Developmental Language Disorder

Pragmatics	May act like younger children developing typically.
	Less flexibility in their language when tailoring the message to the listener or repairing communication breakdowns.
	Same pragmatic functions as chronological-age-matched peers developing typically, but expressed differently and less effectively.
	Less effective than chronological-age-matched peers in securing a conversational turn. Those with receptive difficulties most affected.
	Inappropriate responses to topic.
	Narratives less complete and more confusing than those of reading-ability-matched peers developing typically.
Semantics	First words and subsequent vocabulary development occurs at a slower rate, with occasional lexical errors seen in younger children developing typically.
	Poor fast-mapping of novel words.
	Naming difficulties may reflect less rich and less elaborate semantic storage than actual retrieval difficulties. Long-term memory storage problems are probable.
Syntax/ morphology	Co-occurrence of more mature and less mature forms.
	Similar developmental order to that seen in children developing typically.
	Fewer morphemes, especially verb endings, auxiliary verbs, and function words (articles, prepositions), than younger MLU-matched peers. Learning related to grammatical function as in children developing typically.
	Tend to make pronoun errors, as do younger MLU-matched peers, but tend to overuse one form rather than making random errors.
Phonology	Phonological processes similar to those of younger children developing typically, but in different patterns—that is, occurring in units of varying word length rather than in one- or two-word utterances.
	As toddlers, vocalize less and have less varied and less mature syllable structures than age-matched peers developing typically.
	Poor nonword repetition.
Comprehension	Poor discrimination of units of short duration (bound morphemes). Ineffective sentence comprehension.
	Reading miscues often unrelated to text graphophonemically, syntactically, semantically, or pragmatically.

frequently should be theoretically easier to learn. When we compare children with DLD to peers with TDL, we find that children with DLD have disorders in both word segmentation or breaking a word into phoneme components and in fast mapping or the ability to determine a word's meaning quickly from use (Haebig et al., 2017).

Pragmatics. Preschool children with DLD demonstrate a reduced ability to resist distracting input and to inhibit it (Spaulding, 2010). In conversation, where most language is learned, many things are occurring at once that require both of these abilities in order to focus on language.

Children with DLD have deficits in their ability to recognize the impact of and to express emotions compared to typically developing age-matched peers (Brinton et al., 2007). Social perception skills, such as understanding the thoughts and emotions of others, affect children's communication abilities in everyday situations. Children with DLD demonstrate difficulties in their social perception abilities. Syntax and pragmatic aspects of the language impact **theory of mind** (ToM) understanding in school-age children with DLD (Spanoudis, 2016).

You may recall from your language development course that ToM is the knowledge that others have minds, perceptions, and ideas that differ from your own. Although not as severely affected as children with ASD, children with DLD do perform significantly below their peers with TDL on verbal ToM tasks (Loukusa et al., 2014).

The conversational behaviors of children with DLD compared with those of mental-age-matched peers with TDL are marked by both qualitative and quantitative differences. For example, qualitative differences, such as difficulty initiating interaction and inappropriate responses, lead to increased interruptions by other children.

Not surprisingly, given their other deficits, children with DLD use less expressive elaboration in oral narratives than their age-matched peers with TDL, producing narratives that resemble those of younger children (Ukrainetz & Gillam, 2009). The stories of both 6-year-old children with TDL and 8-year-olds with DLD have fewer appendages, such as a preceding abstract; fewer orientations, such as a description of a character; and poorer evaluations. Children with DLD, like younger children with TDL, show poorer performance with simple narrative elements such as character names.

Semantics. Children with DLD often have vocabulary disorders. When we compare the receptive vocabularies of children ages 2;6 to 21 years both with DLD and without, the majority of children with DLD have lower levels of receptive vocabulary throughout the age range (Rice & Hoffman, 2015).

Both semantic and phonological deficits contribute to word-learning difficulties (Gray, 2005). Although word retrieval problems are usually defined as difficulties in accessing words that are already known by a child, the drawings, definitions, and recognition responses of children with SLI are also relatively poor, indicating limited semantic knowledge which, in turn, contributes to their frequent naming errors (McGregor et al., 2002). For example, compared to their peers with TDL, children with DLD recognize fewer semantic aspects of objects and actions, such as physical features (color, shape, size), thematic elements (throw, hit, catch within a game), and/or causation (who caused an action, who or what received) (Alt et al., 2004).

The sparse underlying lexical–semantic representations in children with DLD can be explained in part by **lexical competition**, a significant factor in poorer word definitions (Mainela-Arnold et al., 2010). When we begin to hear a word, based on the initial phonological information, our brains activate our best prediction of what that word will be. Hearing the word spoken confirms or does not confirm our prediction. Choices are limited by the phonemes heard and by semantic sensemaking. For example, you're in a fast-food restaurant with a friend and she says, "I'll have a /bI/..." You predict she'll say "Big Mac" not *Big Bird*, *bib*, or *bitter*. The competing words are canceled automatically. Research suggests that the majority of children with DLD experience difficulty inhibiting activations of nontarget competitor words (Mainela-Arnold et al., 2008).

Although the naming abilities of children with DLD are slower than those of age-matched children with TDL, they are similar to those of other children at the same vocabulary level (Sheng & McGregor, 2010). This similarity and the naming errors of children with DLD suggest immaturities in their semantic representations.

A significant subgroup of children with DLD demonstrate deficits in lexical–semantic organization (Sheng & McGregor, 2010). On word association tasks, compared with both age-matched and vocabulary-matched peers with TDL, children with DLD produce fewer semantic responses (e.g., cat–pet), more phonologically based responses (e.g., cow–now), and more errors.

However, for both children with DLD and children with TDL, fast mapping of new words appears to occur in a similar fashion (Gray & Brinkley, 2011). The phonotactic probability or predictability of the new word and previous lexical knowledge affect word learning in similar ways for both groups of children. As you may recall from your language development course, **fast mapping** is rapid assumption of a word's meaning upon hearing it, followed by subsequent use, although the complete meaning is unknown to a child.

A relationship exists between EF and word learning for both children with TDL and those with DLD. **Executive function** is the directing and tuning of the brain for various tasks. Preschoolers with DLD perform worse than peers with TDL on measures of EF and novel word learning (Kapa & Erikson, 2020). These deficits in word learning and EF in children with DLD help account for the difficulties seen in learning new words.

Compared to peers with TDL, school-age children with DLD demonstrate more effortful cognition during language comprehension (Montgomery et al., 2018). For children with TDL, comprehension occurs automatically through pattern recognition and linguistic chunking, suggesting a holistic approach. In contrast, comprehension for children with DLD may occur on a more word-by-word basis.

Language comprehension and processing are active processes in which the listener infers the meaning from the auditory message, contextual information, and stored world and word knowledge. Children with DLD do not appear to employ actively all of this available information. In general, they have difficulty constructing an integrated representation of a series of events, whether the series is presented verbally or nonverbally. Thus, vocabulary growth—which occurs typically as the result of inferring meaning from repeated exposure and without direct reference or prompting from adults—will be very difficult for the child with DLD using limited active processing strategies.

Not surprisingly given what you just read, school-age children with DLD also exhibit significant deficits in spoken sentence comprehension. Most of this difference seems to be explained by memory-based deficits rather than syntax-specific deficits, but additional research is required (Montgomery et al., 2016).

Syntax/Morphology. Children with DLD produce significantly more speech disruptions than their same-age peers with TDL (Finneran et al., 2010; Guo et al., 2008). Speech disruptions, such as inserting pauses or fillers (e.g., *uh* or *well*) or repeating syllables or words, can be a sign of underlying syntactic difficulties, even when the sentences contain no grammatical errors. Underlying lexical and/or syntactic weaknesses may also be seen in the more extensive reliance on gestures to support and supplement speech (Lavelli & Majorano, 2016).

The comprehension and production of complex syntactic structures are restricted in the majority of children with DLD, as we saw with Juan (Frizelle & Fletcher, 2014a, 2014b; Riches et al., 2010). This limitation is related to memory difficulties (Marton et al., 2006) also noted in verbal and nonverbal learning of sequence-specific information (Hsu & Bishop, 2014).

Morphological inflections and shorter words, such as pronouns, are especially difficult. As small units of speech, morphemes receive little stress and may be difficult for a child to identify. Thus, children with DLD often make errors with verb endings, pronouns, and auxiliary verbs. Problems may be related because pronoun selection (*he* versus *they*) determines some verb endings (*walks* versus *walk*).

Auxiliary verbs, infinitives, verb endings, and irregular verbs offer persistent problems for both preschool and school-age children with DLD, as we saw in Juan's speech (Goffman & Leonard, 2000; Redmond & Rice, 2001). The relatively late appearance of tense markers, such as past tense *-ed*, may be an early indication of DLD (Hadley & Short, 2005). Although most tense markers are mastered by age 4 years for children with TDL, the majority of children with DLD take an additional 3 years to achieve the same level of competence. Even as adolescents, the majority of children with DLD continue to struggle with morphological markers and exhibit an ongoing maturational lag compared to age-matched and language-matched peers with TDL (Rice et al., 2009).

Deficits in morpheme use vary. Children with DLD use the regular past tense *-ed* less when temporal adverbs, such as *tomorrow* and *already*, are present in the sentence, suggesting that other sentence elements also play a part in use of the tense marker (Krantz & Leonard, 2007).

In short, the majority of children with DLD have less developed lexical–morphological networks than their peers with TDL and thus less derivational morphology knowledge or less knowledge in root word structure and morphological manipulation. This can have consequences for vocabulary and reading comprehension. For example, one way that vocabulary increases in late elementary school through adolescence is by inclusion of root words (*fortune*) and variations (*fortunate, unfortunate, fortunately, unfortunately*).

Summary. Children with DLD have difficulty (a) learning language rules, (b) registering different contexts for language, and (c) constructing word-referent associations for lexical growth. The result is difficulty in morphological and phonological rule learning and application and in vocabulary development. Pragmatic problems result from inability to use effective forms to accomplish language intentions.

Possible Causal Factors

Causes of DLD are difficult to determine and may be as diverse as the children who have the disorder. With such a diverse population, it is not surprising that several possible causal factors have been identified.

DLD is best characterized as a complex multifactorial disorder caused by a combination of genetic and environmental risk factors of small effect (Bishop, 2009). We discuss three areas of concern: biological, social–environmental, and processing factors.

> ***Food for Thought:*** **What might cause a language disorder with no obvious causal factors. Even if we can find genetic differences, they explain little about what is going on during linguistic processing.**

Biological Factors. The language and learning problems of children with SLI suggest a neurological disorder. Magnetic resonance imaging suggests that compared to children with TDL, those with SLI exhibit different patterns of brain region activation and coordination that suggest reliance on a less functionally efficient pattern (Ellis Weismer et al., 2005). These patterns are presented in Figure 2–3. Note the differences. In addition, those with SLI show reduced activation in the brain areas critical for communication processing (Hugdahl et al., 2004). Recall that children with SLI are the primary group represented in DLD.

Figure 2–3. Neurological processing of children with TDL and SLI. The size of the arrows represents the amount of coordination between brain areas. *Source:* Ellis Weismer et al. (2005).

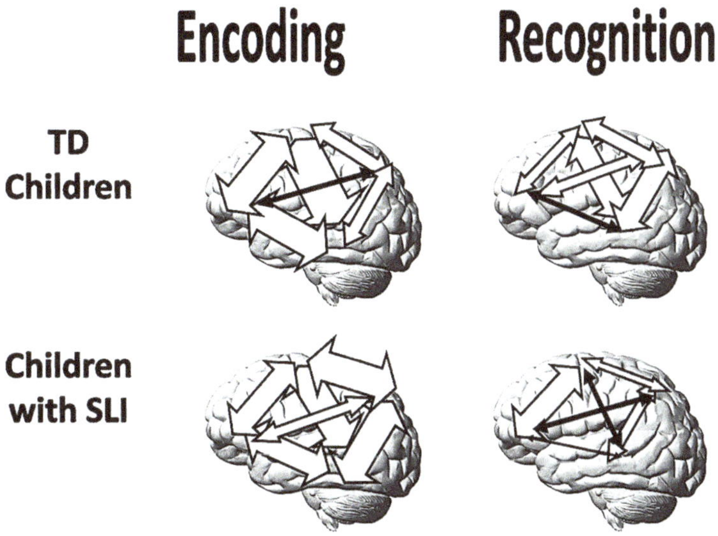

Many children with DLD have a deficit in the neural circuitry responsible for procedural memory (Ullman & Pierpoint, 2005). **Procedural memory** is involved in the learning and execution of sequential cognitive information such as language. The problem is not limited to language expression; comprehension is influenced as well (Tomblin et al., 2007).

There is a predominance of males among children with DLD. In addition, there is increased likelihood of a child having DLD if there is a sibling or parent with the disorder (Whitehouse, 2010).

A biological cause is also suggested by this strong familial pattern (Choudhury & Benasich, 2003). Sixty percent of children with SLI have an affected family member, and 38% have an affected parent. The relationship is particularly strong for children with SLI who exhibit expressive language problems. When language disorder occurs in families with a history of SLI, it is often accompanied by reading disorders (Flax et al., 2003). Further evidence of a biological factor can be found in preterm births. A sizable minority of infants born at 32 weeks or less are at considerable risk for DLD.

These relationships plus the finding of language disorders in twins, even into school age, suggest a genetic link (Rice et al., 2020). Preliminary results indicate a genetic link in some forms of DLD (Andres et al., 2020). For example, family-based linkage mapping has identified a language-associated locus on chromosomes 14q and 15q24.3–25.3.

Social–Environmental Factors. Although the majority of prenatal, perinatal, and neonatal risk factors do not have a clear causal role in childhood DLD, poor neonatal health may signify increased risk. In contrast, input from parents does not play an important causal role (Dale et al., 2015; Warlaumont & Jarmulowicz, 2012). I'm not saying that environment is unimportant, but it's unlikely to be a causal factor in DLD. However, the interactional patterns within parent–child interactions may be subtly modified by the child's language disorder and parents' responses to it.

Processing Factors. Although children with DLD demonstrate typical nonverbal intelligence, they may demonstrate cognitive disorders not exhibited on standard intelligence measures. As mentioned previously, these children do not seem to employ active processing strategies that use contextual information and stored knowledge. Information-processing problems of the majority of children with DLD occur with incoming information, in memory, and in problem-solving. In addition, children with DLD demonstrate slower linguistic and nonlinguistic processing on both expressive and receptive tasks compared to age-matched children with TDL.

These characteristics suggest limitations in cognitive processing capacity in which trade-offs exist between accuracy and speed of responding (Ellis Weismer & Evans, 2002). In the rapid give-and-take of conversation, this trade-off results in reduced processing and storage of phonological information, inefficient fast mapping and novel word learning, slow word recognition, and ineffective sentence comprehension (Ellis Weismer et al., 2000; C. Miller et al., 2001; Montgomery 2000). All have been mentioned previously.

Specific difficulty with morphological markers suggests that the brevity of these morphemes in speech may be a factor. Children with SLI perform considerably below age-matched typically developing children in sensitivity to sound contours and sound

CHAPTER 2 LANGUAGE DISORDERS

duration (Corriveau et al., 2007). In addition, these children demonstrate difficulty in nonword or nonsense word repetition. Taken together, these characteristics may indicate underlying language-processing deficits in working memory, where language is held while processed.

Executive Function and Working Memory Deficits. As you may recall from your language development course, several aspects of memory are important for language learning and use, including the following (Hood & Rankin, 2005):

- Short-term memory (STM)
- Long-term memory (LTM; including semantic and episodic memory)
- Working memory (WM)

STM involves the temporary storage of information, such as immediately recalling items on a shopping list or numbers in a recently heard telephone number or steps in following directions (Alloway et al., 2009; Minear & Shah, 2006). LTM is storage of older information, especially important for word meanings. When you recall what happened on vacation, you're tapping into LTM. Finally, WM is an active process that allows limited information to be held in a temporary accessible state while cognitive processing occurs (Cowan et al., 2005). Information in WM is in an active and/or accessible state and temporarily maintained while a mental operation is completed.

Although all components of WM in children with SLI are below those of their peers with TDL in preschool, by age 7 or 8 years, it's primarily verbal working memory (VWM) that still lags behind (Vugs et al., 2017). It may be helpful to conceptualize VWM as part of EF. EF consists of inhibition, working memory, planning, organization, and regulatory processes that enable us to engage in goal-oriented behavior (Bashir & Singer, 2006; Singer & Bashir, 2018). Complex tasks may require simultaneous storage of information and active processing (Barrouillet et al., 2007; Kidd, 2013; Swanson, 2017).

To date, almost all research on VWM and language disorder is with children having SLI, a disorder subsumed in DLD. I'm uncomfortable characterizing the research differently, so I'll refer to SLI as such or as DLD/SLI. Remember that the overwhelming majority of children with DLD were previously assumed to have SLI.

According to Gillam and colleagues (2017), children with SLI differ from children with TDL in their use of cognitive strategies for processing, organizing, and chunking language in VWM and in their regulation of attention. Although children with DLD/SLI demonstrate significant language disorders despite normal-range hearing and nonverbal IQ, many, but not all, of these children do show marked deficits in VWM abilities (Archibald & Joanisse, 2009). A brain imaging study of children with DLD/SLI found differences in the left-hemispheric VWM tracts and a lack of lateralization in WM tracks compared to children with TDL (Verly et al., 2019).

A model of WM proposed by Gillam, Evans, and Montgomery (GEM) adds some clarity by integrating the structural–functional relationship between WM/LTM and comprehension (Figure 2–4). The GEM model reflects the relationship between cognitive processing and sentence comprehension by representing the indirect influences

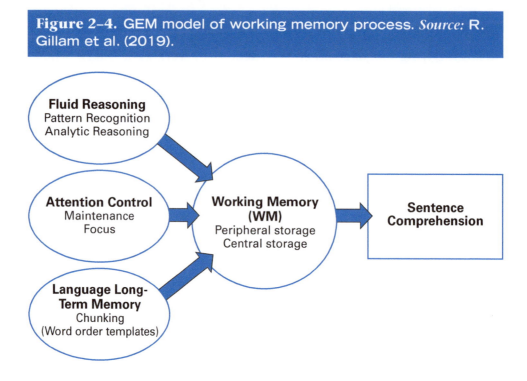

Figure 2–4. GEM model of working memory process. *Source:* R. Gillam et al. (2019).

of pattern recognition, controlled attention, language LTM, and WM to explain how children use word order to build language structure and the importance of the resulting syntax as a foundation to comprehension.

Briefly, the GEM model consists of four cognitive mechanisms (R. Gillam et al., 2019; Montgomery et al., 2021):

- Fluid reasoning is the ability to use logical and analytical reasoning to solve novel problems, such as recognizing and interpreting patterns.
- Controlled attention is necessary for comprehension.
- Language knowledge found in LTM is essential in a chunk-and-pass model of language processing (McCauley & Christiansen, 2015) that includes immediate chunking of the input at lower levels, such as phonological and lexical, and passing these to higher levels, such as multiword units and syntax where a child constructs intermediate structures such as noun phrases, verb phrases, and clauses.
- Working memory.

Fluid reasoning, controlled attention, and language knowledge in LTM all contribute to variation in complex VWM, which in turn causes variation in the comprehension of syntactic structure. The stronger the relationships between each of the cognitive variables and complex WM, the greater a child's ability to comprehend speech and reading (R. Gillam et al., 2019; Motallebzadeh & Yazdi, 2016).

Comprehension requires both (a) sustaining attention to a sentence to enable a child to attend to the incoming words and (b) attention switching to enable a child to shift

CHAPTER 2 LANGUAGE DISORDERS 47

between storing created linguistic chunks in VWM and LTM, which in turn generates new chunks from incoming input (Finney et al., 2014).

> ***Food for Thought:*** **Have you noticed your own ability to attend to communication wavering? Is it more difficult to follow a conversation if you watching Netflix at the same time? Why is that?**

Finally, the chunking that occurs and reoccurs due to LTM continues until all necessary structures are realized, assigned meaning, and combined into a single, meaningful, cohesive unit. As a child matures and has more language processing experiences, chunking units increase in size and become more stable, thus increasing the efficiency of the comprehension system (Thiessen, 2017). In turn, these multiword chunks become building blocks for language production as well (Cornish et al., 2017; Theakston & Lieven, 2017).

These three mechanisms function through WM. Each mechanism relates positively with WM, meaning that better fluid reasoning, controlled attention, and language knowledge correlates with better WM. These mechanisms don't cause WM; they are part of the WM process.

Preschoolers with DLD have deficits in EF. These deficits are related to selective attending, inhibition control, attention shifting, and mental-set shifting or fluid reasoning (Kapa et al., 2017; Yang & Gray, 2017). WM deficits on nonverbal tasks suggest that these deficits in EF are at work here as well (Henry & Botting, 2017). Compared to peers with TDL, children with SLI have difficulty with general inhibition control and fluid reasoning that goes beyond the demands of linguistic tasks (Pauls & Archibald, 2016).

We are constantly bombarded by stimuli. Unable to focus on everything, we attend selectively. Active cognitive control directs the brain toward a relevant stimulus and simultaneously inhibits attention of irrelevant stimuli. For the majority of children with DLD, attention shifting and inhibition are significant predictors of spoken word recognition. Children with SLI have difficulty exerting control over their auditory attention and inhibiting distracting stimuli (Victorino & Schwartz, 2015).

Communication often requires shifting attention from one person to another or to objects mentioned or used to communicate. Preschool children with SLI experience difficulty shifting or changing their attention as efficiently to changing stimuli as their peers with TDL (Aljahlan & Spaulding, 2019). Inefficient attention, especially over an extended period of time, correlates with deficits in VWM and language ability in children with TDL (Jongman et al., 2017; Smolak et al., 2020).

The problem becomes one of where to attend or allocate cognitive resources. Poor resource allocation is a significant factor in complex sentence comprehension difficulties. For the majority of children with DLD, comprehension is mentally demanding (Montgomery & Evans, 2009). Thus, processing capacity limitations and difficulty in inhibition control may explain why children with DLD consistently perform more poorly than their peers with TDL on tasks that tap into the storage and processing components of WM (Brocki et al., 2008; Isaki et al., 2008; Marton et al., 2007; Riccio et al., 2007).

The CEF is responsible for resource allocation or determining where to place energy when tasks become more complicated. With deficits in these areas, children with SLI demonstrate weaker resistance to interference compared to their peers with TDL, which in turn affects their information processing abilities in general (Marton et al., 2014).

VWM is a conduit through which three things—syntactic knowledge in LTM, controlled attention, and general pattern recognition—indirectly influence sentence comprehension and production (Montgomery et al., 2021). Let's briefly discuss VWM and apply it to children with DLD. A listener uses VWM to create structure and meaning in the moment, anticipate upcoming language, and hold earlier parts of a sentence as new sentence information arrives. In other words, sentence comprehension is all about simultaneous processing and storage.

Although listeners are limited in their ability to hold more than a few bits of information, language form aids immediate storage by allowing the listener to group or chunk information into meaningful units. Better language knowledge enables more "chunking" and better comprehension. The process is further facilitated by the meanings of words and by our experiential or world knowledge.

Children with DLD have significant difficulty with syntactic knowledge and general pattern recognition as well as with control of attention, an important aspect of VWM (Archibald & Gathercole, 2007; Evans et al., 2009; Lum et al., 2014; Victorino & Schwartz, 2015). These deficits inhibit the VWM system and, hence, comprehension. Most likely, children with DLD have less strong sentence patterns in LTM and require more cognitive energy for comprehension (Montgomery et al., 2017, 2018, 2021).

Compared to age-matched peers, many children with DLD/SLI show several significant limitations in VWM mechanisms and in processing speed. The cognitive processing factors that influenced children's ability to recognize a target word in a stream of speech differ from those of children with TDL (Evans et al., 2018). Poor updating and receptive vocabulary result in children with DLD having slower speed in spoken word recognition (Evans et al., 2018).

Verbal Working Memory and Language. Verbal working memory deficits may place these children at risk for lexical difficulties (Gathercole, 2006). Difficulty with attention and VWM capacity and speed can mean that small units such as bound morphemes or phonemes are overlooked or not perceived. Morpheme learning may involve

- perceiving an inflected word (*boys*) and comparing it with the uninflected component (*boy*);

- hypothesizing the grammatical function of the morphological marker; and

- placing the marker in a morphological paradigm or model.

Moreover, these operations must be completed with speed to ensure correct morphological analysis.

A child must be able to store the novel inflected word, retrieve from LTM its uninflected component, and simultaneously perform a comparative morphological analysis

CHAPTER 2 LANGUAGE DISORDERS

before the marker decays from memory. The production of newly learned morphemes and sentences may stretch VWM and slow processing speed of children with DLD. This is also true for sentence production and may explain the pauses and fillers in the speech of children with DLD, such as Juan.

The need to access a newly learned morphological inflection and then append it to a word while simultaneously formulating and producing an utterance in a timely fashion may exceed the overall processing capacity of children with DLD/SLI. Thus, many children with DLD are at risk for constructing incomplete or inaccurate morphological representations.

In general, children with DLD also exhibit poorer sentence comprehension compared to age-matched peers with TDL. Comprehension may also represent general cognitive processing limitations in VWM and processing speed (Bishop, 2006; Montgomery & Evans, 2009). Complex sentences place additional processing demands on VWM. Most likely, deficits in VWM interact with past knowledge, the nature of the task, and the strategy used by the child. These influence the outcomes in tasks with significant VWM demands (Minear & Shah, 2006).

Imagine that you have limited WM but communication is occurring at a rapid rate. As the input increases, you are easily overwhelmed, slowing the entire process. Your limited memory makes it increasingly difficult to hold information as more comes in, slowing the process even more. You begin to lose information as more comes in. It's increasingly difficult to relate new information to partially processed old information. Maybe you've experienced this when you've tried to communicate in another language. Now you get some inkling of one aspect of language processing for children with DLD/SLI.

Summary

Many children with DLD will not be detected until the increasing demands of the school curriculum overwhelm their ability to process language. The language difficulties of children with DLD are primarily found in, but not limited to, language form, especially the smaller units, such as morphemes and phonemes, and shorter words, such as pronouns, prepositions, and auxiliary verbs. The cumulative result is poor sentence production and comprehension.

Although effective interprofessional cooperation is important in meeting the needs of children with DLD in school, it's difficult to achieve. A review of the professional literature indicates a lack of shared understanding about DLD (Gallagher et al., 2019). One of the main differences that influences intervention is the nature of DLD. Teachers may see the disorder as primarily requiring increased instruction. Such an approach does not address the core issue of language disorder.

Social Communication Disorder

Social communication disorder (SCD), a neurodevelopmental communication disorder, affects both verbal and nonverbal communication skills in speaking and writing. As such, SCD is a classic example of the overlapping and sometimes conflicting naming of communication disorders. SCD first appeared in the fifth edition of the *Diagnostic and Statistical Manual of Mental Disorders*, the American Psychiatric Association's (2013) classification tome of mental disorders. The complicating factor is that although SCD exists on its own, the characteristics may be seen in other language disorder categories, primarily, but not limited to, ASD. The two disorders, as we'll see, are different.

Social communication includes speech style, perspective taking, rules for verbal and nonverbal communication, and use of language to accomplish goals. Acceptable social communication is determined by one's environment, but there's a wide range of acceptable norms within and across individuals, families, and cultures (Curenton & Justice, 2004; Inglebret et al., 2008).

SCD is characterized by difficulties with the use of both verbal and nonverbal communication for social purposes in both speaking and writing. Deficits are evident in the individual's inability to (American Speech-Language-Hearing Association [ASHA], 2019)

- communicate for social purposes appropriate for the social context;
- modify communication for the context or needs of the listener;
- follow rules for conversation and narration;
- understand abstract, figurative, or ambiguous language; and
- understand what is not explicitly stated.

Thus, SCD can result in difficulty participating in social settings, developing peer relationships, achieving academic success, and employment performance.

> ***Food for Thought:*** **You'll recall that Juan had some interactional difficulties. The difference is that his were secondary to his language disorder and not the primary feature.**

Precise estimates of the prevalence of SCD are difficult to determine because of the inconsistent or ambiguous definition and the validity of the criteria for the disorder (Swineford et al., 2014). Among kindergarteners, pragmatic language disorder occurs in approximately 7.5% of children (Ketelaars et al., 2009). Boys are identified at a ratio of 2.6:1.0 compared with girls. The rate is much higher (23–33%) among individuals previously diagnosed with language disorders (Botting et al., 1998; Ketelaars et al., 2009).

Given the fact that many children with ASD exhibit interactional difficulties, it might be helpful to make a distinction. One characteristic of ASD, which we'll explore later, is the presence of restricted and repetitive interests and behaviors (RRIBs). Children with SCD but no co-occurring disorders will exhibit significant social communication and pragmatic difficulties but without RRIBs (Cholemkery et al., 2016; Gibson et al., 2013; Greaves-Lord et al., 2013; Swineford et al., 2014; Timler, 2018a).

Although the social-interactional behaviors of children with ASD and SCD may look similar, the two disorders are distinct and should be mutually exclusive. As mentioned previously, you still may encounter children with both diagnoses. In part, the confusion stems from similar terms used to describe each disorder and overlapping diagnoses. Some overlap exists because SLPs can diagnose SCD, which is a pragmatic language disorder, but in most states are not authorized to diagnose ASD, which is usually the purview of a psychologist or psychiatrist.

In many cases, the difference between ASD and SCD is one of degree of severity. In addition to RRIBs, children with ASD have difficulty transitioning between activities, may have extreme focus on a few topics, and display over- and undersensitivity to sensory stimuli.

Language Characteristics

Language characteristics of children with SCD vary with a child's age and the communication context and requirements. As a child matures into school age and adolescence, the requirements for social communication increase and behavior that was acceptable at a younger age, such as interrupting others, is no longer so. Although SCD can take several forms, common language characteristics include the following (ASHA, 2019):

- Inappropriate and inadequate greetings
- Lack of flexibility changing language and communication style to fit a setting or partner
- Difficulty producing and comprehending narratives
- Awkward engagement in all aspects of conversation, such as initiating or entering a conversation, maintaining the topic, and turn-taking
- Poor repair of communication breakdowns
- Inadequate, ineffective, or confused use of appropriate verbal and nonverbal signals to regulate conversational interactions
- Misinterpretation of the verbal and nonverbal signals of others
- Difficulty understanding ambiguous or figurative language and information not explicitly stated

As you might imagine, this lack of or difficulty with conversational give and take leads to a child having few, if any, close friendships. Children with SCD are often isolated and lonely.

Although we'll discuss assessment later, it seems appropriate to note the difficulty in measuring the pragmatic deficits mentioned. There is currently no reliable standardized test for SCD, in part because the pragmatic aspects of language are fluid and dynamic (Yuan & Dollaghan, 2018). Unlike syntax, pragmatic rules are context-dependent and less explicit (Adams, 2002; Norbury, 2014; Volden et al., 2009).

In addition, it's important to recognize that what is appropriate communication behavior in one culture may not be acceptable in another. For example, the amount of eye contact varies by culture. Differences related to cultural norms are not disorders, although children with SCD are found across all human cultures.

Possible Causal Factors

Causes are often varied because SCD co-occurs with so many disorders. For example, the causes of ASD and traumatic brain injury, both of which can co-occur with social interactive difficulties, differ greatly. In short, the cause of SCD in the absence of any other disorder is not known.

Conclusion

The language disorders discussed in this chapter are "stand-alone" language disorders. I made up that term, but it's recognition that other disorders are not present. That doesn't negate other difficulties, such as issues with WM, but those alone are not classified as disorders.

The fact that we have no associated disorders does not lessen the impact of a language disorder on the child and their family. As we saw with Juan, a language disorder can greatly influence a child's academic and social interactions and has the potential for lifelong consequences.

We're now about to discuss language disorders that are associated with other disorders. Before we do that, check to be sure that you understand the ones discussed so far.

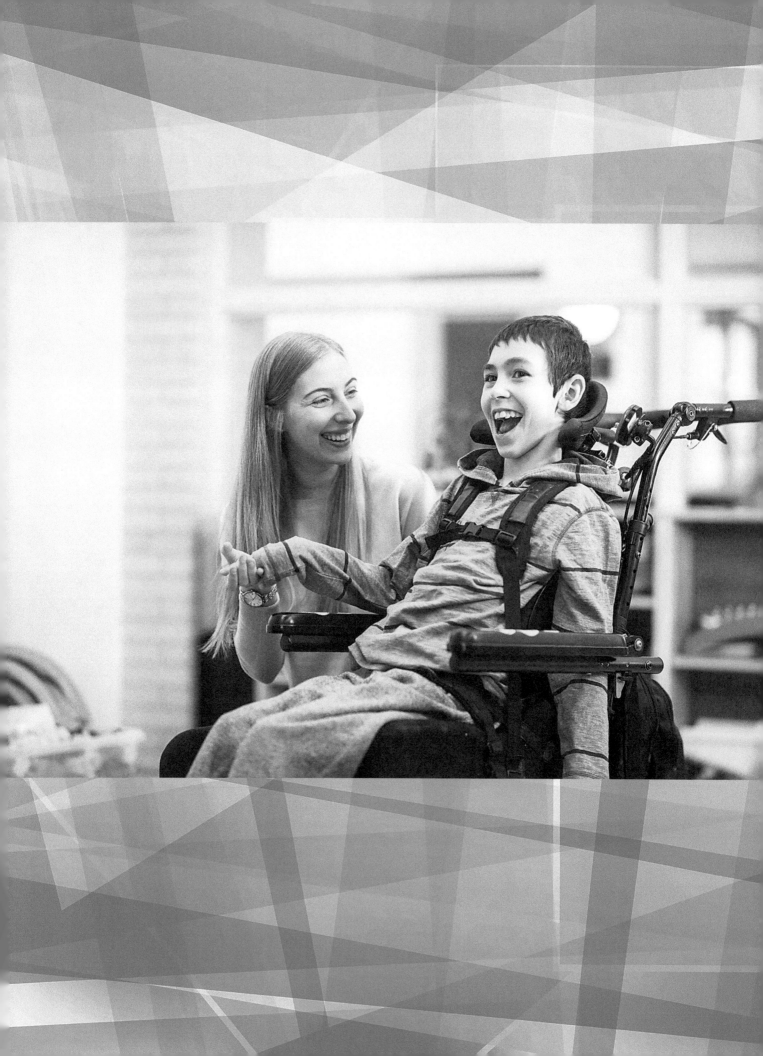

CHAPTER 3

LANGUAGE DISORDERS ASSOCIATED WITH OTHER DISORDERS

Julie is an active, some might say overactive, third grader who is very athletic. She did well in school but shined on the playing field, especially in soccer. Last year, she suffered a traumatic brain injury.

After striking her head when she ran into the goal, she was unconscious for more than an hour and seemed lost and confused when she came to. She was rushed to the hospital. No brain swelling was detected, so she did not have any cranial surgery but was kept in bed for several days.

Initially, her motor functioning was affected, but this returned to normal quickly and physical therapy ceased upon her release. Unfortunately, memory and speech and language took much longer. Even a year after her head injury, Julie cannot recall the accident and has some difficulty recalling directions and remembering words and names.

Her spoken and written sentences are simple. Speech is halting as she tries to recall words and phrases. Her grandmother, with whom Julie lives, reports that "She's different somehow, distant, less personable." Her teacher notes that the other girls avoid her, and she is prone to mood swings and outbursts.

You'll recall from Chapter 2 that we can conceptualize language disorders as those with no obvious cause and those associated with other co-occurring or comorbid conditions. We've discussed the former and now turn our attention to the latter. The following discussion begins with children with language disorders and co-occurring autism spectrum disorder (ASD) and then proceeds to learning disability (LD), intellectual developmental disorder (IDD), neurocognitive disorders such as traumatic brain injury (TBI), and maltreatment and neglect. It finishes with other less frequent disorders. That's a lot to cover, so without further fanfare, here we go.

Language Disorders Associated With Autism Spectrum Disorder

The fifth edition of the *Diagnostic and Statistical Manual of Mental Disorders* (*DSM-5*; American Psychiatric Association [2013]) defines autism spectrum disorder (ASD) as a disorder in reciprocal social interaction that includes restricted and repetitive interests and behaviors. The following behaviors characterize ASD:

- Persistent deficits in social communication and interaction including deficits in social–emotional reciprocity, nonverbal communicative behaviors, and developing, maintaining, and understanding relationships.

    Deficits in reciprocity can range from abnormal social behavior and failure in typical conversation to a seeming inability to initiate or respond in social interactions. Nonverbal deficits can range from poorly integrated verbal and nonverbal communication to a total lack of facial expressions and other nonverbal communication. In other disorders, a lack of verbal communication often means a reliance on nonverbal, which is the opposite of what we might see in children with ASD. Finally, deficits in relationships can range from difficulty adjusting to social contexts to a lack of, or absence of, interest in one's peers.

- Restricted, repetitive patterns of interest, behavior, or activity (RRIBs), seen in at least two of the following:

    - Stereotyped or repetitive motor movements.
    - Insistence on sameness.
    - Highly restricted, fixated interests.
    - Hyper- or hyposensitivity to incoming stimuli or unusual interests in sensory stimuli.

    Repetitive motor movements may be seen in the use of objects or in speech. Children may repeat a sound, sound combination, or word with seeming disregard for the context. The insistence on sameness may be seen in inflexible commitment to routines, or ritualized patterns of verbal or nonverbal behavior, such as rocking continually. Interests, in children with ASD, may be abnormal in intensity or focus. Finally, a child may be extremely sensitive to one stimulus, such as touch, but seemingly insensitive to another, such as pain.

- Some symptoms must be present at an early age.
- Symptoms cause significant impairment in areas of functioning.
- Deficits are not explained by other developmental delays.

Not every child with ASD will exhibit all of these characteristics, and several characteristics, especially in children who have mild or high-functioning ASD (HFA), are present in other disorders. Table 3–1 presents the characteristics of different severities of ASD.

According to the U.S. Centers for Disease Control and Prevention (CDC, 2018c), in the United States, ASD affects approximately 1 in every 44 children across all racial, ethnic, and socioeconomic groups. The CDC further reports that these data are in line with the reported prevalence in Asia, Europe, and the Americas. Forty-four percent of children identified with ASD have average to above average intellectual ability (CDC,

CHAPTER 3 LANGUAGE DISORDERS ASSOCIATED WITH OTHER DISORDERS   **57**

Table 3–1. Severities of Autism Spectrum Disorder

Severity	Social Communication	Restricted, Repetitive Behaviors
Level 1 (requires some support)	Deficits in both verbal and nonverbal communication Limited initiation Minimal responding Unusual communication behavior	Inflexible behavior interferes in one or more contexts Difficulty switching between activities Problems with organization and planning
Level 2 (requires substantial support)	Marked deficits in both verbal and nonverbal communication Social impairment Limited initiation Reduced or abnormal responding Limited, narrow-interest topics Markedly odd nonverbal communication	Inflexibility Difficulty coping with change Restricted/repetitive behaviors that interfere with functioning Difficulty changing focus
Level 3 (requires very substantial support)	Severe deficits in both verbal and nonverbal communication Very limited initiation Minimal responding to direct approaches Unusual approaches to meet needs only	Inflexible behavior Extreme difficulty coping with change Restricted/repetitive behaviors markedly interfere with functioning Great distress/difficulty changing focus or action

Sources: Compiled from information on CDC (2018c) and Autism Speaks (n.d.) websites as well as *DSM-5* (APA, 2013).

2016). ASD is four times as common in males as in females, who tend to have less restricted and repetitive behavior compared to males of similar age and severity (Knutsen et al., 2019).

ASD can co-occur with other disorders. For example, there is a high prevalence rate of ASD in children with Down syndrome (DS). Approximately 20% of children with DS also have ASD (DiGuiseppi et al., 2010; Warner et al., 2014; Wester Oxelgren et al., 2017).

The average medical expense for a family is $4,110 to $6,200 annually per child or adolescent with ASD (CDC, 2019). In addition, intensive behavioral intervention for a child with ASD can cost $40,000 to $60,000 per year (Amendah et al., 2011).

Development

The age of detection of ASD varies with severity and the presence of developmental delay, especially in communication and social interaction. The more intense the symptoms, the poorer language and overall development (Pry et al., 2005). Children with more severe ASD are often diagnosed in preschool, whereas many of those with high-functioning ASD will go undiagnosed even into adulthood. Previously called **Asperger's syndrome**, HFA has been a characteristic of some of the most brilliant minds, especially in science and technology.

We should be cautious with generalizations about development given the seeming varied paths in development among children with ASD and the fact that many studies are based on parental memory. However, infants with severe ASD have been described as either lethargic, preferring solitude and making few demands, or highly irritable, with sleeping problems and screaming and crying. In the first 6 months, children with severe ASD reportedly show normal acquisition of developmental milestones (Davidovitch et al., 2018). By 9 months of age, however, children with severe ASD begin to fall behind in language and communication, as well as motor skills.

Although it is rare that ASD is identified prior to 18 months of age, usually, between 18 and 36 months the signs become more pronounced, including more frequent tantruming, repetitive movements and ritualistic play, extreme reactions to certain stimuli, lack of pretend and social play, and joint attention and communication difficulties including a lack of gestures. In approximately 20% of children with severe ASD, parents report typical development until 24 months, especially among girls.

Early identification is often difficult because of the lack of obvious medical problems and the early typical development of motor abilities. Infrequently, onset occurs in later childhood. Recent data suggest that young children with severe ASD exhibit impairment in joint or mutual attending, symbolic play, and social affective communication.

Development often proceeds in spurts and plateaus, rather than smoothly. Most areas of development are affected, although occasionally one area, such as mechanical or mathematical abilities, is typical or above. I have worked with children well above average in mathematics but unable to dress themselves or to participate in meaningful conversations.

Characteristics

The *DSM-5* description is very thorough, so I won't repeat each portion, but I think some comments are in order. Relational disorders may be the most distressful aspect of ASD, especially for parents. Children with ASD often avert their gaze or stare emptily and lack a social smile, responsiveness to sound, and anticipation of the approach of others. Parents often are treated as "things" or, at best, no different from other people.

Children with ASD exhibit sensory modulation dysfunction (SMD). Sensory modulation occurs within the central nervous system (CNS) as it attempts to balance excitation and inhibition inputs within the sensory mechanism with external stimuli. Typically, sensations are detected and responded to in a routine manner that is appropriate and adaptive (Lane, 2002). SMD is a mismatch between the external demands and a person's internal system characteristics, resulting in behavior that is underresponsive or overresponsive (Hanft et al., 2000). For children with ASD, stimuli must be within the limits of a child's tolerance and expectation. Children with ASD fluctuate between the two extremes, exhibiting overresponsiveness until overload occurs that results in shutdown and a defensive or withdrawal response. Behaviors such as tantrums do not seem to be related to communication ability (Mayes et al., 2017).

Over- and underresponsiveness to stimuli may be found in the same child. For example, loud noises may get no response from a child, whereas whispering results in a catastrophic response.

CHAPTER 3 LANGUAGE DISORDERS ASSOCIATED WITH OTHER DISORDERS

Children with severe ASD tend to prefer shiny objects, especially those that spin; things that can be twirled; and noises they produce themselves, such as teeth grinding. Children with ASD seem to prefer routines and may become extremely upset with change. Individual children may have very definite preferences in taste, touch, and smell. I worked with one child whose only food preference was dill pickles. Self-stimulatory behaviors may include rocking, spinning, and hand flapping.

Risk Factors

A wide range of risk factors have been found for ASD (CDC, 2019; Tager-Flusberg, 2016). These include the following:

- Demographic factors
  - Being male. Males are affected four times as often as females.
  - Having a family history of ASD. Among identical twins, if one child has ASD, then the other has a 36% to 95% chance of also being affected. In addition, families who have a child with ASD have a 2% to 18% chance of having a second child who is also affected.
  - Having a chromosomal disorder. Approximately 10% of children with ASD are also identified as having Down syndrome, fragile X syndrome, or other genetic and chromosomal disorders.
  - Being born to older parents.
  - Being born preterm or with low birth weight.
  - Having other developmental, psychiatric, neurologic, chromosomal, and genetic diagnoses. The co-occurrence of one or more non-ASD developmental disorders is 83%. The co-occurrence of one or more psychiatric disorders is 10%.
- Behavioral factors
  - Lack of early gesturing.
  - The presence of certain repetitive motor behaviors.
- Neurological factors
  - Atypical lateralization for speech.
  - Increased brain growth.

Unfortunately, many of the risk markers are also found with other disorders, making early identification difficult.

Language Characteristics

Communication problems are often one of the first indicators of possible ASD, especially in severe cases. These may include a failure or delay in developing gestures or speech, a seeming noninterest in other people, or a lack of verbal responding. Lack of communication skills is one of the most significant stress factors for families of children with ASD and one of the earliest indicators of the disorder.

Although children with ASD vary widely, we can generalize that the most rapid expressive vocabulary growth is found in children who say and imitate more words; have better pretend-play skills with objects; and use gestures more often to initiate joint attending, such as pointing at entities to direct attention (Smith et al., 2007). Calling attention to entities through gestures and sounds seems to be important for comprehension of new vocabulary words (McDuffie et al., 2005). The importance of these factors is similar to that found in typical development (Watt et al., 2006).

Conventional gesture comprehension increases during the early development of children with language disorders and those with typically developing language (TDL). Although data suggest a reliance on gestures by children with language disorders, those with ASD experience a deficit in both oral language and nonverbal communication (Perrault et al., 2018). In other words, the intention to communicate is not as evident. As a speech-language pathologist (SLP), you may be challenged to help build that intent, as we'll see in Chapter 4.

Poor social interaction and poor language and communication skills are extremely characteristic of children with severe ASD. Speech does not seem to be difficult for those who speak, although speech is often wooden and robotlike, lacking a musical quality. Although children with HFA are able to perceive affective stress (sad, happy) and lexical stress (*HOTdog* versus *hot DOG*) as well as peers with TDL, they have reduced ability to produce natural prosody in their own speech (Grossman et al., 2010), adding to the robotic sound.

Those children using speech and language may demonstrate immediate or delayed echolalia, a whole or partial repetition of previous utterances, often with the same intonation. In fact, many children with more severe ASD who learn to talk go through a period of using echolalia.

Immediate echolalia is variable and increases in highly directive situations; with unknown words; when unable to comprehend; in the presence of an adult; in unfamiliar situations; in face-to-face communication with eye contact; and with longer, more complex utterances. Children with ASD produce less immediate echolalia in a story-telling context than in a play-based one (Gladfelter & VanZuiden, 2020). Immediate echolalia also has been found to signal agreement in some children.

No such data are available for delayed echolalia. One child with whom I worked would repeat many of the utterances directed to him during the day as he lay in bed prior to sleep.

Language characteristics vary widely among children with ASD. At one extreme are children whose language structure is within normal limits, whereas at the other extreme are children who remain essentially nonverbal (Landa, 2000). Even when language structure seems intact, difficulties with appropriate social use of language or pragmatics may persist (Adams, 2002; Tager-Flusberg, 2004; Young et al., 2005). Specific language characteristics of children with ASD are presented in Table 3–2.

Not all children with ASD have language disorder. Those who do are more significantly socially impaired (Bennett et al., 2014).

CHAPTER 3 LANGUAGE DISORDERS ASSOCIATED WITH OTHER DISORDERS

Table 3–2. Language Characteristics of Children With Autism Spectrum Disorder

Pragmatics	Deficits in joint attending.
	Difficulty initiating and maintaining a conversation, resulting in much shorter conversational episodes.
	Limited range of communication functions.
	Difficulty matching form and content to context. May perseverate or introduce inappropriate topics.
	Immediate and delayed echolalia and routinized utterances. Few gestures used; misinterpretation of complex gestures. Overuse of questions, frequent repetition.
	Frequent asocial monologues.
	Difficulty with stylistic variations and speaker–listener roles. Gaze aversion, seeming use of peripheral vision.
Semantics	Word-retrieval difficulties, especially for visual referents. Underlying meaning not used as a memory aid.
	More inappropriate answers to questions than age-matched peers.
Syntax/ morphology	Morphological difficulties, especially with pronouns and verb endings.
	Construction of sentences with superficial form, often disregarding underlying meaning.
	Less complex sentences than mental-age-matched peers developing typically.
	Overreliance on word order.
Phonology	Phonology variable within individual child, often disordered. Developmental order similar to children developing typically.
	Least affected aspect of language.
Comprehension	Impaired comprehension, especially in connected discourse such as conversations.

Pragmatics

Across nonverbal and minimally verbal toddlers with ASD, we find uneven communication profiles with relative strength in phonology and significant weakness in pragmatics (Bean Ellawadi & Ellis Weismer, 2015). Thus, deficits in pragmatics are central to any discussion of ASD.

Preverbal children with ASD exhibit deficits in joint or shared attending and attending to people. Joint attention, an early social interactional behavior, is sharing the attention of another person, as when a caregiver and child play with or explore the same toy. A child's ability to establish joint attention and express intentional communication, in addition to parental linguistic responding, are positive predictors of both expressive and receptive spoken language growth in children with ASD (Shumway & Wetherby, 2009; Yoder et al., 2015).

As you might expect, 18- to 24-month-old children with ASD communicate via gestures, vocalizations, and verbalizations at a lower rate than either children with TDL or those with other developmental disabilities. Compared to children with TDL, those with ASD use a significantly lower percentage of communicative gestures, instead relying on more primitive gestures.

Children with ASD who are more verbal have difficulties in initiating a conversation and in responding to initiations of others. Once the conversation has begun, they have difficulty with the give-and-take of conversation and with taking turns appropriately (Botting & Conti-Ramsden, 2003). Speakers with ASD may fail to contribute new, relevant information to the topic and may repeat previously mentioned topics or previous utterances or fail to link their utterance to prior ones, resulting in sudden and inexplicable topic changes (Volden, 2002).

In part, pragmatic difficulties may reflect deficits in **presupposition** that relate to difficulties with theory of mind (ToM). You may recall from your language development course that presupposition is the pragmatic ability of a speaker to assess what a listener may know or need to know and to adjust the content of speech accordingly. Adolescents with TDL produce shorter narrations when they share knowledge with a listener. This does not seem to be the case in children with ASD, although it does vary with age for children with ASD and with severity of ASD (de Marchena & Eigsti, 2016).

Compared to peers with TDL, elementary school children with HFA do significantly poorer on ToM measures, executive functioning, and pragmatic competence (Berenguer et al., 2018; Bora & Pantelis, 2016; Hutchins et al., 2016). ToM incompetence and poor pragmatic language skills help explain the atypical social functioning of these children.

In addition, the range of expressive intentions may be very limited. Also, intentions may be expressed in an individualistic manner, such as saying "Sesame Street is a production of the Children's Television Workshop" for "Goodbye."

The conversations of children with ASD often contain inappropriate, irrelevant, bizarre, or stereotypical utterances (Adams, 2002; Gilchrist et al., 2001; Volden, 2004). For example, a child might say, "Did you know that the Volt is a type of electric car" in the middle of a conversation about what they had for breakfast.

Finally, children with ASD have difficulties generating the oral narratives that are part of conversation. For example, the narratives of adolescents with ASD are shorter and sentences are less grammatically complex, containing fewer causal statements than those of peers with TDL (King et al., 2014).

Semantics

Semantics may be affected. Definitions tend to be very concrete and may not generalize to similar words. Figurative language is also difficult for many children with ASD, who tend to interpret phrases such as "Hit the roof" in an overly literal manner.

CHAPTER 3 LANGUAGE DISORDERS ASSOCIATED WITH OTHER DISORDERS

Children with ASD also seem to have difficulty matching the content and form of language to the context. Occasionally, children will incorporate rote utterances, such as the child who says "Attention, shoppers" to get the teacher's attention. Even individuals who have acquired language often have peculiarities and irregularities in their communication.

Attention toward the speaker correlates positively with receptive–expressive vocabulary size (Bopp et al., 2009). This fact suggests that variation in attention toward a speaker might in part explain the vocabulary size deficit of children with ASD compared to the vocabulary of children with TDL (McDaniel et al., 2018). If a child is not attending or is doing so poorly, it is difficult to learn words from the language around the child.

You may recall that children with TDL use statistical learning and fast mapping to learn new words. Children with ASD appear to have intact statistical learning, regardless of their language ability, but their fast-mapping abilities differ according to their language functioning (Haebig et al., 2017).

Research has suggested that language comprehension might also be a deficit area in children with more severe ASD. School-age boys with ASD exhibit sentence comprehension delays comparable to their level of receptive vocabulary. However, sentence comprehension is much weaker than nonverbal cognitive abilities would suggest (Kover et al., 2014).

Syntax and Morphology

Language structure is often not disordered. Oral language structure or form is a relative strength for children with ASD, especially those with HFA. Language form errors that do occur seem to represent a lack of underlying semantic relationships.

Although many children with ASD fail to develop verbal communication skills, verbal children are similar in syntax and phonology to other children matched for mental age. In addition, verbal students with ASD appear to develop language form and speech in a typical developmental sequence (Watson & Ozonoff, 2000).

As might be expected with any disorder, but especially for one that has a spectrum of behaviors, the language of children with ASD varies considerably. Researchers have identified two distinct language profiles emerging as children with ASD mature (Tek et al., 2014). When language is measured by the size of a child's lexicon or personal dictionary, morphosyntactic production measured by grammatical morphemes, and *wh-* question complexity, children with ASD and higher verbal skills were comparable to children with TDL on most of these measures. Children with ASD and low verbal skills had less development than either group.

The morphosyntactic profiles of children with developmental language disorder (DLD) and children with language disorders associated with ASD are not significantly different when assessed using both standardized tests and language sampling (Huang & Finestack, 2020). That's not to say the two groups of children are similar. As an SLP, you'll be challenged to accurately assess these children.

> ***Food for Thought:*** **The number of children diagnosed with ASD has exploded worldwide in recent years. Why do you think this has occurred?**

Possible Causal Factors

In the past, children with ASD were classified as having an emotional-, physical-, environmental-, or health-related disorder. The cause may be any, all, or none of these. The primary causal factors are probably biological. Even within this population, neuroanatomical and neurochemical features may differ.

Biological Factors

A high percentage of individuals with ASD have abnormal brain patterns. The incidence of autism accompanying prenatal complications, fragile X syndrome, and Ritt syndrome (a degenerative neurological condition) and among those with a family history of ASD is higher. In addition, ASD is often accompanied by IDD and seizures. All of these suggest a neurobiological basis but do not explain the actual disorder. Other studies have found unusually high levels of serotonin, a neurotransmitter; abnormal development of the cerebellum, the section of the brain that regulates incoming sensations; multifocal or infectious disorders of the brain; and disorder of the neural subcortical structures with accompanying impairment in cortical development.

Although more research is still needed, cross-sectional neuroimaging to date reveals abnormalities in primary sensory areas of the brain (Lainhart, 2015). In addition, abnormally enlarged brain volumes and increased rates of brain growth during early childhood have been found in some, but not all, children with ASD.

Specifically, disorganized development seems to occur in the white matter, which is connective tissue between surface processing neural areas, and in the amygdala, an almond-shaped section of the CNS believed to play a critical role in the way humans experience, recognize, and process emotions (Figure 3–1). The resultant processing changes are unknown. There are also data indicating inefficiencies and dysfunction in posterior cerebral regions.

Studies have suggested a genetic link in ASD, although it seems doubtful that a solitary autism gene exists (Wentzel, 2000). It is more likely that several genes are involved and may be shared with other disorders.

Social–Environmental Factors

Early studies blamed parents for their child's ASD. No basis has been found for this conclusion. In general, parents interact with their children at the appropriate developmental level.

Although mothers of children with ASD and TDL use equal amounts of content words in child direct speech, the content of the mothers with children with ASD consists of significantly more concrete nouns (*doggie*) and active verbs (*run*). Only rarely do mothers of children with ASD use abstract nouns (*fear*), stative verbs (*feel*), adjectives (*big*), and adverbs (*really*) (Tubul-Lavy et al., 2020). The effect of this difference is unknown and may reflect a child's behavior and a child's attention.

Parental behavior can result in positive outcomes. Maternal positive affect and the use of multimodal initiations and responses are associated with more positive affect, vocalizations, gaze to face, and multimodal bids or responses among infants with ASD

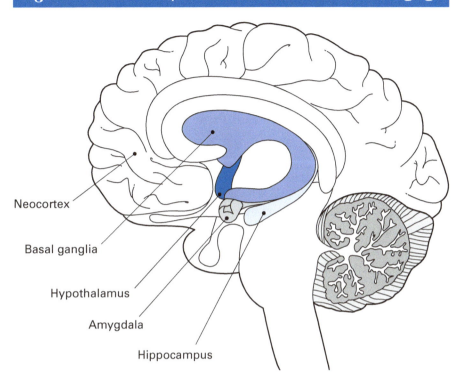

Figure 3–1. Autism spectrum disorder and neural imaging.

(Schwichtenberg et al., 2019). Multimodal behaviors take the form of various communication modalities, such as facial expression, gestures, and speech.

Processing Factors

Children with ASD have difficulty analyzing and integrating information. When attending, they tend to fixate on one aspect of a complex stimulus, often some irrelevant, minor detail. In other words, responding is very overselective. This fixation, in turn, makes discrimination difficult.

Aberrant sensory processing may affect the rate of acquisition of language, social, and communication skills in children with ASD. Specifically, hypo-responsiveness and sensory-seeking behavior, such as self-stimulatory behaviors, are negatively associated with language skills and social adaptive skills.

Overall processing by these children has been characterized as a "gestalt" in which unanalyzed wholes are stored and later reproduced in identical fashion, as in echolalia. In this relatively inflexible system, input is examined in its entirety rather than analyzed into its component parts. Information usually is reproduced in a context that is in some way similar to the initial context. This reliance on unanalyzed wholes could account for the tendency of children with ASD to repeat an agrammatical sentence rather than to correct it as language-matched children with IDD will do.

The behavior of children with ASD suggests that very little of the world makes sense to them. They seem to overload quickly. Information "swallowed" whole, as suggested in the previous paragraph, could quickly "fill" and overload a child's processing system.

Storage of unanalyzed wholes also might hinder memory. Children with ASD reportedly are less able to use environmental cues, such as a word or gesture, to aid memory, possibly because those cues do not exist as separate entities in the child's memory. It is also difficult for these children to organize information on the basis of relationships between stimuli.

In addition, children with ASD have difficulty transferring or generalizing learned information from one context to another. This difficulty reflects the inability of these children to identify the relevant contextual information.

Summary

As with other disorders, children with ASD demonstrate heterogeneity. Great differences are found in severity, especially in communication abilities. In general, these differences affect the pragmatic and semantic aspects of language and may reflect processing difficulties such as stimulus overselectivity and storage of unanalyzed wholes.

Early intervention is critical to maximizing outcomes for children with ASD, but early identification is often difficult. Although SLPs alone do not make evaluations of children for ASD, they are a vital part of the evaluative team (Prelock et al., 2003).

Children with ASD also demonstrate deficits in joint attention and symbolic communication (Wetherby et al., 2000). Given the limitations of current research, it may not be possible at this time to make a definitive diagnosis prior to 24 months of age (Woods & Wetherby, 2003). That's not stopping researchers and clinicians from attempting to find definitive early behaviors.

In closing this section, note that although there is no definitive cure for ASD, up to 70% of children with severe ASD are prescribed psychoactive medications to ameliorate disruptive behaviors associated with ASD. The entire health care team, including SLPs, should be involved in monitoring the behavior for medication efficacy, tolerability, and potential side effects. Self et al. (2010) offer an excellent tutorial on medications prescribed to treat behaviors associated with ASD, including potential side effects.

At this point, it might help further discussion if you make a few notes contrasting DLD, social communication disorder, and ASD. As we proceed, you can add to your list.

Language Disorders Associated With Learning Disability/ Specific Learning Disorder

Most of us are familiar with the term *learning disability*, even if we're unsure of the exact meaning. LD is an educational term defined in U.S. federal education law, the Individuals with Disabilities Education Act (IDEA, 2004). The DSM-5 uses the medical term *specific learning disorder* (SLD). There's considerable overlap in the definitions, although from differing perspectives (Cortiella & Horowitz, 2014).

IDEA defines learning disability as follows (U.S. Department of Education, 2018):

- Involving one or more of the basic psychological processes
- Affects the understanding or use of spoken and/or written language

- May be manifested in the imperfect ability to listen, think, speak, read, write, spell, or do mathematical calculations
- Not primarily the result of visual, hearing, motor disabilities, mental retardation, emotional disturbance, or of environmental, cultural, or economic disadvantage

LD is a general term used primarily in educational settings. Schools often use terms such as *dyslexia* to describe specific learning problems. Dyslexia predates LD and refers specifically to difficulties with accurate or fluent word recognition, poor spelling, and deficits in coding abilities (International Dyslexia Association, 2002).

DSM-5 defines LD somewhat differently and calls it specific learning disorder. The primary differences are those between a medical and an educational usage. *DSM-5* describes SLD as persistent, mentions academic skills below expectation, and states that the disorder begins during the school years. Dyslexia has been replaced with the more awkward *SLD with impairment in reading*. Nothing precludes the continued use of dyslexia or other terms by individuals or support organizations.

As an author, I get to make a few decisions. Given the wording in IDEA, our discussion of children, and the common usage in educational circles, I'll use the more general-use terms learning disability, LD, and dyslexia. In addition, the term "specific learning disorder" sounds a little harsh and too long, especially when we add "with impairment . . . "

Description

Learning disability is a neurodevelopmental disorder that becomes evident during school age and will likely persist into adulthood. Approximately 5% to 15% of school-age children struggle with LD. It's estimated that 80% of those with LD also have a reading disorder (APA, 2018). Approximately one-third of people with LD are estimated to also have attention-deficit/hyperactivity disorder (ADHD). More on ADHD later. Nearly 50% of students who receive special education services fall under the category of LD.

As with other disorders, the severity of LD varies across children. Severity is based on the difficulty a child has with learning and the amount of academic support needed.

Many of you may have LD. I have mild LD, as mentioned previously.

In addition to difficulty with language, characteristics associated with but not central to LD are many and varied. These include motor, attentional, perceptual, memory, emotion, and symbol. We briefly discuss each, leaving the last for our discussion of language.

Motor Difficulties

Motor difficulties usually involve hyperactivity, a condition of overactivity in which children seem to be constantly in motion. Approximately 5% of all children have hyperactivity, but the condition is nine times as prevalent in boys as in girls. The incidence rises to more than 30% among those with LD. It's important to note that not all children with hyperactivity have learning disabilities.

Children with hyperactivity have difficulty attending and concentrating for more than very short periods of time. Other motor difficulties of LD may include poor sense of body movement, poorly defined handedness, poor hand–eye coordination, and poorly defined concepts of space and time.

Attentional Difficulties

Attentional difficulties include a short attention span, inattentiveness, and easy distraction. Although not to the extent found in ASD, some children with learning disabilities may become fixed on a single task or behavior and repeat it. This fixation is called perseveration. Several children with whom I have worked would repeat an utterance over and over, seemingly unaware that they were doing it.

Perceptual Difficulties

Learning disability is not a sensory or reception disorder. It is a perceptual one. Perceptual difficulties are interpretational difficulties. These occur after the stimuli are heard, seen, or received through our senses. As might be assumed then, children with learning disabilities may confuse similar sounds and words and similar printed letters and words.

In addition, these children may have difficulty in figure-ground perception and in sensory integration. Figure-ground perception involves being able to isolate a stimulus against a background of competing stimuli. Sensory integration, on the other hand, involves being able to make sense of visual and auditory stimuli occurring at the same time. Imagine the difficulty for a child with LD perceiving anything in a noisy classroom.

Memory Difficulties

Memory difficulties include short-term and long-term storage and retrieval. Children with LD often have difficulty remembering directions, names, and sequences. Word-finding problems are also common.

Emotional Difficulties

Although emotional problems may accompany LD, they are not a causal factor. Rather, emotional problems are a reaction or an accompaniment to the frustrating situation in which these children find themselves. Children with LD have been described as aggressive, impulsive, unpredictable, withdrawn, and impatient. Some children may exercise poor judgment, have unusual fears, and/or adjust poorly to change. I worked with a child with learning disabilities who was afraid of shoes, which I think you'll agree is a rather unusual fear. In others, poor adjustment to change, another characteristic, may reflect dependence on routines as a way to compensate for difficulty interpreting language in certain contexts.

Language Characteristics

Usually, all aspects of language, spoken and written, are affected to some extent in children with LD. Although hearing or vision difficulties may, as in all of us, be present,

CHAPTER 3 LANGUAGE DISORDERS ASSOCIATED WITH OTHER DISORDERS 69

they are not central to the disorder nor the cause of the language difficulties seen in these children. As mentioned previously, the primary difficulties are attentional and perceptual. Language characteristics of children with LD are presented in Table 3–3.

Pragmatics

Children with LD may have difficulty with the give-and-take of conversation and with the form and content of language. Synthesizing of language rules seems to be particularly difficult, resulting in delays in morphological rule learning and in the development of syntactic complexity. Problems with morphological markers are found both in speaking and in writing, with the most common error being omission of bound morphemes (Windsor et al., 2000).

Semantics

Word-finding is a particular problem, resulting in greater time needed to respond verbally. Retrieval difficulties may result in more communication breakdown, characterized by repetitions, especially before words seemingly difficult to retrieve ("He, he, he . . . John

Table 3–3. Language Characteristics of Children With Learning Disability	
Pragmatics	Little problem with turn taking.
	Difficulty answering questions or requesting clarification. Difficulty initiating or maintaining a conversation.
Semantics	Relational term difficulty (comparative, spatial, temporal). Figurative language and dual definition problems.
	Word finding and definitional problems.
	Conjunction (*and, but, so, because,* etc.) confusion.
Syntax/ morphology	Difficulty with negative and passive constructions, relative clauses, contractions, and adjectival forms.
	Difficulty with verb tense markers, possession, and pronouns.
	Able to repeat sentences but often in reduced form, indicating difficulty learning different sentence forms.
	Article (*a, an, the*) confusion.
Phonology	Inconsistent sound production, especially as complexity increases.
Comprehension	*Wh-* question confusion.
	Receptive vocabulary similar to that of chronological-age-matched peers developing normally.
	Poor strategies for interacting with printed information.
	Confusion of letters that look similar and words that sound similar.

was . . . "), reformulations, substitutions of indefinite pronouns (*it*), empty words (*one, thing*), delays, and insertions ("He was . . . oh, I can't remember . . . ").

Word-retrieval difficulties may be complicated by the deficient vocabularies of children with LD. Young children with LD have poor understanding of literal meanings. As these children age, they experience difficulties with multiple and figurative meanings.

Syntax and Morphology

Overall language development for children with LD may be slow. Their language is often like that of younger children, although children with LD may actually use mature structures less frequently. As preschoolers, these children may exhibit little interest in language and may be unable to follow a story or be uninterested in books.

In general, children with LD have difficulty understanding complex syntax and responding appropriately to questions. They seem to experience problems organizing words to form phrases and sentences. These problems may be related to difficulty attending.

Children with TDL listen to a variety of sentences in everyday interactions and identify statistical regularities that underlie syntax. An inattentive child may not notice the underlying regularities and thus does not benefit from sentence variability.

The linguistic demands of the classroom are often well above the oral language abilities of these children. The well-documented academic underachievement of children with LD demonstrates the link between language deficits and learning disabilities. Oral language skills are the single best indicator of reading and writing success in school. Difficulty with oral language skills among children with LD is evidenced later in written-language problems, called dyslexia.

Possible Causal Factors

Several causal factors may contribute to LD. CNS dysfunction indicates a strong biological basis, but information processing, especially perception, is also important.

Biological Factors

Learning disabilities occur more frequently in families with a history of the disorder and following premature or difficult birth. Children with a parent with dyslexia, especially those with a history of late talking, are at a higher risk for LD (Lyytinen et al., 2001). These facts strongly indicate a biological link in LD. It has been suggested that a breakdown occurs along the neural pathways that connect the midbrain with the frontal cortex, the area of the brain in which executive function, responsible for attention, regulation, and planning, is located.

Several studies have attempted to find a genetic cause for dyslexia. It is doubtful that there is a single dyslexia gene. More likely is a scenario in which several genes are involved in various aspects of the disorder (Grigorenko, 2005). Malformations found in the left hemisphere language-processing areas and between these areas and the visual cortex may be related to these genetic changes and to language-processing deficits (summarized in Galaburda, 2005). Magnetic resonance imaging studies indicate that compared to children with TDL during reading, children with dyslexia exhibit lower

CHAPTER 3 LANGUAGE DISORDERS ASSOCIATED WITH OTHER DISORDERS

activation of the left occipitotemporal region of the brain. There is also heightened activation of Wernicke's area and the frontal lobe areas associated with motor movement, suggesting compensatory use of these areas (Shaywitz & Shaywitz, 2003).

Social–Environmental Factors

Although our definition of LD precluded any environmental causality, certain environmental factors are important. The language and, in turn, interactional difficulties of children with LD certainly will influence a child's development.

As mentioned previously, many of the acting-out behaviors of these children are in response to the very frustrating situations of their lives. Many of the children with whom I have worked had extremely poor self-images. Many were afraid to try anything new; others would do anything for attention and recognition, even if such recognition was negative. The successes or failures that we have as we interact with others have a great influence on our future interactions.

Processing Factors

Children with LD do not appear to function in a manner appropriate for their intellectual level. They seem unable to use certain strategies or to access certain stored information.

Children with LD exercise poor attentional selectivity, concentrating on inappropriate or unimportant stimuli. These children have difficulty deciding on the relevant information to which to attend in both oral and written communication.

In turn, a child with LD has difficulty deciding on the relevant aspects of a stimulus that make it similar or dissimilar to another. Children with LD do more poorly than mental-age-matched peers with TDL on rule extraction or identification following repeated exposures. Poor discrimination skills may also reflect deficits in working memory (Harris Wright & Newhoff, 2001).

Obviously, information that is poorly attended to and poorly discriminated will be poorly organized. These are children for whom the world often does not make sense, especially linguistically. Although children with LD organize information, they may do so inefficiently based on inattention and misperception.

Memory is related to both storage and retrieval. Creation of semantic networks in which words are related and organized occurs later and more slowly among children with LD. One result is less accurate and slower retrieval from long-term memory.

Effective learners actively process, interpret, and synthesize information by using effective strategies to monitor and organize learning. Children with LD often fail to access or use task-appropriate strategies spontaneously. These problems persist throughout adolescence and into adulthood.

> ***Food for Thought:*** **If LD is primarily a perceptual deficit and DLD is a verbal working memory (VWM) deficit, why might we see both disorders characterized by difficulty with morphological markers? Can different causal factors lead to a similar outcome?**

Dyslexia/Specific Learning Disorder With Impairment in Reading and Writing

We'll discuss dyslexia in detail in Chapter 12, but I mention it briefly here. Dyslexia or SLD with impairment in reading and writing is characterized by difficulties in fluent and/or accurate word recognition and in spelling. The disorder is most often associated with difficulties in phonological awareness and sensitivity to and awareness of the sound and syllable structure of words (Lyon et al., 2003). Oral language difficulties are also present (Gallagher et al., 2000). It's estimated that as many as 80% of children with LD have some form of reading problem and that the incidence of dyslexia in the overall population may range from 5% to 17%, depending on how strictly the term is defined (Sawyer, 2006). The disorder is found among males at twice the rate as females. When we compare children with dyslexia to their peers with TDL, the following common elements appear (Sawyer, 2006):

- Comparable verbal IQ and/or listening comprehension
- Below average word reading
- Nonsense or non-real-word reading (word attack) below real-word reading
- Well below average phonological processing scores

Writing lacks organization, and in reading, children fail to understand the underlying organization. Both require active processing skills.

Similar Disorders: Attention-Deficit/Hyperactivity Disorder

Increasingly more children are being labeled with ADHD, characterized by overactivity and an inability to attend for more than a very short period. Although ADHD is not a learning disability, children with ADHD often experience problems in social relations that are explained in part by their accompanying pragmatic problems with language use (Leonard et al., 2011). ADHD is most likely a disorder in executive function that regulates behavior, especially impulsivity.

ADHD is the most common neurobehavioral disorder of childhood, affecting 6.1 million children aged 2 to 17 years in the United States (CDC, 2018a). The expected prevalence of ADHD in the United States is 5% to 7% of all children (APA, 2013; Willcutt, 2012). The diagnosis is based on developmentally inappropriate levels of inattention, overactivity, and impulsivity (APA, 2013). Accompanying these characteristics are poor academic achievement and social interaction.

ADHD may co-occur with other disorders. Approximately one-third of ADHD cases occur without a co-occurring or comorbid disorder, such as language disorder (Sciberras et al., 2014). A nationwide survey in the United States of nearly 15,000 individuals diagnosed with ADHD found that 15.4% have ASD, and 7.9% have IDD (Mohr Jensen & Steinhausen, 2015). In addition, other disorders can mimic ADHD, making differential diagnosis extremely important (Barkley, 2006; Brock et al., 2009; Brown, 2000).

Language Characteristics

Although ADHD is not in and of itself a language disorder, children with ADHD are at increased risk for language disorder, especially in language form and pragmatics. Several studies have reported that approximately 35% to 50% of children with ADHD also have a language disorder (Cohen et al., 2000; Jonsdottir et al., 2005). However, ADHD alone has no independent negative impact on children's language (Redmond et al., 2015). A large study of Scandinavian children aged 7 to 9 years found that language disorder was identified in the majority of those with ADHD and co-occurring reading disorder (Andersen Helland et al., 2016a, 2016b).

Although children with both ADHD and language disorder have increased academic and social challenges (Cohen et al., 2000), language disorder is underdiagnosed (Mueller & Tomblin, 2012). Unfortunately, language disorder accompanying ADHD may be overlooked and assumed to represent a characteristic of ADHD. For a thorough discussion, see Redmond (2016).

Syntactic and semantic difficulties and receptive language deficits are usually observed only among children with ADHD and a language disorder (Andersen Helland et al., 2016). Children with ADHD without language disorder tend to have pragmatic and expressive language deficits (Bruce et al., 2006; Geurts et al., 2004; Geurts & Embrechts, 2008; Helland et al., 2012; Helland & Heimann, 2007). Parents often report that pragmatics is a concern (Bruce et al., 2006).

Pragmatic language disorders include turn-taking difficulties, such as excessive talking or interrupting; lack of coherence and organization in their speech; rambling, often off-topic conversations; and difficulty adjusting their language to different listeners and situations (Green et al., 2014; Redmond, 2004). Mazes, in which a child begins a sentence and then realizes they can't complete the syntax and so tries again and again, are also common.

Among school-age children with ADHD, there is a positive association between verbal ability and good peer interactions, especially for boys. In addition, better verbal ability is associated with higher teacher-reported peer acceptance (Yee Mikami et al., 2018).

Possible Causal Factors

The exact cause of ADHD is not clear. Factors that may be involved in the development of ADHD include genetics, the prenatal environment, or problems with the CNS at key moments in development. According to the U.S. National Institute of Mental Health (2021), possible risk factors include the following:

- Blood relatives, such as a parent or sibling, with ADHD
- Exposure to environmental toxins, such as lead, during pregnancy or at a young age
- Maternal drug use, alcohol use, or cigarette smoking during pregnancy
- Premature birth and low birth weight
- Brain injury

Genetics.

ADHD tends to run in families. A child with ADHD is likely to have another close family member, such as a sibling, with ADHD and has a one in four chance of having a parent with the disorder. Twin studies have demonstrated that there is an 82% chance that identical twins will both have ADHD. The likelihood for fraternal twins is 38%. Geneticists do not find the same rate among adopted children, negating or greatly reducing the influence of environment. Genetics studies are just beginning to identify specific genes associated with ADHD.

Prenatal Environment.

Cigarette smoking and alcohol and drug consumption by a mother during pregnancy can have a detrimental effect on a fetus (CDC, 2020). Specifically, brain anatomy and physiology are affected, resulting in ADHD and other disorders (de Zeeuw et al., 2012).

Central Nervous System Anatomy and Function.

Brain imaging studies have shown differences between children with ADHD and their typical peers in brain structure and organization. Children with ADHD have developmental delays in certain areas of the brain, especially in the prefrontal cortex, which is involved in executive function. Differences also exist in the efficiency of certain parts of the brain in communicating and working with each other.

Seemingly Similar Disorders: Prenatal Drug and Alcohol Exposure

Although neither prenatal drug nor alcohol exposure is in and of itself LD, the behaviors of children with either prenatal history may appear to have LD. There is often another factor, however, that is not seen in children with LD: a poor ability to determine ethical from unethical behavior.

Fetal Alcohol Spectrum Disorder

When a pregnant woman drinks alcohol, the blood alcohol level of her fetus will be the same as her own. Maternal consumption of alcohol during pregnancy can result in fetal alcohol spectrum disorder (FASD). Disabilities associated with alcohol consumption during pregnancy are approximately 6 to 9 in every 1,000 live births (CDC, 2021c). FASD includes, but is not limited to,

- fetal alcohol syndrome, a severe form of FASD characterized by developmental disorders, growth deficiencies, and distinct facial characteristics; and
- alcohol-related neurodevelopmental disorder, which is characterized by significant disorders in several areas of development and distinct facial characteristics.

Exposure to alcohol in utero damages the fetus' CNS development, leading to deficits in cognitive, behavioral, and socioemotional functioning (Streissguth & O'Malley, 2001). Specifically, these children will experience difficulties in attention, memory, executive function, learning, behavior control, mental health, and academics throughout their life spans.

There is a high prevalence of comorbid or co-occurring conditions among individuals with FASD. The most prevalent disease conditions can be grouped as congenital malformations, deformities, chromosomal abnormalities, and mental and behavioral disorders (Popova et al., 2016). The conditions with the highest prevalence include abnormalities of the peripheral nervous system, behavioral disorders, language disorders, and chronic serous otitis media or middle ear infection.

At birth, infants with FASD have a lower birth weight and shorter length. In severe cases, these are accompanied by CNS dysfunction as evidenced in microcephaly or a small head, hyperactivity, motor problems, attention deficits, and cognitive disabilities, including IDD. The left temporoparietal region is especially vulnerable and can result in language disorder (Lindell, 2016).

In general, these children are concrete learners with poor problem-solving abilities who have difficulty generalizing. They are easily distractible, easily overstimulated, impulsive, and perseverative; they have poor memory, interpersonal skills, and judgment; and they exhibit language problems characterized by delayed development, echolalia, and language production that exceeds comprehension. Infants with FASD are irritable and have weak sucking and delayed development. Language deficits include problems with word order and word meaning and difficulties in the give-and-take of conversational discourse (Coggins et al., 2003). Most often, children with FASD are diagnosed as having a learning disability or ADHD.

Predicting the language of others and the use of executive function are disrupted in children with FASD. These children are limited in the amount of linguistic information they can process and have deficits in concept formation, self-regulation, and response inhibition (Jacobson & Jacobson, 2000).

According to parent and teacher reports, children with FASD have poor social communication, characterized by frequent long instances of passive/disengaged and irrelevant behavior. The proportion and average length of time they spend being prosocial are less than those of their peers with TDL (Olswang et al., 2010).

Drug-Exposed Infants

In the United States, 11% to 35% of pregnant women ingest one or more illegal drugs. The effects on an infant vary with the amount and type of drugs, the method of ingestion, and the age of the fetus. Cocaine is especially destructive, with fetal death twice as common as among other non-cocaine drug-dependent mothers, and sudden infant death syndrome three times as high. Cocaine easily crosses the placental barrier, decreasing placental blood flow and fetal oxygen supply, reaching significant blood levels in the fetus, and altering the fetus's neurochemical functioning.

Like infants with FASD, those exposed to crack cocaine also exhibit low birth weight and small head circumference; they are jittery and irritable and spend the majority of their time sleeping or crying. An infant may still be unable to reach an alert state by 1 month of age. Infants exposed to drugs also have hypertonia or poor muscle tone, rapid respiration, and feeding difficulties. Easily overstimulated, these hypersensitive infants actively avoid the human face, which, because of its complexity, may overload them cognitively.

As might be expected, typical mother–child bonding is disrupted, with resultant delays in motor, social, and language development. For her part, an addicted mother may fail to attend to her child, and as a consequence, a cycle of infant passivity and parental rejection may be established.

The language characteristics of children exposed to drugs begin with few infant vocalizations, inappropriate use of gestures, and a lack of oral language. By preschool, these children are exhibiting word retrieval problems, short disorganized sentences, poor eye contact, turn-taking difficulties, few novel utterances, and inappropriate or off-topic responses. In kindergarten, the child uses short, simple sentences and has a limited vocabulary, especially for abstract terms, multiple word meanings, and temporal/spatial terms. School-age years are characterized by problems with word retrieval and word order and by pragmatically inappropriate language. Children with drug exposure are usually diagnosed as having LD or ADHD.

Summary

Learning disability is an extremely complex concept. Although it is relatively easy to describe the outward behaviors of children with LD, it is very difficult to explain the underlying processes. In short, biological or neurostructural differences and functional neuroprocessing differences in children with LD affect their ability to attend to, discriminate, and remember linguistic and other stimuli, resulting in language that may be impaired in all aspects and in all modes of transmission and reception.

At this point, before we add to any possible confusion, it might be helpful for you to stop and jot a few notes on LD, contrasting it to those disorders discussed previously.

Language Disorders Associated With Intellectual Developmental Disorder

Although IDD, previously called *mental retardation*, is a designation found in *DSM-5*, a quick scan of websites doesn't find widespread use of the term. IDD is a neurodevelopmental disorder characterized by intellectual difficulties as well as difficulties in conceptual, social, and practical areas of living. The disorder has three aspects (APA, 2013):

- Deficits in intellectual functioning confirmed by clinical evaluation and individualized standard IQ testing
- Deficits in adaptive functioning that significantly hinder an individual's independence and ability to meet their social responsibilities
- Onset during childhood, hence the word "developmental"

Although IQ scores are de-emphasized, *DSM-5* maintains a vague criterion of functioning two or more standard deviations below the general population in intellectual functioning, which is below an IQ of approximately 70. We'll save the discussion of standard deviation for later in the text. I've worked with individuals with IQs measured in the teens and single digits. In general, a child with IDD is slower in all areas of conceptual or intellectual development and social and daily living skills.

The American Association on Intellectual and Developmental Disabilities has been a driving force in shifting the focus of diagnosis and classification from IQ scores to the types and intensities of supports needed by an individual to lead a normal and independent life. This positive approach moves us from focusing primarily on an individual's deficits. This is reflected in DSM-5, which supports the notion that intellectual functioning reflects several different components—such as verbal comprehension, working memory, perceptual reasoning, quantitative reasoning, abstract thought, and cognitive efficacy—not just IQ.

In educational settings, the more common term is intellectual disability. This can be confusing given that the term in a medical sense applies to other cognitive impairments, such as dementia and traumatic brain injury. For that reason, we'll stick with IDD.

Not every child with IDD is similar. Differences in severity occur, and other factors, such as amount of home support, living environment, education, type of IDD, mode of communication, and age, must be considered. I've worked with very social, very verbal preschoolers and with adolescents and adults who have severe multiple disabilities and very few usable communication behaviors. Other individuals function well in society, have employment, and are married.

As with other disorders discussed, there is a range of severity of IDD from mild to profound. The overwhelming majority of individuals with IDD are classified as having mild intellectual disabilities. Severities of IDD are presented in Table 3–4. Although these classifications are based on daily living skills, the criteria are somewhat nonspecific. For that reason, I've taken the liberty to include older IQ scoring because in a practical sense, these criteria are still used.

As we move from mild to profound IDD, we find an increase in co-occurring disorders. Children with profound IDD often have multiple disorders. The most frequent co-occurring disorders are cerebral palsy and seizure activity. In addition, children with severe to profound IDD more often have chromosomal syndromes, such as Down syndrome (DS) and fragile X syndrome (FXS), which are discussed later in this section.

IDD manifests in childhood and persists throughout a person's life. Children with severe and profound IDD are more likely to be diagnosed early in life, whereas those with mild to moderate IDD may not be identified until preschool or school age.

The exact number of individuals who have intellectual disability is unknown. Estimates vary from 1% to 3% of the population, or approximately 3 to 9 million people in the United States. Males are more likely than females to have IDD. This difference is explained, in part, by X-linked chromosomal causes, such as FXS (Durkin et al., 2007).

In the United States, socioeconomic status (SES) is a determinant of health. In general, those with a low-SES background have poorer health overall, poorer nutrition, poorer access to education and health care, and a higher incidence of disabilities (Graham, 2015). The prevalence of mild to moderate IDD among children from low-SES backgrounds is more than twice as high as that among children from middle- or high-SES backgrounds.

Table 3–4. Severity of Intellectual Developmental Disorder

Severity Classification	Approximate Percentage of Those With Intellectual Developmental Disorder	Daily Living Skills	Older Classification Based on IQ Scores
Mild	85%	Can learn practical life skills Able to function in ordinary life and live independently with only minimal levels of support	52–68
Moderate	10%	Can take care of self with moderate support Basic communication is adequate Independent living with moderate support Able to learn basic skills related to safety and health	36–51
Severe	3.5%	Can learn simple daily routines and engage in simple self-care with supervision in social settings and care in daily living settings such as a community residence Major delays in development Able to understand speech but have limited communication skill	20–35
Profound	1.5%	Cannot live independently and requires close supervision and help with self-care Physical and severe communication limitations Dependent on others for all aspects	Below 20

The association between SES and race/ethnicity and mild IDD is especially strong. Severe IDD tends to be more random in relation to race, ethnicity, and SES. Among non-White Latino/Latina and African American individuals, rates of mild IDD may be twice as high as for White children (Bhasin et al., 2006; Boyle et al., 2011; Van Naarden Braun et al., 2015). Race and ethnicity are not causal factors as much as factors related to low SES. And yet, these same children are less likely to receive educational services (Gary et al., 2019).

We must also add that language and dialectal differences and poverty contribute to the racial and ethnic differences found in performance on cognitive tests, which in turn relate to the differences in prevalence of IDD. Furthermore, evidence exists that test and diagnostic bias contribute to the different rates of the diagnosis of IDD.

Language Characteristics

Language is often one of the most impaired areas for a child with IDD and may be the single most important characteristic of the disorder. Children with IDD often exhibit poor language skills.

Although some of this language difference may be attributed to low intellectual functioning, this factor alone does not fully explain the phenomenon. In addition, the cognition–language relationship is an inconsistent one among individuals with IDD. Differences between the language of children with ID and those developing typically are presented in Table 3–5.

It cannot be stressed enough that children with IDD vary greatly in their communication abilities. Given the heterogeneity of individuals with IDD, research is most often limited to readily identifiable subgroups. Although we discuss general language characteristics associated with IDD, we focus on two genetic disorders—DS and FXS—because of the available data.

Down syndrome, sometimes referred to as trisomy 21, is a chromosomal disorder related to the presence of three strands of genes at chromosome 21. Typically, each parent contributes one strand and thus a typical child has only two strands, not three. FXS is likewise a chromosomal disorder that is sex-linked, which means it is found on the chromosomes that determine biological sex, in this case the X or female chromosome. Females receive one X from each parent, and males receive one X from their mother and a Y from their father. In FXS, the X chromosome is damaged and genetic material is missing. Because males have only one X, the disorder is typically more severe in males than in females.

In general, through middle elementary school, the overall sequence of communication development of children with IDD is similar to that of children with TDL, but the rate is slower. This pattern can be seen in development of intentions, role taking, presupposition, sentence forms, morphological markers, and phonological processes.

Children with DS and those with FXS have moderate to severe delays in all areas of language (Roberts et al., 2001). Some children with FXS also exhibit behaviors associated with ASD and exhibit more severe language disorder than those without these ASD characteristics (Flenthrope & Brady, 2010; Philofsky et al., 2004).

Pragmatics

Boys with FXS perform differently in conversation than boys with DS. Although both groups make more noncontingent, or off-topic, responses than boys with TDL, those with FXS use more perseverative or overly repetitious speech (Roberts, et al., 2007).

As with other children with ASD, children with FXS demonstrate impaired pragmatic language. Although language use is impaired in both groups, children with comorbid FXS and ASD reportedly demonstrate poorer pragmatics in a semi-naturalistic conversational context (Klusek et al., 2014). Boys with ASD and boys and girls with FXS co-occurring with ASD have more noncontingent or off-topic language and perseveration or repetitions than those with TDL and FXS without ASD (Martin et al., 2018).

Table 3–5. Language Characteristics of Children With Intellectual Developmental Disorder

Pragmatics	Gestural and intentional developmental patterns similar to those of children developing normally. Delayed gestural requesting.
	May take less dominant conversational role.
	No difference in clarification skills from mental-age-matched peers developing typically.
	Able to infer communication intent from gestures.
Semantics	More concrete word meanings. Slow vocabulary growth.
	More limited use of a variety of semantic units.
	Children with Down syndrome able to learn word meanings from exposure in context as well as mental-age-matched peers developing typically.
Syntax/ morphology	Length–complexity relationship similar to that of preschoolers developing typically.
	Same sequence of general sentence development as children developing typically.
	Shorter, less complex sentences with fewer subject elaborations or relative clauses than mental-age-matched peers developing typically.
	Sentence word order takes precedence over word relationships. Reliance on less mature forms, although capable of more advanced.
	Same order of morpheme development as preschoolers developing typically.
Phonology	Phonological rules similar to those of preschoolers developing typically but reliance on less mature forms, although capable of more advanced ones.
Comprehension	Poorer receptive language skills, especially children with Down syndrome, than mental-age-matched peers developing typically.
	Poorer sentence recall than mental-age-matched peers.
	More reliance on context to extract meaning.

Feedback to speakers in the form of eye contact, head nodding, and vocal and verbal behavior signals that the listener is paying attention and comprehending or not comprehending the message. Thus, feedback is a vital pragmatic behavior that facilitates communication and ensures comprehension. Late school-age children and adolescents with FXS are less likely to signal noncomprehension than younger, cognitively matched children with TDL (John Thurman et al., 2017). Likewise, although capable of requesting

CHAPTER 3 LANGUAGE DISORDERS ASSOCIATED WITH OTHER DISORDERS

clarification when communication breaks down, children with IDD are less likely to do so within conversations.

Although both oral and written narratives of children with DS are significantly shorter than those of reading-level matched peers with TDL, school-age students with DS exhibit many oral and written narrative abilities that are comparable in terms of linguistic complexity, narrative structure, spelling, and punctuation (Kay-Raining Bird et al., 2008). The use of linguistic devices and cohesive ties are poorer. The predictors of narrative abilities differ. Vocabulary comprehension is the best predictor for children with DS, and age is the best predictor for children with TDL.

Semantics

In general, children with DS produce fewer words, fewer different words, and shorter utterances while engaging in more verbal perseveration compared to mental-age-matched peers with TDL. Males with FXS perseverate more than children with DS and exhibit more jargon, or meaningless unintelligible speech, and more echolalia, or repetition of a partner's speech.

A longitudinal study of vocabulary development in children with DS found a wide range of internal and external predictors for vocabulary development (Deckers et al., 2017). Receptive vocabulary development was best predicted by the level of adaptive skill functioning and by early receptive vocabulary skills. In contrast, expressive vocabulary development was best predicted by the adaptive functioning and by receptive vocabulary, maternal educational level, level of communicative intent of the child, attention skills, and phonological/phonemic awareness. In general, these predictors resemble those for younger peers with TDL.

Syntax and Morphology

Even when children are matched for mental age, children with IDD seem to use more immature language forms than do their peers with TDL. For example, in phonology, boys with FXS make errors similar to those of younger children with TDL. Those with DS have more significant phonological differences than might be expected by delayed development alone (Roberts et al., 2005).

When the syntax of boys who have FXS with and without ASD is compared to that of boys with DS and boys with TDL matched for developmental age of 2 to 6 years, although the two FXS groups do not differ in utterance length or syntactic complexity, both the FXS groups and the boys with DS produce shorter, less complex utterances overall with less complex noun phrases, verb phrases, and sentence structures than do boys with TDL (Price et al., 2008). Overall, both FXS groups produce longer, more complex utterances compared to the boys with DS.

Children with FXS show significant syntactic growth during the preschool years but seem to plateau or, in some cases, decline during early school age (Komesidou et al., 2017). Longitudinal studies indicate that language challenges persist for children with FXS (Brady et al., 2020). Mean or average length of utterances does not appear to change significantly from late elementary school into adolescence. Although boys score lower on standardized testing, language sample results are similar to those of girls with FXS.

Although children with IDD are capable of learning syntactic rules, they tend to rely on less mature word-order rules and a less mature and simpler method of interpretation. Finally, some children with IDD, especially those with DS, exhibit poorer receptive language skills compared to their mental-age-matched peers with TDL.

Possible Causal Factors

Causal factors for IDD are many and varied, including, but not limited to, biological and social–environmental causes and information-processing differences related to language comprehension and production. I caution that for many children, the cause of IDD is unknown. In addition, more than one causal factor may be at work. In any case, causal factors rarely are related directly to the performance level of the child in question. Causal factors for IDD are presented in Table 3–6.

Depending on its cause, IDD may be stable and nonprogressive or it may worsen with time. The disorder usually lasts an individual's lifetime, but the severity may change some with age. For example, visual or hearing difficulties, seizure activity, childhood psychological or head trauma, substance abuse, and other medical conditions may affect the course of the disorder. Conversely, early intervention may improve adaptive skills.

Biological Factors

Biological causes are most likely a factor for a majority of children with IDD. These include one or more of the causes in Table 3–6. In general, a strong correlation exists between biological factors and severity of IDD. Although biological factors help explain IDD, they tell us very little about development, especially language acquisition.

Social–Environmental Factors

Social–environmental causal factors of IDD are more difficult to identify and may involve many interactive variables. Deprivation, poor housing and diet, poor hygiene, and lack of medical care can affect the development of the child adversely, although the exact effect of each is unknown and varies with each child.

Despite the fact that children with IDD display less mature behaviors, there is no evidence that their mothers interact with them less. In general, maternal behavior varies with the child's language level, whether the child has IDD or is developing typically.

Mothers of children with IDD talk more to their children. By attributing more meaning to their children's less frequent behaviors, these mothers are able to interact more frequently. In short, mothers of children with IDD interpret more of their children's behaviors as communicative than do mothers of children developing typically.

Mothers of children with IDD match their verbal behavior to their child's language ability while adopting a teaching role. Although they exert more control in play than do mothers of children developing typically, mothers of children with DS are equally or more responsive to their children. Their control behavior includes trying to elicit more responses from their children.

CHAPTER 3 LANGUAGE DISORDERS ASSOCIATED WITH OTHER DISORDERS

Table 3–6. Causes of Intellectual Developmental Disorder*

Type	Examples
Prenatal	
Chromosomal	
Errors in number	Down syndrome Klinefelter syndrome
Chromosome deletion	Cri du chat syndrome
Chromosomal defects	Fragile X syndrome
Single gene disorders and genetic abnormalities	
Metabolic disorders	Phenylketonuria Tay–Sachs disease
Neurocutaneous syndromes	Tuberous sclerosis
Brain malformations	Hydrocephalus Microcephalus Cerebral malformation
Maternal infectious processes	Craniofacial anomalies
Maternal toxins and chemical agents	Maternal rubella Congenital syphilis Fetal alcohol syndrome Drug-exposed fetus
Maternal nutrition	Severe malnutrition during pregnancy Various amino-deficiencies
Trauma	Intracranial hemorrhage in fetus
Perinatal	
Third-trimester problems	Complications of pregnancy Diseases in mother such as heart and kidney disease and diabetes Placental dysfunction
Labor and delivery problems	Extreme prematurity and/or low birth weight Birth asphyxia Difficult and/or complicated delivery Birth trauma
Neonatal problems	Severe, prolonged jaundice

continues

Table 3–6. *continued*

Type	Examples
Postnatal	
Brain infections	Encephalitis
	Bacterial meningitis
Head injury	Traumatic brain injury
Toxins	Chronic lead exposure
Nutritional issues	Severe and prolonged malnutrition
Gross brain disease	Tumors
	Huntington disease
Psychosocial disadvantage	Subnormal intellectual functioning in immediate family and/or impoverished environment
Sensory deprivation	Maternal deprivation
Prolonged isolation	
Unknown	Perhaps the largest category of causes

Note: *Causes are not mutually exclusive, and a child may have more than one or mixed causes.

Sources: Information taken from Luckasson et al. (2002), U.S. National Library of Medicine (2010, December 15), and World Health Organization (2010).

> ***Food for Thought:*** If low SES is a factor in IDD, could we lessen the impact on society by decreasing the numbers of those living at low-SES levels?

Processing Factors

There may be differences in the cognitive, or information-processing, abilities of the IDD population that cannot be attributed to low IQ alone. Children with IDD do not seem to process information in the same manner as mental-age-matched peers with TDL. This difference is especially critical for learning. Note that the information presented here is based on individuals with mild and moderate IDD.

Attention. In general, individuals with IDD can sustain attention as well as mental-age-matched peers with TDL. Difficulty comes for the individual with IDD in the scanning and selection of stimuli to which to attend. Persons with severe or profound IDD have more limited attentional capacity and are less efficient at attention allocation.

Discrimination. Individuals with IDD have difficulty identifying relevant stimulus cues. This difficulty reflects, in part, the tendency of individuals with IDD to attend

CHAPTER 3 LANGUAGE DISORDERS ASSOCIATED WITH OTHER DISORDERS

to fewer dimensions of a task than do typically developing individuals. If the stimulus dimensions chosen are not the salient or important ones, the individual's ability to discriminate and to compare new information to stored information is limited. When dimensions of a stimulus are explained, individuals with IDD can apply this information to discrimination tasks as well as typically developing individuals.

In general, discrimination ability and speed are related to severity of IDD. The more severe the IDD, the slower and less accurate the discrimination.

Organization. Individuals with mild to moderate IDD have difficulty developing organizational strategies to aid storage and retrieval. They do not seem to rely on either categorical or associative strategies or to use these strategies efficiently. In categorical strategies, a word or a symbol forms a link between two entities. Thus, dogs and cats are pets. In associative strategies, one word or symbol aids in recall of another, as in "bacon and . . . " or "salt and . . . "

Individuals with mild IDD exhibit both simultaneous and successive coding; however, these individuals may use these processes differently from typically developing individuals, especially in complex tasks. Individuals with DS seem to have greater difficulty with successive processing than do other mental-age-matched individuals with IDD. This deficit may be explained in part by the poor verbal auditory working memory abilities of individuals with DS. Processing both language form and content as information comes in is an especially challenging task.

Memory. In general, individuals with IDD demonstrate poorer recall compared to individuals developing typically. The more severe the IDD, the poorer the memory skills. Individuals with mild to moderate IDD are able to retain information within long-term memory as well as typically developing individuals, but the retrieval process is slower. No doubt, organizational deficits contribute to difficulty retrieving information.

More obvious differences can be seen in short-term memory. Poor performance by individuals with mild IDD may reflect a limited use of storage strategies mentioned previously. Memory may also be affected by a rapid rate of forgetting, especially within the first 10 seconds.

VWM deficits of individuals with DS do not seem to impact the learning of novel words (Mosse & Jarrold, 2011). In fact, novel word learning by children with DS exceeds what their VWM capacity would predict. It's possible that the vocabulary acquisition of children with DS doesn't rely on VWM to the same extent as in children with TDL. In other words, new word learning may rely on another memory process.

Information is retained by rehearsal. It appears that individuals with IDD do not spontaneously rehearse and need more time compared to typically developing individuals. The need for repeated input and practice retrieval is supported in studies of vocabulary learning among children with DS (Chapman et al., 2006).

In general, individuals with IDD do more poorly with auditory information than with visual information. Sentence recall involves reproduction from memory and editing of the recalled text. For individuals with mild IDD, difficulty probably is encountered in the second stage. Deficits in auditory short-term memory for words are implicated in the poor performance of children with DS in sentence memory tasks (Miolo et al., 2005).

Transfer. Transfer, or generalization, is an area of processing especially difficult for individuals with IDD. In general, the more severe a person's IDD, the weaker that person's transfer abilities. In addition, persons with IDD have difficulty with both near and far transfer, in part because of an inability to detect similarities. Thus, generalization deficits may reflect discrimination and organization problems mentioned previously.

How does IDD differ from the other disorders discussed? Take a minute to consider each one.

Language Disorders Associated With Neurocognitive Disorders

Children with brain injury differ greatly as a result of the site and extent of lesion, the age at onset, and the age of the injury. In general, the smaller the damaged area, the better the prognosis or chance of recovery. Brain injury in children may result from trauma; cerebrovascular accident (CVA) or stroke; congenital malformation of the neural blood vessels; convulsive disorders; or encephalopathy, such as infection or tumors. *DSM-5* places most of these under the category of Neurocognitive Disorders. This large category includes many disorders, such as Parkinson disease, that rarely, if ever, affect children. Only the most prevalent types of childhood neurocognitive disorders are discussed here.

Traumatic Brain Injury

Traumatic brain injury is the leading cause of disability and death in children and adolescents in the United States. According to the CDC (2021d), the two age groups at greatest risk for brain injury are those aged 0 to 4 years and 15 to 19 years. According to emergency room data, an average of 564,000 children sustain brain injury annually. Of these, 62,000 require hospitalization.

TBI is diffuse brain damage as a result of external physical force. Recovery ranges from nearly full recovery to a vegetative state in some very severe cases. Although the chances of survival have improved greatly in recent years, long-term disability is a continuing public health problem.

The Brain Injury Association of America (2022) estimates that between 3.2 and 5.3 million individuals in the United States are living with TBI-related disability. Approximately 1 million of those are children and adolescents.

The leading childhood causes of TBI are falls (35%), motor vehicle-related injuries (17%), and strikes or blows to the head (17%), such as in sports injuries (CDC, 2015). Among children, those aged 0 to 4 years experience the highest incidence, mostly from falls and vehicular accidents. Adolescents experience high rates of TBI from sports and recreational activities, motor vehicle accidents, and firearms (CDC, 2018b). Overall, males account for approximately 59% of all reported TBI-related medical visits in the United States (Faul et al., 2010).

Although TBI is a leading cause of acquired disability in children, the TBI category is not widely recognized in special education (Nagele et al., 2019). In fact, few school-based SLPs report having students with TBI on their caseloads (ASHA, 2018).

Students who have experienced a TBI may not receive SLP services, even when their deficits affect communication. For example, young children with TBI often perform

CHAPTER 3 LANGUAGE DISORDERS ASSOCIATED WITH OTHER DISORDERS   **87**

within average limits on traditional standardized language tests and thus do not qualify for school services (Anderson et al., 2000; Cermak et al., 2019). These same children may show differences later in more complex language skills impacted by cognition, such as reading comprehension and pragmatics (Haarbauer-Krupa et al., 2018).

According to DSM-5, TBI results from an impact to the head causing rapid movement or displacement of the brain within the skull, with one or more of the following consequences:

- Loss of consciousness
- Posttraumatic amnesia
- Disorientation and confusion
- Neurological signs, such as, but not limited to,
  - Injury evident on neuroimaging
  - Onset of seizures or a marked worsening of a preexisting seizure disorder
  - Visual field limitations
  - Hemiparesis or weakness on one side of the body

Often, the individual experiences a neurocognitive disorder immediately after the TBI. This condition may continue to some degree after recovery and last beyond the acute post-injury period. Neurocognitive disorders are characterized by severe and modest cognitive deficits in one or more cognitive domain, including the following:

- Attention
- Executive function
- Learning and memory
- Language
- Perceptual–motor
- Social cognition

In major neurocognitive disorder, there is also significant interference with the activities of daily living.

Common symptoms of TBI according to DSM-5 include disturbances in the following:

- Emotional function. These may include irritability, easy frustration, tension and anxiety, and emotional lability.
- Personality changes. These may include social disinhibition, apathy, suspiciousness, and aggression.
- Physical symptoms. These may include headache, fatigue, sleep disorder, vertigo, tinnitus, and anosmia or a loss of sense of smell.
- Neurological symptoms. These may include seizures, visual disturbance, and cranial nerve deficits.
- Orthopedic injuries.

Emotional lability refers to rapid, often exaggerated changes in mood, including strong emotions or feelings, such as uncontrollable laughing or crying, or heightened irritability or temper. Social disinhibition is an inability to inhibit one's behavior. For example, I once evaluated a young man with TBI who kept insisting on kissing my hand.

Many individuals with TBI also suffer from posttraumatic stress disorder (PTSD). Personality changes can be extreme, including acting without considering the consequences. As a result, the prevalence of TBI among incarcerated youth is substantially greater than in the general population. This difference becomes more pronounced with the severity of the injury. Reported prevalence rates of TBI among incarcerated youth range from 16.5% to 72.1%, with a rate of 100% reported among a sample of young people on death row (Williams et al., 2015).

Cognitive deficits include perception, memory, reasoning, and problem-solving difficulties. Deficits may be permanent or temporary and may partially or totally affect functioning ability. Other characteristics include lack of initiative, distractibility, inability to adapt quickly, perseveration, low frustration levels, passive–aggressiveness, anxiety, depression, fear of failure, and misperception (CDC, 2021d; Clegg et al., 2005; Conti-Ramsden & Botting, 2008).

Severity may range from a mild concussion, defined as a loss of consciousness for less than 30 seconds, to moderate TBI (a loss of consciousness or posttraumatic amnesia for 30 minutes to 24 hours, with or without skull fracture) and severe TBI (consisting of a coma for 6 hours or longer). Severity of symptoms is not directly related to the deficits mentioned previously, nor is it the sole prognostic indicator (Cermak et al., 2019).

> ***Food for Thought:*** **Have you or a friend or family member had a mild concussion? If so, how did it affect immediate and long-term cognitive functioning?**

Variables that affect recovery are extremely independent and are complicated. These include degree and length of unconsciousness, duration of posttraumatic amnesia, age at injury, age of injury, and posttraumatic ability. In general, shorter, less severe unconsciousness, shorter amnesia, and better posttraumatic abilities indicate better recovery. However, neural recovery over time is often unpredictable and irregular.

Age at the time of injury is a factor because a child is still developing when the injury occurs. Skills developing at the time of the injury, such as language, are most susceptible to disorder (Cermak et al., 2019). Although younger children have less to recover, they also do not have the benefit of as much past learning as older children.

Language Characteristics

Meta-analysis indicates that, unfortunately, standardized, norm-referenced language assessments are not sensitive to the language disorders accompanying TBI (Cermak et al., 2019). Yet, language deficits are usually evident even after mild injuries. Many of the challenges a child with TBI faces are pragmatic in nature. This is especially evident in individuals with severe TBI and resultant deficits in executive function (Douglas, 2010). Table 3–7 presents the language characteristics of children with TBI.

CHAPTER 3 LANGUAGE DISORDERS ASSOCIATED WITH OTHER DISORDERS

Table 3–7. Language Characteristics of Children With Traumatic Brain Injury

Pragmatics	Difficulty with organization and expression of complex ideas. Off-topic comments. Ineffectual, inappropriate comments.
	Frequency of eye gaze is appropriate during conversation.
	Less complex narratives, containing fewer words, shorter less complex sentences, and fewer episodic elements.
	Short narratives include story grammar and cohesion, as do those of typically developing peers.
Semantics	Word retrieval, naming, and object description difficulties, although vocabulary relatively intact.
	Automatized, overlearned language relatively unaffected.
Syntax/ morphology	Sentences may be lengthy and fragmented.
Phonology	Few phonological difficulties, but there may be some dysarthria or apraxia due to injury.
Comprehension	Some problems due to inattention and speed of processing. Poor auditory and reading comprehension.
	Difficulty with sentence comprehension due to difficulty assigning meaning to syntactic structure.
	Most routinized, everyday comprehension unaffected.
	Vocabulary comprehension usually unaffected, except for abstract terms.

Some deficits will remain long after the injury even when overall improvement is good. Although there is considerable variability among children with TBI, many subtle deficits remain, especially in pragmatics. The language difficulties may also be seen in literacy problems (Catts, Adlof, et al., 2005; Nation et al., 2004).

Pragmatics. Children may have difficulty regulating the amount and manner of conversational participation as well as the relevance of their contributions. This can be noted in the narratives and conversation of these children. Utterances are often lengthy, inappropriate, and off-topic, and fluency is disturbed. A child may lose their train of thought in conversations, and in narratives the same child may not retain the central focus of the story, thus deleting important information.

Semantics. Concrete vocabulary may be relatively undisturbed, although word retrieval, naming, and object description difficulties may be present. Language comprehension and higher functions such as figurative language and dual meanings also may be affected.

Syntax and Morphology. By comparison, language form is relatively unaffected. The majority of children with TBI regain the ability to manipulate language form and content. Surface structure may seem relatively unimpaired. A child's language may be relatively effective in school until the third or fourth grade, when students are required to use higher language abilities to analyze and synthesize.

Possible Causal Factors

Obviously, biological and physical factors are involved in TBI. More important is the manner in which informational processing is affected. Children with TBI are often inattentive and easily distractible. Attention fluctuates, and they may have difficulty focusing on a task. I worked with a high school honor student who post-TBI couldn't seem to settle down to study. Her attention wandered, and she was easily distracted.

All aspects of organization—categorizing, sequencing, abstracting, and generalization—may be affected. Children with TBI seem stimulus-bound—unable to see relationships, make inferences, and solve problems. They evidence difficulty formulating goals, planning, and achieving. This deficiency often is masked by intact vocabulary and general knowledge.

Finally, children with TBI exhibit memory deficits in both storage and retrieval. Long-term memory prior to the trauma is usually intact.

Individuals with neurodevelopmental language deficits may have difficulties in executive function, social cognition, perception, and motor control (e.g., Brumbach & Goffman, 2014; Ferguson et al., 2011; Hill, 2001; Kapa & Plante, 2015; Marton et al., 2005).

Cerebrovascular Accident

A **cerebrovascular accident** occurs when a portion of the brain is denied oxygen, usually because of a blockage or rupture in a blood vessel serving the brain. Most frequently, damage is specific and localized, unlike the diffuse damage found in a TBI. Patterns of recovery, especially in young children, suggest that adjoining portions of the cortex, the surface of the cerebrum, augment the functioning of the damaged portion.

CVAs usually are found in children with congenital heart problems or arteriovenous (blood vessel) malformations in the brain. One of my grandsons experienced a CVA in utero.

For most children, prognosis is generally good. Naturally, the variability will be great, depending on the site and extent of the lesion. Language problems often accompany left hemisphere damage, although any brain damage has the potential to disturb language functioning.

Language Characteristics

Long-term subtle pragmatic difficulties are common. Language form usually returns quickly, although performance may deteriorate when demands increase. Word retrieval may be extremely difficult at first, with deficits in both speed and accuracy. Language comprehension also is affected initially. Children usually recover, although higher level academic and reading difficulties may persist.

Summary

The underlying relationship between cognition and language varies with age and with the aspect of language studied. At many points in development, we are not able to describe the exact relationship. Although we cannot fully explain the mechanisms at work when the brain is injured, we can predict that vocabulary and structural rules will return more easily than higher order functions, such as conversational skills that require complex synthesis of language form, content, and use. Even children who seem to recover may continue to exhibit long-term subtle pragmatic difficulties.

Language Disorders Associated With Maltreatment: Neglect and Abuse

In the United States, in the last year for which data are available, at least 1 in 7 children experienced **child abuse and/or neglect** (CDC, 2021c). Even the government states that this figure is likely an underestimate. Nearly 75% of victims are neglected, 17.5% are physically abused, and 9.3% are sexually abused. This amounts to approximately 656,000 children abused. In addition, 1,840 children died of abuse and neglect.

Although children who are abused and neglected may suffer immediate physical injuries, they are also highly likely to experience more long-term emotional and psychological problems, such as anxiety and impaired social–emotional skills. Exposure to violence in childhood increases the risks of injury, future violence victimization and perpetration, substance abuse, sexually transmitted infections, delayed brain development, lower educational attainment, and limited employment opportunities. Chronic abuse may result in toxic stress, which can change brain development and increase the risk for problems such as PTSD and learning, attention, and memory difficulties. Until recently, these children were not identified as having distinct language problems.

For children, individual risk factors for abuse and neglect include

- age younger than 4 years; and
- special needs that may increase caregiver burden, such as disabilities, mental health issues, and chronic physical illnesses.

Unfortunately, children younger than age 1 year have the highest rate of victimization. A study of more than 50,000 typically developing children found that 9% had been maltreated (Sullivan & Knutson, 2000). The same study reported that 31% of children with disabilities and 35% of children with speech/language disorder had been maltreated.

Caregiver risk factors include drug or alcohol overuse and abuse; mental health issues, including depression; low education or income; and attitudes of acceptance and justification of violence or aggression. In addition to these factors are a lack of understanding of children's needs and of development, a history of abuse and neglect as a child, being a young or single parent, parental and economic stress, and use of corporal punishment as a disciplinary tool. Relationship violence, low SES and an immediate community of high unemployment and low wages, and social isolation are also factors (CDC, 2021c). Although maltreatment occurs across the income spectrum, children from low-SES families are much more likely to be abused (Kapp et al., 2001). Communities with the greatest income inequity also have higher rates of child abuse (Eckenrode et al., 2014).

Neglect and abuse are extreme examples of a dysfunctional family and are a sign of the type of social environment in which the child learned language. Although neglect and abuse are rarely the direct cause of the communication problem, the context in which they occur directly influences a child's development.

Children exposed to both prenatal alcohol and postnatal abuse and neglect have lower intelligence scores and more severe neurodevelopmental deficits than traumatized children who are not prenatally exposed to alcohol (Henry et al., 2007). Developmental deficits occur in language, attention, memory, visual processing, and motor skills.

Children who have been traumatized experience biological brain changes as a result (Atchison, 2007). Characterized as hyperarousal, these changes are associated with acceleration in nervous system areas responsible for perception and processing of potentially threatening sensations. The accompanying release of certain stress hormones influences thoughts, feelings, and actions.

In a state of fear-related activation, the child responds to perceived threats with primitive, reflexive, and aggressive reactions. Over time, the hypervigilant state of the child leads to apprehension, fear, attention difficulties, and restlessness (Lane, 2002). Persistent activation of this response can result in a maladaptive, persistent state of fear.

> ***Food for Thought:*** **As a young abused child, how might you interact with your abuser? How would this affect your language development?**

Language Characteristics

Maltreated children have less complex language compared to non-maltreated children (Eigsti & Cicchetti, 2004). All aspects of language are affected; however, it is in pragmatics that these children exhibit the greatest difficulties (Cobos-Cali et al., 2018). Table 3–8 presents the language characteristics of children who are abused and neglected.

We must be somewhat cautious in making definitive statements about maltreated children given that children with disorders are more likely to be abused and maltreated. In other words, language disorders may have surfaced even without abuse and neglect.

Pragmatics

In general, children who are neglected and abused are less talkative and have fewer conversational skills than their peers. Utterances and conversations are shorter than those of their peers. They are less likely to volunteer information or to discuss emotions or feelings.

Children who are victims of substantiated maltreatment may have compromised ability to provide narrative accounts of their experiences (Snow et al., 2019). This highlights the importance of police and human services training on the best practices for forensic interviewing.

CHAPTER 3 LANGUAGE DISORDERS ASSOCIATED WITH OTHER DISORDERS

Table 3–8. Language Characteristics of Children Who Are Abused and Neglected

Pragmatics	Poor conversational skills.
	Inability to discuss feelings. Shorter conversations.
	Fewer descriptive utterances.
	Language used to get things done with little social exchange or affect.
Semantics	Limited expressive vocabulary.
	Fewer decontextualized utterances, more talk about the here and now.
Syntax/ morphology	Shorter, less complex utterances.
Phonology	Similar to peers.
Comprehension	Receptive vocabulary similar to peers.
	Auditory and reading comprehension problems.

Semantics, Syntax, and Morphology

Maltreated children have consistently poorer expressive and receptive language skills and poor receptive vocabulary (Lum et al., 2014). In addition, there is a high correlation between deficient verbal and reading ability and neglect and abuse.

Possible Causal Factors

Certainly, negative social–environment factors are important in the development of language by children who are neglected and abused, but biological factors should not be overlooked. Medical and health problems among those with low-SES backgrounds also can contribute. Direct effect is difficult to determine because of the multiplicity of overlapping factors, especially among those from low-SES families.

Biological Factors

Poor maternal health, substance abuse, poor or nonexistent pediatric services, and poor nutrition can all affect brain development and maturation. Physical abuse also may cause lasting physical or neurological damage, such as TBI.

Social–Environmental Factors

As in all children, the early language experiences of a child with a history of maltreatment influence the underlying social cognitive behavior of the infant or toddler (Lohmann & Tomasello, 2003). When children are repeatedly exposed to violence and stress, they compensate through behaviors that ensure their survival. These strategies can interfere with critical brain development in areas of socioemotional learning.

As a result, these children have limited ability to predict and interpret the intentions of others and to self-regulate their own language use. Some maltreated children exhibit **alexithymia**, difficulty in the identification, regulation, and understanding of feelings in others and, in extreme cases, in themselves. It is hypothesized that traumatic experiences result in a disassociation between right-hemisphere emotions and left-hemisphere expression (Schore, 2001). As a result, children with alexithymia may have behavioral problems or outbursts of aggressive behavior.

Either or both parents may be neglectful or abusing, but it is a mother's or primary caregiver's everyday responsiveness to a child that has the most effect on language development. The quality of the child–caregiver attachment is a more significant factor in language development than is maltreatment, and it can moderate or exacerbate the effects of neglect or abuse.

Several factors, including childhood loss of a parent, death of a previous child, pregnancy complications, birth complications, current marital or financial problems, substance abuse, maternal age, and/or illness, can disturb maternal attachment. In turn, mothers or caregivers may adopt two general patterns of interaction: controlling or negligent.

Most abusive mothers or caregivers are controlling, imposing their will on the child. As controllers, they tend to ignore a child's communication initiations, thus decreasing the amount of verbal stimulation received by that child. Neglecting mothers or caregivers are unresponsive to their infant's behaviors and have low expectations of deriving satisfaction from their infant. Either situation includes a lack of support for the development of meaningful communication skills and little active interaction, such as playing games, hugging, patting, or nuzzling, and little nurturing maternal speech toward an infant.

The result is insecure attachment on the part of a child. The child may be apprehensive in the presence of the parent or caregiver and may avoid interaction to lessen the chance of hostile responses. Early stimulus–response bonds—an infant's notion that their behavior results in an adult reinforcing response—may be nonexistent, further depressing the child's behavior. Obviously, this is not an ideal language learning environment.

Summary

Only now are we beginning to understand the effect of caregiver behavior on an infant. Although it seems intuitive that neglect and abuse would cause language and communication problems, especially in language use, the data are only correlational, not cause and effect.

Language Disorders Associated With Less Frequent Disorders

Although we've touched on some of the more prevalent language disorders, we have by no means exhausted the discussion. I've omitted several forms of language disorder or related conditions for the sake of brevity. Let me at least familiarize you with some category names and brief descriptions. In order, we explore late language emergence,

CHAPTER 3 LANGUAGE DISORDERS ASSOCIATED WITH OTHER DISORDERS

childhood schizophrenia, selective mutism (SM), otitis media, and children with deafness. Disorders specifically related to literacy have been left for discussion in the chapter on literacy disorders. No doubt, your professor will have others to add to the list.

Late Language Emergence

Approximately 10% to 15% of young children are late talkers. These children are said to have late language emergence (LLE). Approximately half of these children will catch up to their peers with TDL. The remainder may go on to have continued language delays and to eventually be diagnosed with specific language impairment (SLI) or some co-occurring disorder. Although a significant number of late-talking children have persistent language problems throughout the preschool years, it is difficult to predict the effect of early delay on later development (Dale et al., 2003). However, impaired syntactic comprehension among 24-month-old children who have LLE is predictive of DLD/SLI by age 4 years (Chilosi et al., 2019). Early identification is crucial for early intervention services.

Late talkers, even those with more typical development, may have ongoing challenges in language. For example, late talkers identified at age 2 years have significantly lower syntactic complexity at age 5 years compared to their peers with TDL. In general, children with LLE are more likely to be in the low normal range in mean or average utterance length (Rescorla & Turner, 2015).

Unfortunately, being a late talker increases a child's risk of having a smaller vocabulary at 48 months and low school readiness at 60 months (Scheffner Hammer et al., 2017). Smaller vocabularies may relate to a child's ability to acquire new words rapidly. For example, children with LLE require more exposures to novel words to show the same advantage for fast mapping (MacRoy-Higgins & Dalton, 2015).

As mentioned previously, approximately half of late talkers seem to have more typical development as they mature. Some children with LLE continue to remain behind their peers in preschool, whereas others appear to have more typical language development with maturity (Matte-Landry et al., 2020). Children with persistent language delay continue to have language difficulties throughout elementary school. Both those with persistent delays and those with transient delays have psychosocial difficulties, such as ADHD behaviors, peer difficulties, and externalizing behaviors including being physically aggressive or disobeying rules.

Children who seem to have recovered by age 4 years are at modest risk for continuing difficulties, but at no higher rate than that for other 4-year-olds with equivalent language test scores (Dale et al., 2015). The lesson to take from this is that for all children with low normal language at age 4 years, SLPs would do well to continue monitoring their progress.

Although child health is an important factor in early delay, most early language delay is environmental in origin. Environmental factors persist for children whose parents do not seek professional help such as SLP services (Bishop et al., 2003). The risk of being a late talker at 24 months is significantly associated with the following factors (Scheffner Hammer et al., 2017):

- Being male
- Being a non-singleton

- Being from a lower socioeconomic background
- Having moderately low birth weight
- Having a very young mother
- Having lower quality parenting
- Experiencing attentional difficulties
- Receiving less than 10 hours of day care per week

Several of these factors are related. For example, a child is less likely to attend a day care program if the family has a low-SES background.

According to the results of meta-analyses, significant predictors of expressive-language outcomes among late talkers are toddler expressive-vocabulary size, receptive language, and SES (Fisher, 2017). Family SES has the largest effect on a child's readiness for school and highlights the need for universal preschool or expanded programs such as Head Start.

> ***Food for Thought:*** **Many children experience LLE. Should we, as a society, commit to intervention with all of them?**

Many children in homeless shelters exhibit language delays, but there is no common pattern. In fact, although the majority of both mothers and children in homeless shelters have some type of language disorder, the lack of a pattern of language disorder means that they do not form a distinct diagnostic category (O'Neil-Pizozzi, 2003). We'll discuss extreme poverty more in Chapter 8.

Childhood Schizophrenia

Childhood schizophrenia, a serious psychiatric illness that causes strange thinking, odd feelings, and unusual behavior, is uncommon, occurring in approximately 1 of every 40,000 children younger than age 13 years (Gochman et al., 2011). Although the disorder is difficult to recognize in its early phases, it may result from a combination of brain changes and biochemical, genetic, and environmental factors.

Schizophrenia can be controlled by medical treatment. Still, it is a lifelong disease that currently cannot be cured. Symptoms may include seeing and hearing things that are not real (hallucinating), confusing reality and fantasy, exhibiting odd and eccentric behavior, confused thinking and extreme moodiness, and severe anxiety and fearfulness. Behaviors may change slowly over time.

Although there are slightly more males than females with the disorder, it is observed only rarely in children younger than age 5 years. In general, the earlier the symptoms appear, the poorer the prognosis. Among preschool children, approximately 30% who will develop schizophrenia have behaviors similar to those associated with ASD, such as rocking and arm flapping. It is not until early school age or later that a child begins to display symptoms of hallucinations, delusions, and disordered thinking.

CHAPTER 3 LANGUAGE DISORDERS ASSOCIATED WITH OTHER DISORDERS

Approximately 55% of children and adolescents with schizophrenia have language abnormalities, including language delay (Mental Health Research Association, 2007). Although there are few studies of the language of children with schizophrenia, data from adults suggest difficulty with pragmatics, especially in content relevancy (Nicolson et al., 2000). Specifically, adults with schizophrenia have problems with appropriateness of topics and intentions, turn-taking, vocabulary, and nonverbal behaviors (Meilijson et al., 2004).

Selective Mutism

Selective mutism is a relatively rare disorder in which a child does not speak in some situations, such as in school, although they may speak normally in others. From 0.2% to 0.7% of all children may have SM at some time, with girls nearly twice as likely as boys to be affected (Bergman et al., 2002; Kristensen, 2000). SM sometimes happens at times of transition or in stressful situations, such as being repeatedly bullied.

I worked with a young boy whose verbal communication completely shut down when he entered kindergarten. Although he continued to talk at home, he engaged with no one, not even other children, in school.

Related factors include social anxiety, extreme shyness, and language disorder or second language learning. Although 30% to 50% of children with SM are reported to have language disorder, the nature and extent of this disorder remain undetermined.

Otitis Media

Many young children suffer from **chronic otitis media**. In general, the cumulative effect of recurrent hearing loss can be a significant factor in delayed language development (Feldman et al., 2003). Although otitis media is a factor in language disorder, children with otitis media do not constitute a separate category. Otitis media may co-occur with categories discussed previously, such as DLD.

Deafness

Although limited space precludes discussion of the language of children with deafness, it is important to note the effects of early intervention and cochlear implants. Children born with deafness who receive both speech and sign intervention in infancy can often become proficient, if not perfect, speakers or develop language through sign or both. Interestingly, children exposed to sign will express their first word in sign at approximately 8 months, whereas hearing children often don't speak their first word until 4 months later. Infants who sign will continue to develop language.

Those who receive cochlear implants develop language in a manner similar to that of typically developing children. In general, those implanted as infants show more rapid growth in language than those implanted later (Tomblin et al., 2005). Although those implanted later have an initial advantage of maturity that enhances language growth, this advantage seems to disappear later as children who received implants at an earlier age begin to develop spoken language at an ever-increasing rate (Ertmer et al., 2003; Nicholas & Geers, 2007).

Implications

Many language disorders are not outgrown. Even with intervention, they are rarely "cured." Typically, language disorders change and become more subtle. Children with preschool language disorder may continue to have trouble with linguistic and academic tasks. Language disorders in kindergarten are likely to persist well into elementary school (Tomblin et al., 2003). Reading performance may be affected. Children with language disorders may continue to do poorly in speech and language as adults, although nonlinguistic skills seem unaffected. With or without intervention, certain aspects of language disorder affect academic performance and social acceptance.

Poor oral language usually results in poor reading and writing ability. Poor reading often reflects the child's lack of language awareness skills, called metalinguistic abilities. This awareness is crucial for reading.

Within the classroom, children with language disorders form a separate subgroup that interacts increasingly less with their peers with TDL. Because children with language disorders are poor communicators overall, they are increasingly ignored. In general, children with language disorders exhibit more behavior problems and poorer social skills than do their peers with TDL (Qi & Kaiser, 2004). Their poor ability to infer emotional reactions in social situations may contribute to the social difficulties they encounter (Ford & Milosky, 2003). Teachers rate children with language disorders significantly below their peers in impulse control; likability; and social behaviors such as helping others, offering comfort, and sharing. Increasing reticence to talk leads to withdrawal, especially among prepubescent and adolescent boys (Fujiki et al., 2001).

Children with language disorders often continue to have poor vocabularies and poor higher level semantic skills. These include difficulties with abstract meanings, figurative language, dual meanings, ambiguity, and humor.

Their syntax and morphology are usually characterized by the continued use of less mature forms. Word formation processes, consisting of a free morpheme plus one or more bound morphemes, are less mature. Similarly, phonological patterns usually reflect those of younger children.

Finally, language comprehension difficulties, especially at higher levels, such as detection of ambiguity and ability to summarize, may persist. These difficulties reflect underlying language difficulties. Evidence suggests that expressive language deficits are usually accompanied either by limitations in language knowledge or by difficulties in processing of language input (Leonard, 2009).

SLPs are responsible for intervening to correct some language difficulties, to modify others, and to teach compensation skills for still others. In the chapters that follow, we explore a model that proposes to do this in the most natural way possible. It's called a functional approach.

Conclusion

At this point, most likely, you are in need of a one-sentence summary that once and for all distinguishes each language disorder from the others. Unfortunately, I don't have one. Still, we need to make some sense from the wealth of information presented.

CHAPTER 3 LANGUAGE DISORDERS ASSOCIATED WITH OTHER DISORDERS

At the risk of generalizing too much, let's try. Table 3–9 presents a summary of the disorders discussed.

It will be your challenge as an SLP to unravel the language of each individual child. Although we can speak of categories of language disorder, no child will resemble the composite characteristics listed in this chapter. Nonetheless, the categories give us a place from which to begin. The process of assessment and intervention begins here and is the topic of the next chapter and the remainder of the text.

Table 3–9. Language Contrasts in Children With Language Disorders		
Disorder	**Primary Area**	**Characteristics**
DLD	Morphosyntax	Difficulty with small units of language (morphemes, phonemes), syntactic rules. Cause: Deficit in working memory.
SCD	Pragmatics	Difficulty with both verbal and nonverbal.
		Awkward and lack flexible in conversation.
Associated with		
ASD	Pragmatics	Difficulty with pragmatics (from child who will not interact to child with HFA who misinterprets nonverbal communication.
		Lack of gestures in extreme case.
LD	Morphosyntax	Although many areas are affected, the primary is language form.
		In contrast to ASD, rely on nonverbal. Cause: Perceptual deficits.
IDD	All areas	In general, all areas of language are affected.
TBI	Pragmatics	Language form often returns but lingering pragmatic difficulties.
		Difficulty with executive function.
Maltreatment	Pragmatics	Difficulty with pragmatics, especially emotions.
		Alexithymia, possible PTSD.
LLE	Morphosyntax	Seen mostly in young children. Approximately half will have later communication disorders, usually DLD or LD.
Selective mutism	Pragmatics	Affects girls more than boys.
		Prolonger mutism, especially in educational and social settings.

Note: ASD, autism spectrum disorder; DLD, developmental language disorder; HFA, high-functioning autism; IDD, intellectual developmental disorder; LD, learning disability; LLE, late language emergence; PTSD, posttraumatic stress disorder; SCD, social communication disorder; TBI, traumatic brain injury.

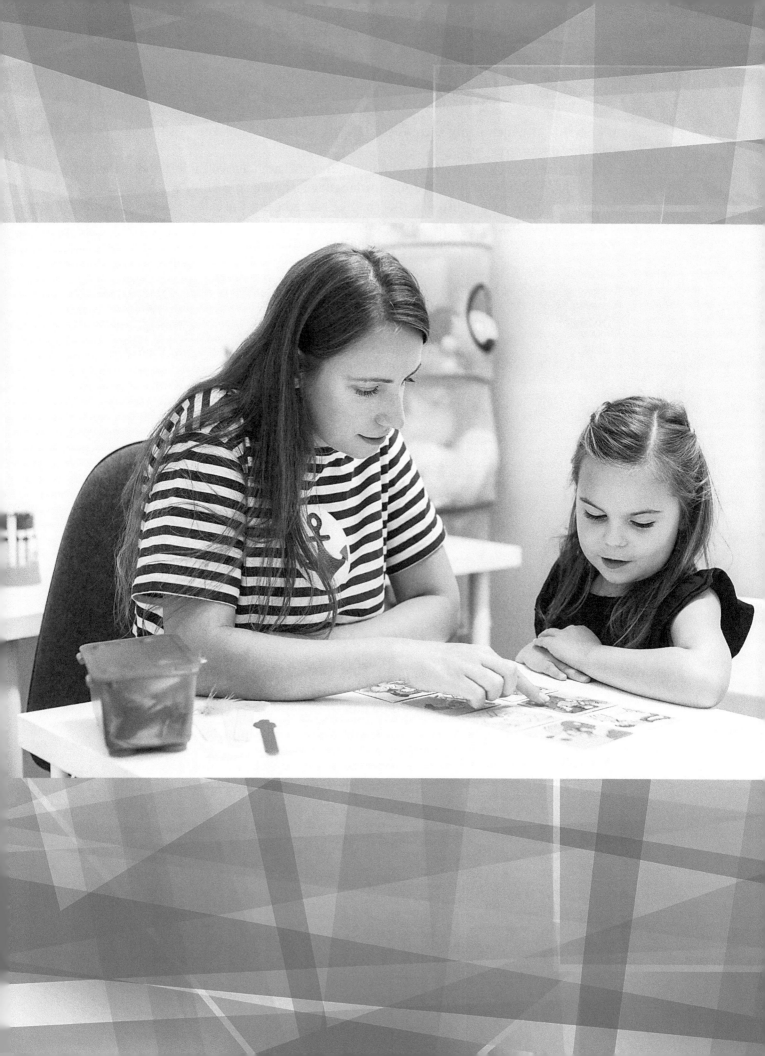

CHAPTER 4

EARLY COMMUNICATION INTERVENTION

Kaylee was born preterm and weighed less than 3 pounds at birth. She spent nearly 3 months in the local hospital's neonatal intensive care unit (NICU) and experienced breathing and feeding difficulties. Her mother visited daily but had interacted very little with Kaylee by the time Kaylee was released to go home.

Kaylee's development was slow, and she seemed younger than her age suggested. She walked by 15 months with a stiff rocking gait that has continued. When she hadn't said her first word by age 20 months, she was brought to an infant health clinic for a communication evaluation. During the interview portion, Kaylee's mother admitted that she was unsure how to proceed. Her daughter seemed so frail to her and had experienced a number of health incidents, including two seizures shortly after release from the NICU. No seizures have occurred since.

Kaylee is very social, making eye contact and sharing toys with her parents. She smiles easily and makes sounds and gestures in an attempt to communicate. Her mother reports that Kaylee makes some sound patterns over and over again, often insistently, as if she is trying to get the other person to understand. These sound patterns, CVCV in nature, are approximately three in number, and most of her communication is described by her parents as "grunts." At this time, she is not enrolled in any day care or early intervention program.

In the United States, approximately 15% of children, including one of my grandsons, have a **developmental disability** (DD) (Centers for Disease Control and Prevention [CDC], 2018b). U.S. Public Law (PL) 106-402, The Developmental Disabilities Assistance and Bill of Rights Act (2000), defined developmental disability as a severe, chronic disability that

- is attributable to mental or physical impairment or a combination of impairments;
- is manifested before the age of 22 years;
- is likely to continue indefinitely;
- results in substantial functional limitations in three or more areas of life activity, such as self-care, receptive and expressive language, learning, mobility, self-direction, capacity for independent learning, and economic self-sufficiency; and

- reflects the individual's need for a combination and sequence of special, interdisciplinary, or generic services, individualized supports, or other forms of assistance that are of lifelong or of extended duration and are individually planned and coordinated (American Speech-Language-Hearing Association [ASHA], n.d.).

Communication deficits among very young children with DD can range from reduced or atypical babbling through limited use of communicative gestures to slow growth of or regression in vocabulary (ASHA, 2008b), as we've seen with Kaylee. Many of the children described in Chapter 3 may also be said to have DD.

These and other children younger than age 3 years, more than 300,000 in all, are eligible for early intervention services as mandated by Part C of the Individuals with Disabilities Education Improvement Act (IDEA, 2004). **Early intervention** (EI) is an educational approach for young children, ages birth to 3 years, who have or are at risk for DD. EI's purpose is to provide both remediation and prevention of future difficulties. The focus is on both the child and family. When the primary focus of intervention is speech, language, and/or feeding, the child's program is referred to as **early communication intervention** (ECI).

The model for ECI is a functional one, focusing on the child and family members within the context of everyday communication. This model of intervention may seem different from what you've seen in the public schools with older children. Let's start our exploration with the legal basis for EI, and then we'll explore children who qualify, followed by a model for assessment and intervention, and end with a discussion of augmentative and alternative communication (AAC).

Legal Basis for Early Intervention

Significant predictors of children's outcomes include an early learning environment, early receipt of speech-language intervention, and the amount of time spent in intervention (Cunningham et al., 2018). But EI isn't just a good idea. In the United States and other developed countries, it's mandated by several laws.

PL 99-457, passed in 1986 and called the Education of the Handicapped Act Amendments, mandates that states establish comprehensive service for infants and toddlers with DD and for their families. The law requires that both assessment and intervention be provided by a multidisciplinary team of professionals. The purpose of the assessment is to confirm the presence and extent of disability and to identify

- a child's unique needs, accomplishments, and strengths;
- a family's strengths and needs as they relate to the child's development; and
- the nature and extent of early intervention services appropriate to the child and family.

Eligibility for services varies by state. Determiners include birth weight, gestational age at birth, and medical diagnosis.

CHAPTER 4 EARLY COMMUNICATION INTERVENTION

Four years later, the U.S. Congress passed the Individuals with Disabilities Education Act (IDEA). Part C of IDEA specifies programs for infants and toddlers. In 1997, IDEA was reauthorized and strengthened the requirement that services be provided within the context of family. Family members are part of the interdisciplinary team and primary decision makers in the collaborative effort. Reauthorized again in 2004 as the Individuals with Disabilities Education Improvement Act (IDEIA), the law mandates that these individualized programs be offered in the natural environment or the least restrictive environment (LRE).

Several principles of intervention outlined in the legislation are important (ASHA, 2008a, 2008b, 2008c, 2008d). Services should be

- comprehensive, coordinated, team-based, and transdisciplinary in nature to optimize the participation of children and their families and integrated to meet the needs of children and their families;
- family-centered and responsive to families' priorities as well as the culture and values of the family, including each families' unique situation, culture, language(s), preferences, resource, and priorities;
- individualized for the child and family;
- developmentally supportive and promote children's participation in their natural environment;
- developmentally appropriate for children's age, cognitive level, strengths, and family concerns and preferences;
- provided in the least restrictive and most natural environment for the child and family; and
- based on the highest quality and most recent research evidence on intervention effectiveness merged with professional expertise and family preferences.

These elements are also supported by the EI guiding principles of ASHA (2008b). Let's explore some of these further.

In addition, the World Health Organization (WHO) endorsed a new model of disability that considers health and disability in relation to each other and to participation in daily life activities (World Health Assembly, 2001). Like the functional model discussed throughout this text, concern is for how and with whom the individual communicates on a daily basis. Daily activities and routines offer learning opportunities that restricted participation can limit. Participation requires communication, and that's where you'll come in.

The Early Intervention Model

Now that we have an idea of the overall EI approach, let's take it apart and briefly look at the individual pieces. Some of you will thrive in this model and find that ECI is for you.

Team Approach

A team is responsible for selecting the most appropriate service delivery based on the individualized needs of a child and family. In a transdisciplinary team approach, parents/caregivers and professionals from multiple disciplines share responsibility for planning and implementing, while at the same time contributing their own unique expertise. In this way, transdisciplinary teams fully integrate the family and different disciplines. Ideally, the team, including parents or caregivers, develops an integrated service plan through consensus or collaboration.

One professional on the team, often the speech-language pathologist (SLP), may be designated as the primary service provider (PSP). The hope is that this model may avoid fragmenting of services. The PSP provides services across disciplines while other professionals act in a consultative manner and are directly involved as needed.

Importance of Families

Effective early intervention is family centered. Family involvement produces positive effects for children's physical, cognitive, social, and language skills; fosters a parent's sense of personal control and self-efficacy; and increases a parent's overall satisfaction with intervention services (Applequist & Bailey, 2000). In family-centered intervention, parents are partners with professionals, not "add-ons" after the fact.

Successful early intervention depends on quality relationships between all parties—children, parents, and intervention facilitators. These relationships have a direct impact on the quality of intervention. In addition to the individual characteristics of each child, variables include family histories, current circumstances, and the family's reasons for seeking services.

Young children whose caregivers participate in intervention activities make more language gains than children whose families are not involved in intervention (Chao et al., 2006). A meta-analysis of parent-implemented language interventions found these approaches to be effective language intervention methods for young children with language disorders (Roberts & Kaiser, 2011). Working collaboratively, SLPs and families can identify goals and typical daily routines within which these goals might be addressed.

Cultural Concerns

Like all children, a child with DD is part of an ecological unit that includes family members, friends, neighbors, and community agencies. The family is embedded within a broader cultural context.

EI must by its nature reflect respect for individuality and for racial, ethnic, cultural, and other differences found across diverse family backgrounds and be responsive to each family's needs. At the least, materials distributed to caregivers should be in the native language, procedures should be nondiscriminatory and in the language to which the infant has been most exposed, and multiple methods of assessment should be employed.

I know of a case in which a parent who spoke only Spanish was told to only use English with her child, resulting in a year of no spoken communication between the parent and the child. This is the opposite of what is required by law.

Ethnic and cultural groups can vary significantly in their beliefs about disability, the nature of family and community supports, medical practices, and use of professional services. To improve ECI participation, collaboration, and service delivery with families from diverse backgrounds, SLPs must understand and respect these culturally specific beliefs and values (Garcia et al., 2000; Rodriguez & Olswang, 2003; Salas-Provance et al., 2002).

Child and Parent/Caregivers

For young children, the recommended model of intervention is one in which a parent or caregiver and an SLP collaborate in planning and intervention, with the family implementing intervention in the home following training by the SLP. This model has a positive effect on the early language skills of young children, confirmed by an analysis of several intervention studies (Roberts & Kaiser, 2011). Compared to SLP-only models, gains for children receiving parent-implemented intervention were significantly higher in receptive language and expressive syntax.

Even a brief training program of only three sessions has been shown to have an effect on parents' vocal and nonverbal behavior with 12- to 24-month-old children (Rajesh & Venkatesh, 2019). Another result with children who are more verbal is that caregivers increase their proportion of comments, suggestions, and reflections on the child's speech and decrease their use of direct commands and questions. These changes generalize to daily interactions.

It's essential that we pay attention to interactions between a parent or caregiver and the child because this is the filter through which all intervention will pass, regardless of whether we choose to recognize its importance. At the very least, SLPs should explore with parents their beliefs and knowledge about (Kummerer et al., 2007)

- their children's speech and/or language disabilities;
- the difference between and importance of both receptive and expressive language;
- why intervention is recommended;
- the role of speech-language therapy and the SLP;
- why it is important for parents to participate in ECI;
- how clinicians will interact with children and the family;
- how the clinician and family can work collaboratively;
- the amount of time and effort needed to remediate children's difficulties; and
- how the family can generalize strategies to the home setting.

These topics are important because uninformed or discouraged parents may be less effective as agents of change.

The SLP's role is to support caregivers in becoming competent and confident in their ability to help their children develop communication. As an SLP, you'll need to integrate your knowledge of and skill in child-focused intervention with adult education principles needed to guide caregivers to implement intervention.

Individualized for Each Child

As with any good intervention, SLP services must be tailored to the individual child. This requires thorough and ongoing assessment and monitoring of a child's communication behavior and accurate record keeping. Flexibility is the key as a young child develops and new opportunities to intervene become available. As a group, children who begin receiving intervention services at a younger age require fewer intervention visits than those who begin later, regardless of the type of disorder (Jacoby et al., 2002).

Individualized Family Service Plan

As EI focus has moved from the child with disabilities to the child as part of a family unit, the change is evident in the Individualized Family Service Plan (IFSP). You may be familiar with the Individualized Education Plan for school-aged children. The IFSP is based on this model but addresses both child and family needs that impact a child's development. At the very least, an IFSP should include

- the child's and family's current status;
- the recommended services and expected outcomes; and
- a projection of the duration of service delivery.

It's essential that the family understands the contents and feels some ownership of the plan through participation in the creation process. The plan should be reviewed periodically and updated as needed to accommodate the child's and the family's changing needs.

The IFSP is a collaborative document and should reflect this cooperative effort between families and providers in its description of a child's and family's needs. Families should be included in the planning of the evaluation of their child and encouraged to discuss their concerns and priorities and their resources for promoting the development of their child. To succeed, family-centered and caregiver-implemented intervention must be based on the caregiver decision making regarding the outcomes, activities, and routines to be used for intervention and on when, where, and how interventions strategies will be embedded.

Natural Environment

The term *natural environments* refers to settings that are typical for infants and toddlers. This contrasts with more traditional intervention settings, such as clinics or medical-based sites. Natural environments include family homes, early care and educational settings, and other community settings in which a family spends the majority of its time with the child. The most frequent natural environment for intervention services is the family home.

Although center-based EI has the potential, if not handled sensitively, to be threatening to some caregivers, it also offers an opportunity for children and parents to interact with other children and parents. When carefully guided, these interactions can be an enjoyable way for caregivers to observe other caregiver–child interactions and to enhance their own interactional skills as an adjunct to home-based services.

CHAPTER 4 EARLY COMMUNICATION INTERVENTION

Home-based intervention involves more than just location. The context of a family's daily routines and activities offers an opportunity for children to learn and develop within events occurring naturally within the home environment. Parents can use daily routines and activities as opportunities for teaching. Thus, eating and being bathed offer meaningful and functional opportunities for learning communication. SLPs, working in partnership with families, can coach parents and caregivers on including individualized communication activities throughout the day.

Teaching caregivers to use intervention strategies across routines is necessary to achieve maximal communication outcomes. For example, although a *teach–model–coach–review* instructional approach results in increased use of these language support strategies by caregivers and subsequent positive outcomes for their young preschool children with language disorders, the generalization and maintenance of these strategies can still be limited within the home unless several daily routines are brought into intervention (Roberts et al., 2014).

Young children learn best when participating in an activity while a caregiver mediates the environment and interactions (Hancock & Kaiser, 2006; Wetherby & Woods, 2006). The SLP can help caregivers understand how young children learn to communicate, enabling the caregivers to make decisions about the best times and ways to interact with their child throughout the day. The probability that caregivers will act as effective communication facilitators is increased when they are involved in problem-solving and planning.

Role of the SLP

This may all sound very different from what you assumed to be your role as an SLP. Within the EI model, the SLP wears multiple hats relative to infants and toddlers and their families. These include (Woods et al., 2011)

- team member, possibly the PSP;
- clinician;
- communication facilitator;
- coach; and
- consultant.

Whereas some of these roles are more traditional, others are not.

In coaching caregivers to learn to embed communication strategies into their daily routines, the SLP acts as both a teacher and a learner. Caregivers are not likely to have the expertise or experience they need to support their child's communication learning. For their part, caregivers inform the SLP about the child's strengths, the nature of the child's daily routines and interests, and which strategies are good fits with the family's culture and values. In other words, both the SLP and the caregiver contribute and gain knowledge and skills as partners to support the child's development (Dunst & Trivette, 2009). This bidirectional teaching and learning relationship is the basis for a truly individualized and functional family-centered approach (Woods et al., 2011).

Children Served in ECI Programs

The more limited a child's communication behavior, the more difficult it is for a child to learn the link between communication behavior and results. Within the first few months of life, typically developing children learn that their behavior can affect other people in their environment. Making this connection is a vital first link in developing communication intent. In addition, communication impairment impacts other aspects of a child's development. For example, toddlers with language delays appear to show more social withdrawal relative to toddlers with typically developing language (TDL) (Horwitz et al., 2003; Irwin et al., 2002; Rescorla et al., 2007). There is also a relationship between the presence of communication impairment and behavioral problems in preschool, possibly leading to later behavioral/emotional disorders.

As we know, children with poor language tend to also have poor psychosocial outcomes. Given this relationship, it seems warranted to target both linguistic and psychosocial development in early language intervention (Newbury et al., 2019).

> *Food for Thought:* What factors of birth and early development might potentially lead to communication and later language disorder?

Several factors can contribute to communication impairments. For example, low birth weight and premature birth are both significant predictors of late language emergence (LLE), as we saw with Kaylee. Other significant factors in LLE include a family history of LLE, male gender, and early neurobiological growth. Factors such as parental educational levels, socioeconomic resources, parental mental health, parenting practices, and family functioning are less significant. Predictors of later language impairment among 24-month-olds include problems in gross and fine motor development, poor adaptive and psychosocial development, and negative temperament.

As outlined in PL 99-457, two broad categories of children are served by early intervention programs: those in established risk categories and those in at-risk categories. In established risk, there is a strong link between the condition and developmental difficulties. Table 4–1 presents examples of established risks.

Although a child has an established risk, the child is not precluded from experiencing at-risk factors as well. At-risk factors include anything with the potential to interfere with a child's ability to interact in a typical way with the environment and to develop typically, and they may also be both biological and environmental in nature. At-risk examples are also presented in Table 4–1. Let's look at each risk category briefly.

Established Risk

As a group, established risks are easier to identify and have a strong link with developmental difficulties. Many of these were described in Chapter 3 and are only mentioned briefly here. Examples of established risk include intellectual developmental disorder (IDD), autism spectrum disorder (ASD), cerebral palsy (CP), and deafness and deaf–blindness.

Table 4–1. Established Risk and At-Risk Examples

Established Risk	At Risk
Intellectual developmental disorder	Preterm birth
Cerebral palsy	Low birth weight
Blindness	Physical abuse
Deafness	Severe, chronic caregiver or child illness
Autism spectrum disorder	
Chronic medical illness	Lack of or limited prenatal care
Severe infectious disease	Chronic or acute caregiver mental illness or developmental disability
Chromosomal and genetic disorder	
Neurological disorders	Caregiver alcohol or substance dependence
Congenital malformations	
Inborn metabolic errors	

Intellectual Developmental Disorder

Although almost every child is able to learn, develop, and become a participating member of the community, the cognitive limitations that accompany IDD will result in a child learning and developing more slowly than a typical child. More severe types of IDD and accompanying multiple handicapping conditions may be obvious at birth. My grandson has IDD, accompanied by CP and blindness; not all of these were definitively established during his earliest years.

Autism Spectrum Disorder

As noted in Chapter 3, children with moderate-to-severe ASD are almost always delayed in speech and language acquisition and in communication in general (Tager-Flusberg et al., 2005). Early language ability and social competence are related to positive long-term outcomes, and verbal skills are the strongest predictors of later language functioning (Liss et al., 2001; Lord et al., 2004; Stone & Yoder, 2001).

Emerging research evidence suggests that abnormal brain circuitry in infants with ASD precedes altered social behaviors. It is hoped by some professionals that intervention designed to promote early social engagement and reciprocity could potentially redirect brain development toward a more typical trajectory and thus remit or reduce these behaviors (Webb et al., 2014).

Multiple factors seem to contribute to the development of language skills in young children with ASD. Of importance are the following (Bono et al., 2004; Charman et al., 2003; Stone & Yoder, 2001; Woods & Wetherby, 2003):

- Functional and symbolic use of objects
- The number and type of gestures

- Ability to initiate joint attention
- Presence of verbal imitation skills
- Number of words produced
- Number of words comprehended

Although there is widespread variability, toddlers with ASD tend to have relative strengths in phonology and significant weaknesses in pragmatics (Bean Ellawadi & Ellis Weismer, 2015). Two important factors are joint attention and the use of gestures. Although several studies have stressed the importance of early joint attention for early communication and language development among children with ASD, there does not seem to be a long-term effect that carries into pragmatic development in the school years (Gillespie-Lynch et al., 2015).

As an SLP, you'll face the challenge of determining whether and when a preverbal child with ASD will use spoken language as their primary means of communication. Although I'll summarize the information, I recommend the thorough tutorial by McDaniel and Schuele (2021). These authors provide practical guidance on expressive language predictors.

In early development, children with ASD vary widely in their spoken language skills (Ellis Weismer et al., 2010; Luyster et al., 2008; Pickett et al., 2009). Many preschoolers with severe ASD are not producing words, and approximately 50% to 70% are not producing spoken phrases (Ellis Weismer & Kover, 2015; Thurm et al., 2015). Unfortunately, approximately 25% to 30% of all children with severe ASD remain minimally verbal and do not use spoken language as their primary means of communication (Anderson et al., 2007; Tager-Flusberg & Kasari, 2013; Tager-Flusberg et al., 2005; Wodka et al., 2013).

> **Food for Thought:** How would you go about assessing a young child for possible ASD? What signs would you look for?

A meta-analysis found wide variation in the age of diagnosis for ASD, ranging from 38 to 120 months, although the age has continued to decrease (Daniels & Mandell, 2014). Factors associated with earlier diagnosis include greater symptom severity, higher socioeconomic status (SES), greater parental concern, and family interactions with health care and educational systems prior to diagnosis. Geography is also a factor, suggesting that community resources and state policies and procedures play a role in early identification. You can be an advocate for these children and families, including enhancing parental awareness and service provider education on early detection and intervention options and strategies.

For example, among Latina mothers, there appears to be a general lack of awareness about ASD and a belief, unfortunately supported by misinformed professionals, that exposure to both Spanish and English will increase their children's language difficulties (Ijalba, 2016). Clearly, there is a need to disseminate adequate information about ASD to the Latino/Latina immigrant community through community outreach, home–school connections, and pediatricians.

Cerebral Palsy

Cerebral palsy is a group of chronic brain disorders that affect movement, muscle tone, and muscle coordination in approximately half a million people in the United States. Approximately 8,000 babies and infants are diagnosed with CP annually, with another 1,500 identified during the preschool years. Damage to one or more motor areas of the brain disrupts the brain's ability to control movement and posture because of the faulty signals sent to the muscles. The degree of severity depends on where and to what extent the brain is damaged. CP is associated with difficulty in swallowing and problems with both speech and language.

Cerebral palsy is not a disease, and it doesn't worsen with time. The majority of newborn brain injury cases, approximately 70%, are attributed to events occurring before labor begins. Estimates of the incidence of CP are 2 per 1,000 live births. Risk factors for CP are low birth weight, preterm birth, placental disorders, rubella or other infections of the mother during pregnancy, Rh or other blood incompatibility factors, prolonged loss of oxygen, and stroke or bleeding in the infant's brain.

The three main types of CP are spastic, athetoid, and ataxic. These are rarely seen in their pure form, and many individuals have mixed CP. In addition, many young children initially exhibit what is termed flaccid or hypotonic CP characterized by poor muscle tone and a floppy posture. The majority of these children manifest one of the other forms of CP as they mature. Characteristics of the types and causes of CP are presented in Table 4–2.

Table 4–2. Characteristics and Causes of Cerebral Palsy

Type of Cerebral Palsy	Characteristics	Area of Brain Affected
Spastic	Spasticity, increased muscle tone in opposing muscle groups Rigidity and exaggerated stretch reflex Jerky, labored, and slow movements Infantile reflex patterns	Motor cortex, pyramidal tract
Athetoid	Slow, involuntary writhing Disorganized and uncoordinated volitional movement Movements occur accompanying volitional movement	Extrapyramidal tract, basal ganglia
Ataxic	Uncoordinated movement Poor balance Movements lack direction, force, and control	Cerebellum

An early sign of CP is often failure to develop motor skills similar to other children. My grandson at age 2 years moved about by either rolling or "combat crawling"—pulling himself along—on his stomach, and although he could get to his knees, he seemed incapable of crawling independently.

Deafness and Deaf–Blindness

Hearing impairment occurs when there is a full or partial decrease in the ability to detect or understand sounds. The degree of impairment can be viewed as a continuum from typical hearing to profound hearing loss or deafness. Severity is measured by the degree of loudness or the intensity level, measured in decibels, that a sound must attain before being detectible to an individual. A profound hearing loss is a 90-dB threshold or greater. This means that sounds that are quieter than 90 dB or the level of very loud music are not detectable auditorily.

Although the previous definition of deafness is technically correct, it may be more appropriate to think of deafness in more practical terms. For example, ability to benefit from auditory information is situationally dependent on the type of sound, interfering noise, and the context.

The age at which the hearing impairment develops is crucial to spoken language acquisition. Development of hearing loss either prenatally or during infancy can interfere with both social development and the development of spoken language because a child is unable to access audible/spoken communication from the outset. In general, among children receiving EI services, those whose hearing loss is identified by 6 months of age demonstrated significantly better language than children identified later. For this reason, nearly all infants in the United States are screened as neonates for hearing loss.

The prevalence of deafness in newborns in the United States is approximately 1.7 per 1,000 live births (CDC, 2021b). Another 6 to 8 per 1,000 have severe loss of 70 to 90 dB (Cunningham & Cox, 2003; Kemper & Downs, 2000). For most children, hearing loss is present at birth, although some types of degenerative hearing loss may not become evident until later.

Young children with major impairments in both auditory and visual abilities have unique communicative, developmental, emotional, and educational needs. Sensory deficits can lead to communication impairment and frequently lead to behavioral challenges.

Total blindness is the complete lack of form and visual light perception. A child described as having only "light perception" can distinguish light from dark but nothing more. In the United States, Canada, and most of Europe, legal blindness is defined by a visual acuity with the best possible correction of 20/200 or less in the better eye compared to 20/20 for typical vision. The 20/200 value means that a person standing 20 feet from an object would see it with the same degree of clarity as a typically sighted person at 200 feet. Approximately 10% of those deemed legally blind have no usable vision. Visual field may also be affected. Typical vision includes 180 degrees of field. Those with legal blindness may have a visual field of less than 20 degrees.

Having a child with a dual sensory impairment or with other multiple impairments, such as a child with deafness, visual impairment, and CP, can create emotional and financial stress on a family. If we consider the family as a unit, then having a child

At-Risk Children

Unlike children in established risk categories in which there is a strong link between their condition and developmental disability, those in at-risk categories may or may not experience developmental difficulties, although the possibility exists. In the following sections, we discuss some of the more common at-risk categories, including international adoption, low SES, maltreatment/neglect and fetal alcohol spectrum disorder, and premature birth and low birth weight.

International Adoptions

In 2018, there were 4,059 international adoptions in the United States (U.S. Department of State, 2019). The largest number of adoptions came from China, India, and Colombia. Infants and toddlers adopted from countries with a different language and culture undergo a unique language learning experience. Usually, development in the birth language is arrested and replaced by development of the adopted language because adoptive families usually are unable to maintain the birth language (Glennen & Masters, 2002).

Potentially complicating language acquisition is the large percentage of these children initially raised in orphanages. It is estimated that children raised in orphanages lose 1 month of linear growth for every 3 to 5 months in an orphanage (Johnson, 2000; Miller & Hendric, 2000). In addition, many of the countries from which children come have low personal income, poor nutrition, and limited access to health care. These risk factors create a less-than-optimal environment. Thus, many adoptees are among the lowest for height, weight, and head circumference.

The heightened incidence of several conditions and diseases, such as fetal alcohol spectrum disorder (FASD), iodine insufficiency, hepatitis B and C, tuberculosis, and intestinal parasites, among international adoptees may also adversely affect development of young international adoptees (Johnson, 2000; Miller & Hendric, 2000). Other factors include poor maternal health care, high-risk pregnancy or delivery, and premature birth.

Although children adopted at early ages catch up more quickly than children adopted at later preschool ages, 3 years after adoption, there is no significant difference in language test scores between most international adoptees and children with TDL. In addition, the percentage of children with language or speech delays is also similar to that of children with TDL (Glennen, 2014). However, international adoption is still a risk factor.

Low Socioeconomic Status

Risk of communication impairment is associated with socioeconomic factors such as economic deprivation. Many children with language disorders come from homes lacking in stable and continuous child care, adequate nutrition, and even rudimentary medical care.

Beginning at conception, poverty significantly heightens a child's risk for the following (Halpern, 2000):

- Birth complications such as fetal alcohol syndrome
- Physical health problems such as asthma and malnutrition
- Mental health problems
- Inattentive or erratic parental care
- Neglect and abuse
- Removal from the home and placement in foster care
- Deficits in cognitive development and achievement

Children from low-SES backgrounds may be exposed to multiple risks. An accumulation of risk factors can increase the negative effects of poverty and increase the risk for developmental disability (Stanton-Chapman et al., 2004).

Family stress related to poverty also affects the language skills of toddlers reared in homes experiencing socioeconomic disadvantage. As a group, these children's receptive language skills are in the low normal range, related most directly with caregiver–child interactions and indirectly with maternal distress (Justice et al., 2019).

Late Language Emergence

In a large, representative population sample, researchers found approximately 13% of children began language development at a late age and growth was slower than expected. This delay is termed **late language emergence** (Zubrick et al., 2007). These children were almost twice as likely to have language disorders at age 7 years than children without a history of LLE (Rice et al., 2008). In fact, LLE may be the single strongest predictor of later language disorder. Even children who "outgrow" LLE and subsequently develop language at a more typical pace may have lingering deficits that place them in the low normal range. Approximately half of children with LLE will subsequently be diagnosed as having DLD.

Maltreatment/Neglect and Fetal Alcohol Spectrum Disorder

As noted in Chapter 3, there is a clear interaction between language disorder and the factors of caregiver maltreatment/neglect or fetal alcohol spectrum disorder (FASD) (Hernandez, 2004; Hooper et al., 2003). Although the United States spends more money fighting child abuse than any other country, it has the highest rate of child abuse in the industrialized world (Lindsey, 2003).

There is a direct relationship between the amount of language input a child receives and the amount of language a child produces. Very socially depriving circumstances will affect language development. In addition, some children who experience extreme deprivation show behaviors, such as rocking, self-injury, and atypical sensory interests, similar to ASD, although the underlying causes are distinctly dissimilar (Beckett et al., 2002; Fombonne, 2003; Rutter et al., 2001).

CHAPTER 4   EARLY COMMUNICATION INTERVENTION

For some children, maltreatment begins in utero when they are exposed to the negative impact of maternal alcohol abuse, resulting in FASD. Each year in the United States, approximately 40,000 infants are born with FASD, with as high as 8,000 of these born with fetal alcohol syndrome, the most severe form (American Academy of Pediatrics, 2022). At least 2,000 may experience severe medical concerns (Braillion & DuBois, 2005).

Preterm and Low-Birth-Weight Infants

Preterm birth and low birth weight are major challenges in early health care. Most neonatal or newborn deaths occur in preterm and low-birth-weight infants. However, most preterm and low-birth-weight infants develop typically.

Preterm Birth. Preterm birth is an important risk factor for neurological impairment and disability (Tucker & McGuire, 2004). Preterm birth in the United States is a public health problem with significant consequences for families, and it costs U.S. society at least $26.2 billion or $51,600 per infant annually (Institute of Medicine, 2006).

Although treatment of preterm infants in NICUs or special care nurseries (SCNs) can greatly improve their survival, as it did for Kaylee, these infants remain vulnerable. Long-term problems may include CP, intellectual disabilities, visual and hearing impairments, behavior and social–emotional problems, learning difficulties, and poor health and growth.

> ***Food for Thought:*** **Were you or someone you know a preterm or low-birth-weight newborn? Did this affect development in any way?**

Most pregnancies last 37 to 42 weeks, and infants born during this window are called full term. Preterm births occur before week 37. Eighty-four percent of preterm infants are born between 32 and 37 weeks of gestation. Approximately 10% are born between 28 and 31 weeks and are labeled very preterm, whereas only 6%, called extremely premature, are born prior to 28 weeks of gestation (Martin et al., 2006).

Most mortality and morbidity affect very preterm and extremely preterm infants. Morbidity is illness or disability. Although survival is possible for infants born as early as 22 to 27 weeks, most likely these children will face a lifetime of health problems. The age of viability or the age at which a fetus can survive outside the womb is currently approximately 21 or 22 weeks in the United States.

Low Birth Weight. Although birth weight and gestational age are positively related, they are not interchangeable. Categories for low birth weight are as follows:

- Low birth weight: Less than 2,500 g or 5.5 lbs
- Very low birth weight: Less than 1,500 g or 3.3 lbs
- Extremely low birth weight: Less than 500 g or 1.1 lbs

Only approximately two-thirds of low-birth-weight infants are preterm. Full-term infants may be of low birth weight because they are "small for gestational age," usually defined as in the lowest 10% for birth weight. Infants may be small for gestational age as a result of intrauterine growth restriction (IUGR). Fetal growth restriction is the second leading cause of perinatal morbidity and mortality, with prematurity being the first. The incidence of IUGR is estimated to be approximately 5% in infants.

Incidence. During the past 20 to 30 years, the incidence of preterm birth in most developed countries has been approximately 5% to 7% of live births (Tucker & McGuire, 2004). According to the WHO (2018), the rate of preterm birth varies by country from 5% to 18%. Low birth weight rates are 15% to 20% globally.

The incidence of preterm birth in the United States is 10.1% (CDC, 2021d). Factors include increasing rates of multiple births; greater use of assisted reproduction techniques, such as in vitro fertilization; and more obstetric intervention, such as the increased use of cesarean section (Tucker & McGuire, 2004). In the United States, the highest rates for preterm births are among African American women (14.4%) regardless of SES background.

Causes and Consequences. Most preterm births, approximately 70%, are a result of spontaneous labor, either by itself or following spontaneous premature rupture of the membranes (PROM) of the sac inside the uterus that holds the fetus (Goldenberg et al., 2008). All causes are presented in Figure 4–1. PROM may be triggered by the body's natural response to certain infections of the amniotic fluid and fetal membranes.

The most important predictors of spontaneous preterm delivery are a history of preterm birth and low SES. Medical and health conditions during pregnancy, such as intrauterine infections and maternal high blood pressure or diabetes, also may increase preterm labor and delivery (March of Dimes, 2007).

The remaining 30% of preterm births result from early induction of labor or cesarean delivery due to pregnancy complications or health problems (Iams, 2003). In most of these cases, early delivery is probably the safest approach for both mother and infant.

Complications from preterm birth or low birth weight may be any of the following (Bromberger & Permanente, 2004; March of Dimes, 2007):

- Respiratory. Approximately 70% of infants born before 34 weeks of gestation have some type of respiratory difficulty.
- Circulatory. Circulatory problems may be related to immaturity of the heart, internal bleeding, and anemia.
- Immunological. Neonatal immunological problems can lead to many forms of infection because of immature immune systems and may include pneumonia or lung infection, blood infection or sepsis, and meningitis, an infection of the membranes surrounding the brain and spinal cord.
- Feeding and digestive. Preterm or small infants are not able to suck and swallow until they reach approximately 32 weeks of gestational age and may experience

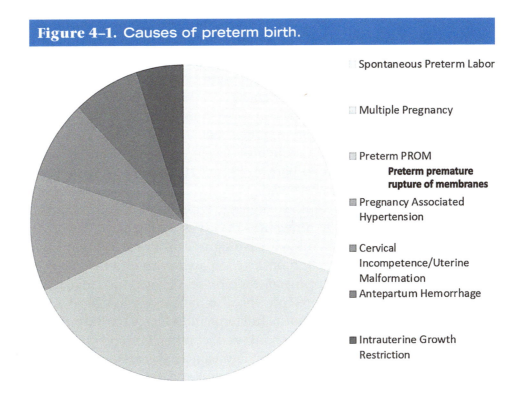

Figure 4–1. Causes of preterm birth.

serious digestive problems, such as necrotizing enterocolitis, in which the child experiences temporary or permanent necrosis or death of intestinal tissue.

These complications can range from mild to severe.

Premature infants tend to need the most care immediately after birth. As might be expected, the most preterm generally require the greatest attention. Many families find the experience to be an emotional roller coaster that can be extremely difficult.

Initially, the infant is kept in the NICU/SCN on an open warmer—a bed that keeps the infant warm by heating the surrounding air. Once the infant's breathing rate is stabilized, the infant is usually placed in an isolette—an enclosed plastic incubator with controlled air temperature. When it is easier for an infant to maintain its own temperature and the infant weighs approximately 4 pounds and if there are no serious complicating factors, the infant is placed in an open crib.

Infants extremely preterm are at greatest risk of neurological disabilities and cognitive dysfunction. Although approximately 80% of infants born at 26 weeks and 90% of those born at 27 weeks survive to 1 year, approximately a quarter of these infants will develop serious lasting disabilities, and up to half may have milder problems such as learning and behavioral difficulties (American College of Obstetricians and Gynecologists, 2002).

At age 5 years, 49% of children born at 24 to 28 weeks of gestation or extremely preterm have some disability (Larroque et al., 2008). CP is present in 9% of all children born very preterm, and 32% are intellectually disabled. In the very preterm group, 5% have severe disability, 9% moderate disability, and 25% mild disability. Special health care/education resources are used by 42% of children born at 24 to 28 weeks and 31% born at 28 to 32 weeks, compared to only 16% of those born full term.

Significant predictors for language, motor, and cognitive delays are lower maternal education and a younger gestational age at birth (Frome Loeb et al., 2020). At 30 months following birth, preterm children tend to have an overall language ability, especially expressive language, significantly lower than children with TDL and those with other health conditions. In addition, preterm children with LLE are significantly more likely to have delays in cognitive or motor development or both.

Compared to children born full term, those born preterm and with motor delays perform even more poorly on language measures. Cognitive deficits seem to contribute to the difference in receptive language, while both cognitive and motor deficits independently contribute to differences in expressive language (Ross et al., 2018).

Extremely preterm children have significant lower communication, cognition, and motor performance at 30 months compared with children born full term (Månsson & Stjernqvist, 2014). In general, even by school age, the language abilities of children born extremely or very preterm who also have a very low birth weight are significantly below those of children who are full term and average birth weight (Zimmerman, 2018). Throughout the elementary school years, children born prematurely, at less than or at 32 weeks or less than 1,500 g, display significantly lower test scores in semantics and syntax even though most are within low normal limits (Mahurin Smith et al., 2014).

Children with expressive vocabulary delays by 24 months of age are more likely than other children to continue to need speech/language services into school age (P. Morgan et al., 2016). African American children and those from low SES backgrounds and/or with a primary language other than English, however, are less likely to receive these services, clearly indicating a need for more culturally and linguistically sensitive practices related to access to needed EI services.

ECI Assessment

Assessment of very young children is not like any other type of communication evaluation. Young children are very independent when it comes to cooperating and responding to standardized testing, and some may have multiple handicapping conditions. It's safe to say, "I don't think we're in Kansas anymore, Toto!" By the same token, for those of you who are creative, curious about the world, and think you might like the challenge, early communication assessment and intervention may be just the right fit.

Currently recommended practices within EI focus on providing a clear picture of the child's overall development and identifying the child's relative strengths and challenges (Crais & Roberts, 2004). In addition to being required by law, this type of developmental "profiling" is thought to provide the best overall portrait of the child and to help families and professionals make the most informed decisions.

A child's speech and language are built on a foundation of prelinguistic skills that not only serve as an indicator of the child's current skill level but also are a strong predictor of the child's potential for language competence later. For very young children, especially those who are not talking, it is important to identify the key components of prelin-

CHAPTER 4 EARLY COMMUNICATION INTERVENTION

guistic communication, such as vocalizations, vocabulary comprehension, gesture use, initiating and responding to joint attention, parental interactions, and familial history of language and/or learning impairments (Hadley & Holt, 2006; Mundy et al., 2007).

Our charges—the infants and toddlers we serve—are small, often sick or with multiple handicaps. Similar to Kaylee's mother, caregivers may be confused and overwhelmed by their child's needs. I've had parents begin to cry as soon as I ask the first question about their child. We must be sensitive to all these issues.

Your assessment may be the child's and family's introduction to EI. The manner in which we as professionals interact with the family and the child can mean all the difference between a satisfying and fruitful experience that can lead to future collaboration and a situation that leaves a family confused, frustrated, and possibly hostile.

Part H of IDEA specifies that an evaluation must be conducted to determine a child's eligibility for services, identifying a child's level of developmental functioning in a comprehensive and nondiscriminatory manner. Traditionally, evaluations are more structured and formal and rely on the use of standardized instruments.

In contrast, assessment is the ongoing process of identifying a child's unique needs; the family's priorities, concerns, and resources; and the nature and extent of the EI services needed by both. As such, assessment activities are usually less formal and rely on the use of multiple tools and methods with the close cooperation of families and professionals. Typically, assessments focus not on what is wrong with a child but on identifying what can be done to help. In this way, an assessment is truly a first step in intervention and essential for progress monitoring.

Transdisciplinary Model of Assessment

A transdisciplinary team approach is one in which there is a conscious effort to pool expertise and freely exchange insights and ideas. This is best accomplished if caregivers and professionals observe the entire evaluation and simultaneously assess the child, a method dubbed *arena assessment*. Instead of the child being separately assessed by each discipline, a common sample of the child's behavior is collected and recorded as all observe and participate in the process.

The format is often play-based. Compared to more formal, structured, discipline-specific methods, play-based assessment is more

- naturalistic;
- ecologically sound;
- context-based; and
- child-centered.

The word *play* does not imply an open-ended or haphazard free-for-all. This is play with a purpose. A good evaluation requires planning, training, and considerable expertise. Through play, the SLP attempts to elicit specific behavior. For example, while playing, an adult, either a professional or a parent, may play an imitation "game" to see if the child will follow suit. Throughout, the *process of interaction takes precedence* over the product or result.

> *Food for Thought:* If caregivers are members of the transdisciplinary team, how do we empower them in the assessment process?

As mentioned previously, EI should be family-centered. As an SLP, you'll want the family's full engagement in the assessment process and in the possible intervention to follow.

Assessment serves as their introduction. In order for families to be empowered, they must be full participants and real decision makers (Dunst, 2002). Our behavior at that time determines the extent to which a family becomes invested in their child's communication development program. If your recommendations are to be "owned" by families, these proposals must match their notions of appropriateness and importance.

Family Concerns, Priorities, and Resources

IDEA 2004 requires that programs provide an opportunity for a family to identify their concerns, priorities, and resources related to enhancement of their child's development. Six key objectives may guide the gathering of family information (ASHA, 2008b; Bailey, 2004):

- To identify the family's concerns and what they hope to accomplish through their participation
- To determine how the family perceives the child's strengths and needs relative to their family values, structure, and routines
- To identify the family's priorities and how service providers may assist with these priorities
- To identify the family's resources related to their priorities
- To identify the family's preferred role in the service delivery and decision-making processes
- To establish a supportive, informed, and collaborative relationship

Each of these outcomes should be addressed in an assessment and throughout the intervention process.

Informal Communication Assessment

Students approaching the topic of ECI often assume there's little to assess in young children because they may not be talking yet. Actually, the opposite is true. The difficulty comes in trying to winnow down all the possible behaviors and to note only the most important ones. Currently, researchers are attempting to identify the most significant early communication developments. One of the values of evidence-based practice is that we are beginning to recognize those child behaviors that seem to have the greatest

CHAPTER 4 EARLY COMMUNICATION INTERVENTION 121

impact. Let's explore the information that we hope to gain from an evaluation of both the child and caregivers.

> ***Food for Thought:*** **Assume that you're working with preverbal children. They seemingly lack usable speech and language. What should you assess?**

Description of Communication

The SLP and other team members should attempt to describe as thoroughly as possible the present communication system of the child and caregiver. Of importance are the forms/means of communication and communication success.

Successful communication depends on more than just the child. Success requires a responsive partner.

Forms/Means of Communication. Communication forms are intentional or unintentional behaviors performed by a child in the presence of a partner. The means may be physical, vocal, or both. Physical or nonvocal signals may include eye contact, facial expression, communication distance, body movements or contact, gestures, and even aggression to self or others. Vocal signals can range from soft sounds to screaming and crying. The key is the intention to communicate.

A relationship exists between the early use of various means of communication, such as eye gaze, gestures, and vocalizations, and later language skills in children with communication delays, especially those with ASD (McCathren et al., 2000; Zwaigenbaum et al., 2005). It is important, therefore, that all forms of communication be identified in an assessment.

Communication Success. Stated simply, communication success occurs when a communicator's goal is attained. The success of a child's communication depends as much on the communication partner and the environment as on the child.

Communication efficacy improves with the advent of intentional or goal-oriented behavior, demonstrating that the child understands that objects and persons can be used to obtain a desired outcome. Compared to unintentional behaviors, intentional nonsymbolic communication, such as gesturing, is less ambiguous, more efficient, and more successful. Our task as SLPs is to describe communicative or potentially communicative behaviors as best we can and to attempt to determine how they are used by the child and/or interpreted by caregivers as communication.

Caregiver–Child Interactions

In addition to a caregiver's membership on the team, their behaviors are also evaluated within the context of interacting with the child. It is within this interaction that most of the work of intervention will occur, so the quality of that interaction is an important factor. I once asked a mother to play with her child, and she sat in her chair and directed the child. Clearly, I had work to do.

Part of any evaluation is determining the sensitivity and responsiveness of and the interpretation of intent by caregivers in response to the behavior of the child, especially attempts to communicate. Sensitivity includes noticing the often-subtle behavior of the child as they display interest or attempt to interact with an object or a person or to communicate in some way.

A child can learn the impact of certain behaviors through the responsiveness of others. This requires caregivers to be more than just sensitive. A contingent caregiver response is one based on the perceived intent of the child. Caregiver responses provide consequences that encourage or discourage behaviors. Responsiveness includes

- contingency or the relatedness of the response to the behavior of the child;
- consistency of the adult response; and
- timeliness or the quickness with which the adult responds.

Presymbolic Behaviors

During the presymbolic period, a typically developing child learns to initiate communication for a variety of purposes and to attend jointly with a partner. Communication becomes purposeful and increasingly symbolic. Of most importance are the following presymbolic behaviors:

- Joint attention and attention-following of gazing and pointing (Yoder et al., 2015).
- Intentional communication and the use of gestures and vocalizations (Yoder et al., 2015). The use of gestures correlates with later receptive language abilities (Watt et al., 2006). Gestures may, in fact, serve as a bridge from understanding language to actively producing language.
- Complexity of presymbolic vocalizations, including the variety of consonants and syllable structures (Yoder et al., 2015).

These behaviors and parent responses have been shown to predict expressive language skills. This is also true for most children and for those with ASD (Yoder et al., 2015).

Given the nature of ASD, it's important to assess gesture function, which is a better measure than frequency for discriminating at-risk infants from low-risk infants at 12 months of age (Hughes et al., 2019). In general, these infants and those with fragile X syndrome (FXS) display significantly fewer social interactional gestures. Social interactional gestures emerge at approximately 8 or 9 months of age and are used to attract a person's attention and to engage in social interaction, such as initiating a social game or routine, provide comfort to another, tease, obtain permission, or show off.

Communicative intent may be difficult to determine. For intent to be present, three observable things should occur:

CHAPTER 4 EARLY COMMUNICATION INTERVENTION

- The child performs a signal or behavior in the presence of another.
- The signal is directed toward another person.
- The signal appears to indicate some communication purpose.

The last one can be particularly difficult to judge. Changes in either the rate or the magnitude of behavior can signal intentionality, especially in children with neuromuscular deficits.

In addition to the behaviors mentioned, other presymbolic behaviors may be important for later communication training. Chief among these are

- functional use of objects as a way of learning concepts, such as *spoon-ness*; and
- motor imitation.

Although neither behavior is sufficient for communication growth, each can provide a method for enhancing teaching and learning.

> ***Food for Thought:*** Here's a new challenge, the early use of symbols. Now what would you be interested in assessing and describing?

Symbolic Assessment

Once a child is using symbols, whether through words, signs, or some other form of AAC, the focus of an early communication assessment changes somewhat. In addition to some of the previously mentioned areas of concern, such as caregiver responsiveness, we now focus on symbols and the ways in which a child uses them to communicate. The areas of a communication assessment that are particularly relevant for a young child using symbols are gestures in combination with speech, symbolic play, receptive language or comprehension, and form and pragmatic functions of expressive language (Lyytinen et al., 2001).

For speech or another means to qualify as communicative, it should be produced for the purpose of conveying a message to a partner. For speech to be functional, it also should be frequent, flexible, and purposeful. In other words, perseverative speech or saying the same word repeatedly, imitation of the speech of others, or echolalia is not functional in most cases.

Through several means, the SLP will attempt to collect data on the child's

- phonotactic abilities or range of production of sounds, sound combinations, and syllable structures;
- ability to imitate words;
- expressive vocabulary;

124 LANGUAGE DISORDERS: A FUNCTIONAL APPROACH TO ASSESSMENT AND INTERVENTION IN CHILDREN

- multiword combinations;
- word combination patterns; and
- pragmatic functions or intentions.

Recall from your development course that single symbols or symbol combinations reflect the intentions previously expressed through gestures. Words are acquired to fulfill the intentions previously expressed through these gestures. Possible early intentions of symbolic communication are presented in Table 4–3.

Intentions are part of pragmatics or the uses to which we put language. But there's another aspect to this. What is a child talking about and how is it constructed? A child's

Table 4–3. Early Preverbal and Verbal Intentions

Gestural/Vocal Intentions	Early Verbal Intentions	Examples
Requesting (reach with persistence)	Demanding	*Cookie* (accompanied by a reach)
	Requesting	*Me do?* *Help* (possibly accompanied by holding object up to adult)
Protesting (push away, shake head side to side, become uncooperative)	Protesting	*No* (accompanied by pushing away or being uncooperative)
Labeling (point)	Naming/labeling	*Doggie* (accompanied by a point)
	Declaring/stating	*Fall* (commenting on event) *Eat* (commenting on dog barking)
	Exclaiming	Squeals with delight when picked up
	Expressing state	*Hungry*
Asking (point and/or use rising intonation)	Content questioning	*Wassat?* (What's that?)
	Hypothesis testing	*Doggie?*
Answering	Answering	*Car* (in response to "What's that?")
	Replying	*Eat* (in response to "The doggie's hungry.")
Accompanying	Accompanying	Uh-oh (when something spills) *Whee?* (when pushing car)
Greeting (wave)	Greeting	*Hi* or *Bye*
Calling	Calling	*Mommy!*
Repeating/practicing	Repeating	*Cookie, cookie, cookie*
	Practicing	*Doggie* (in response to "Let's walk the doggie.")

CHAPTER 4 EARLY COMMUNICATION INTERVENTION

multiword combinations describe the child's current language and can be used, in part, to plan the direction of intervention, including new word combinations and expansion of older ones.

An older, more traditional way of describing early child language is to use what's been called semantic–syntactic rules. As linguists began to study early child language in the 1970s, they found syntactic categories, such as verbs and nouns, to be inadequate for describing how children were initially combining words. For example, how do we describe "Mommy sock"? Noun + noun? That doesn't give us much to work with.

In the 1970s, several linguists decided that children used semantic categories. More recently, linguists have decided that this too is not adequate to describe what children are doing. I don't even mention semantic–syntactic rules in my language development course.

The semantic–syntactic rules were always adult categories to describe child language. I'm an adult, so I'm going to crawl out on a limb and suggest that we can still use them to help us characterize a child's language if for no other purpose than to categorize and keep track of the building units a child is using. Therefore, semantic categories are presented in Table 4–4. I'll explain how these constructions might be used when we discuss symbolic intervention.

Constructionism, a newer school of linguistics, examines child language developmentally, hypothesizing that a child builds their language one construction at a time rather than using rules such as those suggested in the last paragraph. Thus, a child builds "Mommy eat," then may substitute "Daddy eat" and so on, only later seeing commonalities with other utterances that we might call "rules." Levels or steps in constructionism are presented in Table 4–5. I hope you were exposed to constructionist theory in your language development course.

Let's combine the two theories. If you hear a child say "Mommy eat," you could describe the utterance by the semantic categories *Agent + Action*. As you collect more data, you might hear "Doggie eat," "Daddy eat," and "Baby eat." There is now a pattern of *Agent + Action* that appears to be at the constructionist pivot schemes level of development. This is the beginning of *noun + verb*. Thus, you have a method for mapping a child's language to determine which semantic constructions are developing and at what level. If we add to this the child intentions mentioned previously, we have a rich picture of a child's language at a moment in development. Isn't that what we're trying to describe in an assessment?

Another possible measure is a list of the action words (*up, out, eat, go*) used by a child. We could call this list a "verb lexicon" or a child's personal verb dictionary. Verb lexicon measures, especially diversity or the number of different verbs in spontaneous speech, are better predictors of grammatical growth than noun lexicons. At 24 months, the child with TDL has approximately 50 verbs and is adding roughly 8 verbs or verb-type words (*up, out*) per month, although the rate decelerates with age (Hadley et al., 2016).

> ***Food for Thought:*** **Do you truly understand the different word categorization schemes? This is a good place to stop and ponder and to review.**

Table 4–4. Semantic Patterns of Early Language

Function	Description	One- and Two-Word Examples
Nomination	Naming a person or object using a single word or in the form *Demonstrative + Nomination*	*Choo-choo, Kittie* *That horsie, This book*
Location	Marking a spatial relationship with a single word or in the form *X + Location*, in which X may be any word	Adult: *Where's kittie?* Child: *Bed* *Kittie bed, Throw me, Come here*
Negation	Marking nonexistence, rejection, and/or denial with a single word or in the form *Negative + X*, in which X may be any word	*No, Allgone* *No ride, No ni-night, Allgone juice*
Modification	Modify noun-like words or concepts with single words or in the form *Modifier + Modified*	
Possession	Marking that an object belongs to or is frequently associated with an individual	*Mine, Mommy* *My kittie, Mommy sock, Baby ball*
Attribution	Marking properties not inherently part of an object	*Big, Hot* *Yukky peas, Little doggie*
Recurrence	Marking reappearance or expected reappearance of an object or event	*More, 'Nuther, 'Gain* (again) *More juice, 'Nuther cracker*
Notice	Attempting to gain attention or signal some event in single words or in the form Introducer + X	*Hi, Bye-bye* *Hey Mommy, Hi man*
State	Mark feeling with single word or in form *Experiencer + Stat*	*Tired* *I tired, Doggie sleepy*
[Action] Agent	Marking that an animate entity initiated or caused an action	*Mommy* (throwing)
Action	Marking an activity	*Eat, Jump*
[Action] Object	Marking that an animate or inanimate object was the recipient of action	(Throwing) *Ball*, (Eating) *Cookie*
Agent + Action		*Daddy eat, Doggie bite*
Action + Object		*Eat cookie, Ride bike*
Three-word combinations can recombine the two-word rules. Thus, Agent + Action could be combined with X + Locative (remember that X can be anything).		
To form		
Agent + Action + Locative		*Mommy throw* (ball to) *me.*

Note: Although linguists no longer believe this is the way young children organize their language, the semantic system is a convenient way for SLPs to group and track young children's single words and early combinations.

CHAPTER 4 EARLY COMMUNICATION INTERVENTION 127

Table 4–5. Constructionist Patterns

Level	Explanation	Examples
Word combinations	Equivalent words that encode an experience, sometimes as two successive one-word utterances	*Water hot, Wave bye, Juice cup*
Pivot schemes	One-word or one-phrase structures the utterance by determining intent. Several words may fill the "slot," as in "Want + Things I want."	*Want up, Want juice, Want go, Want car*
Item-based constructions	Seem to follow word-order constructions based on specific rules. May contain morphological markers.	*Daddy driving, Drive car, Drive to Nana's* *Baby eat, Hug baby, Baby's bed*

Notes: At the word combinations level, words are treated independently and only combined with some words but not with others. In other words, *water* and *hot*, in the examples, would be combined together but not with other words. Noticing other possibilities, at the pivot schemes level, a child can expand the number of combinations by keeping one word constant but adding many others to it. Notice that *want* can be combined with several other words, as can *eat, no,* and *more,* to name a few. Now armed with several combinations, at the item-based constructions level, the child will try to change word order and add new words and morphemes. A variety of constructions are introduced. As the child notices patterns, syntactic rules begin to take shape.

Early Syntax. First phase syntax (FPS; Ramchand, 2008) is a model that can help SLPs conceptualize early syntactic constructions. I'll do my best to highlight the main points, but I refer you back to the excellent tutorial by Rispoli (2019) for more detail and real-life examples. FPS can also offer a course for intervention with early verbal children.

At the one-word level, children are unable to join verbs to other single words that are primarily nouns. Interpreting a child's utterance, therefore, is dependent on context. Among one-word utterances, as noted previously, are verb-like words called particles, such as *up, down, on, off, in,* and *out.* Particles are preposition words tacked onto a verb to complete it. Examples include the following:

- I looked *up* the meaning.
- Check *out* this video.
- You take *after* your mother.

Particles are not used as prepositions. For example, we're not saying "up the meaning" or "out this video." In a child's one-word utterances, *particles serve as verbs.* When a child stands at your feet, looks up, raises their arms, and says "Up," most likely you interpret that to mean "Pick me up."

At the early two-word level, state verbs, such as BE or WANT, are not spoken but can be assumed from what a child says, as in "Soup hot" or "Hat off." Models for these utterances may occur in child directed speech, such as "Take your *hat off.*"

Later combinations include high-frequency, early acquired, intransitive verbs. Intransitive verbs do not need a direct object to act upon. Examples are "Baby fall down" and "Mommy go out."

By the first true syntactic level, the child adds a direct object, as in "Put block in" or "Want coat on." Within these utterances are the kernel of a complete adult sentence, such as "Mommy put the block in" or "I want my coat on."

I see great possibilities here as a way of describing early word combinations. There is no one way to do this as long as we're thorough. Your professor may have additional ideas.

Formal Assessment

Formal normative tests of language development are usually inappropriate for measuring language comprehension and production in children younger than age 3 years, especially those with ASD (Mirenda et al., 2003). Standardized tests, for example, adhere to inflexible performance criteria that are often difficult for young children. In addition, children with ASD may have difficulty understanding testing tasks, and social deficits may interfere with their performance (Barokova & Tager-Flusberg, 2018).

Alternative parent-completed vocabulary checklists, such as those in the *MacArthur–Bates Communicative Development Inventory* (MCDI; Fenson et al., 2006), have proven to be both valid and cost-effective for assessing vocabulary size and development (Dale et al., 2003). The MCDI also contains a list of play behaviors that parents can check off. My text *Early Communication Intervention* (Owens, 2018) also offers a list of possible early words in Appendix D.

Although standardized measures may be inappropriate, those that incorporate play or accept observation and parent reports can be very useful and may be required in order to qualify a child for EI services. A list of early communication tests is presented in Appendix A. Although published assessment can provide useful information, substantial time may be required to understand the administration procedures, gather all of the supplies, and score and interpret.

Two measures that seem more appropriate for children with ASD are the Communication and Symbolic Behavior Scales Behavior Sample (CSBS-BS; Wetherby & Prizant, 2003) and a parent-report measure, the Early Screening for Autism and Communication Disorders (Wetherby et al., 2007, 20021), when used together (Stronach & Wetherby, 2017). Children with ASD score significantly lower on the CSBS-BS than peers with TDL, indicating poorer social communication skills, and higher on the Early Screening, indicating the presence of ASD features.

> *Food for Thought:* Now that we have all the pieces, how would you put together a thorough assessment that includes all these elements?

Organizing an Early Language and Communication Assessment

Now we need to organize our assessment in a logical manner to describe how an individual child communicates within their environment.

Communication Screening

In the United States, children in the established risk category are eligible for services under IDEA 2004 Part C. This is not true for children in the at-risk category, and states have varying criteria for eligibility. It is the responsibility of SLPs to integrate knowledge of at-risk factors with the results of screening tests and, if needed, with more thorough communication assessment (ASHA, 2008b).

Screening is a process for determining whether a child is likely to show deficits in communication and/or feeding and swallowing development. For young children at risk, further evaluation can establish eligibility and determine the appropriate in-depth assessment. As in all assessment, the measures used must be valid, reliable, sensitive, specific, and representative (ASHA, 2008b).

Screening measures include direct assessment of the child and/or parental report on a standardized instrument. Of course, the validity of the screening process increases with a combination of measures.

Increasingly, the process for initial identification is an interview, often based on a questionnaire focusing on the child's interests and behavior and on caregivers' priorities (Wilcox & Woods, 2011). The interview process is described later. For Spanish-speaking families or any family who may lack transportation, telehealth and e-health observation have proven to be possible alternatives to a face-to-face screening visit (Guiberson, 2016).

Results of the screening should be shared with the family, who in turn should be encouraged to ask questions. If a child passes the screening, the SLP should make sure the family understands that (ASHA, 2008b)

- screening is only a general estimate of the child's performance at a point in time;
- continued monitoring of the child's progress over time is important; and
- further screening or a full evaluation may be needed if concerns persist or new concerns arise.

When a child fails a screening, an evaluation is typically conducted to determine if the child meets eligibility for services criteria under IDEA and state guidelines.

Assessment Steps

Typical ECI assessment encompasses in-depth observations and information gathering. Ideally, the assessment is completed within a transdisciplinary context that assesses a child across all developmental domains. Within a transdisciplinary context, team members work collaboratively, pooling members' knowledge and skills across discipline boundaries and including the family's concerns and expertise. Before each task, professionals can explain its purpose to parents, and as each is completed, families and professionals can share their impressions and discuss their findings.

Thorough assessments include several sources of information and multiple methods of collection and will most likely not be obtained in a single sitting. Assessment tools and procedures should be individualized for the child and family, age-appropriate, and culturally sensitive. Because our goal is to obtain the best description possible of a child's functional communication abilities, we are interested in the observations of both professionals and caregivers.

The SLP is interested in the entire communication dynamic of the child, the caregiver(s), and their shared communication environment. Our overall assessment goals are to

- describe the child's communication abilities;
- relate those abilities to partners in familiar environments/contexts;
- describe the communication behaviors of the child's partners;
- identify the child's responses to various facilitative prompts; and
- discover promising intervention techniques.

At the very least, the assessment process should include the steps presented schematically in Figure 4–2. The order reflects an efficient way to accomplish the evaluative task. It is hoped that, like any good detective, the assessment team discovers more and more as they advance. Each step informs the next. Specific procedures are presented in *Early Communication Intervention* (Owens, 2018).

Preplanning and Preliminary Data Gathering. In pre-assessment collaborative planning, the process by which families and professionals set the parameters of the upcoming individualized assessment, professionals actively listen to family members' concerns and appreciate the family members' knowledge of the child.

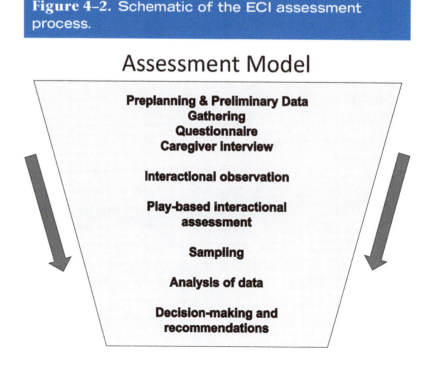

Figure 4–2. Schematic of the ECI assessment process.

Questionnaire. Ideally, questionnaires consist of open-ended questions that allow caregivers to elaborate and describe behaviors within everyday routines and contexts, reinforcing the notion that communication is part of each family's day and that intervention can occur in the context of everyday events. Sample questions are presented in Table 4–6.

Caregiver Interview. Through open-ended interview questions, parents are asked to identify (a) ways their child communicates basic needs; (b) the communicative forms and functions or uses that the child routinely exhibits; (c) problem or challenging behavior and its possible communication function; (d) the family's attitudes, concerns, and desires; and (e) successful and unsuccessful ways to motivate communication in the child. The process provides the SLP with an opportunity to introduce the concept of daily activity- and routine-based intervention and participation-based outcomes, laying the groundwork for a collaborative team process.

Interactional Observation. Through observation of the primary caregiver's communicative interactions with the child, the SLP and team (a) identify situations in which a child communicates most, (b) document the frequency of communication opportunities and the responsiveness of the child's communication partners, and (c) record the forms and functions of the child's intentional communication. A key component of this process is gaining understanding of contextual factors and how they may enhance or constrain participation (Wilcox & Woods, 2011).

Table 4–6. A Sample of Open-Ended Assessment Questions
What are things your child is really good at doing?
How does your child let you know they are . . .   Angry? Sad?   Confused? Surprised?   Happy? Tired?   Hungry or thirsty? Uncomfortable?
How does your child let you know they need . . .   Assistance?   Toileting?
How would you feel about your child using other means of communication either as a replacement for or an addition to speech?
What do you and your child mostly communicate about?
What are the biggest obstacles to others understanding your child?
What are the biggest obstacles to others communicating with your child?

Formulating Hypotheses. Collaboratively, team members, including the family, begin to formulate hypotheses about (1) the communication observed and (2) the quality of the parent–child interaction and its potential as a vehicle for change while setting parameters for the play-based assessment to follow.

Play-Based Interactional Assessment. Within a play mode, the SLP and parent(s) use "communication temptations," such as eating a treat in front of the child, and manipulating the context, such as pausing in the middle of a fun activity, to attempt to elicit communication from the child.

Testing and Structured Probes. After the more unstructured, child-initiated play portion, the SLP can conduct testing and structured probes, such as dynamic assessment, strategically embedded in natural routines and play. Test or portions of test can be used to gain more insight and possibly obtain a developmental level for the child's communication. As you know, testing is required by many government entities for qualification for services.

Dynamic assessment, discussed in more detail in Chapter 5, is an adult-mediated strategy that attempts to probe "teachability" of a behavior and may take a *test–teach–test* format. After observing how the child responds without assistance (*test*), the SLP provides limited assistance over several trials until the child's behavior changes (*teach*) and then withdraws the assistance and returns to the original situation to determine if learning has occurred (*test*).

For example, as an SLP, you might try to elicit physical imitation by modeling and saying "Do this." If the child does not respond, you might try again and then physically assist the child. Such prompts are introduced and withdrawn as needed by the child to be successful. You then return to your original request. If the child is successful the second time, you might assume that a physical prompt is a helpful teaching device with this child. Of course, this is a greatly simplified example.

Sampling. For children using vocal and/or verbal communication, spontaneous language samples can be useful as a method for assessing language problems, developing a sound inventory and a babbling analysis, establishing semantic and pragmatic inventories, describing early syntax, categorizing sound and/or syllable patterns, and making judgments about intelligibility.

Analysis of Data. After obtaining information, the team attempts to determine (a) the caregiver's priority activities and routines, (b) ways to enhance the child's communication and participation, (c) possible use of augmentative or alternative communication or other forms of assistive technology to enhance the child's participation, (d) activities and routines that can provide a context for embedding learning opportunities for more complex communication skills, and (e) skills needed for children to successfully participate (Wilcox & Woods, 2011).

Decision Making and Recommendations. The team members, including the family, review the results and discuss different intervention options while continuing

CHAPTER 4 EARLY COMMUNICATION INTERVENTION

to build consensus between families and professionals. When families and professionals work collaboratively during the assessment, they set the tone for future collaborative interactions.

> *Food for Thought:* Did this discussion of assessment in ECI challenge your notions of what an assessment involves? Can you see why SLPs require special skills?

Considerations for Infants With Culturally/ Linguistically Diverse Backgrounds

One element of an EI assessment may be asking caregivers to complete a checklist of the words their child understands and says. Because many children in bilingual homes or homes in which a language other than English predominates are exposed to varying degrees of the heritage language and English, it's best to include word checklists in both languages (Peña et al., 2016). MCDI checklists (Fenson et al., 2006; Jackson-Maldonado et al., 2003) are available in several languages. These are adaptations and not translations because some items in American English are not applicable to other cultures.

Other culturally sensitive tools might include the *Language Exposure Assessment Tool* (De Anda et al., 2016) to measure children's exposure to Spanish, English, and other languages, such as the indigenous languages of Mexico. If possible, recordings in the home can provide a naturalistic measure of a child's language that can be analyzed using tools such as the *Language ENvironment Analysis* (2015–2021).

ECI Intervention

Language skills emerge out of multiple shared social experiences. Intervention is similar. For example, we know children with FXS who have more joint engagement with parents also have more advanced expressive language skills in preschool and kindergarten (Hahn et al., 2016). This data supports early intervention that uses joint engagement as a means for promoting and teaching language and social communication.

As a child matures and intentionally communicates, the form of that communication evolves from presymbolic to symbolic and from gestural and vocal to verbal. It seems logical, therefore, that intervention should also focus on placing symbolic forms of communication onto existing prelinguistic functions or intentions. If you as an SLP target these intentions, your intervention becomes functional, fulfilling the child's need for communication while at the same time building on communication uses already in place. If ECI targets both child presymbolic communication behaviors and parental responses to these behaviors within everyday events, then we can facilitate a child's language development.

The SLP and parent can collaborate on developing gestures as a child's initial means of communication. Enhanced natural gestures (Calculator, 2016), such as reaching for desired items or looking at interesting entities, could be modified into requesting and pointing, respectively. Studies of maternal and child gesturing in children with Down syndrome support focusing on increased parent responsiveness to child gestures (Lorang et al., 2018).

Use of Daily Routines

Within daily routines, parents can be trained in the use of language-facilitating responses to these child communication behaviors. Use of caregiver-identified child interests and activities is associated with the greatest gains by children (Dunst et al., 2007).

Each family's daily routines and activities are unique, creating specific interactions that shape a child's development. Routines, such as feeding and bathing, are an important part of everyday family life and an ongoing natural learning environment. Embedding intervention within home-based daily routines is also consistent with current educational practices and legal requirements that services be provided in the LREs. For example, if a child usually has "floaty" toys in the bathtub, a simple change to requesting them first becomes a vehicle for change.

Once the caregiver and SLP agree that a certain routine is a good teaching milieu, they can identify ways of creating opportunities for the child to use the targeted behavior. They can discuss the plan for intervention and possible methods, followed by an SLP's modeling of techniques, role-playing by the caregivers, and a discussion and critique.

Telehealth

Given the scheduling difficulty a single, working parent may have or the lack of personal transportation of many families with low SES backgrounds, other alternatives to face-to-face interactions may be needed. SLPs are exploring the best, most efficient ways to interact.

Although more research is needed, there is evidence to modestly support the efficacy of a distance delivery format, such as video teleconferencing, along with coaching onsite by the SLP. For example, in one study of a hybrid program using video teleconferencing and naturalistic parent-implemented language intervention targeting mother's verbal responses, there was an increase in maternal utterances that followed the child's focus of attention and prompted child communication acts (McDuffie et al., 2016).

Record Keeping

For progress monitoring during intervention, especially for children with ASD, it may be most useful during therapy sessions to use brief, frequent communication samples that are relatively sensitive to small incremental changes (McDaniel & Schuele, 2021). McDaniel and Schuele (2021) provide examples of data collection documents for monitoring intentional communication, consonant inventory, and responding to joint attention within short communication samples. These documents can be adapted for specific children. If you think you may be interested in working with preverbal children with ASD, I encourage you to note the specific methods for recording data presented in the article by McDaniel and Schuele (2021).

Intervention Strategies

Specific intervention strategies with promising evidence fall into one of three groups: *responsive interaction, directive interaction,* and *blended* (ASHA, 2008b). Responsive interaction approaches typically include models of the target communication behavior without an obligation for the child to respond and include the following:

- Following a child's attentional or conversational lead with a response
- Responding to a child's initiations, both verbal and nonverbal, with natural consequences
- Extending a child's topic in a reply
- Self-talk and parallel talk describing an action
- Providing meaningful feedback
- Expanding the child's utterances with models slightly in advance of the child's current ability within typical and developmentally appropriate routines and activities

Expansion of the child's utterance to a slightly more mature utterance is a powerful strategy because the adult response immediately connects the child's communication to more mature communication that serves the same purpose.

Incidental teaching is a naturalistic child-directed intervention strategy used during unstructured activities. Usually, incidental teaching occurs when a child has shown an interest in something and the adult follows through by interacting around that interest. Such naturalistic interventions have been shown to improve communication skills for young children in the early stages of communication development.

In contrast, directive interaction strategies are best characterized as behavioral. Adults alter cues and prompts ("Say cookie.") that precede the behavior in a systematic way to elicit the behavior ("Cookie!") and also manipulate what follows the behavior to give corrective feedback ("I like the way you said 'cookie.' Here it is.") while strengthening the desired response and weakening others through reinforcement.

Finally, blended approaches have evolved because behavioral strategies frequently fail to generalize to more functional and interactive environments. These are the approaches we've discussed and include teaching in natural environments using strategies for modeling language and responding to children's communication that derives from typical mother–child interactions.

Natural Settings and Partners

Optimal ECI services are provided in natural environments, which offer realistic, authentic, and ecologically valid learning experiences and promote successful communication with caregivers (ASHA, 2008b). Authentic learning has the potential to maximize children's acquisition of functional communication and promote generalization to natural, everyday contexts (Roper & Dunst, 2003). Naturally occurring activities offer opportunities to promote a child's participation and learning throughout the day using familiar activities, materials, and people (Bernheimer & Weismer, 2007; Dunst et al., 2000).

Parents or caregivers are in a unique position in ECI. They are team members and the primary agents of change at the same time that they are clients themselves. The SLP is concerned with changing adult behaviors concurrent with changing those of the child. Not only are parents capable of learning and implementing multiple teaching strategies but also positive outcomes for young children occur when they do (Bibby et al., 2001). Caregiver-implemented intervention with young children has been linked to the following (Kaiser et al., 2000):

- Increases in verbalizations
- More spontaneous speech
- Increased use of target utterances
- Longer intervals of engagement
- More responsiveness in target tasks
- Decreases in disruptive and noncompliant behaviors

Surprisingly, given the importance of parent involvement, there are few studies of children with ASD (Koegel et al., 2020). Inclusion of parents or caregivers as language facilitators maximizes the chance that intervention is consistent and frequent and takes place in functional contexts (Goldstein et al., 2005).

The teaching techniques that caregivers use with their child do not need to be elaborate or formal. Simplicity is best. Daily activities provide the best time for language learning because the child knows the routine, making participation easier, and has experienced the same actions and words repeatedly within each routine.

A parent might be taught to expand on their child's behaviors and to encourage the child to imitate in turn. Nonsymbolic behavior can also be interpreted verbally by the parent, adding meaning to the child's behavior. At a symbolic level, expanding a child's utterance into a longer utterance can stimulate a child's development, while replying in kind can be reinforcing and can keep a child participating, as in the following exchange:

Child: Big doggie.

Adult: I see the big doggie. Do you want to pet the doggie?

Professionals differ on the language adults should use when speaking with young children with language disorders. There is a weak positive correlation between the length of parental input and child language outcomes. On the other hand, there seems to be little difference in comprehension among young children with language disorders whether an adult uses very simple speech (*Mommy eat*, *No juice*, *Go up*), called "telegraphic," or simplified speech but with more grammatical structure (*Mommy is eating lunch*, *No juice in your glass*, *Want to go up*) (van Kleeck et al., 2010).

Although the results of a meta-analysis are not extremely strong, they do suggest that SLPs avoid intervention practices that prescribe shorter, grammatically incomplete utterances for parents of children with ASD (Sandbank & Yoder, 2016). For example, although more research is needed, telegraphic input from parents seems to have a negative impact on language development of these children (Venker et al., 2015).

In early childcare settings, childcare providers (CCPs) can aid children's communication development. For example, CCPs have effectively helped children with low-SES backgrounds establish and use intentional communication through gestures. An effective coaching strategy is for CCPs to model a gesture, then pause to encourage imitation, provide opportunities for children to model gestures, and respond and expand children's gestures (Romano et al., 2021). Gestures can also be used by CCPs within daily routines and activities, such as book sharing.

Teaching Adults

It's easy for SLPs to overwhelm caregivers with too many intervention tasks. Adult learners do better with introduction of one new thing at a time. Feedback should be specific and address the current situation. Parent training should include the following steps (Roberts et al., 2010):

- Teach a specific strategy rather than several strategies, and provide a rationale, examples, and a time for practice.
- Demonstrate, practice, coach, and critique, including asking how parent feels about the training and the strategy being taught.
- Plan together for everyday use of the strategy and stress the importance of home routines in intervention.
- Monitor progress of both the child and the adult through easy-to-use measures of behavior.
- Solicit feedback from the parent by inviting parent questions and comments.

SLPs should be mindful of the need to build caregiver confidence and to help them avoid feelings of inadequacy or failure. Principles need to be presented multiple times and applied to multiple situations in order to help caregivers learn. Information should be meaningful and individualized.

Although we still have much to learn, especially on the optimal amount of intervention needed, we can say with confidence that systematic caregiver instruction on use of language facilitation strategies has positive effects on changes in children's language skills (Roberts & Kaiser, 2015). One promising method of parent teaching is the *teach–model–coach–review* instructional approach of enhanced milieu training (EMT) (Roberts et al., 2014). For example, Spanish-speaking caregivers with low-SES backgrounds have been able to implement the strategies of *EMT en Español* with their young children (Nogueira Peredo et al., 2018).

> *Food for Thought:* Why might an SLP need to consider cultural differences? Can't all parents learn to use the same communication teaching strategies at home?

Culturally Responsive Intervention

It should seem logical that ECI that is culturally and linguistically responsive results in better outcomes (Durán et al., 2016; Larson et al., 2020). A three-stage approach to program design might include the following (Cycyk et al., 2021):

- Self-study and collaboration with the community to understand the cultural foundations
- Initial program adaptation, piloting, and revision
- Finalized adaptation and efficacy testing

The goals of intervention should be congruent with the perspectives of the target population being served (Bernal & Sáez-Santiago, 2006).

Although throughout this text I advocate for following a child's conversational lead or offering choice-making, the culture may prioritize adult-directed activities and place less importance on child autonomy (Cycyk & Huerta, 2020; Peredo et al., 2017). An SLP needs to be flexible. Instead of food choices, which may be inappropriate with some families, a child can be offered a choice of colored plastic dishes to eat from.

Program adaptations should include changes to intervention content, procedures, and/or materials (Stirman et al., 2013). For example, cooking is an everyday routine important in many Latino/Latina communities for transmitting culture and, if appropriate, should be included in intervention.

It's vitally important to use a language comprehensible to the participants (Bernal & Sáez-Santiago, 2006). Written materials need to be translated into the heritage language using a collaborative translation process (Douglas & Craig, 2007). You'll also need to keep in mind dialectal differences. For example, there are many dialects of both Spanish and Arabic.

Recent research with Latino/Latina families indicates varied preferences for the location of early language intervention (Cycyk & Huerta, 2020). As with other program considerations, family preference is important. For example, Mexican immigrant families have reported that participating in groups with other caregivers promotes access to information and emotional support (Mueller et al., 2009).

It's important to recognize that some families may lack transportation, making participation in center-based programs difficult. Undocumented families may not be eligible for a driver's license. Providing bus passes or free transportation for those who express the need can ensure better parent turnout.

Caregiver sessions are best in the heritage language, whereas in child play groups, a combination of English and the heritage language may be best, but is dependent on a child's individual needs (Cycyk et al., 2021). Supporting a child's home language has been shown to yield stronger emotional, cognitive, social, and academic outcomes without any negative impact on English language development (Durán et al., 2016; National Academies of Sciences, Engineering, and Medicine, 2017).

In communities with extended family living arrangements, parents or caregivers may wish to include other family members. It may be helpful to inform parents that they are free to bring other adult caregivers to caregiver group meetings (Cycyk & Huerta, 2020).

CHAPTER 4 EARLY COMMUNICATION INTERVENTION

Some EI programs use cultural–linguistic mediators to aid with effective and mutually satisfying communication between professionals and families (Lynch & Hanson, 2004; Moore & Perez-Mendez, 2006). A cultural–linguistic mediator, knowledgeable about the family's culture and/or linguistic community, can facilitate communication between families and EI agencies and providers. Alternative strategies include (Wing et al., 2007)

- involving more acculturated siblings or others;
- using more structured tasks or group settings for language treatment; and
- using direct training techniques that are consistent with the family's culture.

Finally, many children with special needs also participate in special care nurseries, childcare settings, or preschools. Longitudinal studies have demonstrated children's gains in both receptive and expressive language skills as a result of participation in day care programs offering developmentally facilitative activities, high levels of staff training, and optimal levels of social and linguistic responsiveness to children's communication attempts. These settings offer yet another location within which the SLP can attempt to intervene.

A Hybrid Model

For a number of reasons, a hybrid model has evolved as the most efficacious means of providing ECI services. Such a model might include individual and group services.

The SLP sees the child two or three times per week at home or in a childcare, EI, or preschool program. During these visits, the SLP works with the child and also instructs caregivers in the best methods for training the mutually agreed upon target behaviors. Parents and teachers can be further trained in group or individual meetings.

In groups of parents and children, six to eight caregiver–child dyads may be optimal. Larger groups make it difficult for an SLP to attend easily to each individual caregiver–child dyad and for each adult to participate in discussions and demonstrations. It's best to focus on a narrow range of functional ages or abilities of children. This will facilitate the use of materials and activities that will promote engagement for children in the group.

Individual caregiver–child sessions will have much to accomplish in a short amount of time. Table 4–7 outlines the steps in a typical individual intervention session.

Group sessions with parents will vary in format, sometimes including the child while at other times only parents or other family members. Wilcox et al. (2005) offer a wonderful online resource for structuring of these meetings when the intervention target is single word production. Their website, listed in their bibliography, offers handouts, self-assessments, and other materials for parents. Table 4–8 presents a possible format for successive caregiver meetings. If it is not feasible for parents to meet in groups, the material presented in the following section can also be covered in individual sessions.

SLPs are also expected to participate in consultation with and education of the team's professional members. Other responsibilities include service coordination, transition planning as a child approaches preschool age, advocacy, and awareness and advancement of the community knowledge of EI. In ECI, SLPs work in collaborative partnerships with

Table 4–7. Format for Individual Caregiver–Child Intervention Sessions

- SLP and parent review data kept by the parent on child responsiveness to the intervention.
- Parent models techniques used.
- SLP critiques the parent's teaching.
- SLP and parent decide on targets and methods for the intervening days.
- SLP models methods for the new or revised targets.
- Parent attempts the methods for the new or revised targets.
- SLP critiques the parent's teaching, and revisions are made as needed.
- SLP and parent agree on what data will be kept in the intervening days.
- SLP and parent brainstorm new ways to create even more opportunities for communication.
- SLP models new ways to talk with or stimulate the child.
- Parent attempts these new methods.
- SLP critiques.

families and caregivers and in consultative relationships with team members, including the family and other caregivers, and with other agencies and professionals (Buysse & Wesley, 2006). You'll be busy.

Intervention for Children With Autism Spectrum Disorder

Given the increasing number of children with ASD and the growing academic interest, it seems appropriate to address this topic within a discussion of ECI. There has been a rush to identify children with ASD and to intervene at an early age.

Models of Intervention

A variety of intervention approaches have been developed to address the social communication of children with ASD. The most commonly used intervention options are derived from the field of behavior analysis. Structured **applied behavior analysis** (ABA) approaches have specific intervention targets addressed through grouped multiple trials of *antecedent–behavior–consequence* chains. Adult-selected materials are presented repeatedly to promote success, and adults exercise tight control over the antecedent stimuli, prompt hierarchy, and consequences. Many programs teach individual skills one at a time through drill-based repetition. Although structured ABA procedures are very effective in a variety of areas, the following difficulties exist:

- Gains are often extremely slow.
- Gains often do not generalize.
- Children are often unmotivated to be involved.

CHAPTER 4 EARLY COMMUNICATION INTERVENTION

Table 4–8. Possible Format for Successive Caregiver Group Meetings

Sensitivity: Tuning in to Opportunities for Language Learning

Session 1 Group meeting: *Overview and Introduction: Teaching Your Child*

Session 2 Group meeting: *Creating Opportunities for Teaching*

Session 3 Group meeting: *Using Daily Activities to Teach Language*

Session 4 Individual meetings in your home

Session 5 Group meeting: *Encouraging Communication*

Session 6 Group meeting: *Encouraging Communication During Play*

Contingency: Responding to Children's Communications

Session 7 Group meeting: *Talking to Young Children*

Session 8 Individual meetings in your home

Session 9 Group meeting: *Imitating, Interpreting, and Expanding*

Session 10 Group meeting: *Responding to Your Child's Communications*

Session 11 Group meeting: *Options for Responding*

Session 12 Individual meetings in your home

Consistency: Self-Monitoring Skills and Encouraging More Complex Language

Session 13 Group meeting: *Strategies to Further Enhance Children's Language*

Session 14 Group meeting: *Identifying More Complex Communication and Language*

Session 15 Individual meetings: *Reviewing Progress and Planning Future Goals*

Source: Information from the model presented by Wilcox et al. (2005).

Although EI programs based on ABA principles report promoting social communication development, almost all are based on use of standardized assessments and not on children's language in daily activities (Trembath et al., 2016).

Because of the issues mentioned previously, professionals have devised variations on the ABA model that increase children's responsiveness. These include more child-directed naturalistic behavioral methods and social–pragmatic developmental interventions. One example is pivotal response treatment (PRT) (Ingersoll & Schreibman, 2006; Koegel et al., 1999).

PRT is based on behavioral principles of ABA but incorporates variables known to improve responsiveness, rate of responding, and interactive behavior. These variables include the following:

- Child choice
- Task variation
- Interspersing maintenance and acquisition trials
- Reinforcing attempts that are less than perfect
- Using direct natural consequences

The PRT approach is significantly more effective than ABA alone in improving targeted and untargeted areas of intervention (Mohammadzaheri et al., 2014).

During the past half century, there has been a slow movement to more naturalistic behavioral interventions for children with ASD, especially for very young children. Naturalistic interventions, frequently conducted within the home and everyday activities, promote social development (Morrier et al. 2009). Ideally, parents can easily implement these strategies in the child's natural environment and during ongoing activities such as bathing, meals, and walks to the park (McGee, 2005; Schreibman & Koegel, 2005). Is this beginning to sound familiar and more functional?

Called naturalistic developmental behavioral interventions (NDBIs), these methods have the following similarities (Schreibman et al., 2015):

- Implemented in natural settings
- Involve shared control between child and adult
- Utilize natural contingencies
- Use a variety of behavioral strategies to teach developmentally appropriate and prerequisite skills

See Schreibman and colleagues (2015) for a more detailed discussion. The core components of NDBIs are presented in Table 4–9.

Although there are several overlapping instructional strategies across NDBIs, let's examine just a few that tip toward functional intervention:

- Child-initiated teaching episodes, also referred to as following a child's lead or interest, or child choice, involve the presentation of instruction or the opportunity for a child to respond within the context of a child-chosen or child-preferred activity or familiar routine.
- Environmental arrangement is the way in which the adult structures the environment so that the child must initiate or interact with the adult in order to obtain a desired outcome, *enticing* the child to interact.
- Natural reinforcement related to a child's communication goal, such as receipt of a requested toy.
- Verbal, visual, and/or physical prompting inserted between the instruction and the target behavior in order to elicit a desired response and then gradually faded as a child gains more independence.
- Balanced turns or turn-taking supports the back-and-forth interactional nature of early learning (Harris & Waugh, 2002).
- Adult modeling often follows the child's focus of interest and demonstrates a target skill for the child to display.
- Adult imitation of a child behavior to increase the child's responsivity and attention to the adult, with subsequent imitation of the adult, and continuation of the interaction.

Table 4–9. Core Components of NDBIs

Nature of the intervention targets	Developmental systems approach.
	Cross-domain intervention so that a skill in one domain (e.g., learning a gesture in one activity) is crossed over to development of skills in other domains (e.g., using the gesture with another person and in other activities).
	Generally, skills are taught within a child's typical daily experiences and routines, with multiple materials and while interacting with multiple people.
	Intervention targets focus on precursors of development or enhancers of these achievements.
Contexts	Learning is embedded in active, emotionally meaningful social interactions (Topál et al. 2008).
	Intervention occurs through establishing adult–child engagement activities transformed into motivating play routines or familiar daily routines.
Instructional strategies	Incorporates behavioral strategies into everyday events.
	Adult supports the child's expansion of language through the increasing play, social, and action complexity within the routine.

Source: Information from Schreibman et al. (2015).

In general, NDBIs share a strong research base that supports their use with young children with ASD. Many of the assumptions and methods of NDBIs are supported throughout this text.

> ***Food for Thought:*** **Is it surprising that the functional approach to communication and language assessment and intervention can be used with children with ASD who may offer a challenge to an SLP.**

Intervention Strategies

The intentional communication of a child with ASD can be addressed via multiple approaches and requires attending to how the child communicates (Carter et al., 2011; Green et al., 2010; Hardan et al., 2015; McDaniel & Schuele, 2021; Yoder & Stone, 2006). Many of these strategies are used with other children with language disorders. Children with ASD have also demonstrated benefit from AAC for developing intentional communication and other language skills (Ganz et al., 2012; Kasari et al., 2014).

Success in training responding to joint attention varies. As an SLP, you'll need to attend to the verbal and nonverbal cues of the caregiver. Both developmental and behavioral techniques have shown success in teaching responding to joint attention (Kasari et al., 2006, 2010; White et al., 2011).

Although limited information is available, intentional communication and parental verbal responses facilitate language growth through the vocabulary experienced in the context of communication (Woynaroski et al., 2016). Once a child understands words, the child can be taught to say those words within intentional communication.

Interestingly, expanded consonant use increases intentional communication, which leads to increased expressive language skills (McDaniel et al., 2017). However, we do not know how targeting consonant use improves expressive language skills in preverbal children with ASD.

Augmentative and Alternative Communication

We would be remiss if we didn't consider AAC. Some children, both of my grandsons included, need extra assistance to be able to communicate more effectively, play, eat, or move more freely. Assistive technology (AT) is an essential part of early intervention, consisting of adaptations and devices for children and families that enable children to function more independently.

Augmentative and alternative communication is a form of AT and an intervention approach that uses other-than-speech means to complement or supplement an individual's communication abilities and may include combining existing speech or vocalizations with gestures, manual signs, communication boards, and speech-output communication devices. Thus, AAC incorporates a multimodality ECI approach that enables a child to use every mode possible to communicate.

The use of AAC does not mean that speech is ignored. Speech will be a component of most multimodal AAC systems. In this way, a child makes optimum use of vocal and speech skills for communication as part of a multimodal AAC system.

The breadth of communication behaviors involved in AAC has the potential to enhance communication skill overall. AAC can promote communication development in infants and toddlers by (ASHA, 2008b)

- enhancing both input and output;
- augmenting existing vocalizations and speech;
- replacing socially unacceptable behaviors with a more conventional means of communication (Beukelman & Mirenda, 2005);
- serving as a language-teaching tool (Romski & Sevcik, 2005); and
- facilitating a young child's ability to more fully participate in daily activities and routines.

Typically, AAC intervention focuses on output. Receptive uses are equally important for the very young child beginning to develop communication skills (Romski & Sevcik, 2005).

Approximately 12% of preschoolers receiving special education services require AAC (Binger & Light, 2006). Given these findings, there is a critical need for you as an SLP to be prepared to provide AAC services for EI children (Cress & Marvin, 2003).

Types of AAC

AAC systems are typically divided into unaided and aided based on the non-use and use of external devices, respectively:

- Unaided AAC does not require any equipment and relies on the user's body to relay messages.
- Aided AAC incorporates the use of communication devices in addition to the user's body.

Unaided AAC systems include signs and gestures in addition to vocalizations and possibly verbalizations. One issue for an SLP and the child's family will be which sign language, such as American Sign Language, or sign system, such as Signed English, to use.

Aided AAC can range from low-tech to high-tech. Low-tech non-electronic devices, which may include communication boards with visual–graphic symbols such as photographs that are selected by pointing, are portable, readily accessible, and very adaptable.

In contrast, high-tech electronic devices, which are extremely varied, can consist of commercially available AAC devices, individually designed AAC equipment, or adaptations to existing computers. Electronic AAC devices differ primarily by

- input mode, varying from simple pressure switches operated by a touch with virtually any body part through touchscreen devices accessed by direct selection or scanning and on to position switches such as a computer mouse;
- control electronics; and
- output or display, ranging from single-message voice output devices to speech-generating devices (SGDS). Voice output can effectively gain the attention of others, and partners also find voice output easy to interpret and understand (Hustad et al., 2002).

Although several organizational arrangements are possible on aided devices, schematic designs or organization based on events or contexts offer many advantages for presymbolic young children (Light & Drager, 2007). In a schematic design, a birthday party may contain communication icons for *cake*, *ice cream*, *presents*, and the like. Although visual scene displays have been used with a variety of children, adaptation for those with ASD may be needed. For example, children with ASD take longer to view images if more than two human figures are in the scene (Liang & Wilkinson, 2018).

Evidence-Based Practice

Evidence-based practice on the use of AAC with very young children is thin. Most studies are single subject, making comparisons across diverse clinical populations difficult (Campbell et al., 2006). There is some evidence on the efficacy of AAC intervention for infants, toddlers, and preschoolers with a variety of severe disabilities, but more studies are needed (Cress, 2003; Romski et al., 2001; Rowland & Schweigert, 2000).

Although there may be an initial learning advantage for unaided AAC over aided, there is little difference between the two in generalized communication over time (Schlosser & Lee, 2000). In addition, there is no evidence that either signing or aided techniques are more likely to lead to speech development (Millar et al., 2000).

Even with this less than complete evidence for guidance, we can make some definitive statements. For example, AAC can play many roles in communication development and should be introduced early (e.g., Cress & Marvin, 2003; Reichle et al., 2002). Early access to AAC has been shown to be a means for acquiring some necessary prelinguistic and cognitive skills essential for establishing symbolic communication (Brady, 2000). In other words, AAC is appropriate for a young child just developing both communication and language skills.

We can also say that young children who use AAC exhibit improvement in speech skills, even if only minimal in some cases (Beukelman & Mirenda, 2005; Cress, 2003; Cress & Marvin, 2003; Millar et al., 2006). Use of AAC not only helps a child communicate but also has a positive impact on parental perception of their child's language development (Romski et al., 2001).

Contrary to the notion that AAC may inhibit spoken language, results of early intervention using AAC find that it supports both receptive and expressive spoken language skills (Millar et al., 2006). Compared to children who have spoken language intervention only, children who have spoken and AAC intervention have significantly more spoken target vocabulary words and no statistically significant differences in speech sound errors (Walters et al., 2021). In addition, research data clearly suggest that the introduction of AAC will neither cause a child to abandon speech they may be using nor prevent acquisition of new spoken words.

Assessment

Children communicate along a continuum from prelinguistic through symbolic to fully linguistic. Although one focus of an AAC assessment is to determine the need for AAC, it's more important to explore this continuum and to determine the devices and services that can help a child fully participate in their environment (Romski et al., 2002).

Standardized tests may be of little help in clearly indicating what the nonsymbolic child knows. Of importance is identifying what facilitates and what inhibits communication at each step in the process.

> ***Food for Thought:*** Are you getting the impression that with very young children standardized testing is of limited value? Does this reinforce the notion that you as a knowledgeable SLP are your own best assessment device? Frightening to have all that responsibility?

In addition to the communication assessment process mentioned previously for presymbolic children, an SLP should determine a child's

CHAPTER 4 EARLY COMMUNICATION INTERVENTION 147

- communication methods;
- physical abilities; and
- barriers that affect the child's participation in AAC.

This can be accomplished through family/caregiver interviews and informal observation of the child interacting with family, friends, and caregivers during natural daily routines and in typical settings. Team members then engage in a problem-solving process to determine the most appropriate devices, adaptations, services, and/or strategies that will reduce or eliminate these barriers and enhance participation. Problem solving may include trial-and-error usage of a variety of devices and strategies. Most likely, you'll have an entire course in AAC, and these techniques will be explored in detail.

Some of the elements of a communication assessment mentioned previously take on new relevance in an assessment for AAC. Keeping in mind that AAC is or should be a multimodal communication system, you as an SLP will be particularly interested in current modes of communication. Relevant areas for AAC use include motor skills, visual perception, and sign and symbol recognition. Research data indicate that given the choice, children will use the method of communicating that they find most efficient, and this may vary even by individual symbol (Richman et al., 2001; Sigafoos & Drasgow, 2001). As an SLP, you should not impose your favorite method nor artificially restrict AAC use.

Within reason, SLPs should give the child and certainly the family a choice of their preferred methods of communication. If the family is not comfortable with an AAC device, they may not use it at home. Positive results with AAC are critically tied to a family's participation in both assessment and intervention (Angelo, 2000; Goldbart & Marshall, 2004). One of the best ways to know if an AAC system is a good fit is to try it. If possible, a device on loan may help families adjust to this new technology. To be optimally effective, an AAC system needs to be (Light & Drager, 2005)

- versatile enough to meet a child's communication needs in a variety of situations and contexts and provide the potential for growth;
- appealing;
- easy to learn; and
- dynamic or capable of changing and growing as a child learns new skills and matures.

With aided AAC, there are several specific issues to be addressed, including the symbol system, the method and rate of symbol selection, and the organization of symbols. Navigating a system or moving about a device to find a target symbol can pose a particular challenge for young children. Organization and layout of symbols can either facilitate or impede the accuracy and efficiency of a child's ability to locate, select, and functionally use those symbols.

Potentially important factors that may influence learning and use include grouping and arrangement of symbols, color, background, borders, shape, pattern, texture, size, position, and movement/animation (Beukelman & Mirenda, 2005; Scally, 2001). As mentioned previously, most young children organize concepts by events and context, so it would make sense to organize symbols in this manner (Shane, 2006). We must be cautious because many 2½-year-old children have difficulty regardless of the format, although contextual embedding is easier (Drager et al., 2003, 2004).

Scenes are most helpful when they are displayed so a child may select a scene and then locate the desired symbol within (Drager et al., 2004). For example, in a playground scene, the child can touch the swing or the slide to indicate these items. Actions can be selected by touching children performing these actions. As a child's vocabulary grows, the scene may open a second page containing the actual words to choose.

Color can be used to highlight pictures or items in pictures. SLPs should consider incorporating color in the foreground of line drawings in visual displays. Older typically developing preschool children are able to locate line drawings featuring only foreground item color faster than drawings featuring color throughout (Thistle & Wilkinson, 2009).

AAC Intervention

One popular AAC communication-training program for nonverbal young children with ASD is the Picture Exchange Communication System (PECS). Although PECS holds some promise, it is not yet an established evidence-based intervention for facilitating communication in children with ASD and gains are small (Flippin et al., 2010). A 1-year follow-up study reported that PECS training can have long-term enhancement benefits for some sociocommunicative skills in children with ASD (Lerna et al., 2014). This may be enhanced by use of peers, discussed later.

Each child needs a language system that can facilitate crucial transitions from one level of linguistic complexity to another. Although PECS can help some children begin to use symbols, it offers little on expansion to longer utterance. If these transitions are not inherent in an AAC system, a child cannot expand their communication abilities. Similarly, the choice of communication modes should relate to a child's changing skills, communication contexts, partners, tasks, and intent (Binger & Light, 2006; Blackstone & Hunt-Berg, 2003; Light & Drager, 2005).

Typically, an AAC device is just one part of a child's AAC system. It is not uncommon for children to also use signs, gestures, vocalizations, and speech approximations in different situations with different communication partners (Beukelman & Mirenda, 2005).

AAC systems can be made more appealing for young children in a number of ways. These include incorporating motivating, interactive activities; popular movie, book, or television characters and favorite activities; sound effects, such as laughter, music, and songs; and bright colors and decorations; in addition to offering a child choices. Last, the SLP and family need to make use of AAC systems fun (Light et al., 2004, 2008).

One factor that affects learning and use is response efficiency. Any of the four components of response efficiency—response effort, rate of reinforcement, immediacy of reinforcement, and quality of reinforcement—may have an effect on a child's use of AAC (Johnston et al., 2004). Response effort includes both the physical effort required to communicate and the cognitive effort required to recall or use symbols or a communication system. For example, holding up an empty cup to request more juice may be both physically easier than activating an electronic device and cognitively easier than locating a symbol in an array.

Reinforcement rate is particularly important in teaching a new method of communication. Immediacy of reinforcement would suggest that aided communication devices be present and available for use by children throughout the day. If not, children may simply ignore a communicative opportunity rather than tolerate the delay in reinforcement resulting from finding and using the AAC device.

Reinforcement quality relates to the desirability of the reinforcer. Simply stated, when one event or object is preferred over another, the preferred one has a higher quality of reinforcement.

These variables usually do not function in a vacuum but, rather, interact with each other. An AAC user will determine the most efficient response for the message they wish to send. The notion of efficiency depends on the demands of the communicative context. Because contexts differ, training multiple ways of communicating offers a child options.

Evidence from several studies suggests that aided AAC input can enhance expression and comprehension across all five domains of language (O'Neill et al., 2018). For example, using iPads with a SonoFlex speech-generating device (SGD), nonverbal children with ASD increase their initiated requests, responses to questions, and social comments in both class and recess settings (Xin & Leonard, 2015). Gains are aided by caregivers' use of expectant delay or awaiting a response, direct prompting (e.g., spoken, gestural), contingent responding, and open-ended questions in conjunction with AAC use.

Although more data are needed, we can say with some certainty that several strategies are important for positive outcomes in intervention, especially with children learning to use SGDs. These include (Gevarter & Zamora, 2018)

- creating and using communication opportunities via such methods as time delay and questioning;
- providing feedback via reinforcement of requests, praise, or expansions;
- verbal, physical, and gestural prompting;
- modeling; and
- training communication partners.

Modeling appears to be the primary instructional strategy, although there are many variations.

SLPs report making decisions based on the needs of the child with ASD but do not regularly consider processing differences nor the effects of input during instruction (Clarke & Williams, 2020). For children with ASD using SGDs, improvements in spontaneous communicative utterances, novel words, and comments all favor a blended behavioral intervention that focuses on joint engagement and play skills along with incorporating an SGD (Kasari et al., 2014).

> *Food for Thought:* Intervention with children using AAC is much more than just getting them to imitate touching a symbol. Does this sound frightening or like a wonderful challenge?

AAC, Communication Partners, and Children With ASD

Preschool peers have been shown to be effective agents of change for preverbal and early verbal children. Likewise, preschool peers with TDL can be trained to be communication partners with children with ASD who use SGDs.

Children who receive peer-mediated treatment demonstrate significant increases in rates of communication and have more balanced responses and increased initiations than children with ASD who do not receive peer mediation (Thiemann-Bourque et al., 2018). In addition, generalization improves and the children maintain communication gains, evidenced by greater classroom social participation and interactions with peers.

Peers with TDL can learn to initiate communication with children with ASD within a *Stay, Play, Talk* model using an AAC device, such as GoTalk 4+ (Attainment Company) (Thiemann-Bourque et al., 2017). Stay, Play, Talk is a social skills program that trains children with TDL to initiate communication and model language with teacher monitoring (Ledford et al, 2016). Children can be paired and encouraged to communicate within classroom social activities. Within a model such as this, some children with ASD will improve communication reciprocity and peer engagement. The highest rates of communication for the children with ASD may be around preferred foods and toys.

In a small study, researchers were able to demonstrate the benefits of teaching peers with TDL to be responsive listeners to preschoolers with ASD who were learning to use PECS (Thiemann-Bourque et al., 2016). Peers with TDL increased their communication with the children with ASD, who in turn improved in social engagement.

We can safely assert that communication partners who efficiently use AAC are essential for interactional training and generalization. Important considerations include device training for caregivers and enhancing caregivers' understanding of intervention targets. It's important that communication is supported across different learning contexts and domains of communication over time (Shire & Jones, 2015).

Vocabulary

Although AAC systems offer increased opportunities to participation in activities in their home, school, and community, without the appropriate vocabulary, AAC will not be effective (Fallon et al., 2001). An initial vocabulary for young children should be meaningful, motivating, functional, and individualized; be appropriate to a child's age, gender, background, personality, and environments; and be able to support a range of communicative uses and intentions. This necessitates a detailed understanding of a child's most frequented contexts and the communication expectations of those settings and an appreciation of the individual child's own style of communication.

CHAPTER 4 EARLY COMMUNICATION INTERVENTION 151

When selecting vocabulary, SLPs should be mindful of the need for a core vocabulary of words commonly used in a given situation, such as common verbs and greetings, and a fringe vocabulary of words specific to an individual or activity, such as the SLP's name, song words for "circle time," and favorite treats. A core vocabulary is generally stable across people and contexts, consisting of words that can be combined into longer utterances. Several potential core vocabulary lists exist and can be accessed easily by typing "core vocabulary" into your computer's search engine. Even so, core vocabulary should be adapted to the individual child.

Fringe vocabulary is activity-specific and infrequently used in other environments and contexts. Examples of fringe vocabulary might include action words such as *paint*, *dance*, and *color* that only occur in certain contexts.

There are three main approaches to selecting vocabulary for children: developmental, environmental, and functional—none of which are mutually exclusive. A developmental approach involves the use of vocabulary from children with TDL and may not be appropriate for all children. In contrast, an environmental approach is based on an ecological inventory, in which words are identified for specific communication environments. Finally, a functional approach is pragmatic in nature, and vocabularies are identified based on expressed communication intentions of a child, such as requesting.

Several ecologically sound and individualized methods can be used by SLPs for fringe vocabulary selection. These include

- conducting a survey of the environments and activities in which a child needs to communicate;
- using a communication diary to record a child's attempted interactions;
- compiling a list of words and phrases thought to be potentially useful to a child; and
- completing a caregiver vocabulary selection questionnaire similar to that for other nonsymbolic children.

A fine example of a questionnaire is presented by Fallon et al. (2001).

Children are most apt to communicate if they have vocabulary that allows them to do the things they want to do—a functional vocabulary. Potential words should be selected based on the extent to which they enable a child to talk about the things in the environment and to use each symbol to express a variety of intentions.

New vocabulary items, if learned within the context of events and activities, enable caregivers and teachers to use the AAC system when conversing with the child. As an SLP, you can work closely with the family to select vocabulary and contexts that reflect the family's culture. For example, eating utensils may be inappropriate for Ethiopian American children, whereas *injera*, a doughy flatbread used to bring food to the mouth, is not. The vocabulary should reflect food, clothing, and celebrations from the child's world. Pictures should also depict the child's cultural background in skin color, facial features, and clothing, to mention just a few. Vocabulary choices should also enable a child to express their unique personality.

Early words or symbols are usually learned during routines in which a child matches messages to functional goals within the interaction. Likewise, a child using AAC can learn new concepts and words by using them. By experiencing a word within a routine, the child forms an activity-based concept to which the label may be attached.

Generalization: Role of the Environment

One of the major concerns, an issue I have stressed and will continue to emphasize throughout this text, is generalization. Our focus is newly learned AAC skills. In order for generalization to occur, it must be actively promoted from the onset of the intervention process. Short of this, SLPs are left with a "train and hope" approach, in which, unaware of the variables that affect generalization, they "hope" that it will occur. That's not good enough!

AAC intervention most often focuses on changing the behaviors of AAC users rather than that of partners (Schlosser & Lee, 2000). For children using AAC, most communication partners may have only marginally higher, if not lower, AAC competency.

Teaching Caregivers to Use AAC. The effectiveness of an augmentative communication system depends on communication partners. Without training, partners tend to dominate and take the majority of turns while limiting the child to yes/no answers. In response, AAC users may respond by playing an increasingly passive role; initiating few interactions; responding only when required to do so; producing only a limited range of intentions; and using restricted linguistic forms, such as one-word responses. This situation is less than optimal and works against language and communication development for a child.

Obviously, the key to changing a child's role to a more active one is changing the behaviors of a child's communication partners. For a child's partners, this means learning to facilitate interactions and to use strategies to better support the communication of the child using AAC. You can see how important it is to collaborate with the family. Four interactional skills have been identified as intervention targets for the communication partners (Kent-Walsh & Light, 2003):

- Extending conversational pause time or expectant delay by initiating eye contact with the child
- Being responsive to communicative attempts
- Using open-ended questions
- Modeling of AAC system use

Following instruction, communication partners can learn to lessen conversational dominance and to provide more turns for the AAC user. When this occurs, participation, turn-taking, and the range of communicative functions of AAC users will increase.

Intervention goals related to participation or involvement in life situations are more directly related to a child's communicative functioning (Granlund et al., 2008). Often, adults focus on the mechanics of an AAC device, but this goal will not affect participation

CHAPTER 4 EARLY COMMUNICATION INTERVENTION

153

(Lund & Light, 2006). If we hope to improve participation within family life, we should directly target this area of functioning. In general, children with better AAC outcomes tended to have a more supportive family environment than those with less positive outcomes (Hamm & Mirenda, 2006).

Parents and other family members can be taught techniques to support their child's communication. These include the following (Light & Drager, 2005):

- Planning together with the SLP to integrate the AAC system into the natural environment
- Identifying varied communication opportunities within each context
- Modeling AAC and speech
- Learning to wait and to anticipate the child's communication
- Responding to the child's communication attempts in meaningful ways:
  - Responding in a timely and positive manner when a child attempts to communicate
  - Fulfilling the child's intent, such as providing a requested toy
  - Expanding through AAC and speech to the child's message
  - Replying conversationally
  - Modeling correct forms of immature or incorrect child behaviors
  - Expanding on the child's message

Beginning with the facilitator's current strengths, the SLP can gradually build new knowledge and skills through a combination of explanation, modeling, practice, monitoring, and feedback. That looks like the format for an ECI session mentioned previously.

As an SLP, be mindful of a family's needs and comfort level, and do not introduce too many new things at once. The last thing a family needs is a time-consuming burden, such as endless drills involving AAC.

Building Language System. Building expressive language can be a challenge for the child, the family, and the SLP. The overall goal must be useful communication beyond a basic level. They must be concerned for the expressive language development of children who use AAC. For example, as a child's language matures, graphic symbols can be enhanced by letters that represent verb and noun endings and shorter high-usage words such as *am*, *are*, and *is*. Graphic symbols can represent a single word, a phrase or sentence, or a category or theme. I encourage you to read the thorough article by Binger et al. (2020), who present a detailed framework of phrase and sentence development using graphic symbols.

Although a single picture can be used to meet basic expressive needs, such as touching COOKIE when asked "What do you want?", this limits the child to one intention—requesting. As children mature, they can learn to construct multisymbol utterances that reflect the language of their environment (Binger et al., 2017; Kent-Walsh et al., 2015; Tönsing et al., 2014). Graphic symbols can be a bridge to literacy and truly complex linguistic communication. Requiring a child to adhere to spoken language grammar supports the long-term goal of linguistic competence.

Binger et al. (2020) propose a four-phase model of utterance and sentence development based on the earlier work of Hadley (2014). This model is presented in Figure 4–3. A child progresses from early symbol productions of typically one or two symbols through early symbol combinations and childlike sentences containing both a subject (noun or pronoun) and a predicate or verb and, finally, to adultlike sentences. The authors also offer an analysis method for determining semantic meaning, pragmatic intent, and syntactic maturity.

Summary

To be truly useful for young children, AAC technologies need to be updated and redesigned to increase their appeal, expand functions, and reduce the learning demands (Light & Drager, 2002). For example, the appeal for young children may be increased by (Light et al., 2004)

- integrating play into both AAC design and intervention;
- providing meaningful fun contexts for interaction and intervention;
- expanding output options to include voice or animation;
- enhancing aesthetics to resemble toys in color and design; and
- providing options for personalization.

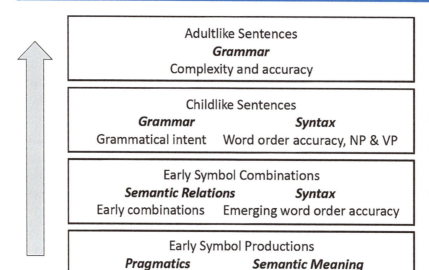

Figure 4–3. Four-phase model of utterance and sentence development. Information taken from Binger et al. (2020)

CHAPTER 4 EARLY COMMUNICATION INTERVENTION

These modifications cannot be accomplished at the expense of ease of learning. Currently, learning AAC systems is extremely challenging for some young presymbolic children, especially given the need to attend to and interact with communication partners at the same time (Light et al., 2002). Add to this the dynamic nature of communication and you get some idea of the challenge for a young child with communication impairment.

Conclusion

As you can see, working with young prelinguistic children is a challenging task. Caregiver-delivered home programs are useful and deliver results if the intervention occurs frequently in the home and parents are directly trained by an SLP (Tosh et al., 2017).

Given the challenge of language teaching with infants and toddlers who may be preverbal, you, as an SLP, can hope to accomplish very little seeing a child an hour or even a few hours each week. It's sad to report, but given recent funding cutbacks, intervention may be even more limited. My grandson was being seen once a month! In my estimation, that's criminal and illegal. If the SLP does not enlist the aid of parents and family members, teachers and classroom aides, and childcare providers, they are missing a valuable opportunity to provide effective intervention in a functional manner that fosters communication and language growth.

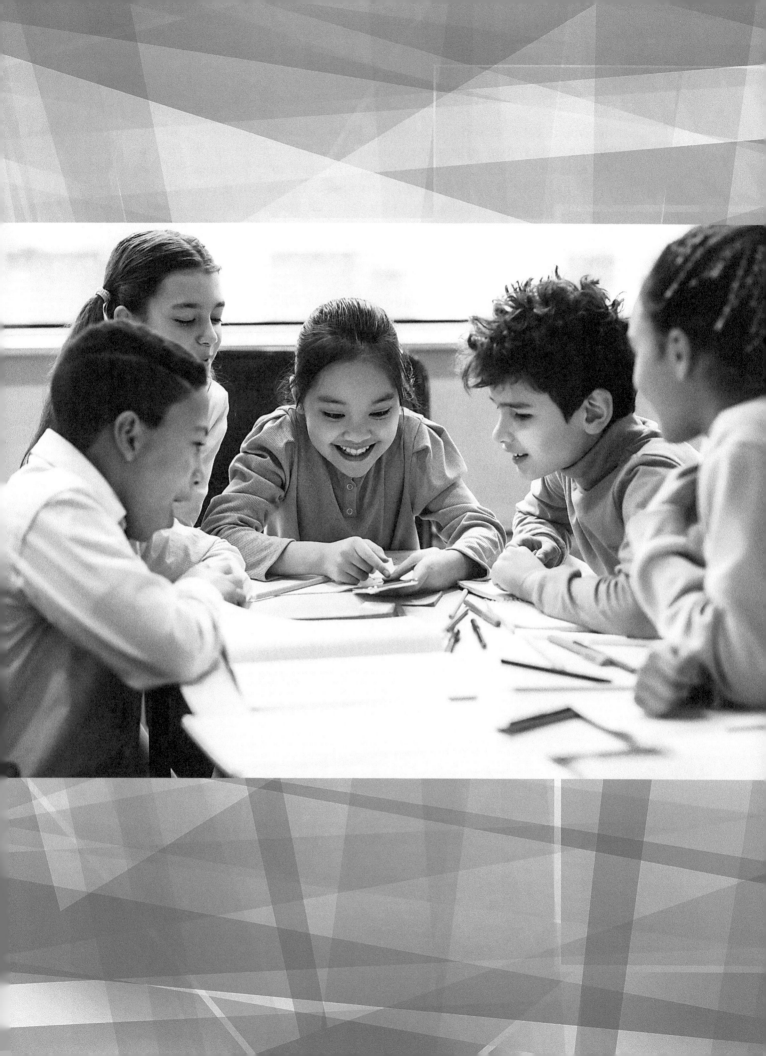

CHAPTER 5

ASSESSMENT OF PRESCHOOL AND SCHOOL-AGE CHILDREN WITH LANGUAGE DISORDERS

Jake is described by his teachers as a sweet boy who is somewhat formal in his mannerisms and in his speech. He prefers to talk with adults rather than children and spends much of his time alone. Rather than engage in small talk, he tends to impart information on his favorite topics, aerospace and computers. It's not uncommon for Jake to descend on a group of children, make a statement on one of these topics, and withdraw with little attempt to engage.

For the most part, Jake is polite and respectful, but he's also easily confused by the behaviors of other children. In part, his preference for adults may reflect his observation that "I find adults more predictable." He seems especially confused by emotional responses of others, gestures, figurative language, and slang.

Similarly, he has difficulty describing the thoughts and feelings of characters in narratives. His writing is syntactically correct and factual, but it lacks engagement with the reader. Like his speech, his writing is delivered in the form of a lecture.

Although only in third grade, Jake has unfortunately attracted the unwanted attention of some older boys. On the playground, they often gather around and tease him. On those occasions, he will cover his ears, scream, and shake his head violently side to side as if to make the sound of their voices disappear. With extreme provocation, he'll strike out, screaming, hitting, and kicking. When that occurs, his teacher or an aide will take him aside to quiet him, often with a book.

Jake's parents are very concerned about the possibility of bullying as he matures. His mother has discussed putting him in a private school when he reaches middle school.

Academically, Jake is very advanced and seems bored by the lessons in class. The teacher has gone out of her way to provide him with more advanced information and assignments, especially in math and science. Here again, his parents worry that the school may not be meeting his needs. They consider him to be gifted intellectually, and clearly he excels in most academic areas.

Language assessment with older children is very different from early intervention (EI). You might still have some children in your caseload who are presymbolic or early symbolic, but for the most part, preschool and school-aged children will be using language to communicate through speech, augmentative and alternative communication, or in print. Most assessment and intervention will occur in a preschool or school unless you work in a clinical setting or in private practice. In all these settings, you'll either be working alone or with a team consisting of yourself along with the school or district psychologist, classroom or special education teacher, and others as needed.

The American Speech-Language-Hearing Association (ASHA) **Scope of Practice** outlines our responsibilities and what we can and cannot do as speech-language pathologists (SLPs). Other regulations are part of state certification requirements and those of state departments of education and school districts. For example, it won't be within your scope of practice to diagnose and designate children as having autism spectrum disorder (ASD) or learning disability (LD), but you will be assessing for language disorders in these children, most likely as part of a team. For example, you might diagnose the pragmatic difficulties of children with ASD and describe the other behaviors you observe. Descriptions of these patterns of behaviors can then be used by another professional designated to make a diagnosis of ASD (Timler, 2018a). In addition, as a member of an interdisciplinary diagnostic team, you'll be expected to contribute in-depth information that describes a child's communication abilities.

Likely, most of your caseload will consist of children with developmental language disorder (DLD) and/or social communication disorder. No matter the child, your responsibility is to systematically gather data through an individualized, well-designed, and thorough assessment of a child's communication skills and deficits.

Before we begin, note that in the real world, no clear line exists between assessment and intervention. Both are part of the intervention process, and portions of each are found in the other. Ideally, assessment and measurement are ongoing throughout intervention. No clinical goal should be determined or modified without first having obtained data on the communication performance of a child.

Adequate evaluation of a child is one of the most difficult and demanding tasks you'll face as an SLP. The goal—much more complex than providing a score or a diagnostic label—is to describe the very complex language system of each child and their unique pattern of language rules and behaviors. Along the way, you'll make decisions that determine the path your assessment of a child will take. You'll want to be certain that your assessment is unbiased and as accurate as possible. Figure 5–1 presents some of the paths you might take in an assessment. We discuss this information in detail throughout this chapter.

As an SLP, keep in mind three words: *why*, *what*, and *how*. Considering *why* a child is being assessed helps you clarify the purpose of your assessment. This clarity, in turn, enables you to decide *what* specific behaviors to assess. The reasons for assessment can be grouped as (a) identification of children with potential language problems, (b) establish-

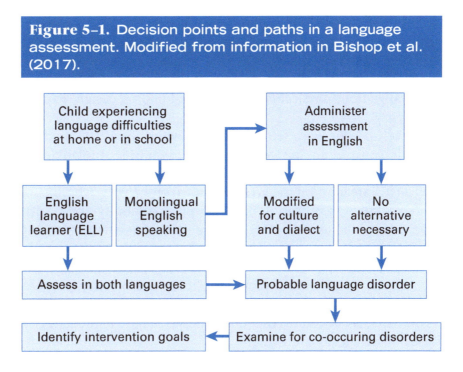

Figure 5–1. Decision points and paths in a language assessment. Modified from information in Bishop et al. (2017).

ment of baseline functioning, and (c) measurement of change. Baseline functioning and measuring of change are usually considered steps in intervention and are discussed later. Finally, you'll need to decide *how* to best evaluate for the purpose of identifying behaviors. How will you collect the data needed to make informed decisions? Your clinical intuition is an important factor throughout this process, especially when determining which aspects of language to evaluate and summarizing the data.

The data-gathering process is scientific in nature in that it must be unbiased and objective. This collection process should be precise and measurable, with very little intrusion by an SLP's premature conclusions. It is important not to lose the child in the mass of data you'll collect. This is a real person, not just a set of data.

It may be helpful to consider assessment procedures as existing along a continuum from formal, structured protocols to informal, less structured approaches. In general, the more structured the elicitation session, the less variety of structures and meanings expressed by the child. Language elicited in more structured tasks is usually shorter and less complex, especially with younger children, than language sampled in less controlled situations. Generally, the more specific the information desired, the more structured the approach. Even formal tests or portions of tests, however, can be used in an informal way as a probe of specific behavior. More on these modifications later.

I would be remiss if I didn't at least mention the World Health Organization's International Classification of Functioning, Disability and Health (WHO ICF, 2001), an international classification framework for describing and organizing information on health and health-related areas, including communication disorders (WHO, 2001). Stated simply, the WHO notion is that a disorder does not reside solely in an individual but, rather, in what that individual must do to get through each day.

An individual's level of functioning is dynamic, an interaction between health conditions, environmental factors, and personal factors. Thus, the ICF focuses on both the positive and the negative aspects of functioning in everyday life that we cannot infer solely from an individual's disorder. Environmental factors that affect daily functioning can range from physical factors, such as building design, to social factors, such as attitudes and laws.

Even if your work setting isn't following the WHO model, it's important to keep in mind that as an SLP, you will want to consider the environment in which a child functions, home and school, and the demands of each. Two excellent overviews of the WHO ICF are found at the WHO website (https://www.who.int/standards/classifications/international-classification-of-functioning-disability-and-health/who-disability-assessment-schedule) and the ASHA website (https://www.asha.org/slp/icf/). Remember also that I defined a functional approach as one similarly concerned with how a child must use their language to navigate their environment.

In this chapter, we explore the differences between psychometric and descriptive assessment paradigms and describe a combined, or integrative, approach that attempts systematically to address the shortcomings of both approaches while describing a child's use of language in context.

As we go, think about Jake and the *why*, *what*, and *how*. This process is about children and their language.

Psychometric Versus Descriptive Procedures

The goals of communication assessment are to identify and describe each child's unique pattern of communication and, if that pattern signifies a language disorder, to recommend treatment, follow-up, or referral. Through this process, an SLP determines

- whether a problem exists;
- the causal-related factors; and
- an overall intervention plan.

There are two major philosophical approaches to this task. The normalist philosophy is based on a norm, or average performance level—usually a score—that society considers typical functioning. In contrast, the neutralist approach compares a child's present performance to their past performance or to that of other children and is descriptive in manner.

The two methods are not mutually exclusive. For example, the results of normative testing can be reinterpreted to provide more descriptive information. Test items on which a child is unsuccessful can be probed to determine other methods that result in a correct response.

More descriptive approaches, such as language sampling, can highlight the individualistic nature of a child's communicative functioning. In contrast, psychometric normative testing imposes group criteria on an individual. Each method of assessment

CHAPTER 5 ASSESSMENT OF PRESCHOOL AND SCHOOL-AGE CHILDREN WITH LANGUAGE DISORDERS 161

has its strengths and weaknesses, as well as possible applications within the clinical setting. These are described in the following sections.

Normalist Assessment Measures

Tests are usually standardized and normed. Standardized means that there is a consistent or standard manner in which test items are to be presented, and the adult is to respond to the child's responses. For example, the test manual may direct an SLP to give the following instructions:

> I am going to read a sentence to you. When I'm finished, I want you to select the picture that best illustrates what I have said. Listen carefully, because I can only read each sentence once.

The test is to be administered in this manner.

Most standardized tests are also normed, which means that the test has been given to a group of children that supposedly represent all children for whom the test was designed, giving us a criterion for measurement. Ideally, the norming group has the same characteristics as these children. In other words, gender, racial and ethnic, geographic, and socioeconomic differences in the norming group mirror those of the target population, such as all first graders.

Even these constraints do not ensure that the test will be appropriate, especially with children from culturally and linguistically diverse backgrounds or children represented by a very small portion of the norming group. It might surprise you that children with language disorders are rarely included in the norming group. This has ramifications that we describe later.

If we put standardization and norming together, you'll see that the test must be administered in only one way and not haphazardly in order to compare children. Every child in the norming group took the test in the standard or prescribed manner, and so must our child in order to make comparisons.

Traditional language assessment procedures heavily emphasize the use of standardized norm-referenced tests. In general, there are very few standardized measures for toddlers and adolescents and an abundance of measures for preschoolers and early school-age children.

Statistical Characteristics

Ideally, a standardized test has demonstrated high reliability, validity, sensitivity, and specificity. Reliability is the repeatability of measurement. More precisely, reliability is the accuracy or precision with which a sample of language taken at one time represents performance of either a different but similar sample or the same sample at a different time. Very limited samples of language usually result in unstable scores. Thus, a test must include enough language to be reliable but not so much as to be unwieldy.

One measure of reliability is internal consistency. *Internal consistency* is the degree of relationship among items and the overall test. If a test has high internal consistency, children who score well or poorly overall should tend to have the same performance on individual items and to perform similarly among themselves.

Other measures of reliability include test–retest reliability, alternate-form reliability, and split-half reliability. In test–retest reliability, a child is administered the same test with a time interval between each administration. With alternate forms, a child is administered equivalent or parallel forms of a measure. Finally, a test may be divided into equivalent halves with each used separately. In each case, two test scores are compared, and the consistency of scores is measured.

In addition, an SLP is concerned with the probability of two judges scoring the same behavior in the same manner. This value is called *interjudge reliability*. If two judges were scoring the test, what is the probability of them giving a child the same score.

Validity is the effectiveness of a test in representing, describing, or predicting an attribute of interest to the tester. In short, it is a measure of the test's ability to assess what it purports to assess. Professionals should be cautious when choosing tests. For example, some tests do not report validity.

To assess language knowledge, test designers must select concrete performance tasks very carefully. It's important to remember that tests are merely samples. From the tests, SLPs will make inferences about an attribute or behavior. If the samples are not valid measures, the inferences will be incorrect.

Validity is not self-evident and must be proven. Three types of evidence are criterion validity, content validity, and construct validity. *Criterion validity* is the effectiveness or accuracy with which a measure predicts performance. This usually is calculated as the degree to which a measure correlates with some other suitable measures assumed to be valid.

Content validity is the faithfulness with which the sample or measure represents some attribute or behavior. In other words, the sum of the tasks involved should define or constitute, at least in part, the attribute or behavior being measured. Measures should reflect the professional literature, research, and expert opinion on the constitution of the attribute or behavior tested.

Finally, *construct validity* is the extent to which a measure describes or measures some trait or behavior. Construct validity usually is determined by comparing the measure with other acceptable measures assumed to be valid. If children failed one language test but passed another, it could indicate that the two tests assessed different aspects of language.

Sensitivity and specificity are collectively called *diagnostic accuracy*. Sensitivity is the ability of a test to identify children with a language disorder. Specificity is the ability of a test to determine children with TDL. This is what valid testing should do—determine who has a disorder and who does not.

All four measures—reliability, validity, sensitivity, and specificity—compare two values, such as test–retest performance or scores on one test that signify a disorder and those on another that do the same. In every case, one thing is compared with another.

This type of statistical analysis is termed *correlational*. For example, we compare your height today with your height in a week. Are the two similar. If similar, we have a 1:1 match. If not, the match is something less. If two tests are exactly the same, the value is 1.0. If not, it is less, such as 0.82. The four variables will be less than 1.0 but should be

CHAPTER 5 ASSESSMENT OF PRESCHOOL AND SCHOOL-AGE CHILDREN WITH LANGUAGE DISORDERS 163

above 0.8 to be strong enough to accurately measure a child's language. Values should be given in the test manual and should be considered by an SLP when purchasing or using a test.

Test Considerations

Language assessment instruments differ widely even when purported to measure the same entity. Even tests that seem to be significantly correlated, suggesting an interrelationship, may seem less so when subtests or various portions of tests are compared. In addition, tests can differ markedly in their levels of difficulty, yielding different results for the same child for the same skill.

For these and other reasons, tests should be researched carefully by SLPs before being used. In the following sections, we explore some of these differences, specifically test content, and some of the common misuses of tests. Finally, the variables that should be considered in test selection are discussed.

Content. A major criticism of existing instruments is the inadequacy of the content covered in both breadth and depth. Two issues relative to content validity—relevance and coverage—must be addressed in test construction. Content relevance is the precision with which a certain aspect of language is delineated or defined. This is necessary to determine the dimensions of that aspect to test.

A child's knowledge of language, called competence, is measurable only as test behavior or performance, which is affected by the complexity of the task. Thus, poor performance may indicate an underlying deficit or difficulty with the assessment procedure rather than a child's language disorder.

Content coverage is the completeness with which an aspect of language is sampled. Theoretically, coverage of language features should reflect general use. If coverage is inadequate, more subtle language impairments may go undetected.

Testing produces data on minimal portions of behavior, thus reducing language to simple, possibly irrelevant dimensions that may not reflect the qualities of a child's language overall. By fragmenting language into observable and measurable features, tests tend to emphasize structural components of language form that are easy to observe. Although structured testing may reveal the child's ability to use language in the test context, it may also reveal very little about the child's language as it is needed and used in everyday communication. For example, a child may use interrogatives throughout the day to obtain information, desired objects, and needed assistance but may be unable to form interrogatives on an isolated test item.

In addition, the test situation may be so foreign to a child or that child's everyday communication environment that it influences the language the child produces. Performance may be affected also by factors as diverse as a child's state of health on the day the test is administered, attention level and comprehension of the instructions, and perception of the test administrator.

Misuse of Normative Testing. Norm-referenced tests should be used with caution. The best advice is to be an "informed clinician" and a wise consumer.

Keep in mind that when we reduce complex behaviors to a number or score, much of the subtlety of difference is lost, as is the richness and complexity of language. However, numbers and scores can enable you, as an SLP, to compare language performance across children and to establish developmental norms that can be used to compare a child to similar children. We just need to be careful in the assumptions we make.

As an SLP, you should be mindful of the possible misuse of these instruments, such as

- use of scores as a summary of a child's performance;
- use of inappropriate norms;
- inappropriate assumptions based on test results;
- use of specific test items to plan intervention goals; and
- use of tests to assess therapy progress.

Let's discuss each briefly.

Misuse of Scores. When does difference become disorder? Where do we draw the line? For example, are the 1% of the population who are blood type B-negative considered deviant or disordered? Or just different? How do we decide? This is not a philosophical question. We're dealing with real people. Let's take just a moment to explore some of the statistical values used by test makers.

When plotted, the number of children in the norming group receiving each score will form a bell-shaped curve, represented in Figure 5–2. Height of the curve indicates the number of individuals at each point. The most frequently used score on standardized measures is the mean, or average, score. Test makers assume that the average score for a

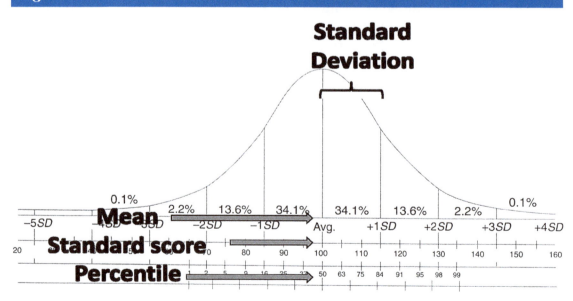

Figure 5–2. Parameters of the normal distribution.

CHAPTER 5 ASSESSMENT OF PRESCHOOL AND SCHOOL-AGE CHILDREN WITH LANGUAGE DISORDERS 165

sample population is the "normal" score for the larger population. An individual child's score can be described relative to the mean, such as below the mean.

A wide scoring area around the mean is considered to be the *normal range*. The distance from the mean is mathematically calculated and called standard deviation (SD). You'll learn more about this in a research design, statistics, or assessment course. Approximately two-thirds of the scores are within 1 SD on either side of the mean score (±1 SD), approximately 33% above and 33% below. Within 2 SDs are approximately 95% of the scores, leaving approximately 2.5% to 3% above and 2.5% to 3% below 2 SD. States and school districts set the point at which typical and disordered categories fall.

Another way to describe points on the curve is standard score. This value is shown below the curve in Figure 5–2. This is a statistical value in which 100 is applied to the mean, and based on the distribution of the scores, other values are added below and above the mean. The best example is IQ. Here, the mean has been arbitrarily assigned a standard score of 100. Notice in Figure 5–2 that –1 SD has a value of 84.

Deep breath. Only one more.

Percentile is a fourth value reported by tests. Don't confuse percentile with percent. Percentile is an ordinal number, a rank, a place in a series. Based on the distribution of the scores, percentile is a rank in a theoretical group of 100. For example, among 100 people, where is a child with a certain score located?

Let's see if you follow. If a child's score is on the mean, right in the middle, the standard score would be 100. It follows then that the percentile would be 50, in the middle of 100 children.

Scores at either end of the distribution represent a quantitative difference. Where we draw the boundary between typical and disordered is relative and somewhat arbitrary. Tests offer guidance and governmental entities set boundaries, but an SLP must describe the difference—a difference that is great enough to impair a child's ability to use language to get through the day or to *function*. There's that word again!

Let's spend just a moment more to consider some aspects of test scores that may be overlooked. First, numbers establish equalities and inequalities. For example, 2 is twice 1 and half of 4. It would seem, therefore, that a child with a score of 4 correct has twice the skill of one with a score of 2, but this is only a measure of the number of responses, not the quality of those responses.

Second, all test items are statistically of equal importance because each has the same weight. If there is one item each for the verb BE and past-tense *-ed*, they each receive the same score even though they are not of equal importance developmentally.

Third, the equality of scores does not translate to an equality of behavior nor describe that behavior. A child who achieves the same score as another child may not make the same kinds of errors. Two children with the same error scores even on the same test items could have answered very differently. Imagine that the test asks two children to provide a word definition and you understand what I mean about differing responses.

As an SLP, you should habitually check a value called the standard error of measure (SEm). Found in the test manual, SEm aids an SLP in knowing the confidence they can have in a child's scores. Because tests are less than perfectly reliable, a certain amount of error is reflected in each score. The larger the SEm, the less confidence one can have in the test's accuracy.

Assume that a child received a score of 25 and that the SEm is ±2. This means that the child's score is most likely in the range of 23 to 27. This value is especially important when comparing scores.

None of my remarks mean that you, as an SLP, should avoid using tests. The use of scores is not inherently bad as long as measurement is meaningful and functional and reflects accurately the entity being evaluated. It is important therefore that an SLP read, understand, and evaluate the information in the test manual and be knowledgeable about test construction and administration. Evidence-based practice (EBP) requires that a test be studied thoroughly before it is used.

Inappropriate Norms. The norming sample should represent the population for whom you are using the test. Otherwise, the norms are inappropriate and should not be used.

Use of inappropriate norms occurs most frequently with children from culturally linguistically diverse, rural, or low-socioeconomic-status backgrounds. In these cases, local norms may need to be prepared by an SLP by following the norming procedure described in the test manual. Test manuals should explain this process in detail.

Incorrect Assumptions. Test scores may represent only scores and not actual differences in linguistic ability. Therefore, as an SLP, you must analyze each child's performance in order to obtain descriptive information. For example, subtest scores can be interpreted independently from each other.

An SLP also should be cautious in extrapolating global language development from scores on language tests, especially those that sample only one or two aspects of language. For example, although the Peabody Picture Vocabulary Test is a good receptive vocabulary test, it does not address other aspects of language or indicate overall language use.

Identifying Intervention Goals. A thorough description of a child's behavior is needed before an SLP can identify areas needing intervention. Individual test items or subtests do not provide an adequate sample of that behavior. Because test items represent only a small portion of language, they do not provide enough information on which to base therapy goals. At the very least, more than one psychometric assessment procedure should be used because of the variability of some children across tests. Only through the use of a number of different assessment protocols, including sampling and dynamic assessment, can an SLP hope to determine intervention goals.

Measuring Therapy Progress. The continued use of a norm-referenced test to assess therapy progress may result in a child learning the test, thus producing artificially high results. Descriptive measures, explained later in the chapter, are more appropriate for measuring individual progress.

Variables in Language Test Selection. As an SLP, you should be a wise consumer of assessment materials and should base test selection on several factors. Of particular interest are test reliability, validity, sensitivity, and specificity discussed previously. Even language tests that meet very stringent psychometric or measurement criteria may not be very precise discriminators of a language disorder.

CHAPTER 5 ASSESSMENT OF PRESCHOOL AND SCHOOL-AGE CHILDREN WITH LANGUAGE DISORDERS

The results for any child must be weighed against the test's accuracy in four areas:

- Correctly detecting impairment that is present (a true positive result)
- Detecting impairment when it is not present (a false-positive result)
- Correctly identifying typical language (no language disorder) (a true negative result)
- Identifying a child as having typical language when language disorder is present (a false-negative result)

If, for example, a test has a high false-positive rate, the SLP must consider the accuracy when a child is found to have language disorder. In this situation, it's easy to see the value of giving more than one test. Unfortunately, not every test manual will give all four values.

Other considerations in test selection include appropriateness of the test for a particular child, the manner of presentation and comprehensiveness, and the type and sensitivity of the test results. A test should be appropriate to the child's age or functioning level. In addition, the norming population should be sufficiently large and varied to include representatives of the child's racial, ethnic, geographic, and socioeconomic background. If the child is from an identifiable group, such as bilingual children, the SLP should check to determine if the norming information gives specific or separate data by that group.

Appropriateness may relate also to the manner of presentation, the number of items, and the content coverage discussed previously. Some children perform better under certain conditions. For example, in general, children with LD perform better if visual input accompanies verbal.

Some tests offer a computerized version for children with motoric problems or those who may perform better on this format. It is still in its infancy, but some professionals are exploring the provision of language assessment via the internet (Waite et al., 2010). Although some language tests yield virtually the same scores whether administered by an online or face-to-face SLP, these results will vary across children.

The type of statistical data resulting from test scores is also a practical consideration in test selection. Depending on the test, the interpretive value of such scores may be very limited. For example, if first graders and fourth graders are likely to receive similar scores, the test is of little value in identifying developmental differences.

When given a choice of tests, SLPs display a remarkable similarity in the relative importance they attach to different tests. For example, there is an overreliance on vocabulary and omnibus language tests that may be too narrow or too broad, respectively, to adequately describe a child's language. Familiarity with the test procedure, EBP, an SLP's overall opinion of the measure, and their clinical experience are all factors in test or task selection and in the relative importance attached to data obtained from different measures.

Summary

Many professionals have decried overdependence on and poor interpretation of the results of testing. Yet, SLPs often are required to incorporate standardized and normed results into their assessments. It is important for you as a future SLP to recognize that tests are informative but not the be-all and end-all of evaluation. Awareness of a test's shortcomings can greatly aid an SLP's interpretation of a child's performance.

Norm-referenced approaches offer a prepackaged assessment with little consideration for the individual needs of the child with whom they are used. Tests are *a priori* and product oriented and may offer little information on the appropriateness of the language features being tested.

Although norm-referenced tests play an important role in identifying children with language disorders, they should not be the only tools used. Simply using a −1 SD or even a −2 SD criterion without considering other factors, such as cultural and linguistic diversity, may be doing a disservice to a child (Oetting & Garrity, 2006).

At the very least, you as an SLP should consider test results from a combination of measures. For example, one study found that in evaluating oral story comprehension, a combination of the Joint Story Retell task and the Expectancy Violation Detection task (Dempsey et al., 2002; Skarakis-Doyle, 2002), and the use of comprehension questions resulted in 96% accurate identification of children with language disorders (Skarakis-Doyle et al., 2008).

The issue of testing is central to the purpose of assessment. Data gathered in an assessment should be relevant to the initial clinical concern, to the determination that a problem exists, to individual differences and individual processing, to the nature of the problem, to prognosis, to intervention implications, and to accountability. Otherwise, it is just a numbers game. Norm-referenced tests seem appropriate for determining if a language impairment exists, but they are inconsistent in determining the specific area(s) of deficit required for intervention.

Although normed tests are potentially valid, reliable, sensitive, specific, and precise in measurement, it is difficult to find a language test that is acceptable in all ways. In addition, normed tests do not easily accommodate cultural and individual variation, nor do they begin to provide a true picture of the richness and complexity of the child's communication behavior.

By their nature, tests are less complex than the language being assessed. Although normative tests may be good for measuring isolated skills, they provide very little information on overall language use. But we can't just fault tests; language is multidimensional and its use individualistic, making it difficult to measure.

As a final word, we cannot totally blame psychometric measures for doing what they do. Nor can we lay all the blame on test authors who often go to great lengths to ensure that test content reflects our best knowledge about language and language development and disorders. In the hands of a skilled SLP, tests can yield valuable information, especially when combined with more descriptive measures.

Descriptive Assessment Approaches

In contrast to testing, descriptive approaches are based on other methods, such as observation, dynamic assessment, and conversational sampling of a child's language. Descriptive approaches have the potential of allowing SLPs to regard the language process while maintaining contextual integrity and individual differences.

CHAPTER 5 ASSESSMENT OF PRESCHOOL AND SCHOOL-AGE CHILDREN WITH LANGUAGE DISORDERS **169**

The advantages of the descriptive approach are that an SLP can apply their own theoretical model to the assessment process and can probe and assess areas that seem most difficult for a child. Thus, the clinical process can remain flexible and attuned to the child's needs. To do this, an SLP must understand the complex interaction of constitutional—biological, cognitive, psychological, and social—and environmental forces.

Let's be honest even though my heart is with descriptive approaches because of their adaptability, there are disadvantages with the descriptive approach, including

- the level of language expertise needed by an SLP to elicit and analyze a child's language;
- the amount of time needed to collect and analyze the child's language; and
- the reliability and validity of the sample.

Although a number of descriptive protocols exist, an SLP may not feel sufficiently well versed in all aspects of language to choose those appropriate for each child. None of these issues are inherent in descriptive approaches and each will be discussed in the following chapters.

All aspects of descriptive evaluation will be addressed in detail, but for now, let's just examine language sampling and the issues inherent in the process so that I don't present descriptive approaches as "the great panacea."

Language Sampling

Spontaneous sampling can be used as an indicator of a child's overall language functioning rather than as a device for noting specific language problems. More specific data can be obtained by probing the child's knowledge. Nor is sampling a one-size-fits-all. There are variations.

A language sample has several advantages over more formally structured testing, which, as we've discussed, reveals little about the use, content, and form of a child's language as needed and used in daily living. Some language features are more sensitive to the linguistic and extralinguistic factors of conversational give-and-take.

In contrast to language sampling, standardized assessments often don't identify deficits in social communication and language pragmatics (Condouris et al., 2003; Tager-Flusberg, 2000). These aspects of language are difficult to measure without engaging in a conversational exchange. Better measures of language may be variables such as the range of intentions, average or mean length of utterance in morphemes, and the number of utterances produced in a given time or turn (Casenhiser et al., 2015). These functional language measures, derived from children's language samples, are very important in making intervention decisions. In addition, data from language samples correlate significantly with results from elicited imitation and sentence completion tasks, adding to the validity of sampling as a language collection and analysis method.

Sampling Considerations. Good samples don't just happen; they take planning and consideration of several issues, not least reliability and validity, which are influenced by productivity, intelligibility, representativeness, and reactivity. Let's take a look.

Validity. Language samples are more susceptible than standardized measures to SLP bias. As an SLP, you must attempt to collect and analyze a language sample in the most objective manner possible. Objective procedures, measurements, and descriptions are generally more reliable and unbiased than subjective judgments. Base decisions on the data.

Reliability and validity are addressed, in part, by the manner of collection and analysis. In a series of studies using a language sample analysis (LSA) method called SUGAR (Sampling Utterances and Grammatical Analysis Revised), Owens and Pavelko reported strong reliability across varying sample sizes (Pavelko et al., 2020) and strong diagnostic accuracy, thus validity, measured by sensitivity and specificity (Pavelko & Owens, 2019a).

Some threats to validity are found within the sample itself. For example, preschool children vary in their attentiveness and disposition to talk moment by moment. As mentioned previously, possible threats to validity in a sample, even with older children, are productivity, or the amount produced; intelligibility, or the amount understood by the listener; representativeness, or the typicality of the sample; and reactivity, or the response of the child to differing stimuli.

Productivity. The uncommunicative child or the child who says very little will not give an SLP a productive sample for LSA. In the child's defense, such a sample may reflect accurately the child's typical output. The child may have little language with which to talk.

The key to greater production is for the SLP to plan a variety of elicitation tasks that serve the purpose of gathering the sample. Avoiding *yes/no* questions in favor of "Tell me about . . . " techniques is more likely to yield longer responses.

Intelligibility. Intelligibility is the amount of agreement between what a child intended to say and what the SLP interpreted from the sample. If much of the sample is unintelligible, few utterances will be suitable for analysis. In general, intelligibility can be increased with increased SLP control over the content of the child's utterances. In short, the SLP who knows the topic can determine more easily what the child said.

In a study of LSA with more than 300 children aged 3 to 7;11 years, Pavelko and Owens (2019b) found that unintelligible words fell into specific categories. These included the names of friends, movie and TV characters, and action figures.

Representativeness. A sample should represent a child's typical behavior. This may not occur if the language sample is collected in an atypical context—for example, a clinical room with an unfamiliar SLP as the conversational partner. Three issues relative to representativeness are *spontaneity*, *variability of context*, and *stability of the structure/ function* sampled.

Spontaneity is increased if the child is allowed to establish the topic and/or the activity. Interesting and varied stimulus materials can provide an excellent basis for spontaneous conversation and can elicit a variety of forms and functions.

Variability in the context and stimulus items will elicit a greater variety of child behaviors theoretically more representative of the child's everyday behavior. Data

CHAPTER 5 ASSESSMENT OF PRESCHOOL AND SCHOOL-AGE CHILDREN WITH LANGUAGE DISORDERS **171**

collected in a variety of settings, with a variety of partners, and on a variety of child-based conversational topics ensures versatility. Because quantity and complexity vary with the task, no lone task is likely to yield a representative sample of a child's language.

Unrepresentative samples may reflect other-than-normal usage by a child. In this situation, the structures or functions sampled may vary widely from one situation to another. Everyday situations are most likely to elicit typical use and thus provide some stability across situations.

A tug-of-war exists between eliciting typical and maximum production from a child. This debate is fueled by the often-reported gaps between what children with language disorders are capable of doing with their language and what they typically do. This makes it doubly important for an SLP to decide on the appropriate sample collection tasks and methods. For example, storytelling tasks yield longer utterances, whereas picture interpretation tasks elicit greater language quantity. Various elicitation tasks are discussed in detail in Chapter 6.

Reactivity. A child's reaction to the SLP and to techniques and materials also will affect the overall validity of the sample produced. For example, although a directed style of collecting in which an SLP uses a questioning technique allows the examiner more control over the content and may, in turn, increase intelligibility, it may sacrifice productivity and representativeness. In general, too much control restricts a child's output.

Although a more open-ended conversation may yield a more representative sample, it may be less intelligible and difficult for some children with language disorders. For example, children with LD exhibit as much difficulty with conversations as with other assessment protocols, such as testing. Likewise, specific stimulus items may increase a specific pattern of responding. For example, a doll may elicit a "baby talk" style.

The items chosen and the directions given also may affect validity. For example, although pictures can be used to elicit language, the instructions given often affect the quantity of language. The directive "Tell me about this picture" elicits less language than a more directive style, such as the following:

> I'd like you to make up a story from this picture. Tell me a whole story that has a beginning and an end. Start with "Once upon a time."

The best advice for any SLP is to remain flexible in order to shift between different contexts and different content in an attempt to elicit the language desired. It doesn't come automatically, but as a seasoned SLP, you'll have a variety of go-to stimulus materials and be skillful in a range of topics potentially interesting to a child.

Narratives. Narratives are a special form of language, self-initiated, self-controlled, and decontextualized. As such, narratives are an important part of the language assessment, especially for school-age children and adolescents, because they provide an uninterrupted sample of language that ideally, a child or adolescent modifies to capture and hold the listener's interest. The narrative speaker is responsible for ordering and providing all of the information in an organized whole.

Narratives differ in several ways from conversation:

- Narratives are extended units of text.
- Events within narratives are linked with one another temporally or causally in a cohesive, predictable, rule-governed manner.
- The speaker maintains a social monologue throughout, making relevant contributions to the overall narrative while remaining mindful of the information needed by the listener.
- Narratives have an agentive focus, meaning the characters are engaged in events over time.

Narratives fall roughly into personal and fictional categories. A child's ability to produce narratives is related to their success in acquisition of literacy (Catts et al., 2003; Griffin et al., 2004). For example, a kindergartner's ability to recall narratives is one of the strongest single predictors of reading success.

In the conversations of young children, personal narratives are far more prevalent than fictional ones. Personal stories are more useful to children in social interactions and, therefore, are a better gauge of narrative development than fictional ones. In fact, the structural characteristics of narratives develop initially within personal stories (Losh & Capps, 2003).

As speakers, we use personal narratives to define ourselves, to participate in conversations, and to amuse and teach. In addition, personal narratives play a role in social–emotional development, self-regulation, and academic success. Given the amount of research on fictional narratives and story retells, it's relatively easy to overlook personal narratives in favor of later developing fictional ones. To ensure that you don't make the same error, I urge you to read the very comprehensive article on personal narratives by Carol Westby and Barbare Culatta (2016).

Ignoring personal narratives may be shortsighted (Catts et al., 2003; Griffin et al., 2004; McCardle et al., 2001). The Common Core State Standards (National Governors Association Center for Best Practices and Council of Chief State School Officers, 2010) address students' ability to access and recount life experiences and to write personal narratives.

A few years ago, a first-grade teacher came to me concerned that a child in her class was having great difficulty with reading comprehension although his passing of a language screening test suggested he did not have a language disorder. In addition, he had no misarticulations, thus the assumption of no underlying phonological issues that might affect phonological awareness. I asked her to inquire of the child what he did over the weekend. To her surprise, he replied in one-word responses, even when asked for a longer explanation or a series of events. The child could not relate simple event narratives, leaving him seemingly unable to interpret the stories he read.

Both oral and written narratives should form a portion of every child's language assessment. The results can be compared with a child's other linguistic abilities prior to making judgments on the adequacy of the child's language system.

Narratives and Language Disorders. The personal event narratives of children with language disorders are often so disordered that these stories negatively impact the social interactions of these children (McCabe & Bliss, 2004–2005). The shorter personal narratives of children with language disorders often omit key information and violate chronological sequences of events. For example, compared with age-matched children with TDL, children with ASD have lower narrative production in terms of both macrostructure or overall organization and microstructure or internal linguistic structures, such as sentences (Hilvert et al., 2016).

In general, the narratives by children with ASD are less cohesive and coherent. The narratives of children with ASD are syntactically less complex, contain more ambiguous pronouns, and include fewer story grammar elements (Banney et al., 2015). In addition, school-age children with ASD and those with DLD produce similarly simple narratives, lacking semantic richness and omitting important story elements (Frazier Norbury et al., 2014).

In both story retelling and story generation tasks, school-age and young adolescent children with ASD demonstrate more ambiguous pronoun use than their peers with TDL (Novogrodsky & Edelson, 2016). Although pronoun errors would be rightly called syntactic problems, these errors demonstrate a pragmatic issue as well—a cognitive deficit in monitoring the listener's mental model of the story.

A storyteller must monitor what the listener knows. Children with TDL help bring their listeners along by monitoring their own production and noting listener responses. Children with ASD are less successful, relating, in part, to deficits in theory of mind.

In contrast. school-age children with attention-deficit/hyperactivity disorder (ADHD) recall less information from the stories they hear compared to their peers with TDL (Papaeliou et al., 2015). In addition, they are less sensitive to the importance of the information they recall and have difficulty answering factual questions. These deficits in narrative comprehension may be related to problems in attention and working memory.

Although we still lack definitive markers in the language of children with fetal alcohol spectrum disorder (FASD) that enable us to differentiate these children from others with language disorder, narratives offer a clue that needs further investigation. School-age children with FASD exhibit elevated grammatical error rates during narration compared to peers with TDL that may reflect the central nervous system abnormality associated with prenatal alcohol exposure (Thorne, 2017).

I hope that this information has alerted you to the need for narrative assessment. An SLP can accomplish this within a conversational sample or as a separate portion of a diagnostic assessment.

Summary

As we've seen, descriptive approaches, such as sampling, are not without problems. Although they are potentially more representative of a child's everyday performance than formal testing, this potential is not guaranteed. In addition, descriptive approaches require that an SLP have considerable knowledge of language and of the variables that affect children's language performance.

An Integrated Functional Assessment Strategy

Repeatedly, I and others have recommended a combined assessment approach. The purpose of an assessment should influence its design; thus, the approach should be an integrated whole. Almost universally, SLPs would agree that no single measure or session is adequate. Ideally, a functional language assessment will consist of multiple assessment techniques in a variety of relevant linguistic and nonlinguistic contexts.

Some behaviors are context dependent. For example, parent and teacher perceptions of specific social behaviors in children with ASD don't always agree (Murray et al., 2009). Parents seem to note more initiating interactions, whereas teachers note responding behaviors and maintaining interactions. This difference heightens the importance of multiple informants and settings.

Child variables to consider when designing and implementing the assessment process include the following:

- Chronological and functional age
- Background information, such as vision, hearing, and health concerns and/or other handicapping conditions
- Cultural and linguistic background
- Cognitive functioning
- Interests and materials available
- Activity level
- Ability to attend to stimulus items

The SLP readily adapts the methods to each child and is mindful that children will respond differently to different adults. In addition, caregiver concerns must be taken into consideration.

At this point, it might be good to add a note of caution. It is hoped that when you have completed an assessment, you'll be able to comment on a child's language ability and predict success with intervention. However, it can be difficult to identify which preschool children with late language emergence (LLE) are likely to have long-term problems (Reilly et al., 2010). Prognosis is also poor for children with comprehension deficits (Ellis & Thal, 2008). Although a family history of language or literacy problems is an additional risk factor (Rudolph & Leonard, 2016; Zambrana et al., 2014), prediction using LLE is still weak.

By age 4 years, the more areas of language disordered, the greater the likelihood that the problems will persist into school age. Sentence repetition tasks have been identified as a relatively good measure for predicting outcomes (Everitt et al., 2013).

For older children with language disorders, the problems are likely to persist. Given that the best predictor of how a child will do in school is the child's oral language skills, children who start school with language deficits are at risk for both reading problems and poor academic attainment (Catts et al., 2002; Thompson et al., 2015). Prognosis is especially poor when receptive language is impaired and when nonverbal ability is relatively low (Catts et al., 2002; Clark et al., 2007; Johnson et al., 2010; Rice & Hoffman, 2015).

CHAPTER 5 ASSESSMENT OF PRESCHOOL AND SCHOOL-AGE CHILDREN WITH LANGUAGE DISORDERS **175**

If you feel sufficiently cautioned, we're ready to begin. It's always good to be careful when we're affecting the lives of others.

A combined or integrated assessment approach might include a referral, questionnaire and/or caregiver interview, an environmental observation, an SLP-directed formal psychometric assessment, and a child-directed informal assessment consisting of dynamic assessment and a language sample. The actual components will differ with each child. Each component is discussed in the remainder of this chapter.

At each diagnostic step, objectives should be derived from the information collected to this point. Thus, each step becomes more focused, and the possible language problems are highlighted. Figure 5–3 presents a possible stage process of collecting data. As you proceed, data moves the process forward. The following discussion deals with a number of assessment steps, both formal and informal, that are aspects of an overall integrated functional model.

Referral, Screening, Questionnaire, and Interview

Caregivers—parents, teachers, and others—are central to a functional assessment and intervention process. Their input can be helpful on several levels.

Referral

Teachers can be a valuable referral source and should be encouraged to be alert for children with potential language problems. I've received referrals from parents and other family members and caregivers; social services agencies; grandparents and babysitters; nurses and physicians; teachers and aides; pastors, priests, and rabbis; and family friends. However, I cannot go forward with an evaluation without the express permission of a child's parents or legal caregivers.

Figure 5–3. A model of the assessment process.

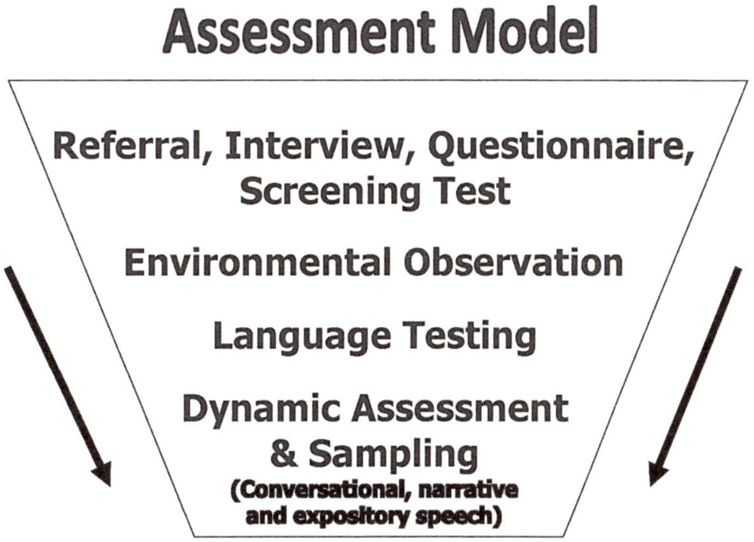

Assessment Model

Referral, Interview, Questionnaire, Screening Test

Environmental Observation

Language Testing

Dynamic Assessment & Sampling
(Conversational, narrative and expository speech)

Teachers will only be a good referral source if they are aware of the manifestations of a language disorder. This means that you will need to provide in-service training and appropriate materials for referral.

In a classroom, teachers may notice other variables in addition to language (Wittke & Spaulding, 2018). For example, preschool children with DLD, whose teachers perceive them as having poorer executive functioning, are more likely to receive language intervention services. We'll discuss teacher identification of children at risk for language disorder in Chapter 12.

Parents and medical professionals can also be effective referral sources for children with more severe language disorder; however, they are less reliable in identifying mild impairment (Conti-Ramsden et al., 2006). This is especially true for children with DLD who, by definition, lack other obvious disabilities.

Screening Tests

Some children will also be identified by screening tests. Currently, in most districts, all preschool, kindergarten, and first and second graders are screened annually.

Unfortunately, current language screening measures do not meet psychometric standards for identifying language disorder. Problematic issues include consideration of a child's socioeconomic background status, language status and dialect, the presence of hearing impairment, and test characteristics, all of which can affect results (Dockrell & Marshall, 2015). In addition, the language development paths of preschool children vary considerably, which may negate screening test results. Composite measures of language are better than single measures, even when screening for language disorder.

The difficulty in identifying children with ADHD and language disorder is illustrative. Subtle pragmatic difficulties may be missed in standard screening procedures. The Children's Communication Checklist–2 (CCC-2; Bishop, 2006) was developed, in part, to identify children with pragmatic language disorder and can be used for language screening. The CCC-2 has demonstrated sensitivity and specificity rates of 100% and 85.29%, respectively, when used as a screening tool with children with ADHD and language disorder (Timler, 2014).

Questionnaires and Interviews

A caregiver interview or questionnaire can be another valuable source of initial information on child functioning and on the perceived problem from the caregiver's perspective. Caregiver expectations for a child also provide an indication of a caregiver's willingness and perceived need to work with the child. Caregivers should be encouraged to ask questions and to participate further, especially with preschool children.

In face-to-face interviews with parents and teachers, it is best to ask questions in a straightforward manner, with no hesitation that might signal embarrassment or discomfort. It's also good practice to avoid tag questions (e.g., "You don't . . . , do you?") that seek agreement, rather than information. Responses should be treated matter-of-factly with little comment that might discourage a caregiver from talking.

CHAPTER 5 ASSESSMENT OF PRESCHOOL AND SCHOOL-AGE CHILDREN WITH LANGUAGE DISORDERS **177**

As an SLP, you'll be interested in the child's prenatal, perinatal, and postnatal medical history; family medical and educational history; the child's educational and social history; and descriptions of the child's behavior. A list of possible language questions is presented in Table 5–1.

Caregiver responses are analyzed and hypotheses are formed before deciding on the strategy for the remainder of the assessment. Potential language problems are researched thoroughly.

Observation

To gain an idea of a natural interaction, an SLP will want to observe caregiver(s) and peer(s) with the child as conversational partners in such everyday settings as the home and the classroom. In the classroom, an SLP might observe the child participating in a number of different activities. These situations, while ideal, are not always possible. Time may not permit just observation, in which case an SLP may observe closely while collecting a language sample and form tentative hypotheses for later confirmation.

If observation occurs in a more clinical setting, appropriate toys and both structured and nonstructured activities are provided for the child and conversational partner. Caregivers are encouraged to use familiar objects and the child's favorite toys or objects from home or the classroom.

The SLP can instruct caregivers to interact as typically as possible with the child. It is essential that caregivers not quiz or direct the child to perform during the observation. Ideally, the SLP unobtrusively remains in the room or leaves and observes from outside via observation windows or video monitors.

Although the frequency of various forms of behavior, such as conversational initiation, may be important, of most interest are the ways in which a child uses the various features of their language to interact with others.

Routine situations, such as play with familiar toys, may provide a preschool child with a scaffold or frame within which language processing becomes automatized. The SLP needs to assess the child's familiarity with the situation and the degree to which that situation provides a prop for the child's language. Atypical situations will not elicit typical language nor yield a representative sample of a child's language.

As an SLP, you'll gain some notion of what to observe from the caregiver interview. Reliability of observation is increased if your descriptions detail as closely as possible the actual observed behavior. It is best if the observation is digitally recorded for later referral. This can easily be accomplished on your smartphone or your tablet (Olswang et al., 2006).

Table 5–2 provides a list of some features that an SLP might observe. This list is not exhaustive. Each category is discussed in some detail in Chapter 7, where we consider the analysis of a conversational sample. The purpose of observation is to note within the larger scope of interaction the language characteristics to be tested, collected, and analyzed later in the assessment.

The selection of behaviors to be observed will affect the validity of the observation. The behavior should represent the underlying language feature of interest.

Table 5–1. Interview or Questionnaire Format

Questions Relative to Language Uses

How does the child let you know items desired?

What does the child request most frequently?

What does the child do when requesting that you do something?

When wanting you to pay attention?

When wanting something?

When wanting to direct your attention?

Does the child ask for information?

How does the child express emotion or tell about feelings?

What emotions does the child express?

Does the child make noises when playing alone?

Does the child engage in monologues while playing?

Does the child prefer to play alone or with others?

Does the child describe things in the environment? How?

Does the child discuss events in the past, future, or outside of the immediate context?

Questions Relative to Conversational Skill

When does the child communicate best?

How does the child respond when you say something? How does the child respond to others? Does the child interact more readily with certain people and in certain situations, and if so, with whom and when?

With whom and when does the child communicate most frequently?

Does the child initiate conversations or activities with you and with others? What is the child's most frequent topic? Does the child join in when others initiate conversations or activities?

Does the child get your attention before saying something to you? How does the child do this?

Does the child maintain eye contact while talking to you?

Does the child take turns when talking? Does the child interrupt? Are there long gaps between your utterances and the child's responses? Will the child take a turn without being instructed to do so or without being asked a question?

When the child speaks to you, is there an expectation of a response? What does the child do if you do not respond? When the child responds to you, does the response usually match or is it relevant to what you said?

How does the child ask for clarification? How frequently does this occur?

If you ask the child for more information or for clarification, what happens? Does the child demonstrate frustration when not understood?

CHAPTER 5 ASSESSMENT OF PRESCHOOL AND SCHOOL-AGE CHILDREN WITH LANGUAGE DISORDERS **179**

Table 5–1. *continued*

Questions Relative to Conversational Skill *continued*
When the child asks for or tells you something, is there usually enough information for you to understand?
When the child tells you more complex information or relates an event or a story, is it organized enough for you to follow the train of thought?
Does the child have different ways of talking to different people, such as adults and small children? Does the child phrase things in different ways with different listeners? Is the child more polite in some situations?
Does the child seem confused at times? What does the child do if confused?
Questions Relative to Form and Content
Is the child able to understand simple directions?
Does the child know the names of common events, objects, and people in the environment? What types of information does the child provide about these (actions, objects, people, descriptions, locations, causation, functions, etc.)?
Does the child seem to rely on gestures, sounds, or the immediate environment to be understood?
Does the child speak in single words, phrases, or sentences? How long is a typical utterance? Does the child leave out words? Are the child's sentences complex or simple? How does the child ask questions?
Does the child use pronouns and articles to distinguish old and new information?
Does the child use words for time, such as tomorrow, yesterday, or last night? Does the child use verb tenses? Can the child put several sentences together to form complex descriptions and explanations?

Sources: Compiled from Brinton and Fujiki (1989), Lund and Duchan (1993), and Spinelli and Terrell (1984).

Reliability of observation is not fortuitous. Although the SLP has no control over what happens during an observation, reliability can be increased by the following:

- Describing the behaviors to be observed as carefully as possible, and training with another observer to ensure good interobserver reliability. By comparing their ratings, the two observers can sharpen the description of the behavior and note possible confusion.

- Recording data on only one type of behavior at a time. This procedure may require the use of digital recording so the observation can be replayed for data collection with other behaviors.

- Not making summation judgments while observing. Judgments about overall behavior are best left until after the data are analyzed.

Table 5–2. Features to Note While Observing the Child

Form of language. Does the child use single words, phrases, or sentences primarily? Are the sentences of the subject–verb–object form exclusively? Are there mature negatives, interrogatives, and passive sentences? Does the child elaborate the noun or verb phrase? Is there evidence of embedding and conjoining?

Understanding of semantic intent. Does the child respond appropriately to the various question forms (what, where, who, when, why, how)? Does the child confuse words from different semantic classes?

Are there frequent fillers or empty words (*thing, one, that*)?

Are relational words, such as prepositions and conjunctions, used correctly?

Language use. Does the child display a range of illocutionary functions, such as asking for information, help, and objects; replying; making statements; and providing information? Does the child take meaningful conversational turns? Does the child introduce topics and maintain them through several turns? Does the child signal the status of the communication and make repairs?

Rate of speaking. Is the rate inordinately slow or fast? Are there noticeable or lengthy pauses between the caregiver's and child's turn? Are there noticeable or lengthy pauses between the child's adjacent utterances? Does the child use fillers frequently or pause before producing certain words? Are there frequent word substitutions?

Sequencing. Does the child relate events in a sequential fashion based on the order of occurrence? Can the child discuss the recent past or recount stories? Are sequential sentences cohesive and easy to follow?

Formal Language Testing

The transition to more formal testing might be accomplished through the use of a nonthreatening receptive task, possibly one requiring only a pointing response. Such a task allows a child to become accustomed to an SLP and to testing. An annotated list of several current tests is presented in Appendix A.

Assessing All Aspects of Language

It is important as an SLP to perform a thorough assessment of a child's language. This task may necessitate more than one evaluative session. Only rarely is a language disorder limited to one aspect of language. Should this be the case, however, testing thoroughly confirms the absence of problems and provides a holistic image of the child's language. Even when problems in a single area are suspected, more than a single method should be used in order to best describe the language area of concern.

It's difficult to measure the degree of a child's developing language knowledge. Procedures such as tests measure current behavior, but use of language relies on the more subtle processes of retrieval and preparation. Formulation of an utterance is not an insulated process. Language production and comprehension rely on the similar types of

CHAPTER 5 ASSESSMENT OF PRESCHOOL AND SCHOOL-AGE CHILDREN WITH LANGUAGE DISORDERS **181**

knowledge (Bock et al., 2007). As an SLP, you'll be challenged to measure and describe behaviors and also to try to determine the cause of, or the reason for, the behavior. We'll discuss some cognitive issues later in this section.

While trying to take a holistic view of language, an SLP must also decide carefully what to emphasize and which measures to use. Vocabulary tests are especially poor at identifying language disorder. Tests that measure grammatical skills and/or verbal working memory (VWM) are considerably better.

Suspected disorders may require different procedures and measures. For example, measures of verb tensing, nonword repetition, sentence recall, and narrative abilities are good for identifying DLD but are not definitive (Pawlowska, 2014; Redmond et al., 2011). In contrast, young school-age children with ADHD have few difficulties with tense marking or sentence recall (Redmond, 2004).

Omnibus language tests such as the Clinical Evaluation of Language Fundamentals–Fifth Edition (CELF-5; Wiig et al., 2013) will cover many aspects of language. Although the CELF-5 offers a good overview of a child's language, an SLP will still need further assessment measures in areas of concern. In the following section, we discuss each aspect of language. Each has its own issues.

Pragmatics. The pragmatic difficulties of children with ASD or traumatic brain injury (TBI) may be missed on traditional tests, which tend to focus mostly on linguistic structure and meaning rather than on language use (Anderson et al., 2005; Bishop & Baird, 2001; Young et al., 2005). In fact, most of the most common assessment instruments fail to measure pragmatic skills. This poses a special problem for children, such as Jake, with high-functioning ASD (HFA) who may score within normal limits on traditional language measures but are still in need of intervention for dysfunctional social language skills that are evident in conversation and in the classroom (Young et al., 2005).

Pragmatics has proven difficult to assess. Because pragmatics is defined as a context-dependent behavior, the rigid structure of most formal language tests fails to measure a speaker's adjustment to changing circumstances. In addition, the clear instructions in a concrete context, such as a standardized testing situation, may enable children with pragmatic difficulties to perform much better than they do in a naturalistic setting. Although some pragmatic tools, such as the Test of Pragmatic Language–Second Edition (TOPL-2; Phelps-Terasaki & Phelps-Gunn, 2007), do exist, they sometimes fail to capture the full range of deficits, such as those in children with HFA.

A supplemental measure is parent/caregiver descriptions of a child's language observed in the home. Ratings provided by parents are particularly informative because parents have access to their children's behavior across a variety of contexts. Such assessment may represent a child's typical level of functioning more than the child's performance on a one-time test procedure. In addition, some behaviors may be difficult to elicit in test situations.

The CCC-2 (Bishop, 2003, 2006) is an example of a parent/caregiver assessment tool. Respondents are asked to rate the frequency with which a described behavior occurs, such as repeating memorized language. The CCC-2 asks about a range of clinically significant pragmatic impairments that other formal standardized pragmatic test instruments, such as the TOPL-2, may not measure (Adams, 2002; Volden & Phillips, 2010).

Teachers can also be a valuable source of information, although they tend to focus on academic rather than pragmatic issues (Redmond, 2002). One result is that children with ADHD are underidentified.

Standardized, norm-referenced social language tests are of limited value. Tests such as TOPL-2 provide hypothetical language situations that may not mirror a child's daily experience. Although these tests have a place, language sampling is a more promising tool for validating concerns about pragmatic skills (Adams et al., 2011; Norbury, 2014; Paul & Norbury, 2012).

LSA offers the following advantages (Timler, 2018b):

- Provides a baseline of the student's verbal and nonverbal behaviors that can be used to develop intervention goals
- Can be repeated as often as needed to document improvement and identify needed modifications in intervention goals
- May be the only tool to capture concerns noted by parents and teachers

Semantics. Although children with language disorders have a range of semantic difficulties with acquisition, storage, and retrieval, most formal assessments are limited to receptive and expressive vocabulary. Few standardized tests assess multiple aspects of semantic knowledge. At the very least, we are interested in word knowledge, novel word learning, word categories, figurative language, multiple meanings, and word-finding.

Word Knowledge. When has a child learned a word? Tests typically assume word knowledge is an all-or-nothing phenomenon. In reality, acquisition of word knowledge is a gradual process. An individual child's success or failure on a test item may be dependent on several factors, such as the type of task or the manner of eliciting the child's response. Testing tasks are often contrived, out of context, and highly literate.

Typical methods of testing semantic abilities are picture identification, word definitions, and word categories. Comprehension vocabulary usually is measured by having a child point to a picture that best represents the word. Such tests tell an SLP very little about the frequency of use or the depth or breadth of a child's understanding of the concept. Comprehension of longer utterances usually is assessed by having a child follow simple commands or again point to pictures.

When a word is not fully understood by a child, they may rely on other comprehension strategies, such as word order, or on nonlinguistic features, such as the position or size of stimulus items in the picture. During testing, an SLP should note behaviors such as locational preferences in pointing responses and verbal comments that accompany responding and may indicate what influences the child's choices.

Expressive or productive vocabulary usually is tested by having a child supply a name or definition. Scoring is often correct or incorrect. In contrast, scaled scoring (0–1–2) allows for partially correct responses but can be extremely difficult to judge reliably.

As with any test, an SLP's insight or the use of other methods may be more valuable. For example, descriptions of the type of definition given can be valuable in determining the maturity of the child's lexicon. Early definitions often rely on use, as in *An apple is something you eat.* These are followed developmentally by descriptions, then use in context, adding synonyms and explanations, and finally, conventional definitions. The entire developmental process takes years to accomplish.

Novel Word Learning. One way to examine word learning in process is to employ the Diagnostic Evaluation of Language Variance–Norm Referenced (Seymour et al., 2018) subtest of novel word learning. SLPs also may wish to develop their own evaluative instruments (Brackenbury & Pye, 2005). For example, incidental learning can be examined using either unknown words or nonsense words within contexts in which the referent or entity referred to is present but not directly defined. Follow-up testing can determine if the word was learned.

A number of factors, such as word length, syllable structure, and familiarity of consonant clusters, influence VWM, where words are held while processing. For this reason, an SLP designing informal measures should research this area thoroughly (Brackenbury & Pye, 2005). Typically, VWM is assessed through nonword repetition tasks such as those found in the Children's Test of Nonword Repetition (Gathercole & Baddeley, 1996). Assessment of WM is discussed later.

Word Categories, Figurative Language, and Multiple Meanings. Several assessment instruments have subtests of semantic categories and relational words, such as prepositions. Sorting and labeling tasks (*These are all . . .*) and following directions (*Put the red square next to the green circle*) can be used in informal assessment.

Categorical understanding is assessed by asking the child to supply an antonym or a synonym, to name related words in a category, or to identify the category. These types of tasks are important when assessing the language of children from late elementary to high school.

As an SLP, use caution. Word-association tasks such as naming another member of a category (zoo animals) may be ineffectual in differentiating children with language disorders and those without. Responses are dependent more on life experience, the familiarity of the category being asked, and the number of responses possible.

Other semantic-related tasks include stating similarities and differences, telling all one knows about a word, detecting semantic absurdities, explaining figurative language, and noting multiple meanings. Each task requires different abilities—including determining the task demands, focusing on critical semantic dimensions, and interpreting cues—that can be complicated by word-retrieval difficulties.

Word-Finding. Little is known about word-retrieval processes. Children with LD or TBI exhibit word-finding and word-substitution difficulties. Late elementary school children with LD exhibit more visually related word-substitution errors, such as saying *shoe* for *sandal*, than do children with TDL. Additional word-finding substitutions found in children with LD include functional descriptions, such as *book holder* for *shelf*.

Although testing may reveal a deficit in naming skills, such tests rarely indicate the nature of the deficit. Identification of the word-retrieval strategies of these children may aid in the design of remediation techniques directly related to these strategies.

Word-finding difficulties can be assessed formally with measures such as the Test of Word Finding–Third Edition (German, 2014). Informally, an SLP can ask for the names of pictures and categories and can use sentence-completion tasks that include a definition or description (*You call someone on your ___*). An SLP must be flexible here. Getting the correct answer is not as important as using the task to try to discover underlying processes.

It's important to distinguish between words unknown to the child and those known but difficult to retrieve. If a child can identify referents receptively but not name them on a different occasion, word-retrieval problems may be present. In informal assessment, especially in severe cases, such as the initial stage of recovery from TBI, it may be useful to begin with common everyday objects and actions in the environment.

One method for attaining more information from tests is a double-naming technique. In this procedure, a standard naming test is administered twice. The results are examined to identify error response groups that occur once and twice. The errors that occur on both administrations require further analysis.

The SLP can administer a number of prompts with the double-error words to determine if the errors indicate word-finding difficulties and to identify naming strategies. In this procedure, cues can be administered in the following order (Fried-Oken, 1987):

1. *General question.* The child is asked a general, open-ended question, such as "Can you think of another word for this?" or "What is this again?"

2. *Semantic/phonemic facilitator.* If the child is incorrect or unable to answer, two cues, based on additional semantic and phonemic information, can be administered. The order of presentation varies, but the SLP should record carefully the order and the response. The semantic cue describes the object's function, provides a categorical label, or states the location, as in "It's something you sit on," "It's a piece of furniture," or "You find it in the living room." The child's response to each type of semantic prompt should be noted. A phonemic cue includes the initial phoneme of the desired label ("The word starts with a /_/.").

3. *Verification.* If a child is still incorrect, the SLP provides the correct label and asks whether the child has ever seen this object before in order to verify whether the word is in the child's repertoire.

The child's responses and the cues are analyzed to determine the qualitative nature of the errors and the child's naming strategy. Possible naming strategies of 4- to 9-year-old children, regardless of whether you use this assessment method, are listed in Table 5–3, targeting the word "shoe."

Syntax. Syntactic testing can be extremely complicated because of the complexity and diversity of the syntactic system. SLPs may wish to use entire test batteries or portions of several tests. The latter strategy is recommended for in-depth probing of potential problem areas. Naturally, when tests are used in a nonstandard manner or test items are combined from several tests, the norms can no longer be used. No matter the method of data collection, results must be described accurately and interpreted in light of the tasks involved.

CHAPTER 5 ASSESSMENT OF PRESCHOOL AND SCHOOL-AGE CHILDREN WITH LANGUAGE DISORDERS **185**

Table 5–3. Naming Strategy Hypotheses: Target Word Is *Shoe*

Child's Behavior	Possible Naming Strategy
Child says, "Chew."	Word association may be phonological.
Child says, "Show."	Word association may be phonological.
Child says, "Boot" or "Sneaker."	Word association may be categorical or semantic.
Child says, "Heel."	Word association may be part/whole.
Child says, "Foot" or "Walk."	Word association may be functional.
Circumlocution	
Child says, "Looks kind of like a car."	Child is using perceptual circumlocution.
Child says, "You wear it."	Child is using functional circumlocution.
Child says, "It has holes and strings."	Child is using descriptional circumlocution.
Incorrect or non-answer	
Child says, "Sky."	Unrelated. Probe to see if there is a hidden or unperceived relationship.
Child says, "Thing" or "That."	Nonspecific
Child says, "I don't know."	Comment
Child does not respond.	Nonresponse
Child mimes putting on a shoe.	Gestural response

Note: One misnomer does not mean that the child has word-finding difficulties and does not establish a pattern. Always probe behind the child's response. Naming strategies are a key to the way in which a child organizes their world.

Source: Information taken from Fried-Oken (1987).

There is considerable variability across tests in the length of individual syntactic items, the structures tested, and the type of testing tasks used. Test tasks can range from highly unnatural ones, such as ordering of scrambled words into a sentence, to more natural tasks, such as sentence combining. Many mirror the highly decontextualized tasks found in school, such as fill-in-the-blank, but do not reflect everyday language use.

A thorough language assessment should include evaluation of both comprehension and production. Although the receptive procedures used and the structures assessed vary widely across tests, the common element is that a child demonstrates understanding—usually by pointing to a picture or following directions—while producing only minimal language, if any.

Syntactic production typically is tested by using structured elicitation, a sentence imitation format, word-ordering, or correction judging. In structured elicitation, a child might be asked to describe a picture, following a model by the test administrator. The model sentence establishes the sentence form to be used (*She is running*) but differs from the desired sentence by the structure being tested (*Tomorrow, she . . .*).

In sentence imitation, a child gives an immediate repetition of the test administrator's sentence. The underlying assumption is that sentences which exceed a child's WM will be reproduced according to a child's own linguistic rule system, which the child must use as a processing aid. Theoretically, the child's sentence should be very similar to the one the child would produce spontaneously. I once tested a child who did not repeat any articles on the sentence imitation test, and subsequently, in his language sample, he also used no articles.

Given the holistic nature of language, it shouldn't surprise us that sentence repetition tasks measure more than just sentence imitation. Sentence repetition performance reflects an underlying language ability factor that crosses several aspects of language and cognition (Klem et al., 2015).

The validity of elicited imitation has been questioned. Although the performance of children with language disorders on elicited imitation tests can be enhanced by the addition of contextual cues, such as pictures or object manipulation, their imitations are still simpler than their spontaneous language production.

Because the relationship between elicited imitation and spontaneously produced language is very complex, SLPs are advised to use elicited imitation results with caution and to rely on the data from spontaneous samples when the two differ. Elicited imitation responses should be analyzed for the specific ways they differ from the model. Such analysis is much richer than simple correct/incorrect scoring. The SLP needs to understand how a child is responding. For example, other than exact sentence imitation responses may

- maintain the intended meaning;
- change the intended meaning;
- omit a word or phrase;
- substitute a word or phrase;
- add a word or phrase;
- change the word order; or
- produce an ungrammatical sentence.

In addition, the SLP should note the influence of sentence length and complexity, which are related to the child's WM functioning.

Tasks requiring the judging of grammatical acceptability are of two varieties. The first merely asks for a judgment, whereas the second requires the child to fix the errant structure. Although the second is more difficult, both require metalinguistic skill, which does not begin to form until approximately age 5 years. You may recall that **metalinguistics** is the ability to consider language out of context. These types of tasks, as well as making judgments of similarity and difference, are inappropriate for preschool children.

Morphology. Morphological testing usually focuses on bound inflectional morphemes, such as plural *–s* or past tense *-ed*. Most tests emphasize these suffixes because of their high usage and relatively early development. In general, children with good spoken and written language abilities have more morphological awareness and do better on such tests.

Suffixes can be divided into two types: inflectional and derivational. Inflectional suffixes indicate possession, gender, and number in nouns; tense, voice, person and number, and mood in verbs; and comparison in adjectives. They do not change the part of speech of the base word. For example, a noun can be made plural with the addition of the -s marker but remains a noun.

Derivational suffixes are ignored in most tests, although the CELF-5 assesses a few. Derivational suffixes have a smaller range of application and many more constraints and irregularities than inflectional suffixes. Application may be unpredictable, as with -tion, which can be added to some but not all nouns. Also, morpheme meaning may not be explicit. It's estimated that more than 80% of multimorpheme words do not mean what the constituent parts suggest. The development of derivational suffixes is related to oral language production abilities, reading level and exposure, derivational complexity, and metalinguistic awareness.

The two most common expressive test formats for morphology are *cloze*, or sentence completion, and sentence imitation. Most cloze procedure test items give the root word and require the child to respond with the root plus a suffix, as in *teach* and *teacher*. Other testing tasks might include judgments of relatedness of words, such as *hospital* and *hospitable*; ability to deduce meaning from component parts; and ability to form words in different and changing linguistic contexts.

Although several tests have morphological portions or subtests, most have too few items and too narrow a scope to provide much valuable information. In addition, prefixes and derivational suffixes are included on only a few tests.

Narrative Test and Measures

A number of narrative language tests exist, including the Edmonton Narrative Norms Instrument (ENNI; Schneider et al., 2005); the Expression, Reception & Recall of Narration Instrument (ERRNI; Bishop, 2004); the Test of Narrative Language–2 (Gillam & Pearson, 2018); and the Narrative Language Measure (Petersen & Spencer, 2012). The ENNI (ages 4;0–9;11 years) is available at http://www.rehabresearch.ualberta.ca/enni/. Narratives can also be assessed through sampling.

Interestingly, the performance of school-age children with ASD on the ERRNI (Bishop, 2004) is significantly poorer than that of their peers with TDL. These results suggest that the ERRNI may reveal pragmatic difficulties that may not be identified by other measures (Volden et al., 2017).

Test Modification

As mentioned previously, tests can be modified to provide the information sought by an SLP. For example, as an SLP, you may wish to test a child's pronoun use in-depth. No test is available that adequately assesses only these structures. You might construct your own assessment tool from items of other tests. Although this type of locally prepared test may be very useful and is acceptable practice, test standards of administration have been violated and the norms would be invalid.

Occasionally, published tests include subtest norms. In this case, a subtest may be administered in its entirety as directed in the instructions, and the norming information would be applicable.

Test administration may also be modified for a child who cannot perform as required or for further investigation of the child's response strategies. The obvious example is a child with cerebral palsy who may need an alternative way of responding to a pointing task. Similarly, use of pictures or repetition of instructions may enhance the performance of some children.

It's important to remember that nearly all tests are designed for children with TDL. Thus, the child with IDD or ASD may be at a very distinct disadvantage. In such cases, description of a child's performance under modified conditions may be much more useful for intervention planning than a test score.

Testing procedures may also be modified through the use of multiple sessions, increased time to respond, and increased trials. For children with LD or ADHD, an SLP might enlarge materials, use a penlight or pointer, highlight certain information, verbally remind the child to attend, add additional practice items, or have the child repeat the test cue prior to responding.

The performance of children with motor problems, ASD, or LD might be affected also by visual or auditory distractions, placement of materials, temperature, lighting, light and dark contrasts, and positioning. Children who perseverate may need to be reminded that the answer for one item is not the same for another. Children with WM challenges may need to have cues repeated, to repeat cues aloud themselves, or to have cues broken into easily processible units.

Finally, children with TBI may need a longer time to respond. The SLP also should test beyond base and ceiling scores to identify "islands" of learning. Other modifications for children with TBI may include reduction of distractions, different response modes, enlarged print and reduction of print per page, simplified instructions, substituting multiple-choice questions to facilitate recall, giving multiple examples, providing breaks when fatigue is evident, and darkening lines or print in visual displays.

Finally, we cannot assume that norms are stable. They change over time. In addition, changes in the format of the test, such as offering it on computer, may also change the norms. New editions of a test may be based on SLP feedback, efficiency in testing, and new research. New editions require new norms. Part of your SLP responsibility will be keeping current on new editions of tests and EBP on current test use.

Assessment of Related Cognitive Factors

Given the number of language disorders and associated disorders, it seems remiss not to at least mention assessment of information processing and WM concerns. Children with a variety of disorders exhibit difficulty processing verbal information (Chiat & Roy, 2007; Conti-Ramsden, 2003; Haynes & Pindzola, 2012; Kohnert, 2013; Leonard et al., 2007; Munson et al., 2005; Rispens & Baker, 2012).

Although questions about cognitive functioning should be answered by a team that includes at least a neurologist, a psychologist, and an SLP, probing by the SLP can answer some questions and suggest alternative methods of both assessment and intervention.

CHAPTER 5 ASSESSMENT OF PRESCHOOL AND SCHOOL-AGE CHILDREN WITH LANGUAGE DISORDERS 189

Standardized testing is no substitute for comprehension and production of language in real-life contexts. Similarly, assessment of WM might contribute important information about a child's cognitive function over and above information from other measures (Gray et al., 2019).

Information Processing

Difficulty with information processing includes weaknesses in three areas (Kohnert, 2013; Singleton & Shulman, 2014):

- Speed of information processing
- Working memory
- Selective/sustained attention

Based on these deficits, we assume that children with language disorders have difficulties with the mental operations needed to manipulate linguistic information.

In measurement of information processing skill, an SLP may ask a child to do the following:

- Recall lists of words
- Repeat number sequences, such as "5–6–3–8"
- Repeat a series of nonsense words, or "non-words"

These cognitive tasks are especially sensitive to memory problems in children with language disorders (Chiat & Roy, 2007; Hoffman & Gillam, 2004; Laws & Bishop, 2003).

Of most importance are changes in performance under varying task demands. The SLP can assess a child's performance by varying the speed of information using both familiar and unfamiliar words and structures (Ellis Weismer & Evans, 2002). Usually, there is a trade-off between accuracy and timing.

In addition, the SLP should use the *test–teach–retest* form of dynamic assessment, the most ecologically sound manner for assessing cognitive functioning (Gillam et al., 2002). Dynamic assessment, described later, is concerned with the child's ability to learn rather than their level of past learning. The retest phase is focused on the kinds of change that have occurred in response to the teaching. Of interest throughout are the child's ability to attend, perceive, and recall information; understand explanations; relate past information to new; infer; and generalize.

Working Memory

Many measures of language, such as the CELF-5 Following Direction and Formulated Sentences subtests, have inherent WM demands. SLPs should consider the storage and processing requirements of language assessment tools and consider how these demands may influence a child's performance. Tasks that require a child to hold onto multiple pieces of information while engaging in a mental activity, such as determining the correctness of a sentence, require VWM. By analyzing the pattern of a child's errors, an SLP can make standardized testing more informative (Ellis Weismer & Evans, 2002). If the SLP hypothesizes that the test results indicate a possible VWM deficit, they can assess further to determine if this may be the case.

Given the significant role VWM plays in language acquisition and learning, you, as an SLP, should include some measure of VWM in a thorough language assessment, especially for children with developmental language disorder (DLD). This may be warranted especially if memory is a concern, as in children with TBI, if memory difficulties have been implicated by other testing or observation, or if underlying factors seem to be contributing to language or academic difficulties (Boudreau & Costanza-Smith, 2011).

A central task to assessing the language performance of children with DLD and other disorders is determining to what extent a child's language and academic problems are related to deficits in linguistic knowledge, deficient VWM abilities, slower processing speed, or a combination of these and other factors. Performance on standardized tests may also be affected, especially for children with DLD who have poor test performance (Leonard et al., 2007; Montgomery & Windsor, 2007). Although standardized language tests seem especially taxing of VWM abilities for children with DLS, they are not for age-matched peers with TDL.

VWM Assessment. An SLP can perform careful analyses of children's performance on standardized language tests to hypothesize on the effects of VWM abilities on poor language performance. Inability to recall a list of words in order to find a common category or to recall a sentence for sentence imitation can greatly influence language performance.

By informally manipulating factors such as the number of units to be recalled, an SLP can determine whether VWM is a contributing factor. For example, in narrative retelling, poor memory may be inferred based on a child's performance on various probe questions, whereas story retelling can be evaluated for responses that indicate a loss of information.

Other informal assessment techniques might include an SLP systematically varying their speaking rate as well as volume and complexity while presenting language information. This will enable the SLP to observe the degree to which memory and comprehension of material are affected by input rate.

On the output side, systematically varying the time children have to complete language production tasks, such as single word retrieval, sentence production, narrative, description, and explanation, may document how children manage multiple memory and language demands. In this way, the SLP may gain a sense of the conditions under which children have trouble coordinating their language and memory (Montgomery et al., 2010).

WM capacity is more formally assessed using a variety of tasks. Listening span is measured by having children listen to sets of sentences that increase in number. They are then asked to respond to the correctness of each sentence, a processing task, and to recall as many sentence-final words as possible, a storage task.

Nonword repetition (NWR) tasks are designed to measure phonologic processing efficiency independent of lexical knowledge (Gillam et al., 2002). A child must maintain an accurate phonological representation of unfamiliar phonologic information in memory. On both the Children's Test of Nonword Repetition (Gathercole & Baddeley, 1996) and the Nonword Repetition Task (NRT; Dollaghan & Campbell, 1998), a child is required to repeat lists of nonwords, which vary in both the number of nonwords and the number of syllables represented in each.

Tests should be carefully chosen to ensure EBP and appropriateness for different age children. For example, although the NRT has been recommended as an assessment tool for school-age children, its use with preschool children results in children being misidentified as having a language disorder (Deevy et al., 2010). The precise words and materials chosen must be based on a child's linguistic background and experience (Schwob et al., 2021).

A plethora of studies have assessed the diagnostic worth of NWR tasks in detecting DLD in both monolingual and bilingual children. Currently, the factors contributing to differences found across children with DLD and those without are not fully explained, although the diagnostic accuracy of these tasks is generally near acceptable thresholds (Schwob et al., 2021). Furthermore, sensitivity and specificity values, although high, are not significantly high enough to recommend the use of NWR alone. As in any good assessment, other measures are essential for an accurate diagnosis.

Assessment of memory impairment can and should be made independent of other cognitive abilities (Gathercole & Alloway, 2006). This is an area in which an SLP can turn to other team members, such as the school or district psychologist. A variety of standardized tools and informal methods for assessing WM are presented in Appendix A.

For now, the best diagnostic techniques appear to be rote memory tasks, such as counting or sequential digit recall, NWR, rule induction (see description of dynamic assessment of children from diverse backgrounds in Chapter 9), story recall, grammatical completion, especially verb markers, number of different words in a speech sample, and memory plus interpretation tasks while listening or reading. The Language and Working Memory Lab at Western University in Canada offers an online DLD Toolbox with information on differential diagnosis of DLD (Archibald, 2021).

Summary

In the discussion of the GEM model in Chapter 2, four cognitive factors (fluid reasoning, controlled attention, complex WM, and language knowledge in long-term memory [LTM]) were presented. These factors are part of a comprehensive language assessment. Gillam and colleagues recommend the following types of assessment that might be appropriate:

- *Fluid reasoning.* In the Matrices subtest of the Kaufman Brief Intelligence Test (Kaufman & Kaufman, 2014), children are asked to examine abstract designs and complete visual analogy problems that complete a pattern.

- *Controlled attention.* The Test of Everyday Attention for Children (Manly et al., 2016) can be used to assess auditory attention and sustained attention. Children silently count the number of tones heard.

- *Complex WM.* In the Competing Language Processing Task (Gaulin & Campbell, 1994), a child judges the truthfulness of sentences that are heard. In addition, the child tries to recall as many sentence-final words as possible, thus dividing attention between language processing and verbal storage. Other useful auditory

WM measures include the Woodcock–Johnson III Tests of Cognitive Abilities (Woodcock et al., 2001) and the Working Memory Rating Scale (Alloway et al., 2009).

- *Language knowledge in LTM.* Complex tasks such as narration that require a child to manage several aspects of language at once can be used to assess language knowledge.

These four tasks can be used by an SLP to differentiate children with DLD from children with TDL (Gillam et al., 2019).

Dynamic Assessment

More traditional, static assessments, such as standardized testing, focus primarily on learning outcomes or products, characterized by *what was learned*, rather than on learning processes, characterized by *how something is being learned*. In contrast, dynamic assessment focuses on the learning process itself, thus allowing SLPs to measure emerging skills. As such, dynamic assessment involves comparing a child's independent performance with their supported performance.

For example, we know that understanding the morphological structure of words can help older elementary students better determine the meaning of unfamiliar words by means of a morphological–semantic analysis. Targeted assessment, such as SLP-designed testing (*What does X mean?*), can predict how students will respond to morphologically based vocabulary intervention. Dynamic assessment, such as breaking a word into morphemes (*Can you break the word into smaller meaningful pieces?*), can significantly increase the prediction of individual student response to intervention (Gellert & Arnbak, 2020). These data suggest that a combination of assessment methods yields the best predictive information.

Wolter and colleagues (2020) have developed the Dynamic Measure of Morphological Awareness (DMMA), a valid and reliable measure of early school-age morphological awareness (MA) and analysis in children with DLD. The results provide support for the use of dynamic assessment to measure MA in early elementary school children.

Although we don't have space to describe the DMMA in detail, highlighting the levels of prompting may help you understand dynamic assessment better. First, a word is presented verbally, and the child is asked what the word means. If the child is incorrect, the word is repeated, pausing on and emphasizing the morphemic units, and the child is asked the meaning again. An incorrect response or no response would be followed by the SLP providing a verbal repetition of the original word with picture support. Finally, the SLP would provide verbal repetition with pausing and emphasis on the morphemic units and picture support. These prompts are further explained in the appendices that accompany the article by Wolter et al. (2020).

Sampling

Conversational sampling has the potential for providing the most accurate description of the child's language as it is actually used in conversational exchange. Although sampling may include free-play and unstructured conversation, it more often includes structured conversation and probing of language features noted in observation and testing. Other sampling formats are picture descriptions, narrative retells, and expository language. In the next several chapters, we discuss all these ways to maximize the information from this source.

Conclusion

There is no one definitive method for assessing children with language disorders. A combination of interviewing, observation, testing, dynamic assessment, and sampling/probing offers a holistic approach that can incorporate not only the child but also significant others and familiar communication contexts.

It's important as you move through an assessment not to become too absorbed in the minutia of various isolated language features. This "missing the forest for the trees" approach can result in less than adequately describing the holistic nature of the child's communication system. At the very least, SLPs, need to take into account

- the areas of language affected;
- the impact on a child and the effect on the child's communication environment;
- the presence or absence of other impairments;
- the developmental path; and
- the age of onset (Reilly et al., 2014).

Once all the data are assembled, final analysis begins. More data may be needed. If collection can be characterized as somewhat scientific in its approach, analysis, although similar in nature, requires more of the artist in SLPs, as they paint an individual portrait of each child with a language disorder.

Results can be confounded by socioeconomic status, languages spoken, dialect, and test characteristics. Therefore, it's vital that multiple measures of language performance be used rather than single measures (Dockrell & Marshall, 2015).

Another support for multiple measures relates to genetics and the environment. Even among adolescents, both genetic and environmental factors contribute to language abilities, although their influence varies with the area of language assessed and the method of assessment (Harlaar et al., 2016).

Although more research is needed, genetic factors seem to have more influence on formal language test performance, whereas environmental factors have more influence on the results of more informal language sampling, the topic of the next few chapters.

Recall that we briefly mentioned sampling. It's now time to unpack that box.

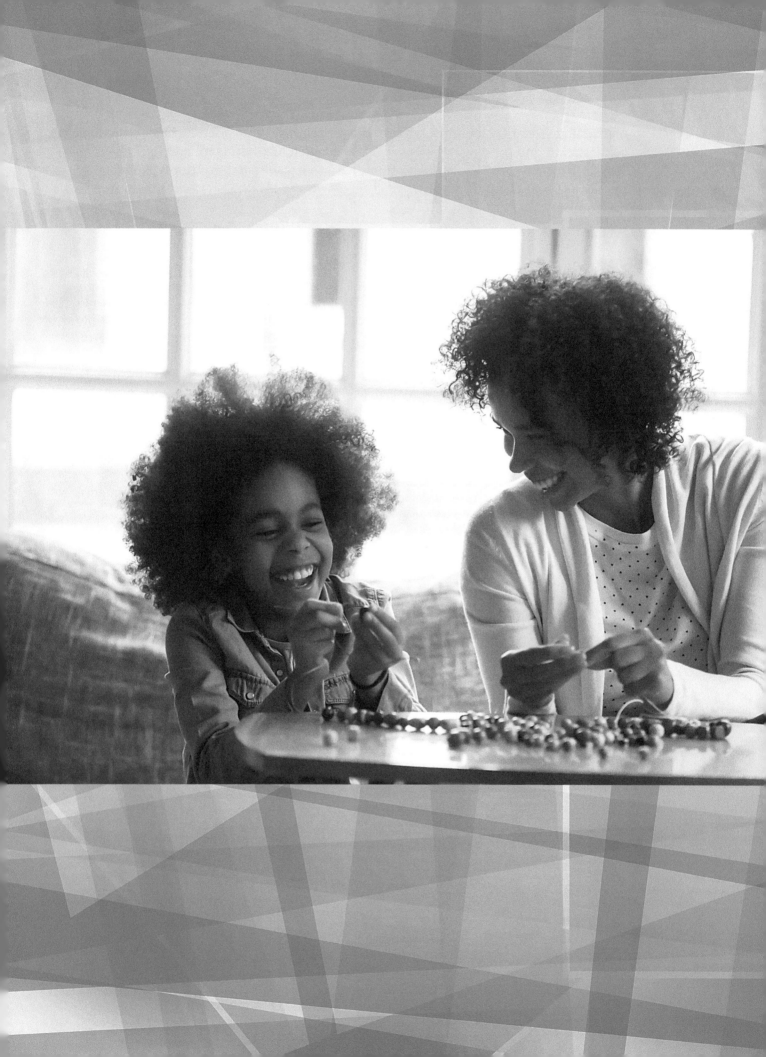

CHAPTER 6

LANGUAGE SAMPLING

Kesha's mother reported that her daughter seemed to be developing typically until she turned age 4 years. According to her mother, Kesha seemed to be less advanced in language. She didn't talk much with other children, showed little interest in group activities such as circle time, and expressed little interest in books.

Her teacher described her language as "truncated" or shortened. Kesha only rarely spoke in full sentences, and when she did, she omitted verb endings and auxiliary verbs.

Although other teachers equated Kesha's language performance to her use of African American English, her teacher was not so dismissive of Kesha's language. Her teacher was more concerned with Kesha's seeming lack of understanding and short sentences.

Language testing revealed that Kesha's language was in excess of –1 standard deviation (SD). She had difficulty imitating complex sentences and remembering directions. The preschool speech-language pathologist (SLP) decided it would be more appropriate to see Kesha's language in context by collecting a language sample.

Although standardized tests of language often figure prominently during evaluations, heavy reliance on these measures is not without its problems, as noted in Chapter 5. For example, if a school district requires a universal cutoff of –1.5 or –2.0 SD below the mean for a child to qualify for services, a child with a language disorder has approximately a 50–50 chance of being identified, depending on the test (Spaulding et al., 2006). This is in addition to the often narrowly restricted range of items tested on many tests. The failure of tests to reflect everyday language use suggests that you, as an SLP, must turn to other measures. One of those is language sampling analysis (LSA). For example. Kesha's testing did not provide enough opportunity for her to express a variety of sentence types in a meaningful context.

Although this chapter is devoted to language sampling, it's important to stress that sampling is only one part of a thorough language assessment and has its own issues. For example, preschool children born preterm perform more poorly than those born full-term when language is measured via LSA rather than by standardized assessment (Imgrund et al., 2019). These findings support the importance of using both LSA and standardized assessment in the evaluation of young children's language skills.

On the plus side, language sampling provides more specific information for planning intervention because it includes both language and the context of language use. If

195

the goal of language intervention is generalization to the language used by a child in everyday situations, it is essential that an SLP collect a language sample that is a good reflection of that language in actual use. And that's what we're going to discuss how to do in this chapter.

Language sampling can be a challenge and is not as prescribed as testing, making it more open-ended. But that's the beauty of language sampling. An SLP gets to see a child's language in operation in real communication situations.

Extent of Language Sampling Use

Unfortunately, not all school-based SLPs routinely sample children's language. Pavelko et al. (2016) surveyed 1,399 school-based SLPs nationwide and found that only two-thirds had used language sampling within the past year. Of these, 55% had collected fewer than 10 language samples, despite having caseloads that were much larger. In other words, LSA was used but not extensively.

When asked, SLPs stated that they didn't sample more because language sampling took too long to accomplish, they had limited resources, they believed they lacked the training, and they had limited confidence that LSA was a valid measure. We address all of these later, but for now let's look at planning, collecting, recording, and transcribing a conversational sample.

Planning a Language Sample

Several issues are of importance when planning a language sample. Among the most prominent are the representativeness of the sample and the effect of the context. These two issues are related to the type of sample desired. In addition, collection of several language forms and functions may require the use of different evocative techniques.

Representativeness

Representativeness or typicalness has always been an issue in language assessment. We might agree that testing is an atypical or extraordinary situation for most children and may not yield everyday language.

One positive aspect of testing is that formal tests push a child to excel and may, therefore, yield a child's best performance or what a child is capable of doing. In a study of assessment of pronouns, a colleague and I found many more pronouns occurring in a test situation than in conversation.

These are the two ends of the sampling continuum: typical versus most mature. This dichotomy has been the focus of professional discussions for decades. Each has its own parameters and characteristics. In the late 20th century, some professionals advocated for collecting in a totally free-play situation, whereas others drafted scripts to be used during collection. Most professionals have softened their position since then.

CHAPTER 6 LANGUAGE SAMPLING

> ***Food for Thought:*** **What might be the rationale for each endpoint on the continuum, free-play vs. scripted? Can you think of times when you might want one over the other? Why?**

In general, samples that are conversational and seemingly more spontaneous elicit a child's most representative language. Representativeness can be increased by ensuring spontaneity and by collecting samples under a variety of conditions.

As an SLP, you can foster spontaneity by relinquishing some of your control over the interaction, lessening the use of contrived elicitation techniques, and shifting the focus from collecting a language sample to achieving a more natural and pleasurable interaction. You can elicit a child's most mature language by controlling the interaction through the use of cues that yield the types of utterances you desire. Let's discuss the variables of control, contrivance, and the child's awareness, and then we'll see if there's a middle ground.

SLP Control

For typical language from a child, an SLP's control of the context should be weak. Otherwise, the SLP may restrict a child's linguistic output in both quantity and quality. Control methods, such as the use of questions and selection of topics by the SLP, may cause a child to adopt a passive conversational role and contribute little.

To lessen adult control, the SLP will want to refrain from leading the interaction or providing excessive support. Instead, the SLP can do the following (Rollins et al., 2000):

- Offer minimally invasive responses, such as "Oh, I see, tell me more about that."
- Ask open-ended questions, such as "What else happened?" or "What happened next?"
- Use topic-continuing questions on the content of the child's previous utterance.

When a child does not participate freely and willingly, other, more structured approaches may be needed. For example, a storytelling task might yield longer, more complex utterances that conversation. The least spontaneous condition involves specific linguistic tasks, such as completing sentences. If the more formal tasks are beginning to sound like formal testing, you're not far wrong.

SLP Contrivance

The sample will be less contrived if the SLP follows the child's attentional lead and adopts the child's topics for conversation. More contrived situations, such as "Tell me about this picture" or "Explain the rules of baseball," don't elicit spontaneous everyday speech but may yield longer, more complex utterances.

It is important for representativeness that sampling be accomplished in real communication situations (Olswang et al., 2001). In general, the cognitive and linguistic processing demands of contrived situations have been shown to be less than in real-life interactions because the adult utterance is very targeted on eliciting a specific child response. In contrast, the increased demands and multiple cues of more natural situations may decrease the language performance of many children with language disorder.

As demands increase, the cognitive and linguistic resources available to process them are stretched. If an SLP's aim is for the language taught in intervention to generalize to a child's natural communication contexts, we should assess within those same contexts.

Child Awareness

If a child is less conscious of the process of producing language, the sample will be more spontaneous. Asking a child to produce sentences containing certain elements, for example, makes the linguistic process very conscious and may be very difficult, especially out of context. Although a child may not be able to produce a sentence with *has been* on demand, the same child may be able to relate the story of the three bears with "Someone *has been* sleeping in my bed." The former task is decontextualized, requiring metalinguistic or abstract linguistic skills that may be beyond the child's abilities.

A child's caregivers can offer suggestions to the SLP on contexts to help obtain a representative or more mature sample. It may also be desirable for caregivers to serve as conversational partners, especially with young children. After the sample has been collected, caregivers can review the data and comment on the typicality of their child's behavior.

Language Sampling Contexts

The sampling environment can contribute to the type of sample collected. Although time-consuming, collecting in a variety of contexts, including various settings, tasks, partners, and topics, will yield the most representative results.

Contexts are dynamic and complex, and the effects are very individualistic. One child may respond well to a certain toy and partner, whereas another child does not. Contextual variables include the task or purpose of the activity, the opportunities to use language, the extent of ritualization in the event, the amount of joint attending, and the responsivity of the partners.

An SLP can design the assessment so that the context fits the purpose of collecting the sample. For example, assume that you're interested in a child's social communication behavior. You might play different roles with dolls or puppets. An interest in a child's inability to comprehend written stories might result in a sample of the child's oral narrative ability.

As an SLP, you'll need to make several decisions before collecting the sample. After studying the interview, observational, and testing results, the SLP decides the context, participants, materials, and conversational techniques to be used.

As noted previously, the task itself can affect both the number and length of the conversational interactions. For example, young children are more referential, attempting to focus the listener's attention in free play, and are more information seeking in book activities. Similarly, parents are influenced by context and engage in more conversation when playing with dolls than they do with cars and trucks.

A child's age can also affect the type of activity that is most facilitative of language production. If we measure complex language by the proportions of multiclausal sentences produced, children younger than age 3 years may use complex language more in free play and script play. In contrast, older preschool children may produce a greater proportion of multiclausal sentences when engaging in script play and narrative retelling (Klein et al., 2010). Note that the previous statements are based on a small study and may not apply to many children.

Pavelko and Owens (2019a) reported vigorous sentence production regardless of age using a robust conversational sampling method that encouraged narrative and expository utterances by children. Called SUGAR, this method is described later.

Two aspects of context are structure and predictability. *Structure* is the amount of adult manipulating of materials and evoking of particular utterances. *Predictability* is the familiarity of the overall task and materials. In general, children will produce a greater frequency and diversity of language features in low-structure situations and more new features in predictable ones. Free-play sampling contexts have both low structure and predictability. Possibly in such low-structure contexts, children assume that the adult knows very little about the situation and needs an explanation. In restrictive, planned contexts, children may assume that the adult knows more, and thus children say less.

The need for language sampling in a naturalistic setting is especially important for young children with autism spectrum disorder (ASD). Much of the data we have on these children derive from non-naturalistic standardized assessments and restricted samples. When we look at samples from these children as a group, we find that the most severe communication characteristics are not as common in naturalistic settings as in standardized assessments (Bacon et al., 2018).

As we know, context effects language performance. This may be especially true for children with ASD. Sampling offers an opportunity for an SLP to view a child's behavior in a typical communication setting. It has been suggested that a potential alternative tool is the Autism Diagnostic Observation Schedule–Second Edition (ADOS-2; Lord et al., 2012). ADOS consists of a series of structured and semistructured tasks that involve social interaction, during which the examiner observes and identifies the child's behavior.

An attentive, responsive partner can elicit more language from a child. In joint, or shared, attention situations, children produce more extended conversation and are best able to determine the meanings and intentions of the partner. Similarly, timely responses by a partner increase a child's understanding.

Variety ensures that the sample will not be gathered in one atypical situation. Instead, variety can reflect the many daily interactional situations of a child. Although variety is desirable, it is not always practical, especially in a public school setting. Audio samples collected by the parent or teacher can provide an acceptable substitute.

Settings and Tasks

Although it's one thing to say that you should design the elicitation context for the language you desire, doing that is quite another thing and there is little evidence-based guidance. For example, the task can be especially difficult if the SLP is attempting to use a naturalistic context—one in which the child can interact freely and express their interests, ideas, and emotions without adult direction. Although a naturalistic elicitation context is the most desirable, it is also the most unpredictable.

A number of studies have examined the effect of context on children's language, especially syntax, and have reported that linguistic complexity is related to characteristics of the elicitation context, but results are inconclusive. Comparisons across studies are also problematic because of uncontrolled differences in these studies.

The best sampling context is a meaningful activity containing a variety of elicitation tasks. In general, a child who is more familiar with the situation will give the most representative sample. Familiar routines provide a linguistic and/or nonlinguistic script that guides a child's behavior. For young children, play with familiar toys and partners is one of these routine situations. Language is a natural part of many routine events.

Different language sample collection contexts place different requirements on children. These might include conversations, personal narratives and fictional narrative retells, and exposition or *how to* explanations. Children tend to use their most complex language in narration and exposition. Timler (2018b) provides brief scripts that model each of the desired discourse types. Scripts such as these are examples and must be adapted to a conversational context.

For most children, conversations are a natural part of each day. This technique is the most common sample collection venue among school-based SLPs with children of all ages (Pavelko et al., 2016). Conversations allow opportunities for use of morphology and syntax in both responsive and initiating utterances, in addition to conversation repairs and topic development and maintenance (Timler, 2018b).

Personal narratives can be incorporated into a conversation by asking a child to tell you about a birthday party or favorite event. Narratives require cohesion or the use of linguistic devices such as verb tenses, pronouns, ellipsis, and conjunctions to tie meaning across utterances and events. Ellipsis is the omission of shared information, as in the response "I do" to the inquiry "Who wants more pizza?" In narratives, children must focus on characters and plot while formulating and organizing a series of consecutive utterances (Miller et al., 2016). We devote much more discussion to narratives later in this chapter.

Similarly, exposition requires language skills needed to create a coherent whole and the logical organization of the steps involved. The conversational partner seemingly does not understand how to do whatever the child is explaining ("How do you play soccer?"), thus requiring the child to bring the listener along, ensuring that each step is clear and leads to the next. Conjunctions such as *before*, *after*, *next*, *if*, *so*, and *because* are important syntactic devices.

Language is used for many purposes, and an SLP may need to provide opportunities for these to occur. Although specific elicitation tasks, described later, may work for older children, they may not be effective with toddlers and preschoolers.

It should be remembered that we can't make children talk but we can offer the opportunity and express interest in what a child has to say. By showing interest and using robust techniques, such as open-ended questions (*What happened at the zoo?*) and responses (*A snowman? Oh, tell me how you make a snowman!*), we can help children produce longer, more complex utterance (Kroecker et al., 2010).

CHAPTER 6 LANGUAGE SAMPLING

Preschool and School-Age Children Sampling. As mentioned previously, an SLP needs to decide whether they want a child's typical or optimal production. Some possible elicitation contexts for preschool and young school-age children include the following:

- *Free play.* Toys with a variety of cars, trucks, and vehicles or a doll house with dolls and furniture are available to encourage expression accompanying play.
- *Role play.* Tasks are designed for enactment of familiar experiences, such as a trip to the market or to a fast-food restaurant.
- *Conversation.* Although conversations can vary, usually the adult attempts to follow the child's lead and maximize the child's talking with prompts, such as "What happened next?" and "Tell me more."
- *Elicited descriptions.* These are more directive and ask the child to describe an ongoing action sequence for the examiner who cannot see the actions.
- *Story retelling.* This can be the most directive, especially if the child is recounting a story from a book that the child can see. Narratives of non-present books or of movies can be more open-ended.

Elicitation Context. Although both narration and conversation result in more complex sentence structure than free play overall, there are differences by age (Southwood & Russell, 2004). Younger preschool children approximately age 3 years produce a greater proportion of complex sentences in the free-play and role-play contexts. In contrast, older preschoolers approximately age 5 years produce a greater proportion of complex sentences while engaging in role play and retelling stories (Klein et al., 2010).

As might be expected, the complexity of the utterances will also vary with age. All of this points to the need to collect in different situations with different partners (DeKroon et al., 2002).

Given the language characteristics of Kesha, mentioned at the beginning of the chapter, her SLP has decided to collect both conversational and narrative retell samples. She will use a popular children's book that is appropriate to Kesha's age for the retell. Her goal will be to elicit as many sentences as possible. If Kesha simply labels pictures, the SLP will prompt with "Tell me what's happening" and "Tell me more."

Conversations can be elicited using introductions such as the following:

- Tell me about . . . (your family, your birthday party, your favorite movie).
- Do you have any . . .? Tell me about your . . . (pets, your brother, your sister). Tell me about how you take care of them.
- I wonder what things you do . . . (in school, on the soccer team, in scouts).

There are additional ideas in the fine writings of Evans and Craig (1992) and Southwood and Russell (2004).

Although question type does not seem to influence mean length of utterance (MLU) in toddlers, preschoolers respond with more multiword utterances following conversationally open-ended (How do you make s'mores?) and topic-continuing questions (Then what happened?) (de Rivera et al., 2005).

In contrast, narratives elicit extended discourse, requiring planning and organization by the child. Thus, narratives are more likely to challenge a child's language system and to reveal an older school-age child's linguistic limitations (Southwood & Russell, 2004).

Familiar, meaningful situations with a variety of age-appropriate and motivating activities provide greater variety and thus are more representative. Good settings for preschoolers include free play, snack time, and show-and-tell. School-age children can be sampled during group activities, class presentations, conversations with peers, and field trips. Generally, a child involved in an activity produces more language than a child who is watching others or conversing about pictures. It is best if the sample consists of at least two different settings in which different activities are occurring.

The challenge for an SLP is to find a context that strikes a balance. Too highly structured methods often are not representative. On the other hand, free play, although low in structure, may be time-consuming and result in very variable data. If nothing else, play can interest a child while the SLP and child engage in a conversation.

For older children, an interview technique may be an effective alternative. For 8- to 9-year-old children with developmental language disorder (DLD), the interview technique yields more and longer utterances, more complex language forms, more temporal adjacency and semantic contingency, and more reliable, less variable results than free play.

In an attempt to elicit more complex language within a conversational context, Owens and Pavelko (2021) compiled a list of adult strategies within their Sampling Utterances and Grammatical Analysis Revised (SUGAR) analysis method that have been shown to result in more robust language samples (Kroecker et al., 2010). By reducing the number of yes/no questions and product *wh-* questions (*what, where, when*) and relying on process *wh-* questions (*how, why*) and statements (*I wonder . . . , Tell me about . . .*), Pavelko and Owens (2017) have been able to increase several quantitative language analyses variables, such as mean or average length of utterance in morphemes (MLU_M). The result of robust sampling is that children produce more narrative and expository utterances within a conversational exchange. The robust sampling techniques are presented in Appendix B along with the SUGAR LSA method.

Even the use of process questions can sometimes limit a child's response. I prefer to use "I wonder . . . " and "Tell me . . . " statements and to comment on a child's utterance, using turnabouts, such as in "Oh, that sounds awful. Then what did you do?" that comment and pass the turn back to the child. When an SLP provides an authentic comment to something said, the child is more likely to provide additional information.

Conversational sampling should be authentic and functional. Authenticity comes from the use of real communication contexts in which the participants convey real information. Functional sampling is most concerned with the success of a child with a language disorder as a communicator. Success can be measured by effectiveness in transmitting meanings, fluency or timeliness, and appropriateness of the message form and style in context.

If certain language features are desired, an SLP must increase the probability of their occurrence by adding more structure. With school-age children, discussion, rather than conversations based on pictures or toys, yields more mature language as measured by clause structure complexity, the ratio of hesitations to words, and grammatical and phonemic accuracy.

CHAPTER 6 LANGUAGE SAMPLING

> ***Food for Thought:*** Can you see why a creative and experienced SLP might be a skillful conversational partner in language sample collection? Do you enjoy talking with children? Are you excited by the challenge?

Materials. The materials used should be interesting, age appropriate, and capable of eliciting the type of language desired. Interest can be piqued if a child is allowed to choose from a preselected group of toys or objects. For young children, parents or caregivers can be invited to bring toys from home.

The selection of materials can affect pragmatic performance by modifying the physical context. When no toys are present, children are more likely to initiate memory-related topics. Toys with construction properties, such as Legos, Play-Doh, or clay, often remove the conversation from the present and are more likely to elicit more displaced topics, especially while objects are being constructed. On the other hand, toys that encourage role-play elicit more verbalizations or vocalizations about the objects, events, and actions performed. Compared with construction-type toys, a toy hospital elicits more discussion of the here and now and more fantasy topics and is more conducive to sociodramatic play and verbal representations of events and actions.

In general, children approximately age 2 years respond well to blocks, dishes, pull and wind-up toys, and dolls and action figures. Children approximately age 3 years prefer books, clothes, puppets, and such toys as a barn with animals or a street with houses and stores that encourage role-playing and language production. Kindergarten and early elementary school children respond best to toys with many pieces and to puppets and action figures. Finally, older children usually converse without the use of objects and can be encouraged to talk about themselves and their interests or to provide narratives.

Toys also can assist in eliciting specific linguistic structures. For example, children are more likely to produce spatial terms in play with objects than in conversation. Object movement and manipulation can serve as nonlinguistic cues for a child. Because children's cognitive knowledge and linguistic performance of spatial relationships may differ markedly, manipulation of toys can also aid an SLP in assessing a child's comprehension. The toys and positions should be varied so as not to suggest answers to children.

Adolescent Sampling. Research data suggest that although narrative language samples and norm-referenced testing are correlated, the relationship is stronger for early elementary age children (6- to 8-year-olds) than for later elementary and early middle school children (9- to 12-year-olds) (Danahy Ebert & Scott, 2014). These data suggest that some other format, such as expository language samples, may be more appropriate for older children.

As children progress through the early school years, they are expected to use different text-level communication genres. In school, children are exposed to factual descriptions and explanations of events. Examples of expository discourse include sharing a news event, explaining the rules of a game, or comparing two events. This discourse genre may be particularly helpful in revealing a child's ability to use complex language structures.

In order to produce expository language, a child needs advanced cognitive abilities and exposure to decontextualized language that contains advanced linguistic structures (Nippold, 2004). In school, children are exposed to expository language through nonfiction books or teacher explanations. In addition to exposure, children are expected to use the more advanced linguistic structures characteristic of this type of discourse.

Research with school-age children has shown that expository discourse improves with age (Berman & Verhoeven, 2002; Nippold et al., 2005; Scott & Windsor, 2000; Westerveld & Moran, 2011). Children show a gradual increase in overall length of their language samples, utterance length, and multiclausal sentences. Early detection may help guide our intervention and prevent some of the problems children face in expository writing tasks in later school years.

Expository discourse can be elicited in several different ways (Berman & Verhoeven, 2002; Nippold et al., 2005; Scott & Windsor, 2000), such as asking a child to

- explain or describe a procedure;
- provide a summary of a short descriptive film;
- discuss the issue of interpersonal conflict after watching a short video; or
- describe a favorite game or sport.

For example, if the child has a favorite game or sport task, the SLP can ask the child to explain using prompts such as "I'm not too familiar with X. Can you explain how to play?" This could be followed with "How do you win?"

Fables can also elicit a high level of syntactic complexity in adolescents (Nippold et al., 2014). In a fables task, adolescents are asked to retell and interpret a fable. The task is effective in prompting teens to use complex language and in encouraging them to express their opinions about the moral messages (Nippold et al., 2017).

Critical-thinking tasks based on the deeper meaning of fables elicit greater syntactic complexity than conversational tasks, making these tasks a potential sampling milieu (Nippold et al., 2015). Adolescents with typically developing language (TDL) produce substantially greater syntactic complexity, measured by mean length and mean number of clauses.

Because of the more complex language required in peer conflict resolution, these problems also hold promise as a language sampling and intervention milieu for adolescents. A peer conflict resolution task consists of a set of hypothetical peer conflicts read aloud by the SLP. After an adolescent has retold the scenario, the SLP poses a series of questions concerning the nature of the problem, how it might be resolved, and what the likely outcome might be. Possible questions include the following (Nippold et al., 2007):

- What is the main problem?
- Why is that a problem?
- What is a good way for Person A to deal with Person B?
- Why is that a good way?
- What do you think will happen if Person A does that?
- How do you think they both will feel if Person A does that?

Conversational Partners

Because as an SLP, you'll be interested in a child's use of language, the conversational dyad is important. For example, when teens talk to peers, they ask more questions, obtain more information, shift to more new topics, use more figurative expressions, and make more attempts to entertain than when they talk with their families (Nippold, 2000). Partners influence all aspects of communication.

Conversational partners for young children should be carefully selected and instructed in their role. As noted in Chapter 3, it is especially important to use familiar conversational partners with children younger than age 3 years because these children often respond poorly to strangers.

With preschool and school-age children, familiar conversational or play situations attain the most typical spontaneous sample in which a child converses as naturally as possible. Interaction may involve one adult or child or a small group of children engaged in sharing, playing, or working in the home or the classroom.

A child should be assessed across several familiar persons, each with their own interactive style. Peer interaction usually involves more equal status between participants. In contrast, adults tend to guide and control the topic when conversing with children. As one might expect, these two conditions can result in very different interactive styles for a child.

The language performance of children younger than age 3 years, of children from culturally linguistically diverse (CLD) backgrounds, and of children with learning disability (LD) may deteriorate in the presence of an authority figure such as an unfamiliar adult. This does not mean that you cannot act as a conversational partner. In many ways, as an SLP, you may be the best conversational partner because of your knowledge of language and of interactions.

The SLP and all other participating adults need to be mindful of the inherent problems in adult–child conversations and act to reduce the authority figure persona. The adult can accomplish this by accepting the child's agenda and topics and by actively participating. The best way to attain a semblance of equal authority is for the SLP and the child to engage in play cooperatively. Instead of being directive, the SLP comments on and participates in their ongoing shared activity. With young children, participation may necessitate using the floor.

As the conversational partner, you can set the tone by being nondirective, interesting, interested, and responsive. An SLP should respond to the content of the child's language, not to the way it is said. At this point, the purpose is to collect data, not to change behavior.

By manipulating the situation skillfully, an SLP can probe for a greater range of information. Initially, it's important for the SLP to get acquainted slowly and in a nonthreatening manner. This task is best accomplished by meeting a child on their terms through play and by following the child's lead.

Children who are reluctant to talk to adults may be more willing to interact with a puppet or a doll. I have found that small animals, such as guinea pigs, make excellent communication partners for children. For example, after explaining to a child that I must leave to run a short errand, I introduce the guinea pig in a cage and ask the child to talk to it so that it will not get lonely while I'm gone. I also caution the child not to open the cage and that we'll hold the guinea pig when I return. The child is observed via one-way glass or on a monitor and their language recorded while I'm absent.

Despite conventional wisdom, neither the race of the conversational partner nor the race depicted in stimulus materials seems to affect language performance as measured by response length and response latency. This is not to say that all children, particularly children with CLD backgrounds, will be unaffected. SLPs should be aware of potential difficulties and approach each child in a sensitive way.

Topics

Children have a wide variety of interests, and the conversational partners must be careful to enable a child to talk about them. Children are more spontaneous and produce more language when they are allowed to initiate the topics of discussion.

An SLP should be prepared to shift topics as readily as activities. Expect to be conversant in topics of interest to children, such as school activities, holidays, movies, television programs, fads and fashions, video games, and music.

Summary

It may be helpful to think of interactional situations along a continuum from relatively nondirected or free to more controlled or scripted. Toys are rather open-ended, especially when a partner has suggested, "Let's talk and play with these things." Books offer more control and can be used to elicit particular words, forms, and narratives. Familiar routines, such as doing the dishes, also can be used, along with such cues as "What are you going to do now?" to elicit more specific language. Interviews, picture labeling, and responding to questions offer the most control but at the sacrifice of spontaneity and representativeness.

Table 6–1 presents contextual variables that can be manipulated in an assessment to influence a child's performance. Each variable can be modified to offer minimal or maximal contextual support. Sampling should engage children in challenging interactions that stretch their language and reveal deficits. This may require a range of interactive situations and discourse types, including conversation, play, narration, and expository or factual/causal communication.

It may seem obvious, but note that although increased structure within the sampling task may be necessary to obtain certain information, it comes at the expense of spontaneity and typical performance. In addition, with increased structure and adult control, the entire interaction slips into probing or informal testing. Probing a child's knowledge certainly has its place in an assessment as another informal data-gathering technique, but it shouldn't be confused with conversational language sampling. As an SLP, you need to be sensitive to when you cross that line.

CHAPTER 6 LANGUAGE SAMPLING

Table 6–1. Continuum of Contextual Support

Minimum Contextual Support	Maximum Contextual Support
Naturalistic interaction	Controlled and contrived interaction to elicit particular structures or behaviors
No prompts, toys, props, or activity	Familiar activities, toys, props, and routines providing scripts
Conversational partner is SLP	Conversational partner is parent, other adult, or child familiar with child
Novel activity	Familiar activity or routine
Indirect language modeling	Elicited utterances and imitation
Neutral responses, such as "Oh" and "Um-hm"	Turnabouts and questions

Source: Information taken from Coggins (1991).

Collecting a Language Sample

Sampling raises a few issues, not least of which is the type of sample, the length of a sample or samples, the method of recording, and methods to explore various aspects of language. For our purposes, I've divided the collection discussion into conversational and narrative samples.

In our discussion, we use the term *utterance*, which may be unfamiliar. An **utterance** is a sentence or less. Thus, "Okay," "In a minute," and "Mommy drove today" are all utterances. Utterances are separated by a pause of 2 seconds or more (even if in the middle of a thought) a drop in the voice, and/or an inhalation. An inhalation alone does not determine a separation of utterances because we often inhale in the middle of an utterance.

Three-year-olds may pause in the middle of a thought, usually because they are searching for a word, as in "I want . . . oatmeal." A pause is a pause, and if 2 seconds in length, we have two utterances. More later when we get to transcription.

Conversational Samples

Although a variety of collection methods can be used, a national survey reported that across all ages, 96% of SLPs use conversation as the primary collection context. As noted previously, conversational samples can be elicited in a variety of ways. For ease of discussion, I'm lumping together conversations, picture descriptions, and expository exchanges.

Sample Length

Both the optimum number of samples and optimum sample length vary. In general, school-based SLPs collect 50 to 100 utterances, recording for approximately 10 minutes (Pavelko et al., 2016). In part, the length is dependent on the purpose, with low-frequency language features, such as double auxiliary verbs (*will have gone*, *could be going*), requiring longer samples.

Although short 1- and 2-minute samples are reliable for measures of verbal productivity and fluency, including total number of words (TNW) and number of different words (NDW), children's grammatical errors are difficult to determine through very short samples, and measures of general performance, including MLU, are not reliable (Tilstra & McMaster, 2007). In contrast, in a narrative retelling task with English language learners who speak both Spanish and English, short narratives averaging 4 minutes in length are reliable in TNW, NDW, MLU_M, and words per minute (Heilmann et al., 2008).

When we compare 1-, 3-, and 7-minute samples, we find that many language sample measures are quite consistent across all three. Measures of productivity, lexical diversity, and utterance length are the most reliable measures when shorter samples are compared with longer ones (Heilmann et al., 2010).

Although the ideal sample length will vary with the type of the sampling and the method of analysis, conversational samples of 7 to 10 minutes are reliable measures of language, even with 3-year-olds (Guo & Eisenberg, 2015). This reported reliability can be seen across categories of analysis such as TNW, NDW, and MLU_M.

Across a larger age range of 3;0 to 7:11 years, Pavelko and Owens (2017, 2019a) reported that nearly all children reached 50 utterances within 7 minutes. This was true for children with TDL and those with language disorders.

Given the less frequent communication of young children, Hadley and colleagues (2018) suggest a 30-minute conversational sample. On average, children produce more than 200 complete and intelligible utterances in that time (Hadley et al., 2018).

Although some professional literature suggests more lengthy samples, these are very time-consuming and not feasible in many clinical settings. The time demand of recording, transcribing, and analyzing is one of the major barriers to the clinical use of LSA (Pavelko et al., 2016).

With time and patience, an SLP can also report valid measures for a child who uses augmentative and alternative communication (AAC; Kovacs & Hill, 2017). Given the slower pace of AAC for some children, an SLP might want to plan on an extended period of several short interactions. Communication attempts should be saved automatically in the electronic AAC device. More research is needed.

Language sampling may even be used with some minimally verbal young children (Binger et al., 2016). Reliable measures, such as average or mean length of utterance in words (MLU_W), mean number of syllables per utterance, and percentage of comprehensible words, can be used to characterize a young child's language.

Occasionally, children fall into repetitive patterns of responding, such as naming pictures in a book. This kind of activity provides very little variation in a child's behavior. It is best either to limit this type of interaction or not to use it for analysis. If, on the other hand, a child frequently exhibits perseverative or stereotypic patterns, they should

CHAPTER 6 LANGUAGE SAMPLING

be recorded for analysis, saved for supporting data, or commented on in the assessment report but possibly not included in the sample.

Evocative Conversational Techniques

Although the sample should represent everyday language use, unstructured samples may have limitations, such as low frequency or nonappearance of certain linguistic features and conversational behaviors. Absence or low incidence does not mean a child lacks these features or behaviors. Therefore, it may be necessary to supplement the sample with evocative procedures specifically designed to elicit them. Test protocols also might be modified to obtain more structured samples.

As an SLP, you may need to plan both the linguistic and nonlinguistic contexts for elicitation of various functions and forms. This requires some forethought. For example, infinitive phrases not only are difficult for children with language disorders but also require specific evocative techniques (Eisenberg, 2005). Infinitives come in two varieties: noun–verb–*to*–verb (*John wants to go*) and noun–verb–noun–*to*–verb (*John wants Fred to go*). An SLP can use play with dolls or puppets and have the child complete sentences within the play in the following manner:

> The cat says, "Can I eat?" The cat wants . . . . You finish the story. The cat . . . ?
>
> The boys says to the girl, "Swim with me." The boy asks . . . . You finish the story. The boy . . . ?

Early developing infinitives accompany verbs such as *ask*, *forget*, *go* (*gonna*), *have* (*hafta*, *gotta*), *like*, *need*, *say*, *suppose*, *tell*, *try*, *use*, and *want*. You can see with this example that as an SLP, you'll need to plan for specific structures.

At first, some procedures may seem stiff and formal, even forced. Initially, you may need to role-play the sampling situation and memorize conversational openers and replies. Once familiar with the many ways of eliciting a variety of functions and forms, an SLP can relax and use the techniques more naturally as opportunities arise within the interaction.

Specific tasks that are within a child's experience also can be used to elicit specific language forms. For example, a mock birthday party can be used to elicit plurals, past tense, and questions. An SLP might elicit plurals by saying the following:

> Today is X's birthday. Let's have a party. What are some things we'll need? (Or, Here are some things we need. What are these?)

In this way, the child's utterances are placed within context in which they make sense. This approach allows a broad range of pragmatic functions to occur.

Pragmatics. An adequate sample of a child's social pragmatic skills will require collecting samples of multiple discourse types, such as story and personal narrative retells, conversation and exposition, or how-to explanations. The different demands placed on children in these situations have been discussed previously. For more in-depth information, I suggest you read the very informative article by Gerolyn Timler (2018b).

It seems especially important in assessment of a child's pragmatic skills that the SLP provide as much freedom to the child as possible. However, specific procedures and activities can be used to elicit a variety of communication intentions, examples of presupposition, and the underlying social organization of discourse within a variety of situations. Table 6–2 presents examples of situations that each elicit a variety of language functions.

Intentions. Most utterances clearly demonstrate the speaker's intent. "What time is it?" demonstrates a desire for information. However, the relationship is not always so obvious. "What time is it?" might be used as an excuse. For example, the speaker who does not wish to do something and knows that time is limited might use this utterance to establish that something is not possible at this time and they may not even expect an answer.

> Well, I don't know . . . , it's getting late. What time is it? Oh, well, it doesn't matter, I really better be going.

Utterances also may express more than one intention. For example, the speaker might respond to a piece of art with "What do you call that *thing*?" Here, the speaker requests information and also makes an evaluation.

Some intentions are responsive in nature—for example, answering a question or following a directive or request for action. In addition to a child's production level of such requests, it is helpful to know the child's level of response.

With responsive functions, an SLP must not interpret noncompliance as noncomprehension. A child simply may not want to comply or may choose to ignore the request. My granddaughter at age 6 years was especially good at ignoring. Come to think of it, so was her mom! An SLP first should be certain that the child can perform the behavior requested. The ages at which children comprehend different levels of requests are listed in Table 6–3.

In some situations, it might be helpful to have another child in ask-and-tell situations to act as a model for the other. Similarly, an SLP and child can switch roles as questioner (or director) and respondent. A puppet or doll can also be a model.

Table 6–2. Situations With the Potential to Elicit a Variety of Language Functions	
Dress-up	Role-playing
Playing house or farm	Playing school
Dolls, puppets, adventure or action figures	Acting out stories, television shows, movies
Farm set or street scene	Imaginary play
Simulated grocery store, gas station, fast-food restaurant, beauty parlor	Simulated TV talk show

CHAPTER 6 LANGUAGE SAMPLING

Table 6–3. Age and Comprehension of Requests	
Age in Years	**Comprehension**
2	I need a _____. Give me a _____.
3	Could you give me a _____? May I have a _____? Have you got a _____?
4	He hurt me. (Hint) The _____ is all gone. (Hint)
4½	Begin to comprehend indirect requests: Why don't you _____ or Don't forget to _____. Mastery takes several years.
5	Inferred requests in which the goal is totally masked are now comprehended. In this example, the speaker desires some juice: Now you make breakfast like you're the mommy.

Source: Information from Ervin-Tripp (1977).

An SLP should note the type of intentions displayed, their forms, the means of transmission, and the social conventions that affect these means. Table 6–4 presents a broad range of intentions and accompanying activities that may elicit language functions or intentions within a conversational or situational context.

Presuppositional and Deictic Skills. Presupposition and deixis underlie the entire conversational interaction. **Presupposition** is the speaker's assumption about the knowledge level of the listener and the tailoring of language to that supposed level. **Deixis** is the production and interpretation of information from the perspective of the speaker. When a speaker says "Come here," this must be interpreted as a point close to the speaker, not as a point with reference to the listener. Deictic terms include, but are not limited to, *here/there*, *this/that*, *come/go*, and *you/me*.

Presuppositional and deictic skills can be assessed in referential communication tasks. In classic referential tasks, one partner describes something or gives directions to the other partner, who is usually on the other side of an opaque barrier or unable to see the speaker, similar to playing the game Battleship. A more practical variation is the use of a smartphone for conversation. Deixis can be elicited by using object-finding tasks in which the child directs the conversational partner toward a hidden object.

In these tasks, an SLP must be alert to the use of direct/indirect reference. In **direct reference**, the speaker considers the audience and clearly identifies the entity being mentioned. **Indirect reference** typically follows direct reference and refers to entities through the use of pronouns or such terms as *that one*. A child with poor presuppositional skills may use indirect reference without prior direct reference, leaving the listener confused.

Table 6–4. Eliciting Intentions

Intention	Elicitation Technique
Answering/ responding	SLP asks child a variety of questions while engaged in play ("Where shall we put the houses?" "Who is that?" "What's in his hand?") and notes the type of question and response. Some question forms may be more difficult.
Calling/ greeting	SLP leaves and re-enters the situation, role-plays people entering and leaving a business, calls on the telephone, or uses dolls, puppets, or action figures to elicit greetings.
	If the SLP turns away with a favorite toy, the child also may call.
Continuance	Continuance is turn filling that lets a speaker know that a listener is attending to the conversation.
	Typical continuants: "uh-huh," "yeah," "okay," and "right"
	SLP notes if child seems to rely on this function rather than contributing anything new or relevant.
Declaring/ citing	Child spontaneously comments on the present action. SLP can model ("Car goes up the ramp") but not attempt to cue a response because declaring/citing is spontaneous.
	SLP also can engage in unexpected or unusual behavior and await the child's comment.
Detailing	SLP presents a child with two objects of different size or color. If child takes one and says nothing, the SLP models ("I'll take the little one" or "Here's a green truck") and presents other objects later.
	SLP does not attempt to cue a response because detailing is spontaneous.
Expressing feeling	SLP models feeling-type responses throughout play.
	Dolls, puppets, or action figures are described as having certain feelings, and the child is asked to help.
Hypothesizing	SLP poses a physical problem for a child, such as "How can we get everyone to the party on time?" or "How can we get Leonardo out of the cage?"
Making choices	SLP presents alternatives, such as "I don't know whether you'd rather have a peanut butter sandwich with jelly or fluff."
Naming/ labeling	SLP presents a novel object or points to pictures in a book and remarks, "Oh, look." If the child does not label the object or picture, the SLP models the response ("Look. A clown.") and goes on. The child may do so on subsequent exposure to other novel objects.
	SLP does not cue a response because labeling, like the other forms of reporting, should be spontaneous.
Predicting	In sequential activities or book reading, SLP can ponder, "I wonder what will happen now" or "I wonder what we'll do next."

CHAPTER 6 LANGUAGE SAMPLING

213

Table 6–4. *continued*	
Intention	**Elicitation Technique**
Protesting	SLP can elicit protesting by putting away toys or taking away snacks before the child is finished. When a child requests an item, an SLP can hand the child something other than what was requested.
Reasoning	SLP attempts to solve a problem, such as "I wonder why the boy ran away" or "I wonder what we did wrong." Child is invited to participate.
Repeating	SLP notes the amount of repetition of self and of the partner. This can take the form of empty comments in a conversation in which a child adds no new information.
Replying	SLP notes occasions when child responds to the content of what the SLP has said. Unlike answers, replies are expected but not required.
Requesting assistance/ directing	SLP presents interesting toys in a way that requires adult help to open or use, such as • placing objects in clear plastic containers or drawstring bags that require help to open; • giving the child one portion of a toy while keeping the other on a shelf; and • letting windup toys run down. The SLP makes such comments as "I wish we could play with this; it would be fun," "Oh, we could use more parts," or "Gee, we need to fix that." SLP also can present child with situations that require a solution, such as toys with missing pieces. During interactions, SLP should note self-directing or self-talk accompanying play. Although this behavior can be modeled, it should be spontaneous on the child's part.
Requesting clarification	This intention can be elicited when SLP mumbles or makes an obviously inaccurate statement.
Requesting information	SLP places novel but unknown objects in front of a child. Naming the object correctly is the naming labeling function, and the SLP should confirm the child's name. The responses "What's that?" or "What?" and those with rising intonation ("Frog?") should be considered requests for information.
Requesting objects	SLP has enticing objects or edibles just out of reach. SLP also might direct child to use an object not present in the situation or not in the expected location. If prompting is required, the SLP can ask, "Do you have the scissors?" When the child answers negatively, the SLP can direct the child by saying, "Ask Sally if she does."

continues

Table 6–4. *continued*	
Intention	**Elicitation Technique**
Requesting permission	SLP hands an interesting object to a child and says "Hold the X for me." The SLP then awaits a response from the child, such as "Can I play with X?" or just "Play X?" Even more effective is to keep the object hidden in an opaque box. SLP peeks into the box and tells the object that it can come out to play when someone wants to play with it. If necessary, a puppet can model the requesting behavior desired.

Additional presuppositional information can be gathered by varying the roles, topics, partners, and communication channels available in the sampling situation. Roles can be varied so that a child has an opportunity to act as listener and speaker. Assessment of both roles is essential. As speakers, these children make limited use of descriptors, provide very little specific information, and are less effective than children developing normally.

The choice of topics also can influence presuppositional behavior and provide for a variety of role taking. Children can be asked to describe events about which the SLP is ignorant, such as a family outing. In this situation, the child must determine the amount of information necessary for the listener to understand the topic.

As the number of communication channels decreases, a speaker is forced to rely more heavily on the remaining ones. For example, the use of a smartphone requires the speaker to rely almost exclusively on the verbal communication channel. This situation is challenging even for some nonimpaired language users.

While gathering the language sample, an SLP can manipulate channel availability systematically. During play, I sometimes turn or look away and then ask the child to describe what they're doing. Whether in this situation or using a smartphone, an SLP is interested in the child's ability to encode the most informative or uncertain elements in a situation.

In general, human beings tend to comment on entities that are new, changing, or unexpected. In the sampling situation, novel items can be introduced. The SLP must attend to the child's behavior to determine how the child refers to the novel stimulus.

I know of one situation in which a kitten was abruptly introduced into the sampling situation. The SLP said nothing but waited to see how the child would comment.

In general, young children with language disorders encode novel information less frequently than do children with TDL. Older school-age children with DLD tend to use more pronouns with less identification of the referent information than do TD children.

Games and stories can also elicit direct and indirect reference. For example, a story can be told and then questions asked to elicit indefinite (*a/an*) and definite (*the*) articles and/or nouns (*girl*) and pronouns (*she*). The child can also retell a story to a second child who has not heard it. Any portion of extended discourse, such as describing a movie, explaining how to accomplish a task, or telling a story, will provide valuable clinical data on referencing.

CHAPTER 6 LANGUAGE SAMPLING

The SLP is interested in both the lexical items used and the ambiguity of the referent. Of interest is the number of times the child mentions the referent by name or by the use of pronouns. Some children overuse the referent name ("The boy . . . , The boy . . . , The boy . . . "), whereas others rely on the pronoun without sufficient return to the referent name to avoid confusion ("He . . . , He . . . , He . . . ").

Finally, specific role-playing activities with older children also can be helpful in assessing presupposition. The child faces very definite behavioral constraints, as in the following:

> Imagine you and a friend are trying to find a drinking fountain. You see a man coming down the street. While your friend remains seated on a park bench, you try to find out about the fountain. I'll be the man. What would you say? (Child responds.) Now, I'm your friend. What would you tell me?

Discourse Organization. Discourse or the verbal exchange of ideas has internal organization based on the type of discourse. For example, a smartphone conversation has a recognizable pattern, as does the telling of a personal narrative or asking for assistance. The organization of discourse can be assessed within familiar activities, such as going to a fast-food restaurant, that provide a scaffold or structure for dialogue. An SLP may be interested in the amount of social and nonsocial speech and a child's awareness of the social nature of speech and language use.

An SLP can provide opportunities for a child to initiate conversation, to take turns, and to repair in response to self-feedback or the feedback of others in different situations. For example, by failing to respond to the child or by responding inappropriately, mumbling, failing to establish a referent, misnaming, or providing insufficient information, an SLP may elicit requests for clarification from a child.

Semantic Terms. Several semantic terms may be of interest and can be assessed through various activities within a conversational exchange. Relational terms, such as *in front of*, *more/less*, and *before/after*, are especially difficult for children with LD. As a consequence, these children use comprehension strategies that may be based on probable location, physical properties of objects, and preferred location. Adjectival relational words, such as *big* and *little*, may be comprehended by using either a preference for amount or similarity of a word's sound. With temporal terms, strategies may include sequential probability and order-of-mention or main-clause-first. Each of these strategies is explained here and may become obvious in an appropriate situation.

It is easier for children to comprehend locational terms and to follow locational instructions when familiar objects are combined in familiar, predictable, or probable ways, such as juice in a cup. Levels of comprehension can be determined by using both the usual context and a neutral context in which object placement is not so predictable, such as block and cup.

The physical properties of an object can also influence responding. For example, a child's rule may be containers are for *in* and surfaces are for *on*. Square containers can be turned on their sides by the SLP and used for both *in* and *on*.

Object characteristics also affect comprehension and production of such terms as *in front of* and *behind*. In general, these terms are easier to use with fronted objects, such as a computer, than with nonfronted objects, such as a ball.

With deictic terms, young children may employ either a child-centered or a speaker-centered strategy, preferring that location as the reference point. Assessing contrastive terms, such as *here/there*, with different speakers, including the child, may help determine if such preferences exist.

Adjectival terms, such as *more/less*, *long/short*, and *big/little*, may be interpreted by the child using a preference for a greater-amount strategy in which a child usually chooses the largest one when in doubt. Assessing both words of the pair in different contexts with different objects and in different word order may help an SLP understand a child's errors. Offering verbal choices to a child (*Tell me which one you want*) requires the use of adjectival comparative terms.

Similarly, the height of objects affects comprehension of such words as *big*, *tall*, *top*, *young*, and *old*. Preschoolers often equate *big* with *tall* and *old* and *little* with *short* and *young*, respectively. Objects can be placed so that their heights are similar by using stands of different heights.

Some children use a strategy in which they interpret contrastive terms such as *deep* and *shallow* to be synonymous or assign one meaning to similar terms. In the latter, *big* becomes synonymous with *tall*, *wide*, and *thick*. Object dimensions can be controlled so that, for example, the tallest objects are not always the biggest overall.

Finally, as mentioned previously, temporal sequential terms, such as *before* and *after*, may be interpreted by using a most probable, order-of-mention, or main-clause-first strategy. In the most probable strategy, a child trusts experience. Among preschoolers, this is the most widely used strategy with familiar, real-world sequences. Order-of-mention, or the first-action-mentioned-occurred-before-the-second, is also popular among preschoolers, whereas children older than age 5 years often use the main-clause-first strategy, in which the main clause of the sentence is assumed to have occurred first. For example, in the sentence, "After we finish school, we can go to the rec center," a child may assume the rec center occurs first. Sequential terms should be noted when used as both prepositions, as in *after school*, and conjunctions, as in *she did X after she did Y*.

With planning, an SLP can work several of these terms into a play context employing conversation. None of this, however, is a substitute for a thorough evaluation of semantics if that is an area of concern.

Language Form. An SLP can manipulate the context to elicit particular forms. For example, the objects and the verbal routines chosen for play may facilitate the use of pronouns or prepositions. Specific syntactic forms, such as verbs, and morphological markers, such as the regular past tense *-ed*, also can be elicited in creative ways. Some intentions discussed previously, such as requesting information, have specific linguistic forms. A few elicitation methods for specific structures are listed in Table 6–5.

Barako Arndt and Schuele (2013), in an adaptation of Hadley's (1998) methods, suggest collecting language samples from preschool children using a play format that keeps the child engaged while diverting the conversation for short periods of time to more complex topics via conversation and narrative and expository tasks. Specific struc-

CHAPTER 6 LANGUAGE SAMPLING

Table 6–5. Elicitation of Morphosyntactic Features

Language Feature	Elicitation Technique
Word classes (nouns, verbs, . . .)	Pull object from a bag and name it. (Nouns)
	Identify actions in pictures, such as sports. (Verbs)
	Ask specific *Wh-* questions: *What's that?* (Nouns); *What's he doing? What will (did) she do?* (Verbs); *Where's X? When's X?* (Prepositions); *How does he feel (look, smell)?* (Adjectives); *How did she do X?* (Adverbs); *Whose X is this?* (Possessive pronouns)
Sequencing preposition and conjunctions	Tell me how to . . . (make a cake, play Chutes and Ladders, talk about your favorite movie)
Comparatives	Pull items from a bag and tell how they differ from some reference item or from the last item. (*This one's longer.*)
Adjectives	Play "I spy." (*I see something and it's X.*)*
	Offer choices with similar objects and ask "Which one do you want?" (*The green one.* or *The big one.*)
Verb tenses	*Tell me what we're we going to do? . . . doing? . . . did?*
Plural *-s* marker	*Let's play camping (birthday party, grocery store)! What do we need to play?*
	Play with Legos or Mr. Potato Head or make crafts and request pieces. (*I want the stickers.* or *Can I have Mr. Potato Head's ears?*)
Possessive pronouns	Pull objects with known owners from a bag and name the owner. (*That's John's.*)
	Play dress-up or with action figures or dolls and have child identify what goes with whom. (*That's X-Man's backpack.*)
Complex sentences	*Your mom says you play soccer. That sounds exciting. But I've never played. Can you tell me how to play?*
Yes/no questions	Play "Twenty Questions." (*Is it . . .?*)

Note: *Also a good elicitor of pronouns.

Sources: Information from Crais and Roberts (1991) and my own clinical experience.

tures can be elicited by manipulating both the nonlinguistic and linguistic context. For example, embedded clauses can be elicited via modeling, as in the following:

> The bear thinks someone is in his bed. I wonder what the girl thinks.

If the child responds with just the embedded clause *She's sleepy*, the SLP can respond, "Who thinks she's tired?" If the child says simply "the girl," I would play dumb:

> I'm confused. The bear thinks someone is in his bed. I wonder who else thinks something.

It's not foolproof, but often the child will help this befuddled adult by stating, "The girl thinks she's tired."

Similarly, the SLP can model *The girl is trying to* . . . or ask *I wonder what the mouse did yesterday?* to elicit an infinitive phrase or past tense verb. Barako Arndt and Schuele (2013) offer a developmental sequence and coding scheme for complex syntax in young children.

Owens and Pavelko (2021) also offer methods for eliciting more complex language from children within a conversational context. These strategies are presented in Appendix B.

> *Food for Thought:* Obviously, eliciting specific forms and intentions will be a challenge. You'll need many techniques in your "bag of tricks."

Narrative Samples

Narration as an expressive language sample has been recommended as a language measure for a variety of language disorders, including intellectual developmental disorder (IDD) (Abbeduto et al., 2012). Narratives are an expression of the organization and interconnection of data in the brain. The storyteller must construct a context within which to relate events, both real and imaginary. Narratives consist of two frameworks: scripts and story frames (Naremore, 2001).

Scripts and Narrative Frames

Scripts consist of typical, predictable event sequences formed on the basis of experience, either real or vicarious. Scripts are not about any one experience but are generalized, organized hierarchically and causally, inhabited by characters, and contain a predictable sequence of events. Each event is represented in the brain and becomes part of a generalized event sequence, such as birthday parties, getting ready for school, or helping wash dishes.

Narrative frames are mental models of story structures. We use them to facilitate production and comprehension of narratives. In short, narrative frames are mental organizers that reduce processing demands.

The narratives of children with language disorders may break down because of linguistic difficulties or because the child doesn't know either the script or the narrative frame. The SLP should be reasonably positive that the child possesses event and script knowledge and a notion of narrative frames prior to beginning a narrative collection and analysis.

If too much mental capacity is used for linguistic processing, the narrative frame and/or the script may collapse. Similarly, poor script knowledge or poorly formed narrative frames may require too much mental "energy," leaving the child little capacity for linguistic processing.

Prior to collecting a narrative, an SLP should attempt to determine if a child has script and narrative frame knowledge. Script knowledge can be assessed by inquiring about a

CHAPTER 6 LANGUAGE SAMPLING

child's experiences, routines, and event knowledge (Naremore, 2001). Assessment of the retrieval of script knowledge can be accomplished by asking a child to act out the script with toys, pictures, or other items. If the child is successful, the SLP attempts to have the child recite an event account with a cue such as "Tell me what you do when you do X" or "Tell me what happened one time when you did X." If the child needs more help, the SLP can ask a few questions to determine the setting and then begin as follows:

You ride the bus to school every day. Last week on the way to school, you . . .

You can assist the child with the event recount by saying, "And then" or "Tell me what happened next." The child's recount should have some logical organization.

Knowledge of narrative frames can be determined by discussing with a child the purpose of narratives and determining the child's experience with narrative frames, either at home or in school and within story reading. Narrative frames will be analyzed in more detail after a few narratives have been collected.

Children will not possess scripts for all possible events. Nor will all children possess narrative frames. Cultural variations are to be expected and are discussed in Chapter 8.

Collecting Narratives

The quality of a child's narrative is influenced by stimuli and topics based on the age, verbal ability, interests, and gender of a child or adolescent. Stimuli may include objects or pictures used for original constructions and heard or read stories used for retelling. In general, the task used to elicit the narrative influences the speaker's adaptation to the listener.

There are many different types of stories and many different contexts within which to tell them. The story type and context affect the eventual narrative form produced. In general, maximally naturalistic topics and contexts elicit the most representative narratives. Other variables that may affect the narrative form are the story type, a child's experiential base, the context in which the narrative is told, the source of the narrative, the topic, the formal or informal atmosphere of the context, and the audiovisual support available.

Several oral narratives should be collected. For older children, the SLP will also want to collect written narratives. A wide variation in narratives is desirable. Prior to collecting, the SLP decides on the type of narratives desired and the stimuli to be used in their collection.

In general, fictionalized narratives may result in incomplete narratives with little emphasis on goals, characters' feelings or motivations, and endings. The pace, action orientation, and frequent commercial interruption found in television form a very different base for narratives than does experience or children's books.

The type of elicitation task will affect the child's performance. Books elicit descriptive information, whereas films elicit action sequences. Films also elicit more causal sequences in retelling than do oral stories. Pictures tend to constrain the form of the narrative and may lead to the production of additive chains (And this . . . and this . . .).

Stories in response to single pictures tend to exclude character information, internal responses, or intentions. Shared information may be omitted and new information treated as old even when the listener has not viewed the picture. In contrast, individual photographs or discussions of familiar events foster event chains.

For some children, wordless picture books seem to be a good resource for eliciting narratives, especially for children, such as those with Down syndrome (DS), who seem to need the extra input (Miles et al., 2006; Schneider & Dubé, 2005). Children with DS express more verbal content in narratives to wordless picture books than might be expected given their formal test results (Miles & Chapman, 2002).

Narratives can be elicited using the following starters:

- Do you know the story of . . . (any popular children's book)? Tell me the story.
- Your mom said that you really liked the movie . . . . I didn't see that one. Tell me the story.
- Look at this [wordless picture] book for a minute. Do you understand the story? Tell the story.

An SLP should do some research beforehand to find out from parents or teachers about the child's favorite book, movie, or television show. When in doubt, I've found that with young girls, it almost always works to say "Tell me the story of your favorite princess movie." Boys will often respond when the cue involves action hero movies.

Narrative Retelling. Narrative retelling and recall can be used to determine a child's memory organization. In narrative retelling, the child listens to a well-formed story and then reconstructs the story orally or in writing. Retelling of short narratives can even serve as a screening tool with young elementary school children. At this age, children should be able to retell the story without deviating significantly from the original in sequence or content.

In story retelling tasks, an SLP must also consider the comprehension skills needed to understand the story, the mode of presentation (oral or written), story length, a child's past experience with the story genre (e.g., fairy tale, mystery), the child's interest in the content, and the degree of story structure. In general, more familiar, more interesting, and more structured stories result in more complete, better organized retellings.

Well-formed stories should be chosen for retelling and should be modified to enhance clarity and organization. Stories can be rewritten to reduce complexity in their oral form and to summarize important sections. Subparts and transitions between parts of the narrative may need to be highlighted. Good narrative models often have repetitive elements.

Narrative comprehension, especially for kindergarten and second grade children with TDL, is affected by the method of narrative presentation. Children have better comprehension when narratives are presented live rather than audio recorded (Kim, 2016). Interestingly, the method of presentation does not seem to affect the comprehension of fourth grade children nor their oral retells.

Children with LD perform much like younger children, recalling less of the stimulus story. In general, children with language disorders produce longer and more complete stories in narrative retelling than in self-generated ones. Clause length is also greater in retold narratives.

A minimal narrative should consist of a sequence of two temporally ordered clauses. In addition, both events should be conveyed in the past tense. Although fictional narratives retold with wordless books are significantly longer than personal stories, they are more frequently not true narratives because they often become picture descriptions that are signaled by a lapse into present tense.

Wordless picture books can be used creatively to assess language across the entire age range from preschool to 18 years of age (Moore Channell et al., 2018). Given the nature of the wordless picture book task, narrative procedures can be standardized for examiner behavior and content.

Abbeduto and colleagues have developed a language-sampling procedure for wordless picture books (Abbeduto et al., 1995; Berry-Kravis et al., 2013; Finestack & Abbeduto, 2010; Kover et al., 2012). In this procedure, the SLP can use either *Frog Goes to Dinner* (Mayer, 1974) or *Frog on His Own* (Mayer, 1973). Without talking, the child first surveys the book. The SLP allows approximately 10 to 12 seconds per page. When this is completed, the SLP asks the child to tell the story while viewing the book a second time. Although a child may seem to have finished describing a page, the SLP should pause for 5 to 7 seconds to allow for additional comments by the child.

It is important to consider the amount of structure inherent in the stimulus and its effect on retold story construction. For example, nondescript dolls or puppets or sets of vehicles provide no structure. In contrast, a sequence of related pictures, such as pictures in a book, provides maximal structure. In general, the more structure found in the stimuli, the less structure the child must provide.

The best narratives, measured by the most complete episodes and the amount of information, occur when children retell a story without picture cues. The task then becomes one of story generation rather than retelling. One additional consideration is that pictures may distract some children with language disorders.

For an SLP, the concern is to keep the narrative sample as representative and natural as possible while prompting the child to continue. An adequate response requiring no further prompting meets one or more of the following (Moore Channell et al., 2018):

- Refers to more than one character or action (e.g., "The bee stung the frog's tongue.")
- Describes an interaction (e.g., "The people are having a picnic and the man gives the woman a drink.")
- Conveys upcoming events in the story (e.g., "They don't see the frog hiding in the basket yet.")

Figure 6–1 presents a graphic representation of narrative prompting.

Personal Event Narratives. Independent, self-generated narrative production requires a child to use their own organizational structure and narrative formulation. Personal–factual narratives may be collected from conversation or prompted. This type of narrative is very common in preschool and early elementary school, especially in show-and-tell activities. Preschoolers naturally create these types of narratives in conversation with each other.

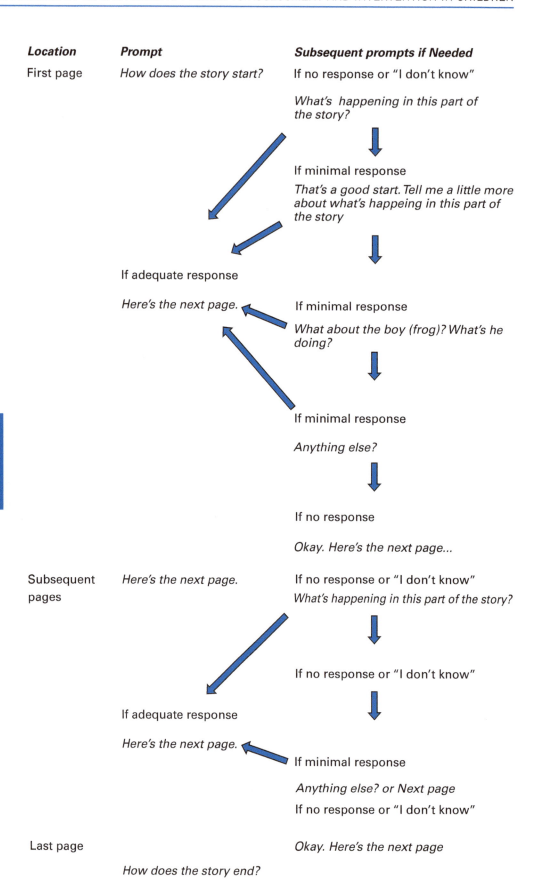

Figure 6–1. Prompting hierarchy for narrative sampling.

Assessment procedures for personal event narratives are related to an SLP's elicitation strategies and the structural analyses that follow. Although personal event narratives typically do not use the types of cues found in retells, this does not preclude using a sample personal story as a model for the type of narrative you desire (Petersen & Spencer, 2012). For example, a child could listen to a recorded narrative by another child or the SLP and then tell their own.

It may be helpful for an SLP to establish some common experience with a child and to share a narrative about this experience as an example for the child. To get a narrative, an SLP often has to give one. Using a combination of narration and probing questions, the SLP can tell a personal story related to a common event, such as going to the market, and prompt the child with leading questions to stir the child's memory of past events ("Have you ever been to the market?"). Experiential topics prompted in this fashion usually result in the longest and most complex narratives.

Topics such as a new sibling or a death usually result in very truncated narratives. Rather, the child can be prompted to relate the scariest or funniest thing that ever happened. With children who are on sports teams, I often cue them with "Tell me about your most exciting game." An SLP can also use other prompts, such as "Tell me about a time . . . " (Noel & Westby, 2014). With older children and adolescents, an SLP can ask that they include thoughts, feelings, and how a solution was found.

With higher functioning adolescents and children, an SLP might elicit a "life story." These narratives may be collected in oral or written form. The child is asked write a half dozen or so important events in their life on cards, arrange the cards in order, and then use the cards to tell their life story (Habermas & de Silveira, 2008). A similar procedure could employ an interview in which the child is asked to think of important events as chapters in a book and to begin with the earliest (Reese et al., 2010).

Children can be asked to support their choices by explaining why each chapter of their life is important. In addition, children can be asked about their reactions and feeling and those of others.

Another method for eliciting life stories is to ask a child to think of the worst things and the best things that have ever happened to them. Subsequently, as they lace these together into a narrative, the SLP can ask how they overcame adversity, what they learned, and how it changed the child's life (Grysman & Hudson, 2010).

An SLP should add nothing to the child's narrative other than feedback in the form of "uh-huh," "okay," "yeah," "wow," or a repetition of the child's previous utterance. These neutral but enthusiastic responses will not influence the course of the story as others might. The narrative can be resumed or the child prompted to continue by such utterances as "And then what happened?"

Stories are enhanced by familiarity with the listener and the location. The SLP should decide ahead of time on strategies for terminating rambling stories and for probing to elicit longer ones.

> ***Food for Thought:*** **It's easy to forget the centrality of narratives in our daily conversation. Step back some and listen to the conversations around you today.**

Recording the Sample

Slightly more than half of SLPs responding to a national survey said they transcribed while the child was talking (Pavelko et al., 2016). Transcribing a child's language while talking violates all norms for a conversation, the most frequently used collection context. It may disrupt conversation or narration if a child is focused on the behavior of the SLP. In addition, it's impossible to write everything a child is saying, so portions of the sample will be missed. This method is not optimal nor is it recommended.

A language sample can be recorded permanently by using an analog or digital recording device such as a smartphone or a tablet. Audio recording is essential because the interaction must be reviewed repeatedly for information. I caution that a smartphone is not a secure device and can potentially violate HIPPA patient privacy regulations if left there. Transfer to a secure device immediately, and erase the smartphone recording. It's wise to consult agency or district policy before recording on a nonsecure device.

Although videorecording can be intrusive, it yields the best data for describing the verbal and nonverbal behaviors observed. You could use the webcam found on most laptops and tablets. Again, if you use a smartphone, transfer the data and erase the file immediately.

Collecting Samples of Written Language

Written samples should also be collected with school-age children and adolescents, especially if literacy is a concern. Underlying language processes make it imperative that an SLP sample all modalities.

In general, if a teacher suspects that a child has a language and/or literacy disorder, they should contact the school's SLP, who can ask the teacher to compile a portfolio of the child's written work. The portfolio should include first drafts of expository writing, narrative fiction, and nonfiction. The SLP can evaluate the sample for phonological and linguistic awareness; word boundaries; vocabulary and usage; ability to communicate thoughts precisely, sequentially, and systematically; generation and organization of ideas; morpheme usage; syntactic usage, semantic awareness, and word associations, such as opposites and synonyms; and handwriting. This assessment is discussed in Chapter 13.

In addition, the SLP should elicit a written sample as they observe the child. As this occurs, the SLP must be mindful of the child's general demeanor, the presence of frustration, the amount of help needed, and the look and quality of the finished product.

The child's written language can be compared to the spoken sample for similarities and differences. Of particular interest will be language features noted in the language of older children, such as cohesive devices, noun and verb phrase structure, illocutionary functions, vocabulary and word relationships, conjoining and embedding, along with spelling and penmanship. These are all be discussed in Chapter 7.

Transcribing the Oral Sample

The oral sample is transcribed as soon after recording as possible. This timeliness ensures that the SLP brings to the task as much memory of the situation as possible.

CHAPTER 6 LANGUAGE SAMPLING

The format of the transcript varies with the purpose of the assessment. For most purposes, the format will be that of a script for a play. There may be situations, however, in which the SLP is interested in other aspects of a child's language. For example, the timing of utterance might be important if the SLP is interested in the effect of the language disorder, such as a word-finding deficit, on the flow of language.

Transcribing is a time-consuming aspect of LSA. If available, trained transcribers or SLP assistants might lessen this burden for the SLP.

Another option is voice-to-text transcription using a method similar to Google Cloud Speech. Google Cloud Speech is significantly more accurate than real-time transcription with narrative samples and is not impacted by the child's speech rate (Fox et al., 2021). These data would seem to suggest that automatic speech recognition shows great clinical utility as an expedited transcription method. Currently, one potential problem is that most voice-to-text programs are not calibrated for the frequency or pitch of child speech and may miss some words and morphemes.

For most SLPs, the simplest way to transcribe is to type the child's and adult's utterances into a text file or word processing document while listening to the recorded sample using an audio player or computer. Transcription may be sped up by using free, downloadable, and user-friendly software such as *Transcriber* (Barras et al., 1998–2008). This software will allow you to divide the audio stream into utterance segments that you can listen to any number of times while transcribing without removing your hands from your keyboard. *Transcriber* displays the transcript in the top portion of the screen and the waveform in the bottom.

To segment into utterances, you press enter on the keyboard while listening to the audio file. After each utterance of the audio file is segmented, you can listen to each one individually using a simple keystroke as many times as necessary to transcribe it. The "export-to-text" feature generates a text file that can then be used for analysis. You can download *Transcriber* at http://www.nch.com.au/scribe/index.html.

Each child utterance should be typed on a separate line and numbered. All of a child's utterances, including false starts, nonfluencies, and fillers, are transcribed. Although these linguistic elements may not be used for calculation of utterance length, they are extremely important in determining language and communication difficulties.

All utterances of the conversational partner(s) also are transcribed. These are important in assessing the manner and style of the conversational partners. The SLP is interested in the amount of control and the amount and type of talking exhibited by the partner.

We've mentioned utterances and utterance boundaries before. Let's explore these is more detail before we close.

> ***Food for Thought:*** **Conversational behavior doesn't resemble the neat dialogues found in most novels. Conversations are messy, filled with half-thoughts, unended sentences, interjections, and the like. Can you see why accurate transcription could be a challenge?**

Utterances

Determining utterance boundaries is often difficult. This is not an exact science, and the artistry of an SLP is needed at this point. Detailed information on utterances is presented in Table 6–6, including examples.

Table 6–6. Utterance Boundaries

A sentence is an utterance.

    Mommy went to the doctor's tomor . . . yesterday.

Run-on sentences with *and* should contain no more than one *and* joining clauses.

    We went in a bus and we saw monkeys and we had a picnic and we petted the sheeps and one sheep sneezed on me and we had sodas and we came home.

        Utterances:

        1. We went in a bus and we saw monkeys.
        2. (And) we had a picnic and we petted the sheeps.
        3. (And) one sheep sneezed on me and we had sodas.
        4. (And) we came home.

Other complex or compound sentences should be treated as one utterance.

    He was mad because his mommy spanked him because he broke the lamp and spilled the doggie's water.

Imperative sentences are utterances.

    Go home.

Pauses, voice drops, and/or inhalations mark boundaries.

    Eat (pause and voice drop) . . . chocolate candy.

        Two utterances: Eat. Chocolate candy.

    Eat (momentary delay) . . . chocolate candy.

        One utterance: Eat chocolate candy.

Situational and nonlinguistic cues help determine boundaries.

    Eat (hands plate to partner insistently) . . . chocolate candy (points to candy dish).

        Two utterances: Eat. Chocolate candy.

    Want (reaches unsuccessfully) . . . mommy (turns to look).

        Two utterances: Want. Mommy.

    Want mommy (reaches unsuccessfully).

        One utterance: Want, mommy.

The linguistic context also helps.

    Partner: Well, what do you want?

    Child: Candy (pause) . . . you get it.

        Two utterances: Candy. You get it.

CHAPTER 6 LANGUAGE SAMPLING

Determining boundaries between utterances is aided by the child's pauses, intonation, and breath patterns. Pauses can be empty or filled ("uh-h-h"), but a pause is a pause, even when filled. If the pause lasts 2 second or more, it separates two utterances.

Declaring sentences to be utterances is easy. Most of what is said, however, is not in complete sentence form. For example, the response to a question often omits shared information and might consist of such responses as "No," "Cookie," and "Okay." Each of these is a complete utterance.

Longer responses, such as "No, later" or "No, let's go later," are also single utterances. This determination might change if the child were to respond with a pause and a drop in the voice after "No":

"No (pause and drop voice). Let's go later."

Now there are two utterances.

Partial sentences or phrases, nonfluent units, and run-on sentences are even more difficult. A partial sentence might consist of the child pointing to an object and saying, "Doggie." This would count as an utterance. Parts of sentences may be strung together, as in the following exchange in which the child makes an internal repair:

Partner: I like to play mommy.

Child: No, you not . . . me the . . . you baby.

The entire unit is an utterance and will be analyzed in different ways by using all or part of what the child said. We'll get to that in a moment.

For run-on sentences of several clauses, there is no rule for how long to go before the utterance ends. Let's assume a child said

I went to the party, and we ate pizza, and we played games, and I won a prize, and we had cake and ice cream.

This type of sentence is common among preschools and it's long but not complicated. I follow a rule that allows two clauses to be joined together in a sentence with *and*. In the following example, using the previous sentence, utterance boundaries have been marked as they might be on a transcript:

I went to the party, and we ate pizza.

[and] We played games, and I won a prize.

[and] We had cake and ice cream.

Children in the late preschool years often make long strings of clauses with *and* meaning *and then*. Counting these as a single utterance inflates the mean utterance length. Young children are less likely to form run-ons with other conjunctions. Other conjunctions form more complex relationships, so I let those stand no matter how long the utterance continues.

Unfortunately, there is no universal rule on run-on sentences, and not everyone would agree with me. Check with your professor on that one.

Although false starts, nonfluencies, and fillers are included with the utterance and do tell us something about where difficulties may be encountered by the child, the SLP does not want to count them in quantitative analysis, such as TNW. For this reason, these elements are placed in brackets as in

So we went, we went to, you know, to the that thing, the the museum.

So we went [we went to, you know,] to the [that thing, the the] museum.

The resulting utterance, *So we went to the museum*, contains six words. The "you know," a filler, and "that thing," an imprecise empty word, may indicate word-finding difficulties.

The use of computers and computer programs for analysis programs, such as the Systematic Analysis of Language Transcripts (SALT; Miller & Iglesias, 2015), requires a consistent transcription format. An SLP will need to conform to the transcription guidelines to obtain the best information from these systems. SALT and other methods are described in Chapter 7 and are also presented in Appendix C.

Once the sample is transcribed, it can be analyzed. Analysis is the focus of Chapter 7.

Conclusion

Collecting a representative language sample from conversation, narration, and/or other means that demonstrates a child's diverse abilities is a difficult task requiring skill. Careful planning and execution are required, as are exacting methods of recording and transcription. Although these procedures may seem difficult and time-consuming initially, they can be accomplished easily and relatively quickly with practice. A properly planned and executed sampling and a thorough transcription will yield an abundance of linguistic and nonlinguistic information.

Guides for collecting a language sample include the following:

- Establish a positive relationship with the child before recording the language sample.
- Reduce your authority-figure persona to ensure more participation by the child. A child is more likely to respond naturally with someone who is more an equal.
- As the conversational partner, you should keep talking to a minimum. Although SLPs may abhor a vacuum, they should wait out the child when possible.
- Avoid yes/no questions and constituent questions (e.g., *What's that?*) that require only a one-word response from the child. Ask *process* questions or comments questions (e.g., *I wonder how you play soccer?*) rather than *product* questions (e.g., *Where do you go on Sunday?*)
- Follow the child's lead in play and in the selection of topic. Determine the child's interests before beginning the collection process. Select those materials at the child's interest level that are likely to stimulate interest.

CHAPTER 6 LANGUAGE SAMPLING

- If the child does not talk or responds in a very repetitive or stereotypic manner, model responses for the child or have another person model.
- Collect more than one sample if needed for a thorough description of a child's language. Remember that language will vary with the task, partner, and topic.

Only through sampling the child's linguistic abilities can the SLP gain insight into how a child's language works daily for that child. This is the first step in designing intervention that is relevant to the child and thus more likely to generalize to everyday use environments. That's called being functional.

CHAPTER 7
LANGUAGE SAMPLE ANALYSIS

Amanda, a school-based speech-language pathologist (SLP), is new in her job and still getting oriented. Several children have been referred by teachers or identified through screening tests as having possible language disorders. Language test scores placed many of these children in the language disorder category, but test scoring and descriptions of each child differ greatly.

Subtests have highlighted various individual aspects of language that seem disordered. The challenge for Amanda is to describe the big picture. How do these individual children function in the classroom and with peers? How does each child's deficit affect language use?

She is especially interested on narration and its effect on literacy. Do these children comprehend oral narratives and can they tell coherent ones? What effect will any oral language deficits have on each child's reading comprehension and the content of writing?

Amanda has decided to collect both conversational and narrative retell samples with each child but is in a quandary. She's unclear how she will analyze the samples. Should she use one method with all the children or tailor the language sample analysis just as she has tailored her overall assessment for each individual child?

She's also wondering how to analyze the narratives beyond morphosyntactic features. Do narratives require different data analysis? She is also concerned about the time it may take to do these analyses.

You probably analyzed a language sample in your language development course . . . and hated it! It may have seemed extremely challenging. After all, you'd never done it before. But your frustration may also reflect the global nature of the assignment: Analyze for everything!

While I'll be reviewing many of the analyses possible with a sample, please remember that if you follow an assessment model similar to that introduced in Chapter 5, by the time you get to language sample analysis (LSA), hopefully you'll have some idea what you're looking for. This fact can greatly shorten the process.

You won't be analyzing for everything and you won't hate it. I promise. Let's begin.

Language is complex, and the analysis methods used in LSA reflect this complexity. For this reason, analysis of a sample should not be a fishing expedition for possible problems. LSA is best used to explore certain aspects of a child's behavior brought into question through other data collection methods.

Traditional LSA has focused exclusively on the utterance or sentence as the unit of analysis. Although this type of analysis is appropriate for many language features, it may not be the best way to assess behaviors that transcend these units. To analyze language only at the utterance level is to miss many of a child's language skills, especially those aspects that govern cohesion and conversational manipulation. Only by going beyond individual utterances can an SLP gain an understanding of a child's use of the many language skills required to communicate. For example, an analysis of a child's use of pronouns necessitates crossing utterance boundaries in order to describe the child's introduction of new information (. . . *a doggie*) and reference to old or established information (*He* . . .) that may have been introduced by the child or the conversational partner.

LSA can range from relatively simple calculations, such as total number of words (TNW), to in-depth intra-sentential exploration, such as noun and verb phrase analysis. In general, quantitative values, such as TNW and mean length of utterance in morphemes (MLU_M), can be accomplished relatively quickly using a laptop computer. An SLP can calculate quantitative values to determine if a child might have a language disorder and then use more in-depth analysis to explore a child's specific difficulties and, hopefully, identify potential intervention targets. In our discussion, I've chosen to place quantitative analyses in the areas of language in which they can be used.

In this chapter, we look at levels of analysis and then discuss other considerations more appropriate for narrative samples.

Levels of Language Sample Analysis

Language sample analysis can occur by communication event, across utterance and partners, and at the utterance level, noting the adjustments a child must make to meet conversational demands. Table 7–1 lists some possible levels of LSA. These are by communication event, across utterances and partners and within utterances. It's important to stress that as an SLP, you'd only analyze areas of concern, not everything. The table may help you conceptualize LSA and provide the big picture view sought by Amanda.

Communication Event

For our purposes, communication event represents an entire conversation or narrative. Within an event, the speakers have a shared or negotiated agenda(s) supported by their utterances and turns. For the teenager who wants to be granted a privilege, such as getting to use the family car, each utterance supports this agenda.

Any difficulty with language will affect overall communication. For some children, such as those with social communication disorder (SCD), pragmatics will be the primary deficit. As you read, you'll note that when examining the communication event, pragmatics is prominent. Many aspects of communication are best assessed by looking at an interaction in its entirety.

An event includes the two roles of speaker and listener. Effective communicators can assume responsibility for both. Assessment variables that might measure a child's ability to participate effectively are the amount of socialized speech and a child's adaptive style; conversation and topic initiation, maintenance, and termination; the completeness,

CHAPTER 7 LANGUAGE SAMPLE ANALYSIS

233

Table 7–1. Levels of Language Sample Analysis
By Communication Event
Social versus nonsocial
Conversational initiation: Method, frequency, and success rate
Topic initiation: Method, frequency, success rate, and appropriateness
Conversation and topic maintenance: Frequency and latency of contingency
Duration of topic: Number of turns, informativeness, and sequencing
Topic analysis format: Topic initiation; type of topic; manner of initiation, subject matter, and orientations; outcome; topic maintenance, type of turn; and conversational information
Turn taking: Density, latency, and duration overlap: type, frequency, and duration signals
Conversation and topic termination
Conversational breakdown Request for repair: Frequency and form
Conversational repair Spontaneous versus listener-initiated Strategy and success rate
Across Utterances and Partners
Stylistic variations Register Interlanguage and code switching Channel availability
Referential communication Presuppositional skills: What is coded and how Linguistic devices: Deictics, definite and indefinite reference
Cohesive devices Reference: Initial and following mention Ellipsis Conjunction Adverbial conjuncts and disjuncts Contrastive stress
Analysis at the Utterance Level

Use
 Disruptions
 Illocutionary functions and intentions
    Frequency and range
    Appropriateness
    Encoding

continues

Table 7–1. *continued*

Analysis at the Utterance Level *continued*

Content
    Lexical items
        Type-token ration
        Over-/underextensions and incorrect use
        Style and lexicon
    Word relationships
        Semantic categories
        Intrasentence relationships
    Figurative language
    Word-finding

Form
    Quantitative measures
        Mean length of utterance
        Mean syntactic length
        T-units and C-units
    Syntactic and morphological analysis
        Morphological analysis
        Syntactical analysis
            Noun phrase
            Verb phrase
            Sentence types
            Embedding and conjoining
        Computer-assisted language analysis

relevance, and clarity of a child's behavior; on-topic exchanges and turn taking; and conversational repairs. We'll discuss all of these.

LSA occurs at two levels: the molar and the molecular. At the molar level, an SLP evaluates each behavior for appropriateness within the conversational context. Inappropriate behaviors may indicate problem areas for further assessment. At the molecular level, an SLP is interested in values, such as frequency, latency, duration, density, and sequence. These values, such as the frequency of interrupting and the density of clauses, can only be determined by looking at the entire event.

Frequency data or the number of occurrences can reveal inordinately high- or low-frequency features. *Latency*, the span of time when an individual does not engage in behavior, is also important. Pauses and hesitations may reveal difficulty decoding the preceding utterance or forming a response. *Duration* is the length of time that a child and a partner are engaged in a certain behavior, such as conversational gaze or conversational turns. *Density* is the number of behaviors within a certain period of time. Of interest are

CHAPTER 7 LANGUAGE SAMPLE ANALYSIS

the density of different conversational topics or specific linguistic structures, such as questions. Finally, *sequence* includes the order of events.

Decisions of appropriateness may be facilitated through the use of a modified ethnographic technique similar to that used in anthropological studies. Each utterance is given a reference frame described by form, content, and use, plus paralinguistic and nonlinguistic behaviors and context. Behaviors are not judged for appropriateness by one aspect alone but, rather, by the totality of the frame. For example, yelling is appropriate in some situations but not in others. Within this frame, behavior is judged for appropriateness. Table 7–2 provides a sample of a dialogue and the accompanying ethnographic analysis. Ethnographic techniques are especially important when assessing children with culturally linguistically diverse (CLD) backgrounds.

Social Versus Nonsocial Communication

Social speech is speech addressed explicitly to and adapted for a listener who has an obligation to respond. For example, a lecture or recounting a story is a social monologue. The speaker's message is delivered as if the speaker expects a listener response.

In contrast, *nonsocial speech* is not addressed explicitly to a listener, and the listener has no obligation to respond. An important measure of communication is the percentage of the child's utterances or the amount of total talk time that can be characterized as social.

Although preschoolers produce many asocial monologues accompanying their play, the amount of time spent in this type of production decreases with age. School-age children with typically developing language (TDL) produce very little nonsocial speech,

Table 7–2. An Example of Ethnographic Analysis

Language Sample	Ethnographic Analysis
Child: What's that? *Partner:* That's a "Thing-a-majibit." *Child:* What it do?	Child does not seem to know the identity of an object and inquires as to its name with an appropriate *wh-* question addressed to the partner. The partner supplies an appropriate answer but does not elaborate. The child seeks such elaboration by asking a second *wh-* question in which he omits the auxiliary verb. Other sentence elements are included in the proper adult word order.
Partner: What do you think it does? *Child:* On the table.	The partner does not answer the question but responds with a second *wh-* question in order to have the child guess at the function from its appearance. The child responds inappropriately to the partner's question, either ignoring the content of the question or miscomprehending the meaning of the *wh-* word.
Partner: YES, on the table. What about "On the table?" *Child:* On the table.	The partner does not pursue the question by restating or reformulating it. Instead, the partner confirms the child's utterance and asks a third *wh-* question incorporating the child's utterance. Again, the child does not respond to the content of the partner's question but repeats the previous utterance with no additional information to aid the partner's understanding.

and their communication becomes more interpersonal as they mature. In contrast, the speech of some children with autism spectrum disorder (ASD) may contain many asocial monologues.

> ***Food for Thought:*** **Many LSA methods focus on utterances. Can you see a need to move beyond this microstructural level?**

Conversations

In conversations, both partners are expected to contribute and to tailor their message for their partner. Within different cultures, the form of a conversation will vary.

Initiation. The most efficient way to initiate a conversation is to gain your listener's attention, greet the listener, and clearly state the topic of conversation or some opener, such as "Guess what happened to me yesterday?" or "Where have you been? I haven't seen you in ages." Openers set the tone of the conversation and the subsequent turns. Opening and closing a conversation is one of the pragmatic problems most frequently encountered in children with language disorders. For example, children with ASD may initiate very little conversational behavior. Of clinical interest is how a child initiates the conversation and how successful they are in having the conversation continue.

Method. It is best to get a potential listener's attention before initiating a conversation. This usually is accomplished by eye contact and a greeting. A child with a language disorder may begin without any greeting or may interrupt an ongoing conversation with "Hey." While in a classroom recently, I became aware that a preschooler was talking to my butt. He had neither sought my attention nor offered a greeting. Some children use the same opener repeatedly (e.g., "Guess what?"), no matter the conversational context. Data may need to be collected over a wide variety of situations or by parental or teacher report to discern a pattern.

Frequency and Success Rate. Children who are withdrawn or unsure, such as those who have a history of abuse, may initiate conversations only rarely. Instead, they adopt a more passive, responsive role. In contrast, other children, such as those with attention-deficit/hyperactivity disorder (ADHD), may interrupt frequently and attempt to initiate conversation indiscriminately. Of interest to an SLP is the density of initiations, or the number of initiations over a given time.

The success rate of children in initiating conversations is also significant. Although children may attempt to begin conversations frequently, they may be ignored or mocked, depending on the audiences they choose. Children who are socially inappropriate may experience more than their share of rejection.

Conversation Maintenance. In effective conversations, the participants seem to adhere to four principles: stay on topic, be truthful, be brief, and be relevant. Children

CHAPTER 7 LANGUAGE SAMPLE ANALYSIS

with language disorders tend to engage in fewer and shorter interactions than do children with TDL. The most frequent challenges for children with language disorders include connecting discourse cohesively, listening and responding to a speaker, knowing when to take a turn, and knowing how to ask and answer questions.

The difference between the turn-taking skills of children with language disorders and of those without widens as language becomes increasingly more complex. Children with ASD may not respond to initiations, whereas other children with learning disorder (LD) or SCD may overuse turn-fillers or acknowledgments (*uh-huh*) to keep the conversation going even when their comprehension is lacking.

Conversation Termination. Conversations end when no new information is added. As with the opening of a conversation, there are often adjacency pairs, such as the following:

Situation 1

Speaker 1: Bye, see ya.

Speaker 2: Have a nice day.

Situation 2

Speaker 1: Thank you.

Speaker 2: You're welcome.

Preschool children or those with language disorders may end the conversation abruptly when they decide it is over, occasionally just exiting the conversational context. Children with LD or traumatic brain injury (TBI) and those with emotional disorders may not prepare the listener for termination and end abruptly or may be unable or unwilling to end the conversation and may perseverate or continue to ask questions that have been answered previously.

Topic

Once a conversation has been initiated, the participants negotiate the topics. Topic is the subject matter being discussed. A topic is sustained as long as each conversational partner cares to continue and can contribute relevant information.

Topic Analysis Format. Several topic analysis formats have been proposed. Each addresses different aspects of topic initiation, maintenance, and change. These are presented in Table 7–3. Topic initiation analysis may include the type of topic, the manner of initiation, the subject matter and orientation, and the outcome. Topic maintenance analysis may consider the type of turn and the ability of the client to further the conversation with the addition of new conversational information.

Initiation. Topic initiations occur when the topic of discussion is changed in some way. One partner introduces a topic; the other partner agrees to adopt that topic by

Table 7–3. Analysis Aspects of Topic	
Topic Initiation	**Topic Maintenance**
Type of topic	Type of turn
Manner of initiation	Conversational information
Subject matter and orientation	
Outcome	

commenting, disagrees by changing the topic, or ends the conversation. Each new topic and directly related utterances can be identified on the transcript.

Mature speakers identify the topic clearly by name and, if in the immediate context, by pointing. Preschool children and those with language disorders tend to rely more on nonlinguistic cues, such as pointing to and holding or shaking objects.

In general, children with language disorders are less adept than both their age-matched and language-age-matched peers in their ability to direct the conversation by introducing topics. This lack of ability might reflect difficulty identifying topics clearly and/or a limited list of potential topics.

Method. As mentioned previously, an effectively initiated topic is identified clearly. Topics are negotiated between speakers based on the shared assumptions of each participant.

In general, the less sure a speaker is that a listener knows the topic, the longer the speaker will take to introduce it. In return, listeners assure speakers that they understand, or they ask for clarification when they do not understand.

A child with a language disorder may not establish topics, preferring to adopt those of others. If a child does introduce topics, there may be little or no background information to aid the listener. A child may also have a very restricted set of conversational or topic openers or may rely on a stereotypic utterance (e.g., "Hey, guess what?"). Some children will not state the topic explicitly and may continue under the assumption that the listener is somehow privy to this information.

As mentioned previously, children with word-finding difficulties or poor vocabularies may rely on nonspecific nouns, such as *one* or *thing*. Nonspecific verbs, such as *do* and *get*, also may be used frequently. "I did it" may not get the topic off to a roaring start.

The child with a language disorder may not be able to identify the speaker's topic or to determine what response is required. Therefore, the child may not respond or provide a noncontingent or off-topic response.

Both the linguistic and nonlinguistic aspects of a sample should be analyzed. The nonlinguistic aspects, such as eye contact, regulate the linguistic ones and are significant in the regulation of turn initiation and termination, topic choice, and interruptions.

Each topic can be rated according to its novelty. Possible rating categories could include *new*, *related*, *reintroduced*, and *rolling*. New topics would be those appearing in the conversation for the first time. Related topics would be linked directly to the previous

CHAPTER 7 LANGUAGE SAMPLE ANALYSIS

239

topic. Reintroduced topics would have appeared in the conversation previously but prior to the preceding turn. Finally, rolling topics are initiated in sequence with no opportunity for the listener to maintain the preceding topic. In addition, the SLP could check with the caregivers to determine whether any of the topics introduced by the child are habitual ones. Table 7–4 presents examples of different types of topic initiation.

Manner of Initiation. The manner of topic initiation might include *coherent changing*, *noncoherent changing*, *branching*, and *shading*. Coherent changing occurs when one topic is terminated and a following topic's content is derived from the preceding topic. Noncoherent changing occurs with the absence of topic termination and/or an utterance signaling transition to a new topic. Branching occurs when the topic being discussed serves as a source for a new topic. Shading differs from branching in that shading is a change of focus on the same topic, rather than a discrete topic change. Table 7–5 presents the different manners of initiation.

Appropriateness and Orientation. The appropriateness of a topic is determined by the context. As an SLP, you'll be interested in determining a child's favorite topics and in assessing their appropriateness in context. Children with SCD may have only limited topics or perseverate on a few. I worked with two brothers with ASD who seemingly could talk only about mathematics. A third child with severe LD seemed limited to discussing—Excuse me—throwing up, a topic with little appeal.

Table 7–4. Types of Topics Initiated

Topic Type	Example
New	*Partner:* Uh-huh, and what else did you see at the zoo? *Child:* Mommy got a new car.
Related	*Partner:* I like monkeys too. What else? Were there any clowns at the circus? *Child:* I don't like clowns. They're scary. *Partner:* Clowns are scary? Why do you think clowns are scary?
Reintroduced	*Child:* And Ernie spilled s'ghetti all over Bert. *Partner:* Was Bert angry? *Child:* Uh-huh. And . . . and Ernie? . . . And Ernie laughed. *Partner:* Poor Bert. That would be yukky. What else happened on *Sesame Street*? *Child:* Big Bird and Little Bird singed a song. *Partner:* Can you sing it for me? *Child:* Uh-huh. I don't like s'ghetti on me.
Rolling	*Partner:* Oh, tell me the story. *Child:* Okay. This little girl? . . . Can you come to my birthday party? I got a new bike yesterday. Do you live here?

Table 7–5. Manner of Topic Initiation

Manner of Initiation	Example
Coherent changing	*Child:* And he chased the dinosaur away. *Partner:* What a great story. Anything else to tell? *Child:* I have a new baby.
Noncoherent changing	*Child:* Let's have toast for breakfast. *Partner:* Let me fix it. *Child:* Those are supposed to go down. *Partner:* You do this one, and I'll do the other one. *Child:* I'm gonna have a bowl of . . . What's that? I think it's a fireman hat. I wanta be a fireman. *Partner:* May I wear it?
Branching	*Partner:* There, I'm gonna make some eggs. *Child:* I don't like eggs. *Partner:* No, why don't you like eggs? *Child:* I want some? . . . some juice. I like juice. *Partner:* What kind of juice do you want?
Shading	*Partner:* Let's have toast. *Child:* Where's the toaster? *Partner:* I'll cook the toast. *Child:* I'll butter it. Where's the knife? *Partner:* You have to find the knife. *Child:* It too sharp for toast.

Orientation might be called the focus and include topics about self, a shared experience or interest with the listener, or a topic seemingly unrelated to the listener or to a shared interest. If the orientation is always the speaker or always unrelated, then SCD or another problem may exist.

Frequency and Outcome. As with conversational initiation, the density and outcome of topic initiation are noteworthy. In general, less dominant speakers will introduce fewer topics and will be less successful in having their topics adopted by their partners.

A success outcome is dependent on the manner of initiation, the subject matter, and the form of the initiation. Success occurs when the conversational partner acknowledges the speaker's topic in some way, responds, repeats, agrees or disagrees, or adds information to maintain the topic. Nonsuccess includes no response, an interruption, initiation of a new topic, or a request for repair. Although there are many variables related to success, the percentage of time that a child is successful can be an important descriptive index.

CHAPTER 7 LANGUAGE SAMPLE ANALYSIS

241

Topic Maintenance. Each partner depends on a response's contingency, or being related to what preceded it. Each response adds new information on the topic that is mentioned frequently enough to enable both participants to recall it.

Topic continuance may be signaled by maintenance devices such as *now*, *well*, *and then*, *in any case*, *next*, and *so*, followed by *I* (*you*, *we*, *they*) did something. Some devices, called *continuants*, maintain the conversation but add little, if any, new information. Examples of this behavior are *yeah*, *uhhuh*, and *okay* used to signal that the listener is paying attention. Other maintenance devices are repeating a portion or all of the previous utterance.

Topic maintenance can be analyzed in all turns subsequent to initiation of a topic. Each turn can be analyzed on the basis of the continuous or discontinuous nature of the turn and on its informativeness.

Contingency. *Semantically contingent* utterances relate to or reflect the meaning of the prior utterance by maintaining the topic and adding to it. For example, in response to the utterance, "We went to Captain Jake's for dinner last night," a second speaker might make the contingent remark, "Oh, did you enjoy the food?" A semantically noncontingent remark would be "My uncle lives on a farm."

The frequency of contingent behaviors by a child is of interest. The child who exhibits few contingent utterances might initiate new topics instead. The SLP can note the percentage of a child's utterances that are on-topic, the relevance of the child's questions, and the child's nonverbal responses, such as following directions or looking at something that was mentioned.

The SLP should look for an underlying contingency that may not be readily obvious. Children with LD may assume that their partners know the underlying relationship and, therefore, may only include unshared information.

A large percentage of off-topic responses may indicate a semantic disorder characterized by difficulty in identifying the topic of discussion. A listener's ability to identify a topic subsequently affects comprehension of comments made about that topic. Imagine responding to "What do you think?" when you can't identify what's being discussed. Some children with language disorders may respond with stereotypic acknowledgments (*uh-huh*, *yeah*) or *what* and *huh*.

Answers should be relevant to the question. For example, the question, "Why is the man eating?" might elicit the following responses from different children:

- Food.
- Because.
- He has to.
- So he won't be hungry.
- He's hungry.

The first answer doesn't answer the question but, rather, tells what the man is eating. The second and third responses are too brief to be accurate. The fourth and fifth answers are relevant and accurate.

If an answer does not fulfill both relevance and accuracy requirements, it is in error and may indicate any number of possible breakdowns in the communication process. I worked with a child with a severe emotional disorder who gave extremely irrelevant replies to emotional or personal questions, although her responses to factual questions were usually acceptable.

A child with a language disorder may not understand what the questioner desires or may not realize that a reply is required. The question form and the specific *wh-* question type also may be confusing. Some *wh-* words and question forms seem easier than others. We can group *wh-* words from easiest to most difficult to comprehend:

Easiest	What + be, which, where
	Who, whose, what + do
Most difficult	When, why, what happened, how

It is easier for children to respond to questions referring to objects, persons, or events that are within the immediate setting.

Most school-age children make contingent responses with little delay or latency. Preschoolers and children with language disorders may allow long gaps to develop. A noticeable latency prior to a child's response may indicate word-finding difficulties, lack of comprehension, or difficulty forming a reply.

Latency can indicate difficulty and is an important measure for both contingent and noncontingent utterances, whether adjacent or nonadjacent. Adjacent utterances are spoken as sequential behaviors by the same speaker. A nonadjacent utterance crosses conversational turns and thus seems out of place. Definitions and examples of these categories are presented in Table 7–6.

Duration. The number of turns taken on a topic is a function of the particular topic and partners involved, the conversational context, and the conversational skill of each participant. In general, a greater number of turns will occur in an adult–child conversation if the child, rather than the adult, initiates the topic. Topics that are sustained longer than others may suggest the child's interest or knowledge or both.

Younger than age 3 years, children rarely maintain a topic for more than two turns. Preschoolers take very few turns on a topic unless enacting scenarios, describing events, or solving problems. More turns generally will be produced when the preschool child is directing the partner through a task or when the child is telling a narrative. Although the number of turns increases slightly with age, the average of two or three turns on a topic remains until mid-elementary school.

A topic suggests words that will accompany it. Thus, the word *hike* suggests *boots*, *woods*, *walk*, and so on. A child who has word-finding difficulties or cannot identify the topic will take few turns and often change the topic.

Topic Termination. Topics usually are terminated by shifting to another related topic. For more mature language users, this process is accomplished by *shading*, in which

CHAPTER 7 LANGUAGE SAMPLE ANALYSIS

243

Table 7–6. Definitions and Examples of Utterance Pairs

Type	Definition	Examples
Contingent	The utterance of one speaker is based on the content, form, and/or intent of the other speaker.	S_1: What do you want for lunch? S_2: Peanut butter. S_1: I hope I don't miss my plane. S_2: Don't worry. Every flight is delayed.
Noncontingent	The utterance of one speaker is not based on that of the other.	S_1: What do you want for lunch? S_2: Gran'ma gots a new car.
Adjacent	Utterances spoken sequentially by the same speaker.	We went to the zoo. I saw monkeys and elephants. But my favorite part was petting the sheeps.
Nonadjacent	Utterances spoken sequentially by different speakers. The utterances may be contingent or noncontingent.	S_1: Here comes the school bus. S_2: Yukk, I was hoping he'd get a flat tire (Contingent)

the speakers shift to another aspect of the topic or to a closely related topic, as in the following exchange:

Speaker 1:   I biked along the canal path yesterday.

Speaker 2:   Oh, I love to bike there at this time of year.

Speaker 1:   I didn't know you bike. What sort of bike do you have?

Speaker 2:   I have an inexpensive 12-speed.

Speaker 1:   I have a 21-speed but it's old.

The original topic of the canal bike path slid into the topic of bicycles. Although we don't possess much normative data, we know that between 7th and 12th grade, the number of abrupt topic shifts in an adolescent conversation decreases from 3.19 to 1.44.

Whether topics are shaded or are changed abruptly, there is normally some continuity, and the new topic is stated clearly. When there is little left to discuss on a given topic, the conversation shifts or ends. The SLP notes the method the child uses to terminate and change topics and to terminate conversations.

Summary. The topic analysis categories presented in this section overlap and are not always mutually exclusive. These are only suggestions, and use will depend on your LSA purpose.

It's difficult to discuss topic without mentioning turn taking. Let's explore this area of possible analysis.

> **Food for Thought:** Imagine a conversation in which one partner could not remain on topic. Each turn resulted in a topic change. What would happen to the overall continuity of the conversation?

Turn Taking

Turn taking is an excellent vehicle for evaluating the interactional framework of a listener and a speaker. The unit of analysis is the dyad (both partners) and the interaction between them.

The minimum number of turns to complete an exchange is three. The person who begins the exchange must have a second turn before an interaction has occurred. Each speaker acknowledges the preceding utterance, contributes, and indicates that the turn is to be shifted:

> *Speaker 1:*   We just returned from Florida.
>
> *Speaker 2:*   Oh, did you go to Disney World?
>
> *Speaker 1:*   No, we were in Fort Lauderdale. Ever been there?

Turns were acknowledged by *oh* and *no*. Indications of turn allocation may consist of questions, intonational markers, pauses, body language, and eye contact.

As an SLP, you might mark exchanges on the transcript, numbering them turn 1, 2, 3, and so on. In this way, a child's ability to initiate, add to, and terminate exchanges can be noted. In addition, an SLP can indicate the frequency, variety or range, and consistency of a child's communication. Within each turn, the SLP notes the presence or absence of the three aspects of a full turn and the average amount of time spent in a turn. The SLP also can examine the effects of adult behaviors on the child's conversational turns and later can help adults develop more facilitative styles.

Turns may be classified as obligation, comment, or reply. An obligation is initiated by the speaker and demands a response. In contrast, a comment does not require a response. A reply can be to either an obligation or a comment. The percentage of each category may indicate active and passive speakers, those that initiate and those that respond.

All responses to obligations can be analyzed further as *adequate, over-adequate, inadequate,* and *ambiguous.* Adequate responses give only the information requested; they are appropriate for the request. Over-adequate responses give more than requested, whereas inadequate responses do not give enough. Ambiguous responses are unclear.

As mentioned in the discussion of topics, turns may also be classified as *continuous* or *discontinuous* on the basis of their linkage or nonlinkage to the topic. Continuous turns continue the topic in some way. Discontinuous turns—ones not linked to the current topic—include new topic initiations, off-topic responses, monologues, and evasion, including inappropriate silence.

This may be difficult to digest given the plethora of terms. Topics continue or do not based on what happens within each turn. The skill in maintaining a conversation is

CHAPTER 7 LANGUAGE SAMPLE ANALYSIS

245

related to how well each speaker uses language. Each turn must be related to the topic and responsive to the partner if the conversation is going to advance. The terms we've mentioned attempt to describe this relationship. Take a minute to be certain that you see this in the previous discussion. Types of turns are presented in Table 7–7.

Analysis includes the frequency and range of each type of turn and the average number of turns per topic. The percentage of continuous versus discontinuous turns also would be valuable data, although no norms exist.

Finally, turns might be analyzed for the extent to which they contribute to the development of the topic. Turns adding new information might include unsolicited conversational replies that add more information or requests and answers to questions that contain new information. Other turns, such as acknowledgments (*uh-huh*), requests for repair (*What?*), and repetitions, generally add no new information. A common strategy when someone does not understand what was said is to respond neutrally with "Uh-huh" or "Yeah." Examples of conversational informativeness are included in Table 7–8.

The SLP can calculate the percentage of turns contributing novel information and thus furthering the topic. Other types of turns may indicate possible problem areas. Specific strategies used by children should be investigated by analyzing the form of the utterances being used.

Density. A low density of turns may indicate that a child's conversational partner dominated the conversation by taking very long turns, relinquishing them to the child only occasionally, or that the child was very reticent. Children with ASD may take relatively few verbal turns, thus leaving the partner to fill the void. In contrast, if a child talked

Table 7–7. Types of Turns

Turn Type	Examples
Obligation	Do you want some cookies?
	What time is it?
	What's that?
Comment	I really love to ski.
	I saw horses in the parade.
Response to comment	I
	It's an old family recipe.
Response to obligation	(Obligation: How old are you?)
Adequate	I'm 25.
Over-adequate	I'm 25, and I have a master's degree.
Inadequate	I go to college.
Ambiguous	None of your business.
	Guess.

Table 7–8. Informativeness of Turns	
Informativeness	**Examples**
New information	*Partner:* Where's Mary? *Child:* She's sick today.
	Partner: We're going to the zoo tomorrow. *Child:* Monkeys live in the zoo.
No new information	*Partner:* And cowboys ride horsies too. *Child:* Ride horsie.
	Partner: Let's play with the stove. *Child:* What?
Problematic	*Partner:* What should we play now? *Child:* A . . . a . . . with a . . . a . . . with a . . . you know.
	Partner: Who's your teacher? *Child:* At school.

for lengthy turns, the density also would be low because the listener would have little chance to reply.

Latency. An SLP can summarize the overall contingent and noncontingent latencies of a child. Longer periods and/or the continual use of fillers and interjections may indicate difficulties with topic identification or word finding.

Informativeness. As mentioned previously, each turn should add to the conversation by confirming the topic and contributing additional information. Children with LD who have difficulty identifying the topic or those with SCD who have difficulty determining what is expected of them may repeat or paraphrase old information, overuse continuants, or use circumlocution, talking around the topic in a nonspecific manner. The SLP can rate each utterance for its contribution to the topic being discussed.

Sequencing. Once a topic is introduced, a sequence follows. In general, more specific information is introduced until a natural termination or a change in topic occurs. Answers or replies follow questions; comments or questions follow comments. New information is introduced and later referred to as old information. A lack of sequencing may indicate a semantic or apragmatic disorder characterized relative to presupposition.

Duration of Turns. There is no ideal length for a turn, although most listeners know when a turn has continued for too long. We all know at least one incessant talker who does not know when enough has been said. A child who talks incessantly may be exhibiting a semantic disorder of not knowing what information is needed to close the topic,

CHAPTER 7 LANGUAGE SAMPLE ANALYSIS

a pragmatic disorder of not knowing the mechanisms for closing a turn or topic, or a processing problem of not being certain what information was conveyed.

The SLP is interested in the average length of the child's and the partner's turns. Different situations, partners, and topics may yield clinically significant differences in turn length.

Overlap. Most turns will be nonsimultaneous. When it occurs, overlap or simultaneous speaking can be very revealing. In general, overlap is of two types: internal and initial. Sentence internal overlaps are used to complete the other speaker's turn and secure a turn. A child with a language disorder may interrupt internally, indicating a lack of understanding of the process, and may add new information or change the topic rather than complete the other speaker's utterance.

Sentence initial overlaps result when a listener interjects between sentences to secure a turn. Continual overlaps of this type may indicate a breakdown in turn taking as a result of the behavior of one or both partners. In contrast, a low incidence of inter-rupting, as noted among some children with specific language impairment (SLI), may indicate passivity or an inability to initiate a "turn grab."

Interestingly, the rate of interrupting increases during the teen years, but the purpose changes. Increasingly, speakers interrupt not to disrupt or change the topic but, rather, to move the discussion forward to facilitate communication.

Data indicate that as a group, children with language disorders exhibit less simulta-neous speech in their conversations. Many children with language disorders are passive in initiating interaction or turn taking.

The adult rules for turn taking state that when an overlap occurs, one speaker will withdraw. Young children or children with language disorders may continue to talk or try to outshout their partner. Some children withdraw habitually. It may help in describing a child's communication to observe this behavior.

Occasionally, a child with a language disorder will respond only to questions. Such children may lack a basic understanding of the expectation to reply. Still others cannot decipher the language code efficiently enough to respond.

Summary. More than one turn type and informativeness category may be present in a turn. A possible analysis format is presented in Table 7–9. Each type of information gives an SLP an additional tool for describing a child's language.

Conversational Breakdown. An SLP's analysis of language is an attempt, in part, to find where a child is ineffectual, where they falter at communication. It is important for an SLP to determine where breakdowns occur and how a child attempts to repair them. The SLP should try to determine the number of conversational breakdowns and, if possible, describe the cause of breakdown, the repair, and the outcome.

Breakdown can occur for a number of reasons, including lack of intelligibility or volume, incompleteness of information, degree of complexity, inappropriateness, irrelevance, and lack of mutual attention, visual regard, or mutual desire. As might be expected, children with language disorders experience a greater number of breakdowns than do age-matched peers with TDL.

Table 7–9. Possible Format for Rating Topics and Turns

Categories	Turns																		Total	% of Total
	1	2	3	4	5	6	7	8	9	10	11	12	13	14	15	16	17	18		
Topic Initiation																				
Type of topic																				
New																				
Related																				
Reintroduced																				
Rolling																				
Manner of initiation																				
Coherent change																				
Noncoherent change																				
Branching																				
Shading																				
Subject matter																				
Appropriate																				
Inappropriate																				
Orientation																				
Self																				
Shared																				
Unrelated																				
Outcome																				
Successful																				
Unsuccessful																				
Topic Maintenance																				
Type of turn																				
Continuous																				
Discontinuous																				
Conversational information																				
New information																				
No new information																				
Problematic																				

CHAPTER 7 LANGUAGE SAMPLE ANALYSIS

Requests for Repair. Requests for repair, called *contingent queries*, signal the listener's attentiveness or understanding and skill in addressing the point of conversational break-down. In general, young children use unspecific requests, such as "What?" More mature speakers try to specify the information desired. Requests for repair may seek repetition of the preceding utterance, confirmation, or clarification.

Appropriate requests for repair and responses by the conversational partner demonstrate an awareness of the cooperative nature of conversation. A child who continually responds with *Huh?* or *What?* may not be attending to the conversation or may have difficulty understanding. The SLP is interested in the degree to which a child requests additional information toward maintaining the conversation and in the form of these requests.

A child with a language disorder may be unaware that a communication breakdown has occurred. In general, children first gain awareness of breakdowns caused by unintelligible words. The order of breakdown awareness development is as follows:

- Unintelligible words
- Impossible commands
- Unrealistically long utterances
- Unfamiliar words
- Question or statement without an introduction and ambiguous, inexplicit, and open-ended statements

Frequency and Form. In general, preschool children and those with LD tend to blame themselves, rather than the speaker, for misunderstanding. Thus, these children use fewer requests for repair than might be expected, especially given the greater likelihood of communication breakdown. The requests produced tend to be less specific, reflecting the difficulty encountered with these forms.

Although there are no norms for the frequency of repair requests, general guidelines do indicate a change in both the frequency and the type of contingent query with age. The earliest requests for repair are repetitions of the partner's utterance with rising intonation (*Doggie go ride?*) or nonspecific requests for repetition (*What?*). With age, requests become more specific and increase in frequency, although both vary according to the conversational partner. With an adult partner, 24- to 36-month-olds use approximately 7 requests an hour, and 54- to 66-month-olds use approximately 14. When the partner is a familiar peer, the mean rate for 36- to 66-month-olds increases to 30 per hour.

Conversational Repair. Conversational repair may be either spontaneous or in response to a request for repair. Preschool children spontaneously repair very little. Even in first grade, children spontaneously repair only about one-third of their conversational breakdowns. Young children or children with language disorders often do not attempt to repair communication breakdowns.

By age 2 years, most children respond consistently to neutral requests such as "What?" although they are more likely to respond if the conversational partner is an adult rather than another child. Two-year-olds also tend to overuse "yes" and thus confirm interpretations even when incorrect, possibly because nonconfirmation requires clarification on their part. By age 3 to 5 years, children respond correctly, even to specific requests, approximately 80% of the time regardless of the partner. Most 10-year-olds are adept at determining breakdown and repairing the damage. Although children with LD at that age can identify faulty messages, they do not seem to understand repair strategies.

Repairs usually focus on the linguistic structure or on the content or nature of the information conveyed. Extralinguistic signals, such as pointing, may be used to clarify. These strategies are not mutually exclusive. In general, successful outcomes are related to the explicitness and appropriateness of the repair strategy chosen.

When a child repairs spontaneously, the nature of the original error and the repair attempts should be noted. The SLP scans the transcript for all fillers, repetitions, perseverations, and long pauses. All of these may indicate word-finding difficulties on the child's part. The original error or repair attempt may be based on any number of relationships with the intended word or phrase, as noted in Table 7–10.

Strategy. Immature speakers usually respond to listener-initiated requests for repair by restating the previous utterance. Continued requests also may result in children providing additional information, although children with language disorders seem less flexible in the use of this strategy.

More mature speakers usually give additional information or reformulate their original utterance. When requested to clarify, children with language disorders tend to respond less frequently and with less complex responses than do their peers with TDL. The responses of children with language disorders usually consist of repetition with little

Table 7–10. Relationship of Word-Finding Errors and Repair Attempts to the Intended Word	
Association	**Examples**
Definition	*the thing you cook food on* for *stove*
Description	*the long skinny one with no legs* for *snake*
	book holder for *bookend*
	fuzzy for *peach*
Generic (less specific)	*do* for *more specific verb*
	hat for *cap, bonnet, scarf,* etc.
	thing or *one* for *name of entity*
Opposites	*sit* for *stand*
Partial	*ball . . . big ball . . . red ball* for *big red ball*
Semantic category	*stove* for *refrigerator* (both are appliances)
Sound	*toe* for *tie* (initial sound similar)
	goat for *coat* (rhyme)

CHAPTER 7 LANGUAGE SAMPLE ANALYSIS **251**

new information included. In contrast, children with TDL seem to have a greater range of repair strategies.

As an SLP, you can prepare a list of the various types of requests for clarification and use them in conversation with a child. Of interest is the child's rate of responding to various requests and the nature of the child's responses.

Frequency of Success. An SLP is interested in how successfully a child identifies breakdowns, repairs them spontaneously, and follows listener requests. In general, children with language disorders make more inappropriate responses to listener requests than do peers with TDL.

Your head may be swimming with terminology. Take a short break and then skim back through the communication event behaviors to be sure that you understand.

Across Utterances and Partners

Let's turn our LSA spotlight on units smaller than the entire communication event but larger than the individual utterance. Although LSA at the utterance level can reveal much about a child's discrete, finite language skills, it can also miss conversational skills overall. Likewise, analysis of the entire event isn't finite enough to examine the use of reference, and individual utterance referencing misses questions of appropriateness to the conversational milieu.

To do all this, the SLP must look across utterances and to the language of a child's communication partner. This level of LSA is appropriate for examining such features as stylistic variation, referential communication, and cohesive strategies.

Stylistic Variations

The style of talking, whether formal, casual, or varied in other ways for the situation, usually does not change utterance by utterance. Rather, it is a manner of talking with a specific language partner or in a specific situation. Different styles also may be seen in role-play. Variation requires a speaker to consider the listener and the situation and the resultant requirements on the speaker.

Register. *Style switching*, the move from one style or register to another, must be judged against the age, gender, and language ability of the speaker and the listener. Styles differ according to role-taking characteristics, dialectal variations, amount of politeness, and conversational control.

Conversational roles can be established by the topics chosen, vocabulary (*dear, sir, honey*), pronunciation, and the discourse style (formal, casual, playful, etc.). Children with LD or SCD often fail to use registers based on differing situational variables.

The most frequent problems with register include providing insufficient information, not knowing when to make a statement, asking inappropriate questions, giving insufficient reason for the cause and effect of a situation, and not adjusting register to the speaker. An SLP can look for a child's modifications in politeness, intimacy, and linguistic code based on the age, status, familiarity, cognitive level, linguistic level, and shared past experience of the listener. Inappropriate styles are those that are too formal, too casual, or include excessive swearing or baby talk. The SLP might also note features such as differing utterance length with various partners. Other variations include vocabulary and topic. More subjective indices include intonational patterns and the use of attention-getting and -maintaining devices.

Channel Availability. Most children younger than age 11 years experience less communication success when they do not visually share the communication environment with their listener, as when on a smartphone. As the number of communication channels decreases, a child with a language disorder should have increasing difficulty communicating. The SLP should note the relative success of the child's communication efforts as the number of channels varies.

Referential Communication

Referential communication is the ability of a speaker to select and verbally identify the attributes of an entity in such a way that the listener can identify the entity accurately. To succeed, the speaker must be able to determine what information the listener needs, deliver that information in a specific manner, make comparisons, and use feedback on message adequacy and breakdown. Whereas "He has brown hair" fails to communicate the referent, "The only boy in my history class has brown hair" succeeds.

Referential communication includes directions, explanations, and descriptions. Deficits in these three essential aspects of classroom discourse may contribute to academic difficulties.

Presuppositional Skills. As mentioned previously, presupposition is a speaker's assumptions about both the context and the listener's knowledge. For most children, the ability to consider a partner's perspective is well established by age 10 years. Children with LD have poor referential skills and are less likely to adjust to the listener and more likely to provide ambiguous and insufficient information.

As an SLP, be alert to the informativeness of a child's utterances and to the social context. The following questions can be applied to the sample:

- What does the child choose to encode?
- Does the child encode what is novel or merely comment on what is already given?
- Does the child encode new information gesturally, linguistically, or both?
- Are messages informative, vague, or ambiguous?
- Are different referents clearly established?
- Does the child talk differently about things present in the context and things that are not?

Noninformative language can take several forms. Table 7–11 presents forms and examples seen in children with language disorders. These types of noninformative

CHAPTER 7 LANGUAGE SAMPLE ANALYSIS

Table 7–11. Types of Noninformative Language

Empty phrases (common idioms, such as *and so on* and *et cetera, excetera*)
Indefinite terms and highly nonspecific nouns (*one, thing, that*)
Deictic terms (*this, that, here, there*)
Pronouns used without antecedent nouns
Comments on task instead of stimulus
Neologisms (*Oh, you know the one that you fly in*)
Paraphrases
Repeated words or phrases
Personal value judgments about the stimulus (*That's pretty dumb*)
Use of *and* alone
Conjunctions *but, so, or,* and *because* alone

language may be especially relevant to the language of children with TBI and LD. The SLP can rate utterances to determine the strategy used by the child.

Linguistic Devices. Several linguistic devices are used to mark informativeness, including deictics and direct/indirect reference. Both of these devices can be used to note referents internal or external to the conversation. Other cohesive devices, listed in Table 7–3, establish relations entirely within the exchange.

Deictics. As mentioned in Chapter 6, deictic terms are linguistic elements that must be interpreted from the perspective of the speaker. Words with deictic meanings appear in several word classes, including personal pronouns (*I/me, you*), demonstrative adjectives (*this, that, these, those*), adverbs of time (*before, after, now, then*), adverbs of location (*here, there*), and verbs (*come, go, give, take*). A child's behavior, especially the errors, should be analyzed to determine confusion or overreliance on one principle or one aspect of a principle.

Definite and Indefinite Reference. A mature language user is able to mark specific or definite and nonspecific or indefinite referents by manipulation of definite (*the*) and indefinite (*a/an*) articles. Article use can be especially difficult for a child with a language disorder. Each article in the sample can be analyzed for appropriate referential use.

Cohesive Devices

Conversational *cohesion*, how language hangs together, can be a useful LSA tool. Any sentence element that sends the listener outside of the sentence for a referent is a cohesive device. For example, a pronoun may require referral to the previous sentence in order to

254 LANGUAGE DISORDERS: A FUNCTIONAL APPROACH TO ASSESSMENT AND INTERVENTION IN CHILDREN

determine the referent. The five types of cohesive relations are reference, substitution, ellipsis, conjunction, and lexical items. We'll touch on some of these.

Cohesion can be expressed through both syntax and vocabulary. For example, a pronoun or a demonstrative, such as *this* or *that*, can refer to the referent, which was identified previously in the conversation. Conjoining—the connection of phrases, clauses, and sentences through the use of such conjunctions as *and*, *because*, and *if*—also is used for cohesion. The major cohesive devices used in English are listed in Table 7–12.

The most frequent problems of cohesion relate to providing redundant information, deleting necessary information, using unclear and ambiguous reference, sequencing old and new information, and marking old and new information with articles and pronouns. In short, errors usually reflect including or excluding information or confusing new and old information.

Reference. Reference is a linguistic device used continuously in conversation to keep information flowing and to designate new and old information. In the process, new information is stated clearly and then subsequently implied by the referral to it as old information. Thus, one utterance presupposes the other. We'll explore all this in the following section. Some children with language disorders, such as children with ASD, have difficulty marking new and old information. An SLP can note the method of introducing new information and the use of following mention.

> ***Food for Thought:*** **Do you find yourself occasionally lost in a conversation. Assuming you were paying attention, could referencing be to blame?**

Initial Mention. In initial mention, mature speakers establish mutual reference clearly, especially if the entity mentioned is not present. Generally, the referent name is stressed

Table 7–12. Cohesive Devices Used in English

Relation	Explanation	Examples
Reference	Initially, the entity is named and may use the indefinite article (*a/an*). Subsequent mention may use a pronoun, words such as *this*, *that*, and *one*, or use the definite article (*the*) with the noun.	*John* went looking for *a car*. He found *one* in the city. I want to buy *a coat*, but *that one* I saw last night is too expensive.
Ellipsis	Subsequent sentences omit redundant or shared information.	Who ate *all the cookies*? I did [eat all the cookies]. I would like to *make a phone call*. May I [make a phone call]?
Conjunction	Conjunctions join clauses to express additive, causal, and other relationships.	We went to the circus, *and* I saw elephants. John's angry *because* I drank his soda.

CHAPTER 7 LANGUAGE SAMPLE ANALYSIS

and preceded by the indefinite article (*a/an*). In English, the referent often is placed at the end of the sentence. In addition, referents that are in the context may be pointed to, touched, or handled.

Children with LD or ASD may not identify new information for the listener. As listeners, these children may have difficulty identifying the new information but will ask few questions to clarify. As speakers, children with word-finding difficulties or poor vocabularies may use empty words, such as *that*, *one*, or *thing*, that do not help clarify the referent. These children may rely on the immediate context and use pointing to specify the referent that their nonspecific vocabulary failed to identify.

Following Mention. In following mention, previously identified referents often are moved to the initial position in English sentences and may be referred to by the use of the definite article (*the*) or a pronoun. Pronoun use is appropriate when the referent is unambiguous or clearly identified. The pronoun should be in close proximity so that there is no confusion as to which noun it refers.

As an SLP, you'll be interested in the way a child introduces new information and refers to that information later. Also of interest is any confusion with article and pronoun use. It is not uncommon for a preschool child or a child with LD to introduce new information with "She did it," leaving the listener to determine who *she* and *it* are.

Ellipsis. Ellipsis is a process in which redundant information is omitted. For example, the response to "What do you want?" may be "Cookie," which omits the shared information "I want." Elliptical fragments are used frequently to keep the conversation moving smoothly and rapidly, but an SLP might miss them if linguistic analysis concentrates solely on full sentences or fails to look across partners. Children with language disorders may not realize that information is shared or may assume that it is shared when it is not. Either assumption interferes with the flow of conversation.

Conjunctions. Conjunctions, such as *and*, *then*, *so*, and *therefore*, are used to connect thoughts. Although preschool children have several conjunction-type words in their vocabularies, they rarely use them to join clauses. In analysis, an SLP notes clausal linking and conjunctions used across utterances, as in the following exchange:

> *Parent:*   We had a great day at the zoo. I liked the monkeys best.
>
> *Child:*   And feeding the deer babies.

Adverbial Conjuncts and Disjuncts. Adverbial conjuncts and disjuncts are conversational devices used for cohesion. **Conjuncts** are across-sentence forms that express a logical relationship, such as the conjunctions *then* or *so*, as in "So we gave up." Conjuncts are of two types: concordant, such as *similarly*, *consequently*, and *moreover*, and discordant, such as *nevertheless*, *rather*, and *in contrast*. **Disjuncts** are used to comment on or to convey the speaker's attitude toward the topic and include words and phrases such as *honestly*, *frankly*, *perhaps*, *however*, *yet*, *to my surprise*, *it's obvious to me that*, and the like.

Conjuncts and disjuncts develop rather late in childhood and, therefore, may be good measures of adolescent language. Children between ages 6 and 12 years use conjuncts infrequently and rely most frequently on *then*, *so*, and *though*. By age 12 years, children use only an average of 4 conjuncts per 100 utterances. In contrast, adults average 12 conjuncts per 100 utterances. Adolescents use the same conjuncts as younger children but also use *therefore*, *however*, *rather*, and *consequently* in both their reading and writing.

Contrastive Stress. Contrastive stress or emphasis can be used to negate or correct the message of a conversational partner. For example, if one speaker said, "Jose brought the cookies," the other might correct, "*Mary* brought the cookies." Again, an SLP must transcend the traditional utterance-level analysis and look across partners.

Conversational Partner

We should note before we move on that language does not occur in a vacuum. Each partner helps form a dynamic context in which a child communicates and learns.

As you know from our discussion of early intervention, caregiver–child interactions usually offer an example of a highly individualized communication process finely attuned to the language skills of a child. For example, caregiver linguistic complexity seems to be related to the language learning child's level of comprehension.

Especially when working with preschool children, an SLP should observe the conversational behavior of the primary caregiver and determine their language learning contributions. Caregiver behaviors can be described and, during intervention, slightly tweaked where needed, and caregivers can become important allies in teaching language to their children.

Within Utterances

Each utterance can be analyzed within use, content, and form categories as previously outlined in Table 7–1 and following a variety of LSA formats. Individual utterances can yield the frequency and range of various features. Some data will be descriptive, whereas other data will be more normative.

A number of computer-assisted LSA (CLSA) and unassisted LSA methods are available. Several are listed in Table 7–13. Although each method yields different data, none presents a total picture of a child's language, something our SLP Amanda was seeking. A few of the more widely used LSA methods are described in more detail in Appendix C. We'll be discussing a more generic analysis method borrowing useful portions from several places.

Language Use

At the utterance level, an SLP can analyze the breakdowns that occur and the intentions of each utterance.

Disruptions. Communication breakdown or disruption can occur for many reasons. The amount and type of disruption will vary with the language task, topic, and partner(s). For example, more breakdowns occur in narration than in conversation, indicating the

CHAPTER 7 LANGUAGE SAMPLE ANALYSIS

Table 7–13. Language Sample Analysis Methods

Unassisted Methods

Pragmatics

Adolescent Conversational Analysis (Larson & McKinley, 1987)

Assessing Children's Language in Naturalistic Contexts (Lund & Duchan, 1993)

Clinical Discourse Analysis using Grice's framework (Damico, 1991)

Language functions (Boyce & Larson, 1983; Gruenewald & Pollack, 1984; Prutting & Kirchner, 1983, 1987; Simon, 1984)

Pragmatic Protocol (Prutting & Kirchner, 1987)

Pragmatic Rating Scale (PRS) (Landa et al., 1992)

Targeted Observation of Pragmatics in Children's Conversations (TOPICC) (Adams et al., 2010)

Syntax/morphology

Assessing Children's Language in Naturalistic Contexts (Lund & Duchan, 1993)

Assessing Language Production in Children: Experimental Procedures (J. Miller, 1981)

Developmental Sentence Analysis (L. Lee, 1974)

Guide to Analysis of Language Transcripts (Stickler, 1987)

Index of Productive Syntax (IPSyn) (Scarborough, 1990)

Language Assessment, Remediation, and Screening Procedure (Crystal et al., 1976, revised 1981)

Language Sampling, Analysis, and Training: A Handbook for Teachers and Clinicians (Tyack & Gottsleben, 1977)

Semantics

Profile in Semantics–Lexical (PRISM-L) (Crystal, 1982)

Analysis of Propositions (APRON) (based on Johnston & Kamhi, 1984; Kamhi & Johnston, 1992; Lahey, 1988)

Narratives

Narrative level (Larson & McKinley, 1987)

Story grammar analysis (Garnett, 1986; Hedberg & Stoel-Gammon, 1986; Roth, 1986; Westby, 1984, 1992; Westby et al., 1989)

Classroom-based

Classroom Script Analysis (Creaghead, 1992)

Curriculum-Based Language Assessment (N. Nelson, 1994)

Descriptive Assessment of Writing (Scott & Erwin, 1992)

Computer-Assisted Methods

Syntax/morphology

Automated LARSP (Bishop, 1985)

Computerized Language Analysis (CLAN) (MacWhinney, 2000)

Computerized Profiling (Long & Fey, 1988, 1989)

continues

Table 7–13. *continued*

Computer-Assisted Methods *continued*

Syntax/morphology *continued*

    DSS computer program (Hixson, 1983)

    Lingquest 1 (Mordecai et al., 1985)

    Parrot Easy Language Sample Analysis (PELSA) (Weiner, 1988)

    Pye Analysis of Language (PAL) (Pye, 1987)

    Sampling Utterances and Grammatical Analysis Revised (SUGAR) (Owens, & Pavelko, 2021)

    Systematic Analysis of Language Transcripts (SALT) (J. Miller & Iglesias, 2015)

relative pragmatic difficulty of each. In addition, the longer the utterance, the more breakdowns present.

Disruptions tend to occur at the developing edge of the child's language where production capacity is "stretched" and there's increased risk of processing difficulty. These utterances are of particular diagnostic significance (Rispoli & Hadley, 2001).

A valuable clue to a child's process of forming an utterance and to the level of cognitive and linguistic demands, disruption analysis isn't needed for all children with language disorders. However, disruption analysis may be helpful for those with word-finding problems or with "tangled," slow, or too long utterances.

Disruption analysis requires that an SLP transcribe all words, word portions, and speech-like vocalizations. All mazes should be identified. A **maze** is a language segment that, like a physical maze, disrupts, confuses, and slows a process. Mazes may consist of silent pauses, fillers, repetitions, and revisions and often indicate where a child is having difficulty.

Intentions. At the individual utterance level, pragmatic analysis can describe the intentions expressed and understood. The appropriateness and form of these intentions are also of interest. Each intention can be analyzed for its form and means of transmission.

Frequency and Range. The paucity of normative data on the frequency and range of intentions reflects the contextual variability of intentions and the lack of agreement by professionals on the intentions expressed at various ages. Intentions are heavily influenced by and heavily influence the conversational context, necessitating several different samples.

A number of taxonomies of intentions are available, reflecting different ages and contextual situations. I have attempted in Tables 7–14 and 7–15 to demonstrate possible changes over time. As an SLP, you may wish to develop a taxonomy based on one or a combination of the available taxonomies.

The range of intentions becomes wider and more complex with increasing age. In addition, with maturity, a child may express multiple intentions within a single utterance, increasing the flexibility of expression.

CHAPTER 7 LANGUAGE SAMPLE ANALYSIS

Table 7–14. Intentions of Children

Early Symbolic (Younger Than Age 2 Years) (Dore, 1974; Owens, 1978)	Symbolic (Ages 2–7 Years) (Chapman, 1981; Dore, 1986; Folger & Chapman, 1978)
Requesting action	Requests (for) Action/assistance/objects Permission
Regulation Protesting	Regulation Protesting and rule setting
Requesting information	Requesting information

Replying
  Continuants
 	
Comments
	Replying
	    Acknowledgments
	    Qualifications
	    Agreements
	Comments
	Assertives

Naming	Identifications and descriptions

Personal feelings	Personal feelings
	    Statements, reports, and evaluations
	    Attributions/details
	    Explanations
	      Hypotheses and reasons
	      Predictions

Declarations
 	
  Choice making
	Declarations
	    Procedurals
	    Choice making and claims

Answers	Answers
	    Providing information
	    Clarification
	    Compliance
	    Conversational organization

Calling/greeting	Attention getters and speaker selection Rhetorical questions Clarification requests Boundary markers Politeness Exclamations
Repeating	Repetitions
Practicing	Elicited imitations

Note: As children become older, they add new intentions and continue to diversify those they already possess.

Table 7–15. Intentions and Age of Mastery

Prior to 24 months	Answering/responding
	Continuance
	Declaring/citing
	Making choices
	Naming/labeling
	Protesting/denying
	Repeating
24–36 months	Calling/greeting
	Detailing
	Predicting
	Replying
	Requesting assistance/directing
	Requesting clarification
	Requesting information
	Requesting objects
After 36 months	Expressing feelings
	Giving reasons
	Hypothesizing

After selecting the most comfortable taxonomy or combination of taxonomies, an SLP can rate each utterance of a child and conversational partner for the intentions expressed. Of interest are the intention, how it is expressed, and the context. No one intention should predominate unless required by the context, such as playing Twenty Questions.

Some children, such as those with ASD, may initiate communication only rarely and respond with minimal replies. Occasionally, a child will fall into a perseverative pattern. Such behavior can skew the data or allow one type of intention to predominate. These patterns should be noted during conversational sample collection, and the situations should be gently changed. The use of different situations and different partners may ensure a better distribution of intentions.

Some children use only a limited range of intentions. If this persists across a number of situations and partners, you, as an SLP, can be reasonably certain that this narrow range represents the child's typical behavior.

Appropriateness. The question of appropriateness of intentions must be judged against other factors, such as age, race or ethnicity, region of the country, socioeconomic status, gender, and, most important, the communication context. Even without norms, LSA can confirm a caregiver's observation that "John seems to ask questions all the time, even when he knows the answers."

CHAPTER 7 LANGUAGE SAMPLE ANALYSIS

Encoding. Intentions can be analyzed by using a means of transmission format, such as verbal/vocal/nonverbal. The transition from nonlinguistic through paralinguistic to linguistic expression can be used to describe a hierarchy of competency or effectiveness. For verbal children, sentence form can be used to describe intentions.

In general, a child with poor linguistic skills will rely on other than verbal means of communicating intentions. Less mature language users tend to depend on nonlinguistic and paralinguistic means more than do mature users. A range of transmission means may be exhibited, which is why we rate each intension.

If a child uses an augmentative form of communication, the form of should be specified along with other means, such as manipulation of an object, moving or touching a partner, gestures, and vocalization and verbalization. Occasionally, intentions are mode-specific; thus, all *yes/no* responses are nonverbal head shakes.

Content

The understanding of word meanings and word relationships is affected by many factors, such as age, gender, and regional and racial/ethnic differences. To know a word is to know more than just what it identifies or its definition. It means a school-age child understands that word's relationship to similar words of meaning and sound and to words of an opposite meaning and also understands the semantic class into which the word can be placed.

Meaning also extends beyond words to larger units of analysis, such as a phrase or sentence. For one child with whom I worked, what was said—for example, "Don't hit me"—was very different from the intended message—"Go away, I don't understand what you want."

Lexical Items. Obviously, all semantic information cannot be ascertained from a single language sample. Word understanding is complicated and may require other collection methods, such as the following:

- Directing a child through a series of tasks
- Playing word-matching tasks
- Making statements with obviously incorrect words
- Playing word games that solicit definitions or antonyms
- Sorting and categorizing words
- Naming members of a category
- Deducing category names from a list of members
- Making ridiculous comparisons ("A mouse is bigger than an elephant") or silly pairings ("The comb goes between his toes")

Although children with language disorders and with LD usually do not have difficulty with referent-symbol tasks, such as matching names to pictures, they may have difficulties with double meanings, abstract terms, synonyms, and nonliteral interpretation.

The physical setting can be especially important because children with language disorders often depend on the context for support. The child may understand a word only given certain physical situations or contexts.

It may be best to assess definitions through formal testing, but word use in conversations may also be important. Between ages 5 and 10 years, the nature of definitions changes from functional (*an apple is something you eat*) to categorical (*an apple is a fruit*), and more elements are added. By second grade, 49% of definitions include categorical membership, increasing to 76% by fifth grade.

Several levels of semantic analysis are possible, although an SLP must keep in mind the individualistic nature of lexical growth. Increases in vocabulary occur at a slow and steady pace. School-age children and adolescents exhibit semantic development in the following areas:

- Comprehension of literate verbs, such as *interpret* and *predict*
- Comprehension of textbook terms, such as *invertebrate* and *antecedent*
- Comprehension of adverbs of magnitude, such as *slightly* and *unusually*
- Comprehension of adverbial conjuncts, such as *meanwhile* and *conversely*
- Comprehension of sarcasm based on its linguistic aspects, as well as intonation
- Comprehension of slang terms used by peers
- Comprehension of complex proverbs and complex metaphors
- Explanation of infrequently occurring idioms, such as to *vote with one's feet*
- Explanation of ambiguous messages
- Definition of abstract concept words, such as *courage* and *justice*

Lexical Diversity. Lexical diversity can be measured in different ways based on the size of the overall language sample, the number of utterances, and the number of words included, but these values can be used to identify children with developmental language disorder (DLD). Therefore, as an SLP, you'll want to carefully note how lexically diverse the sample is (Charest et al., 2020).

Number of Different Words. Although early difficulty in the acquisition of sentence structure is a core diagnostic feature of language disorders (American Psychiatric Association, 2013), some early sentences may be memorized in whole or in part, making assessment difficult. Therefore, Hadley and colleagues (2018) recommend that rather than simple utterance length, SLPs might measure development by the number of different words (NDW) used in different grammatical constructions (Hadley et al., 2017; Hadley & Short, 2005; Naigles et al., 2009). NDW within a sample is sometimes referred to as **lexical density**.

Hadley and colleagues (2017) reported that 30-month-olds use an average of 139 (range: 102–176) different words in 30 minutes of conversation with an adult. We should be cautious in applying this value because Hadley and co-authors are very specific in what constitutes a different word. See Hadley et al. (2018) for a more detailed description, deeper analysis of sentence structure, and norms for number of different words.

CHAPTER 7 LANGUAGE SAMPLE ANALYSIS

Older school-age children should possess a variety of words for describing sensory experiences, such as sight (*clearly*), sound (*loud*), smell (*stunk*), and feelings (*happy, tired*). They should be able to describe the environment in terms of time (*at five o'clock*) and location (*in front of*). Entities should possess physical qualities, such as shape (*sort of round*), size (*big*), number (*two, many, few*), substance (*metal, wood*), and condition (*new, ragged*). There should be terms for relationships, such as comparisons (*bigger than, as big as*) and qualifications (*nearly, not quite, only, enough*); and verbs for describing actions (*run, jump, eat*), states (*am, is, are*), and sensory processes (*feel, hear, see*). Finally, the speakers should be able to describe causation (*because . . .*) and motivation. As noted previously, these terms develop slowly. The full range is characteristic of the mature speaker.

Deictic terms offer a special problem for the child with a language disorder. Children with language learning disability, ASD, or emotional disturbances may lack either the listener or speaker perspective. These children also may refer to themselves by name and may echo the utterances of others, such as referring to themselves as *you*.

TNW increases steadily with age and is a general measure of verbal productivity. Values for TNW are presented in Table 7–16. Significantly lower values for NDW than those in Table 7–16 might suggest either retrieval problems or poor vocabulary.

The validity of TNW as a measure of language development has been questioned by some professionals and is a reminder that no one measure should be used in isolation. For example, although TNW and NDW can be used to differentiate the narratives of monolingual children with TDL and those with DLD, these values do not do so for bilingual Spanish–English preschool children (Muñoz et al., 2003). Other measures, such as syntactic accuracy, may be more appropriate.

Type-Token Ratio. The type-token ratio (TTR) is the ratio of NDW to TNW. TTR has had a checkered past of professional acceptance. This uncertainty reflects recognition that the value may vary widely with the language sample size. Larger samples of 350 words or more and multiple samples from different settings yield more stable values.

Children between ages 2 to 8 years demonstrate TTR values of 0.42 to 0.50, respectively. Children who receive values greater than 0.50 have greater variability and flexibility in their language, whereas those who received values below 0.42 tend to use the same words. Very low values may indicate perseverative or stereotypic behavior, word-retrieval problems, or restricted vocabulary. English language learners (ELLs) also may score lower because of their lack of English vocabulary.

Over-/Underextensions and Incorrect Usage. An SLP should note all inaccurate uses of words that indicate some variation between a child's meaning and the conventional one. In general, meanings mature from the concrete, personal, experiential ones found in preschool children to the shared, conventional, abstract ones of adults.

Some children use words incorrectly because they do not know the shared conventional definition. Others use word substitutions that are incorrect. For example, a recent letter from a young adult with dyslexia included the following:

I wish I could write as good as you. You know where to put paragraphs and how to use *punctuality* [my italics] right.

Table 7–16. Values for TNW and NDW

Age in Months	TNW[1] (20 minutes)	NDW[1] (50 utterances)	TNW[2] (50 utterances), SUGAR
18			
21	240	36	
24	286	41	
27	332	46	
30	378	51	
33 [30–35]	424	56	
36	470	61	192.3
39 [36–41]	516	66	
42	562	71	244.05
45 [42–47]	608	76	
48	654	81	261.4
51 [48–53]	700	86	
53–59			278.71
60–71			299.81
72–83			337.73
84–107			379.63
108–131			421.36

Notes: [1]Klee (1992). [2]Owens and Pavelko (2020); Pavelko and Owens (2017). NDW, number of different words; TNW, total number of words.

Because I am usually late, I assume he meant punctuation. Further testing by an SLP can reveal the basis of a child's substitutions. The child may miss the target word slightly, as in the previous example, or may have word-finding difficulties.

Style and Lexicon. Language sample analysis across contexts might highlight a conversational style shift. These changes can be analyzed further for the vocabulary used in different styles.

A child's literate vocabulary, consisting of words primarily used in common academic contexts, is also important. A good, literate lexicon is needed to achieve academic success, especially among adolescents. Possible lexical terms are *analyze, criticize, deduce, define, infer, interpret, predict, remember,* and *understand.* Classroom teachers can suggest other useful literate terms. Literate language is considered further in our discussion of narrative LSA.

CHAPTER 7 LANGUAGE SAMPLE ANALYSIS

> ***Food for Thought:*** **Does this seem like an area of assessment that might take more than a single 50-utterance sample? If so, you'd be correct. Assessing vocabulary in depth will require more data.**

Word Relationships. Relationships consist of word associations (e.g., *salt and pepper* or *king and queen*), synonyms, antonyms, and homonyms. Some of these associations are expressed in a conversational sample, whereas others need to be probed by an SLP. These associations reflect underlying cognitive organizational strategies.

Semantic Categories. Semantic categories, such as agent, action, and location, introduced in Chapter 4, are described in Table 7–17. Semantic knowledge, the underlying concepts of sentences, may be a better framework than language form for some children, especially those with morphosyntactic errors.

Semantically, a single event may be described by the *agent* that originates the action, the *action* or *state* changes, and/or the recipient or *object* of that action. In English, the agent as a noun or a noun phrase is usually first, followed by the action word or verb, which in turn is followed by the recipient or object of that action in the form of a noun or a noun phrase ("John threw *the ball*" or "Mother ate *the sugar cookie*").

If the agent performs the action for the benefit of some other person, that beneficiary —the indirect object or *patient*—either precedes or follows the noun phrase describing the object of the action. For example, in "He painted the picture *for mother*," *for mother* follows the object of the sentence. Likewise, we could say, "He painted *mother* a picture." Instruments used to complete the action usually are placed after the action and follow the preposition *with*, as in "He painted *with acrylics*."

Intrasentence Relationships. In addition to an interest in a child's word meanings and relationships, an SLP can investigate other relationships expressed in a sentence through the use of conjunctions, negatives, and prepositions and various sentence forms, such as passive voice.

Conjunction. Four types of conjunctive relations are expressed in conjoined sentences: additive, temporal, causal, and adversative. In the *additive* form, two clauses with no dependent relationship simply are joined to one another. In the sentence "Julio ate pie and Brigid drank coffee," neither event depends on the other for its existence.

In the *temporal* form, one clause depends on the other to precede or follow or occur at the same time. In "I'm going to the store before I go to the party" or "I'll rake the leaves while you finish painting the trim," the timing of the clauses is obvious.

Causal conjoining implies a dependency in which one clause is the result of the other—for example, "I went to the party because I was invited." A preschool child may use *because* alone or at the beginning of a clause, as in "Cause I want to," although true causal conjoining with *because* occurs much later.

Finally, in *adversative* conjoining, one clause contrasts with information in the other, as in "I read the article, but I was unimpressed." One clause opposes or negates the other.

Table 7–17. Semantic Categories

Semantic Function	Description	Examples
Action	The predicate expresses action with a transitive or intransitive clause.	We *grew* pumpkins and squash. (Transitive) He *swims* daily. (Intransitive)
State	The predicate makes a statement about the way things are with a transitive, intransitive, or equative clause.	I *want* a hot fudge sundae. (Transitive) Tigers *look* fierce. (Intransitive) My sister *is* now at Harvard. (Equative)
Agent or actor	Animate instigator of action. Sometimes inanimate, especially if a natural force. Usually, the subject but may also be a passive complement.	*Mike* threw the ball. *Termites* destroyed our cabin. *Wind* blew down the trees. The *cat* chased the dog.
Instrument	Usually refers to the inanimate object used by the actor to effect the action stated in the verb. The actor is usually not stated but may be.	The *axe* split the wood. The *building* was erected by a crane. She used the *baseball bat* with great skill. The shaman kept rhythm on his *drum*.
Patient	The entity on which an action is performed. The patient may be a direct object in transitive clauses or the subject in intransitive clauses.	Mike threw the *ball*. *The lighthouse* withstood the hurricane.
Dative	The animate recipient of action. Usually, the indirect object but may also be the direct object if it does not undergo any action but receives something.	Father brought *mother* a bouquet of roses. Our mascot brought *us* good luck. He built a treehouse for his *daughter*. I loved that *movie*.
Temporal	Fulfills the adverbial function of time in response to a *when* question. May also be the subject of a sentence or a complement.	I'll see you *later*. We'll meet at *four o'clock. Then*, I'll know. *Tomorrow* is a holiday. It is *time to leave*.
Locative	Fulfills the adverbial function of place in response to a *where* question. May also be the subject of a sentence or a complement.	Some of us looked *in the old log*. I know it was *right here*. *Chicago* is indeed a windy city.
Manner	Fulfills the adverbial function of manner in response to a *how* question.	We stalked the big cat *carefully*. He worked *with great skill*.
Accompaniment	Fulfills the adverbial function of *with X* in response to *with whom* or *with what* questions.	He swam *with his sister*. She left *with Jim*. He hunted *with his dogs*.
Empty subjects	Serve a grammatical function.	*It* was sunny. *There* may be some rain.

Negatives. Negatives may be expressed in several ways and develop at different stages. The four mature negative forms include (a) *not* and *-n't*; (b) negative words, such as *nobody* and *nothing*; (c) the determiner *no* used with nouns; and (d) negative adverbs, such as *never* and *nowhere*. Again, the more mature language user should have a variety of forms. Those used by the child can be compared with the developmental data in Table 7–25.

Prepositions. Prepositions can be used to mark location (*in the box*), time (*in a minute*), or manner (*in a hurry*) and to make figurative expressions. These small, often unstressed words may be misinterpreted or misunderstood by children with language disorders and those who are ELLs. A strategy they may use is overreliance on one form.

Passive Voice. In general, children with language disorders exhibit difficulty interpreting sentences in which the information might be interpreted in a reverse manner. For example, a passive sentence, such as "The cat is chased by the dog," might be interpreted incorrectly as "The cat chased the dog" by using an agent–action–object interpretation strategy. This example highlights the disconnect between syntax and semantics that can occur for some children with language disorders.

Figurative Language. Nonliteral meanings used for effect are characteristic of school-age and adult language. Examples include metaphors, similes, idioms, and proverbs. Figurative language occurs frequently in oral conversation and written texts. Interpretation of idioms is highly correlated with reading ability.

Children as young as 3½ years are able to comprehend some idioms, especially the more literal ones. In general, figurative interpretation increases with increasing age.

An SLP can consider the range of figurative language used. Some children overrely on well-worn phrases and expressions, with little knowledge of their actual meaning. Idiomatic expressions may be interpreted literally. These forms can be probed by an SLP to determine a child's actual knowledge.

Word Finding. Word-finding difficulties relate to several aspects of the target words, such as word frequency, age of acquisition, familiarity, and lexical neighborhood (German & Newman, 2004). Neighborhood density, or the number of words that differ from the target word by only one sound, is particularly important. Words such as *rat* have many neighbors: *cat, bat, fat, gnat, sat, hat, mat, rap, ran, rot, wrote/rote, write/right, rate,* and so on. The neighborhood is dense. It's easier to produce and remember words that are phonologically similar to words already known. If neighbors are high-frequency words, recall is enhanced even more. In contrast, word substitutions tend to be words that have a higher frequency, are learned earlier, and also reside in dense neighborhoods with other high-frequency words. Blocked words, or those a child is unable to retrieve, tend to reside in sparse neighborhoods.

Other variables include the context, syntactic requirements, type of stimulus and manner of presentation, priming, and use of categories. Priming occurs when preceding words aid recall, as in "salt and _____" or "For his birthday, he hoped he'd receive many wrapped _____."

The effect of these variables can be very important and difficult to assess in a language sample. It is important, therefore, to use familiar partners, topics, and situations to facilitate retrieval and to probe word recall.

Form

Language form includes syntax, morphology, and phonology, or the means used to encode the intentions and meanings of a speaker. Many children with language disorders experience difficulty with syntax and morphology. Although most LSA methods concentrate on morpho-syntax, few normative data are available. A discussion of phonological analysis is beyond the scope of this text.

Quantitative Measures. Quantitative measures include mean length of utterance (MLU), mean syntactic length (MSL), T-units and C-units, and the density of sentence forms. Each is discussed in the following sections.

An SLP must be cautious with all word and morpheme counts. Careful editing of utterances is required so that interjections, false starts, fillers (*you know*), imitations, and the like are not included in the count. Circumlocutions, or talking around an unretrievable word, actually may increase the length of the child's utterances.

It is recommended that an SLP follow consistent rules for counting. For example, incomplete words, nonessential repetitions, revisions not containing a complete thought, unintelligible words and phrases, and fillers should be offset in brackets and not counted. These structures are retained, however, for disruption analysis.

Quantitative measures may present some problems. In general, there can be wide variability across children and situations. In addition, many values change only slowly with age. However, average words per sentence (WPS) increases from 7 to 14 between grade 3 and grade 12.

Combinations of quantitative data may yield better information than individual bits of information. For example, MLU, the percentage of utterances containing one or more errors of morphology or syntax, and chronological age seem to be optimal for predicting clinical diagnosis of DLD/SLI. Structural errors might include word ordering difficulties; omission or incorrect use of a morpheme; omission of articles, auxiliary verbs, or contractions; use of telegraphic or truncated speech (*Mommy ride bike*); or incorrectly selected negatives.

You may or may not recall that Pavelko and colleagues (2016) reported that one reason SLPs don't sample more is because they question the validity of the LSA method. Owens and Pavelko (2017) found that four quantitative measures correlated best with test results: TNW, MLU_M, clauses per sentence (CPS), and WPS.

Mean Length of Utterance. Mean length of utterance is the average length of a speaker's utterances in morphemes (MLU_M) or words (MLU_W). Although some studies report that up to a value of 4.0, MLU_M is a good measure of language complexity, the reliability of MLU_M has been questioned and the values have been found to vary in response to SLP input. Others report that MLU_M is both a reliable and a valid measure of general language development through age 10 years for children with TDL and those with SLI (Owens & Pavelko, 2020; Pavelko & Owens, 2017; Rice et al., 2006).

To calculate MLU_M, you count the number of morphemes in each utterance and total them for the entire sample. Traditional rules for counting morphemes are included in Table 7–18. Note that these rules are based on the language of very young children.

CHAPTER 7 LANGUAGE SAMPLE ANALYSIS

Table 7–18. Rules for Counting Morphemes

Structure	Examples	Count	Rationale
Each recurrence of a word for emphasis	*No, no, no*	1 each	
Compound words (2 or more free morphemes)	*Railroad, birthday*	1	Compound words learned as a unit by preschoolers.
Proper names	*Bugs Bunny, Uncle Fred*	1	Proper names, even those with titles, learned as a unit by preschoolers.
Ritualized reduplications	*Choo-choo, Night-night*	1	
Irregular past tense verbs	*Went, ate, got, came*	1	Verb tense learned as new word by preschoolers, not as verb + *ed*.
Diminutives	*Doggie, horsie*	1	Phonological form CVCV easier than CVC for preschoolers and does not denote smallness.
Auxiliary verbs and catenatives	*Is, have, do; gonna, wanna, gotta*	1	Preschoolers do not know that such words as *gonna* are *going to*.
Contracted negatives	*Don't, can't, won't*	1–2	Because negatives *don't, can't,* and *won't* develop before *do, can,* and *will,* count as one until the positive form appears. Then count the negative forms as two morphemes. All other negatives— *couldn't*—count as two.
Possessive marker (-*'s*)	*Tom's, mom's*	1	
Plural maker (-*s*)	*Cats, dogs*	1	
Third-person singular present tense marker (-*s*)	*Walks, eats*	1	
Regular past tense marker (-*ed*)	*Walked, jumped*	1	
Present progressive marker (-*ing*)	*Walking, eating*	1	
Dysfluencies	*C-c-candy, b-b-baby*	1	Count only the final complete form.*
Fillers	*Um-m, ah-h*	0	

Note: *In the example "I want can . . . I want can . . . I want candy," only the last full reduction is counted, being three morphemes.

The total number of morphemes for the entire sample is divided by the number of utterances from which it was derived to determine the MLU_M. This value then can be compared to the age data in Table 7–19. It is obvious from the table that a wide variability and a wide range of ages are considered within the normal range. If data have been collected in two or more settings, the MLU_M values from each can be compared to assess the stability of the overall data. If a child falls below one standard deviation (SD) and we're reasonably sure that we have captured their typical performance, we should consider that the child has a possible language disorder.

Within the Sampling Utterances and Grammatical Analysis Revised (SUGAR) method of LSA (Owens & Pavelko, 2021), robust sampling methods and modifications in morpheme counting to accommodate older children, plus the calculation of 14 additional bound morphemes frequently used by older school-age children, result in continued significant growth in MLU_{SUGAR} or MLU_S until age 10;11 years (Owens & Pavelko, 2020; Pavelko & Owens, 2018). Appendix B presents SUGAR modifications, including the 14 additional morphemes counted in SUGAR.

As with any single measure, MLU alone is a poor diagnostic tool, and the validity and reliability of results may vary with the sample size (Eisenberg et al., 2001). However, Pavelko et al. (2020) reported no significant difference in MLU_S in 25- and 50-utterance samples.

As with all data, an SLP must be cautious. A low MLU_M doesn't necessarily indicate a language disorder. Utterance length may vary with the situation, and some very talkative children may have inflated MLU_M.

Mean Syntactic Length. Mean syntactic length is the mean length in words of all utterances of two words or more—those utterances with some internal grammar. This measure eliminates all one-word responses, such as *yes/no* answers. MSL seems to correlate more strongly than traditional MLU_M with age. Values for MSL are listed in Table 7–19 (Klee, 1992).

T-Units and C-Units. Expressive language syntax of older children and adolescents can be measured in T-units or minimal terminal units, consisting of one main or independent clause plus any attached or embedded subordinate clause or nonclausal structure (discussed later). Note that the unit has shifted from utterances to the sentences.

A simple (one main clause) or complex (one main clause and one subordinate clause) sentence would be one T-unit, but a compound sentence (two or more independent clauses) would be two or more T-units. For example, the sentences "I want ice cream" and "I want the one that is hidden in the blue box" each constitute one T-unit. "I want the ice cream in the picture and he wants a shake" consists of two independent clauses and thus two T-units. Examples of T-units are given in Table 7–20.

The T-unit is more sensitive than MLU_M to the types of language differences seen in older children. A children's language can be described in words per T-unit, clauses per T-unit, and words per clause. A gradual and progressive increase in words and clauses per T-unit and in words per clause in spontaneous speech occurs with increased age throughout childhood and adolescence, although the values change only gradually during early school years (Table 7–21).

Table 7–19. Quantitative Measures of Language

Age in Months	MLU_W (SD)[1]	MLU_M (SD)[2]	MSL[3]	MLU_{SUGAR} (SD)[4]	Words/ Sentence[4]	Clauses/ Sentence[4]
18		1.1				
21		1.6	2.7			
24		1.9	2.9			
27		2.1	3.1			
30		2.5*	3.4			
33 [30–35]	[2.91 (0.58)]	2.8 [3.23 (0.71)]	3.7			
36		3.1	3.9			
39 [36–41]	[3.43 (0.61)]	3.3 [3.81 (0.69)]	4.2	4.24 (1.37)	5.27 (1.39)	1.09 (0.13)
42		3.6	4.4			
45 [42–47]	[3.71 (0.58)]	3.8 [4.09 (0.67)]	4.7	5.41 (1.28)	6.24 (1.17)	1.15 (0.11)
48		3.9	4.9			
51 [48–53]	[4.10 (0.65)]	4.1 [4.57 (0.76)]	5.2	5.79 (1.53)	6.48 (1.37)	1.19 (0.13)
54		4.3				
57 [54–59]	[4.28 (0.72)]	[4.75 (0.79)]		6.18 (1.32)	6.97 (1.26)	1.21 (0.11)
60		4.4				
[60–65]	[4.38 (0.63)]	[4.88 (0.72)]				
[66–71]	[4.47 (0.61)]	[4.96 (0.70)]		6.66 (1.35)	7.33 (1.21)	1.29 (0.13)
[72–77]	[4.57 (0.66)]	[5.07 (0.75)]				
[78–83]	[4.70 (0.66)]	[5.22 (0.71)]		7.60 (1.60)	8.05 (1.42)	1.36 (0.14)
[84–90]	[4.72 (0.83)]	[5.22 (0.91)]				
[90–95]	[4.92 (1.03)]	[5.35 (1.13)]				
[96–101]	[5.08 (0.84)]	[5.67 (0.97)]				
[102–107]	[4.99 (0.71)]	[5.51 (0.79)]		8.59 (1.40)	8.87 (1.19)	1.34 (0.14)
108		8.8				
108–131				9.61 (1.52)	9.70 (1.40)	1.37 (0.15)

Notes: [1]Rice et al. (2010). [2]Combined data from four different studies (Klee et al., 1989; J. Miller, 1981; Scarborough et al., 1986; Wells, 1985). [3]MSL (mean syntactic length), words per sentence, and clauses per sentence extrapolated from tables in Klee (1992). [4]Owens and Pavelko (2020); Pavelko and Owens (2017). Robust sampling and additional morphemes. *Hadley et al. (2018) reported 2.9 (SD = 0.66).

Table 7–20. Examples of T-Units and C-Units

Sentence Structure	Examples	Number of T-Units and C-Units
Simple—one clause	They watched the parade on TV.	1 T-unit, 1 C-unit
Complex—embedded clause	Washington has the horse I want.	1 T-unit, 1 C-unit
Compound—conjoining of two or more clauses	They went to the movie, but I stayed home.	2 T-units, 2 C-units
	Mom went to work, I went to school, and my sister stayed home.	3 T-units, 3 C-units
Partial sentences		
Elliptical answers	(Who went with you?) Marshon.	1 C-unit
Exclamations	Oh, wow!	1 C-unit
Aphorisms	A penny saved.	1 C-unit

A variant of the T-unit is the C-unit. C-units are similar to T-units but also include smaller units, such as elliptical utterances, that are more characteristic of speech (see Table 7–20). C-unit values are also given in Table 7–21.

Percent Grammatical Utterances. Grammaticality or the percentage of grammatically correct utterances (PGU; Fey et al., 2004) is determined by using your own language knowledge. Determine if the utterance follows the rules of English grammar as used commonly in your daily communication. Semantic errors such as the wrong name or action word are ignored. Ratings of grammaticality correlate with other LSA measures, such as MLU_M (Hoffman, 2013).

To calculate PGU, an SLP codes each utterance as grammatical or ungrammatical and then calculates the PGU as a percentage of the total sample. As you might expect, PGU is considerably lower in children with language disorders in comparison to their peers with TDL. Eisenberg and Guo (2013) report a cutoff PGU score of 58.32% for children aged 3;0–3;11 years, with most children with language disorders scoring below this point. Older children have a higher PGU score. For example, Guo and Schneider (2016) report 91% and 95%, respectively, for 6- and 8-year-olds. In comparison, children with language disorders have 64% and 78%, respectively.

The percent of grammatical responses (PGR) is a similar measure. PGR is collected in response to questions from pictures and correlates well with standardized tests (Eisenberg & Guo, 2018). It is hoped that further research will lead to normative data, although this lack does not preclude using the measure, especially to chart intervention progress.

Quantitative measures can be useful tools that are relatively easy to calculate. For example, preterm children born at less than 30 weeks score lower than term-born peers on multiple metrics, including MLU_M and MLU_W, NDW, and Index of Productive Syntax sentence structures, discussed later (Sanchez et al., 2020).

CHAPTER 7 LANGUAGE SAMPLE ANALYSIS

Table 7–21. T-Units and C-Units by Age and Grade

Unit	Age 4	Age 6	Age 6–7*	Grades 3–4	Grades 6–7	Grade 9	Grades 10–12
Words/T-unit							
Spoken			8.67	7.8	9.7		11.4
Oral Spanish		5.64					
Written				9.5	9.4–11.8		10.6–14.3
Words/C-unit							
Oral					9.82	10.96	11.7
Oral AAE	3.14	3.81					
Written					9.04	10.05	13.27
Clauses/T-unit							
Spoken		1.26	1.33	1.31	1.5		1.5
Written				1.3	1.6		1.6–1.8
Subordinate clauses/C-unit							
Spoken					0.37	0.43	0.58
Written					0.29	0.47	0.60
Words/clause							
Spoken	7.14		7.75				
Written					7.26		8.82

Note: *Use expository task.

Sources: Adapted from Nippold et al. (2008), Crowhurst and Piche (1979), and Scott et al. (1992).

SUGAR, mentioned previously, calculates MLU_S, TNW, WPS, and CPS. These values, especially MLU_S and CPS, have very high sensitivity (.98) and high specificity (.83) with children aged 3;0 to 7;11 years (Pavelko & Owens, 2019a).

Morphological Analysis. With preschool children, the SLP will want to analyze five inflectional morphemes for correct production. These are listed in Table 7–22 and include *-ing*, plural *-s*, possessive *-'s*, regular past *-ed*, and third person *-s*. For older children, the SLP may be interested in a variety of morphological prefixes and suffixes. Called derivational suffixes, these morphemes are used to change word classes, as in adding *-er* to a verb such as *teach* to create the noun *teacher*. Derivational suffixes are more common in written than in oral language, making them important in LSA with school-age children. Common affixes are included in Appendix D. In part, the high sensitivity and specificity of SUGAR reflect inclusion of some of these in calculation of MLU_S.

Table 7-22. Inflectional Morphemes and Age of Mastery

MLU	Morpheme	Examples	Age Range of Mastery* (in Months)
2.0–2.5	Present progressive -ing (no auxiliary verb)	Mommy driving	19–28
	Regular plural -s	Kitties eat my ice cream Forms: /s/, /z/, and /lz/ Cats (/kaets/) Dogs (/dɔgz/) Classes (klaeslz), wishes (/wɪʃɪz/)	24–33
2.5–3.0	Possessive 's	Mommy's balloon broke. Forms: /s/, /z/, and /lz/ as in regular plural I throw the ball to daddy.	26–40
3.0–3.5/3.75	Regular past -ed	Mommy pulled the wagon. Forms: /d/, /t/, and /ɪd/ Pulled (/pʊld/) Walked (/wɔkt/) Gilded (/gɪldɪd/)	26–48
	Regular third person -s	Kathy hits. Forms: /s/, /z/, and /lz/ as in regular plural	26–46

Note: *Used correctly 90% of the time in obligatory contexts.
Sources: Adapted from R. Brown (1973) and J. Miller (1981).

The percentage of correct morpheme use is determined by dividing the number of correct appearances by the total number of obligatory or required contexts. In a context such as *three dog*, a child might use the morpheme correctly, make a substitution, or omit the morpheme. Although useful, the percentage correct alone will not describe the types of errors.

Pronouns offer a special case of morphological analysis because of the complex nature of the underlying semantic and pragmatic functions. If the child's strategy is "when in doubt, use the noun," then it will be difficult to find errors in pronoun substitution. The types of errors, such as gender or subjective–objective confusion, may reveal a child's underlying rules.

Syntactic Analysis. For meaningful syntactic analysis, it's best to exclude imitations and stereotypic or rote responses because these types of utterances are not usually clin-

CHAPTER 7 LANGUAGE SAMPLE ANALYSIS

275

ically significant. Syntactic analysis can occur at both the phrase and the clause level as well as overall sentence formation.

Let's begin with noun and verb phrase development and progress to sentence types and embedding and conjoining. These analyses will be especially important for school-age children and adolescents. As an SLP, you'll need to be alert to word-order errors and cohesive difficulties that may become evident in analysis of units larger than just the individual sentence. The sample as a whole may be your best evidence.

Noun Phrase. Although noun phrase (NP) word order is relatively fixed and the noun or pronoun is somewhere in the middle of NPs, as shown in Table 7–23, we should say a few words about this noun/pronoun element first.

The noun function can be filled by subjective pronouns, such as *I, you, we,* and *they;* objective pronouns, such as *me, you. us,* and *them;* genitive pronouns, such as *mine, yours, ours,* and *theirs; reflexive myself, yourself, herself, himself, itself, ourselves, your selves,* and *themselves;* nouns, such as *boy* and *woman;* and mass nouns, *sand* and *water.* When a pronoun is used, the NP is relatively simple, such as *all of us* or *them in there.* The noun function also may be complex or may consist of a phrase, as in *Statue of Liberty, need to succeed,* and *city of Los Angeles,* or a compound, as in *Jim and Bob.*

Thirty-month-old children use pronoun subjects much more than noun subjects (Hadley et al., 2018). Although there is little elaboration, an SLP should record the pronoun types and any errors.

NP elaboration is assessed by describing the number and variety of elements. This is especially appropriate for children in late childhood or adolescence. Briefly stated:

- Initiators limit or quantify the phrase that follows, as in *just* and *at least.*
- Determiners include the following, in order of mention:
  - Quantifiers express quantity not in exact numbers, but as in *both, half,* and *one of.*
  - Articles include *a, an,* and *the.*
  - Possessive pronouns express relationship, as in *my* and *our.*
  - Demonstratives are interpreted from the perspective of the speaker, as in *this, that, these,* and *those.*
  - Numerical terms are specific numbers, such as *one, ten,* and *sixty.*
- Adjectivals more closely describe the noun or pronoun.
  - Possessive nouns express a relationship, as in *mommy's.*
  - Ordinals express rank, as in *first* and *next.*
  - Adverbs serve to emphasize the following adjective, as in *very* and *really.* As an SLP, be mindful that only very few adjectives will be present as in **very** *big dog* and **really** *hot cocoa.*
  - Adjectives describe, as in *little, important,* and *blond.*
  - Descriptors are nouns used to describe, as in **hot dog** *stand* and **cowboy** *hat.*
- Noun or pronoun.

Table 7–23. Elements of a Noun Phrase

Initiator	+ Determiner	+ Adjectival	+ Noun	+ Post-Noun Modifier
Only, a few of, just, at least, less, nearly, especially, partially, even, merely, almost	**Quantifier:** All, both, half, no, one-tenth, some, any, either, twice, triple	**Possessive noun:** Mommy's, children's	**Pronoun:** I, you, he, she, it, we, they, mine, yours, his, hers, its, ours, theirs	**Prepositional phrase:** On the car, in the box, in the gray flannel suit
	Article: The, a, an	**Ordinal:** First, next, next to last, final, second	**Noun:** Boys, dog, feet, sheep, men and women, City of New York, Port of Chicago, leap of faith, matter of conscience	**Adjectival:** Next door, pictured by Renoir, eaten by Martians, loved by her friends
	Possessive: My, your, his, her, its, our, their	**Adverb:** Very, usually		**Adverbial:** Here, there (embedded)
	Demonstrative: This, that, these, those	**Adjective:** Blue, big, little, fat, old, fast, circular, challenging		**Clause:** Who went with you, that you saw
	Numerical Term: One, two, thirty, one thousand	**Descriptor:** Shopping (center) baseball (game), hot dog (stand)		
Examples				
Nearly . . .	all the one hundred . . .	old college . . .	alumni . . .	attending the event
Almost . . .	all of her thirty . . .	former . . .	clients	
Just . . .	half of your . . .	brother's old baseball . . .	uniforms . . .	in the closet

- Post-noun modifiers may take many forms.
  - Prepositional phrases, as in *in my class*. (Note that my class is an NP.)
  - Adjectivals further describe and will be infrequently used, as in *girl **next door*** and *friend **loved by all***.
  - Adverbials will also be infrequent and almost exclusively consist of *here* and *there*.

CHAPTER 7 LANGUAGE SAMPLE ANALYSIS

○ Embedded clauses, called relative clauses, describe in more detail and will most likely only be seen in older elementary school children, as in *who goes to my school*.

By now, your head is probably swimming with new terminology and categories. You won't see all the NP elements in a single sample. Development takes years for most children with TDL.

With increasing age, children add more elements, although the typical elaboration is one or two elements through elementary school. Table 7–27 offers some developmental guidelines from 50-utterance samples. The SUGAR website (Owens & Pavelko, 2021; https://www.SUGARlanguage.org/) has easy-to-use subanalysis forms based on the NP elements seen in 80% of children's 50-utterance samples (Owens et al., 2018).

Children with language disorders can be expected to have simpler, less elaborated NPs. Pronouns offer a special problem, as discussed previously.

> ***Food for Thought:*** **Do you understand what a noun phrase is? Do you also understand that many of the words in the different elements can have multiple purposes, some not in noun phrases? For example, "one" is a numerical term, but it can also be a noun, as in "I want that one."**

Verb Phrase. As mentioned in Chapter 2, verb morphology can be especially challenging for children with DLD. Verb phrase (VP) word order can be similarly daunting.

VPs consist of the verb and associated words, including noun phrases used as complements or as direct or indirect objects. An SLP is concerned with the verbs used and those that are missing or incomplete. Other elements of the VP that are present or absent are also important and reflect the maturity of the speaker's language system.

Predicate or verb relationships take three forms: intransitive, in which the verb cannot take an object, as in *she **walks***; transitive, in which the verb can take an object, as in *mommy **bought** candy*; and equative, which consists of the copula (*to be*) plus a complement of a noun (*She is a doctor*), adjective (*He is sick*), or adverb (*They were late*). Verb phrases can be described by the length, type, and elements, as demonstrated in Table 7–24.

Simple transitive (*Mommy throw*) and equative verb phrases (*Doggie big*) appear at an MLU of approximately 1.5. At this level, the verbs are unmarked for tense or person, and the copula is omitted. As language becomes more complex, verbs become marked, the copula appears, and intransitive VPs appear.

By an MLU of 2.0 to 2.5, the progressive *-ing* marker and semi-infinitive forms such as *gonna, wanna, gotta,* and *hafta* appear. As an SLP, don't assume a child is functioning at this level just because these forms are present; they are frequently used in several dialects. Being from a low-socioeconomic status and middle Atlantic background, I use *gonna* frequently.

The perfective form (*have + verb-en*) and the passive voice begin to be used when the MLU reaches 3.0 to 3.5/3.75. Adverbial phrases (*in a minute, together, quickly*) also begin to appear.

278 LANGUAGE DISORDERS: A FUNCTIONAL APPROACH TO ASSESSMENT AND INTERVENTION IN CHILDREN

Table 7–24. Elements of the Verb Phrase

Modal Auxiliary	+ Perfective Auxiliary	+ Verb BE	+ Negative*	+ Passive	+ Verb	+ Prepositional Phrase, Noun Phrase, Noun Complement, Adverbial Phrase
May, can, shall, will, must, might, should, would, could	Have, has, had	Am, is, are, was, were, be, been	Not	Been, being	Run, walk, eat, throw, see, write	On the floor, the ball, our old friend, a doctor, on time, late

Examples

Transitive (May have direct object)

May.................have...wanted.........a cookie

Should...not...throw..........the ball in the house

Intransitive (Does not take direct object)

Might.................have...............been...a doctor

Could...not...talk............with a doctor

Equative (Verb BE as main verb)

....is..............not...a doctor

....was...late

....were...on the sofa

May...be...ill

Note: *When model auxiliaries are used, the negative is placed between the model and other auxiliary forms—for example, "Might not have been going."

Late childhood and adolescent language development is characterized by increasing verb complexity and correct use of auxiliary verbs (*do, have*), modal auxiliaries (*may, should*), and perfective forms, such as *have been going*. There is also increasing use of adverbs and adverbial phrases, such as prepositional phrases of manner (*in silence*), place (*in the city*), and time (*in a week*). In general, many children with language disorders exhibit these more complex structures but tend to use them less frequently than do children with TDL.

Tense markers are used to describe the temporal relationships between events. For example, if the event being described is taking place while the speaker mentions it, the speaker uses the present progressive verb form (*auxiliary + verb-ing*) to indicate an ongoing activity (*am walking, was eating*). In contrast, the perfect form of the verb (*have + verb-en*) indicates that the action is being described in relation to the present.

CHAPTER 7 LANGUAGE SAMPLE ANALYSIS

Thus, "I have been working here for 2 years" implies that this action is still occurring, whereas "I have eaten my dinner" implies that the action is now complete. Table 7–25 identifies the ages at which most preschool children acquire auxiliary and modal auxiliary verbs.

Irregular past tense verbs are a special challenge for children with language disorders (Shipley et al., 1991). English contains approximately 200 irregular verbs, and although many are used infrequently, others, such as *went, saw, sat,* and *ate,* are among the most frequently used verbs. Development begins in the preschool years and extends into adolescence. Table 7–26 presents the ages at which 80% of children are able to use different irregular verbs in a sentence completion task.

Modal auxiliary verbs, such as *can, could, will, should, shall, may, might,* and *must,* express the speaker's attitude. Syntactically, modals function in the formation of questions (*Can we go tonight?*) and negatives (*I shouldn't go out in this weather*). They are used also in such statements as "I'll do it tomorrow." Modals represent a complex interaction of form, content, and use that is reflected in the slow rate of acquisition, which usually lasts from age 2 years to age 8 years.

Modals associated with action, such as *can* and *will,* are acquired first, often before age 4 years. After this age, the child clarifies the different forms and their uses. In general, children with language disorders have more difficulty with infinitives, modals, and auxiliary verbs than their overall language would suggest.

Sentence Types. Sentences can be grouped by length or categorized by structure. For example, declarative sentences can be categorized as subject–verb, subject–verb–object (S-V-O), subject–verb–complement, and multiple clauses, either embedded or conjoined. The form of a preschool child's sentences can be compared with normative data, such as those in Table 7–25, to best determine the child's development, although descriptive data are also valuable.

Sentences that differ from the predominant subject–verb–object format of English may be difficult for the child with a language disorder to decipher and form. Often, overreliance on the S-V-O strategy is not noted until the child begins school. The child may resist rearrangement or interruption of this form and may attach other structures only at the beginning or the end. Yes/no questions may be asked with rising intonation, rather than through relocating the subject and verb elements (*He is sick?* versus *Is he sick?*). Passive sentences, which use a S-V-O (*The pencil was replaced by the pen*) form but an object–action–agent semantic makeup, may be misinterpreted.

As an SLP, you should note the range of internal sentence forms and different sentence types. Sentence types include positive and negative forms of the declarative, interrogative, and imperative. The range of sentence types and the maturity of form are of interest. For preschool children, these were presented in Table 7–25.

Embedding and Conjoining. Both embedding and conjoining involve relationships between clauses. In addition, embedding involves the relationships between phrases and clauses. It's sometimes difficult for SLP students to identify multiclausal sentences as either conjoined or embedded. I suggest that you refer to the excellent tutorial by Steffani (2007). Her descriptions and identification flowchart are extremely helpful.

Table 7–25. Preschool Language Development

MLU	Approximate Age (Months)	Sentence Types	Intrasentential/Morphology
1–1.5	12–21	Single words *Yes/no* questions use rising intonation. *What* and *where* *Negative* + X	Pronouns *I* and *mine* Isolated nouns elaborated as *art./adj.* + *noun.* Serial naming without *and*
1.5–2.0	21–26	*S* + *V* + *O* appears. Negative *no* and *not* used interchangeably. *Yes/no* question form is *This/that* + X?	*And* appears. *In* and *on* appear.
2.0–2.25	27–28	*Wh-* question form is *What/where* + *noun?* *BE* appears as main verb*	Present progressive (*-ing*), no aux. verb mastered by 90%. Pronouns *me, my* and *it, this* and *that* Nouns elaborated in object position only [(*art./adj./dem./poss.*) + *noun*].
2.25–2.5	28–29	Basic *SVO* used by most. Negative element (*no, not, don't, can't* interchangeable) placed between noun and verb.	*In/on* and plural *-s* mastered by 90%. *Gonna, wanna, gotta, hafta* appear.
2.5–2.75	30–32	*What/where* + *N* + *V?* Inversion in *What/where* + *be* + *N?** *S* + *aux. verb* + *V* + *O* appears. Aux. verbs include *can, do, have, will.*	Pronouns *she, he, her, we, you, your, yours,* and *them* Noun elaboration in the subject and object position [*art.* + (*modifier*) + *noun*]. Modifiers include *a lot, some,* and *two.* Select irregular past (*came, fell, broke, sat, went*) and possessive (*-'s*) mastered by 90%.
2.75–3.0	33–34	*S* + *aux. verb* + *be* + X appears. Negative *won't* appears. Aux. verbs appear in interrogatives: inverted with subject in yes/no type.	*But, so, or,* and *if* appear.

CHAPTER 7 LANGUAGE SAMPLE ANALYSIS

281

Table 7–25. *continued*

MLU	Approximate Age (Months)	Sentence Types	Intrasentential/Morphology
3.0–3.5	35–39	Negative appears with aux. verb + *not* (*cannot, do not*). Inversion of aux. verb and subject in *Wh-* questions.	Uncontractible copula (verb BE as *main verb*) mastered by 90%. Pronouns *his, him, hers, us,* and *they* Noun phrase elaboration includes *art./dem. + adj/poss./mod. + noun.* Clausal conjoining with *and* appears. Clausal embedding as object with *think, guess, show, remember,* etc.
3.5–3.75	39–42	Double aux. verbs in declaratives Add *isn't, aren't, doesn't,* and *didn't* Inversion of *be* and subject in *yes/no* interrogatives Add *when* and *how* interrogatives	Articles (*the, a*), regular past (*-ed*), and third person regular (*-s*) mastered by 90%. Infinitive phrases appear at end of sentence.
3.75–4.5	42–56	Indirect objects appear in declaratives. Add *wasn't, wouldn't, couldn't,* and *shouldn't* Negative appears with other forms of *BE.* Some simple tag questions appear.	Pronouns *our, ours, its, their, theirs, myself,* and *yourself* Relative clauses appear attached to object. Infinitive phrases with same subject as main verb
4.5+	56+	Add indefinite negatives (*nobody, no one, nothing*), creating double negatives. *Why* interrogatives appears in more-than-one-word interrogatives. Negative interrogatives after 60 months	Irregular past (*does, has*), uncontractible auxiliary to be and contractible auxiliary *BE* and copula (*BE* as main verb) mastered by 90%. Remaining reflexive pronouns added. Multiple embedding; embedding + conjoining Relative clauses attached to subject appear.

Note: *Copula.

Table 7–26. Irregular Verbs and Age of Acquisition	
Age (Years)	**Irregular Verbs**
3;0–3;5	Hit, hurt
3;6–3;11	Went
4;0–4;5	Saw
4;6–4;11	Ate, gave
5;0–5;5	Broke, fell, found, took
5;6–5;11	Came, made, sat, threw
6;0–6;5	Bit, cut, drove, fed, flew, ran, wore, wrote
6;6–6;11	Blew, read, rode, shot
7;0–7;5	Drank
7;6–7;11	Drew, dug, hid, rang, slept, swam
8;0–8;5	Caught, hung, left, slid
8;6–8;11	Built, sent, shook

Source: Information taken from Shipley et al. (1991).

Although school-age children with language disorders are often able to construct sentences using a range of verbs, their sentences are more restricted in their use and they produce fewer semantically accurate complements (Eisenberg, 2004; Steel et al., 2016). Let's take a moment to review some complicated syntactic structures, including complements.

An infinitive phrase (*to + verb*) can share the subject with the main verb, as in *Juan wants to eat*, or have a separate noun, as in *Juan wants Domonique to eat*, which is more difficult for children to comprehend and produce. You may recall from your language development course that infinitives appear around age 3 years and are the earliest form of more complex sentences to develop (Diessel, 2004; Diessel & Tomasello, 2001).

Around age 4 years, children begin to embed clauses to form multiclausal sentences. Clausal embedding initially develops in the object position at the end of the sentence (see Table 7–25). Called *object noun complements*, these dependent clauses take the place of the object following such words as *know*, *think*, and *feel* (*I know that **you can do it***).

Object noun complements using *that* (*I think **that I like it***) appear at an MLU of 4.0, most frequently following the verb *think*. By an MLU of 5.0 to 5.9, this type of embedding accounts for only 6% of children's two-clause sentences. Object noun complements using *what* (*I know what you did*) account for 8% of these sentences. The embedded clause completes or complements the verb phrase and is used with the following (Diessel, 2004; Owen Van Horne & Lin, 2011):

- Mental-state verbs, as in *I **know** what you did*.
- Verbs of desire, as in *I **want** what Keisha has*.

CHAPTER 7 LANGUAGE SAMPLE ANALYSIS **283**

- Verbs of perception, as in *I **heard** what you said.*
- Manipulation verbs, as in *I **hope** you'll do it.*
- Communication verbs, as in *Mommy **said** we can go.*

Notice that these verb phrases could also take the earlier infinitive form, as in *I know how to do it* and the previously mentioned *Mommy said to stop.* The nature of the verb in the main clause determines whether it can take an embedded clausal complement as the object of the main clause. Transitive verbs, such as *kick, want, need, have,* and *remove,* take a direct object, as in *I want help,* and can take an embedded clausal complement, as in *I want what you're eating.*

Relative embedded or subordinate clauses attached to nouns develop next, beginning in the object position, as in "I want the dog *that I saw last night.*" Finally, the relative clause moves to the center of the sentence, describing the subject, as in "The one *that you ate* was my favorite." During late childhood and adolescence, an increase occurs in relative clauses either attached to the subject or serving as the subject, as in "*Whoever wishes to go* should come to the office." This type of clausal embedding is more common in written than in oral language.

Relative clauses appear at approximately 48 months initially as post-noun modifiers for empty nouns, such as *one* or *thing.* The most common relative pronouns for preschoolers are *that* and *what.* During the school years, relative pronouns expand with the addition of *whose, whom,* and *in which.* Among preschoolers, relative clauses appear less frequently than other forms of clausal embedding, although by school age, 20% to 30% of two-clause sentences may be of this type.

Phrases also may be embedded in clauses. As in clausal embedding, phrasal embedding usually develops initially at the end of the sentence. SLPs are interested in the number and type of embeddings. Some developmental data are included in Table 7–25.

Clausal conjoining appears relatively late in preschool development, although some conjunctions appear much earlier. Around 30 months of age, children begin to sequence clauses, using *and* as the initial word in each sentence (***And** we saw ponies*). As noted in Table 7–25, *and* is also the first conjunction used to join clauses. Among school-age children, 50% to 80% of all narrative sentences begin with *and.* With age and an increase in written communication, use of *and* decreases. Between ages 11 and 14 years, only 20% of spoken narrative sentences begin with *and.* In written narratives, the rate is only approximately 5%.

Other conjunctions may express a causal relationship (*because*), simultaneity (*while*), a contrasting relationship (*but*), and exclusion (*except*). The most frequently used conjunctions through age 12 years are *and, because,* and *when.*

An SLP is interested in the range and frequency of the conjunctions used and in the amount of conjoining present in the sample. This information is especially important in narratives analysis.

An SLP also should note multiple embeddings and embedding and conjoining that occur within the same sentence. Again, this usage is much more characteristic of school-age language than of preschool language. The narratives of children aged 10 to 12 years are easily distinguishable from those of preschoolers by the presence of multiple embedding and conjoining within the same sentence.

284 LANGUAGE DISORDERS: A FUNCTIONAL APPROACH TO ASSESSMENT AND INTERVENTION IN CHILDREN

> ***Food for Thought:*** Be honest with yourself. If grammar seems overwhelming, you'll need to get as much extra instruction as possible. Continuing education once you graduate may be something to pursue.

Summary. As an SLP, you'll be interested in the range and frequency of the NP and VP elements and the types of verbs a child exhibits. The development of NPs and VPs takes years for most children with TDL and continues into adolescence. With increasing age, children's VPs become increasingly complex.

Table 7–27 offers some developmental guidelines from 50-utterance samples. As with NPs, the SUGAR website (Owens & Pavelko, 2019; https://www.SUGARlanguage.org/) has easy-to-use subanalysis forms based on the VP elements seen in 80% of children's 50-utterance samples (Owens et al., 2018).

Narrative Analysis

Narratives, as connected conversational units, offer a glimpse into all aspects of language. This may be why Amanda, the SLP mentioned previously, is interested in LSA using narratives.

Narrative skill can be broken down into two interrelated aspects of narration: *macrostructure* and *microstructure*. Narrative macrostructure includes causal networks, event

Table 7–27. New Structures Likely to Appear in a 50-Utternce Sample*

Age (Years)	Noun Phrase	Verb Phrase	Clausal
3;0–3;5	Article, possessive pronoun, noun	BE copula, irregular past, infinitive phrases, prepositional phrases	
3;6–3;11	Adjective, descriptor	BE auxiliary	Conjoining
4;0–4;5		*Do/does* + verb	Embedding
4;6–4;11		Adverbs, adverbial phrases	
5;0–5;11	Quantifier		
6;0–6;11		Modal auxiliaries, metacognitive verbs	More than 2 clauses
7;0–8;11	Demonstrative, numerical		
9;0–10;11	Relative clauses, more than 3 noun phrase elements		Relative clauses, more than 3 clauses

Note: *Based on appearance in more than 80% of 50-utterance samples.
Source: Owens et al. (2018).

CHAPTER 7 LANGUAGE SAMPLE ANALYSIS

representations, and story grammar elements; thus, analysis is more global or conceptual, which is difficult to measure. Narrative organization skills are positively related to advances in use of grammatical forms, such as verb tense; lexical forms; and lexico-grammatical features, such as relational words (Bowles et al., 2020). That's microstructure.

Narrative microstructure involves specific words, phrases, clauses, and sentences. Analysis of narrative microstructure may follow more traditional LSA methods described previously in this chapter. Given the language demands of narratives, analysis might also involve cohesive devices, such as pronoun use, reference, coordinating and subordinating conjunctions, and other morphosyntactic devices in more detail.

Given the relationship between microstructure and macrostructure, it should come as no surprise that children with language disorders have difficulty with both aspects of narration (Manhardt & Rescorla, 2002; Pearce et al., 2003; Reilly et al., 2004). This difficulty, in turn, suggests that these language deficits may be due to broader information-processing deficits, possibly reduced processing capacity (Boudreau, 2007; Colozzo et al., 2006). Given the use of narratives in conversation, a child's difficulty with narrative organization can have a serious impact on their everyday language use. This can further impact school performance because narratives are a major component of the school curriculum.

Before we dive into analysis, we discuss a few assessment tools that are available. The Narrative Assessment Protocol–2 (Bowles et al., 2020), an easy-to-use tool designed to assess the narratives of children aged 3 to 6 years, uses event-based frequency scoring. A child's narrative is recorded on video, and language features are scored without transcription. In event-based frequency scoring, the scorer identifies occurrences of specific structures, such as infinitives, that reflect an aspect of narrative skill. Each occurrence is awarded a point.

The CUBED Narrative Language Measures (NLM; Petersen & Spencer, 2016) is a freely available LSA method that also eliminates transcription. NLM has good validity compared to other language measures. A free download is available at https://www.languagedynamicsgroup.com/cubed/cubed_download/

Finally, the Test of Narrative Language–Second Edition (TNL-2; Gillam & Pearson, 2017), a preschool measure, involves retelling and two narrative generations using a wordless five-panel comic strip. Although relatively expensive, TNL-2 has good evidence of diagnostic accuracy for children with DLD.

Macrostructure Analysis

Macrostructural analysis can occur in several ways, such as narrative levels, high points, and story grammars. Narrative levels are concerned with the structural relationship of the narrative parts to the narrative as a whole.

Narrative levels do not have a goal-based organization, whereas story grammars (what happens in the story) do. Narrative-level LSA is most appropriate for the stories of 2- to 5-year-olds and for school-age children with limited verbal abilities; story grammar analysis is best for those older than age 5 years. The narratives of preschool children may be evaluated also by using high-point analysis to determine the type of narrative structure.

Narrative-Level Analysis

Children use two strategies for organizing their stories: centering and chaining. **Centering** is the linking of attributes or objects to form a story nucleus. The links may be based on similarity or complementarity of features. Similarity links are formed by perceptually observed attributes, such as actions, characteristics, and scenes or situations. **Chaining** consists of a sequence of events that share attributes and lead directly from one to another.

Most stories of 2-year-olds are organized by centering. By age 3 years, however, nearly half of the children use both centering and chaining. This percentage increases, and by age 5 years, nearly three-fourths of children use both strategies.

These organizational strategies can result in six basic developmental stages of story organization (Applebee, 1978), presented here in developmental order:

- *Heaps* are unrelated statements about a central stimulus. The statements identify aspects of the stimulus or provide additional information. The common element may be the similarity of the grammatical structure, but there is no obvious organizational pattern.

  Dogs wag their tails and bark. Dogs sleep all day. A dog chased a cat.

- *Sequences* include events linked on the basis of similar attributes or events that create a focus. Sentences may be moved without altering the narrative.

  I *ate* a hamburger. And Johnny did *too*. Mommy *ate* a chicken nuggets. Daddy *ate* a fries and coke.

- *Primitive temporal narratives* are organized around a center with complementary events.

  I go outside and swing. Bobby push swing. I go high and try to stop. I fall. And I start to cry. Bobby pick me up.

- *Unfocused temporal chains* lead directly from one event to another, while linking attributes, such as characters, settings, or actions, shift. As a result of the shifting focus, unfocused chains have no centers.

  The man got in his boat. He rowed and fished. He ate his sandwich. (Shift) The fishes swimmed and play. Fishes jump over the water. Fishes go to a big hole in the bottom. (Shift) There's a dog in the boat. He's thirsty. He jump in the water.

- *Focused temporal or causal chains* generally center on a main character who goes through a series of perceptually linked, concrete events.

  This boy, he found a jellybean. And his mother said not to eat it. And he did. And a tree growed out of his head.

- *Narratives* develop the center as the story progresses. Each incident complements the center, develops from the previous incident, forms a chain, and adds some new aspect to the theme. Causal relationships may be concrete or abstract and move forward toward the ending of the initial situation. Children with language disorders often omit causal links to tie together the elements of the script (Hayward et al., 2007). There is usually a climax.

CHAPTER 7 LANGUAGE SAMPLE ANALYSIS

There was a boy named Juan. And he got lost in the woods. He ate plants and trees. And he was friends with all the animals. He builded a tent to live in. One day, he builded a fire, and the policemen found him. They took Juan home to his mommy and daddy.

Each narrative can be divided into episodes that are analyzed according to this scheme. Table 7–28 contains examples of narratives and their analysis by narrative level.

High-Point Analysis

High-point analysis is revealed through an event's meaning to the narrator. The accompanying structure has developmental significance.

It is best for high-point analysis to use narratives that describe events in which the child was present. An SLP should select the longest personal event narratives for analysis. Length and complexity have been shown to be related.

The high point of a narrative is marked by children in many ways. These markings include paralinguistic features, such as emphasis, elongation, and use of environmental noises ("The dog went 'Ruff-ruff'!"); and linguistic features, such as exclamations ("Wow!"), repetition, attention getters ("Here's the best part"), exaggeration, judgments, or evaluative statements ("This is my favorite"), emotional statements, and explanations.

Different types of high-point structures are presented in Table 7–29. Next to each is the approximate age at which these structures are most common for Caucasian, English-speaking, North American children. You can use this table to determine whether the child is using narrative structures typical of their age group. After age 5 years, fewer than 10% of children produce one-event, two-event, leapfrog, and miscellaneous narratives. Obviously, a small sample of a few narratives will be needed for an adequate evaluation.

Table 7–28. Narrative-Level Analysis

Examples	Classification
Simple frames	
Granma lives on a farm. There are horsies and piggies. The cows moo. I can ride on the tire swing in a tree. And the calf licked me. That's all.	Sequence
Once there was two kids, Cassidy and . . . and Fred. Fred's a funny name. And they was fighting. Their mom said, "Why are you fighting?" Cassidy and Fred doesn't know why. They stop and be friends.	Focused chain
Complex narrative frame with episodic development	
The kids all went to Burger King on Halloween. Supper Zhiming–that's me–got a cheese-burger. My sister got a Whopper. Mommy and Daddy got nuggets and salad bar. They were eating when a big ghost came out of my milkshake. He threw the milkshake on everyone and got them mad. Super Zhiming stuck the ghost with a fork and he went flat. All the air came out. Daddy was so happy that he buyed ice cream cones for all the kids.	Sequence narrative

Table 7–29. High-Point Narrative Structure

Narrative Structure	Characteristics	Expected Age (Years)
One-event narrative	Contains one event	Below 3½
Two-event narrative	Contains two past events but no logical or causal relationship in the real world or in the narrative	3½
Miscellaneous narrative	Contains two or more past events that in the real world are logically or causally related	Very low frequency at all ages (3½–9)
Leapfrog narrative	Contains two or more related past events, but the order does not mirror the real-world relationship	4
Chronological narrative	Contains two or more related past events in a logical or causal sequence without a high point	Present at all ages (3½–9)
End-at-high-point narrative	Contains two or more related past events in a logical or causal sequence with a high point but no following events (resolution)	5
Classic narrative	Contains two or more related past events in a logical or causal sequence with both a high point and a resolution	6+

Source: Information from McCabe and Rollins (1994).

Variations are to be expected within and across children. Many young children will "test the waters" by stating the high point first ("I got stung by a bee") and then, if it is accepted, will proceed with the narrative. This is not an example of impaired narration and can still be analyzed by using high-point analysis when the entire narrative is told.

Other structural elements might include openers, orientation (who, what, when, where), action descriptions or how something happened, evaluations or why things happened, emotional responses, and closings. Evaluations convey the significance of the event for the teller. These can be expressed through both verbal and nonverbal means.

High-point analysis tends to draw sharper distinctions between narratives of children with TDL and those with language disorders. When we use high-point analysis, the oral personal narratives of early elementary school children with language disorders, although still below those of TD children, are more mature than their fictional narratives from pictures.

Story Grammar Analysis

Story grammars describe the internal structure of a story, including its components and the rules underlying the relationships of these components. By serving as a framework, story grammars may facilitate information processing, narrative comprehension, and memory. The competent storyteller constructs the story and the flow of information in such a way as to maximize comprehension.

A narrative consists of the setting plus the episode structure (story = setting + episode structure). Each story begins with an introduction contained in the setting, as in "Once upon a time in a far-off kingdom, there lived a prince who was very sad . . . " or "On the way to work this morning, I was crossing Main Street . . . ," or simply "We went to the zoo."

An episode consists of an initiating event, an internal response, a plan, an attempt, a consequence, and a reaction. An episode is considered to be complete if it contains an initiating event or response to provide a purpose, an attempt, and a direct consequence (Stein & Glenn, 1979). Episodes may be linked in several ways, forming a coherent narrative.

The seven elements of story grammars occur in the following order (Stein & Glenn, 1979):

- *Setting statement* (S) introduces the characters and describes their habitual actions, along with the social, physical, and/or temporal contexts that introduce the protagonist or main character.

- *Initiating event* (IE) induces the character(s) to act through some natural act (e.g., an earthquake), a notion to seek something (e.g., treasure), or the action of one of the characters (e.g., arresting someone).

- *Internal response* (IR) describes the characters' reactions, such as emotional responses, thoughts, or intentions, to the initiating events. Internal responses provide some motivation for the characters.

- *Internal plan* (IP) indicates the characters' strategies for attaining their goal(s). Children rarely include this element.

- *Attempt(s)* (A) describe the overt actions of the characters to bring about some consequence, such as attain their goal(s).

- *Direct consequence* (DC) describes the characters' success or failure at attaining their goal(s) as a result of the attempt(s).

- *Reaction* (R) describes the characters' emotional responses, thoughts, or actions to the outcome or preceding chain of events.

Two narratives with very different story grammar are presented in Table 7–30.

> ***Food for Thought:*** **Notice the stories used in conversation. Do they follow the story grammar pattern? Do the narratives of children have missing pieces?**

There is a sequence of stages in the development of story grammars (Glenn & Stein, 1980). Certain structural patterns appear early and persist, whereas others are rather

Table 7–30. Story Grammar Examples

Narrative	Story Grammar Elements
Single episode	
There was this girl, and she got kidnapped by these pirates.	Setting statement (S) Initiating event (IE)
So when they were eating, she cut the ropes and got away.	Attempt (A) Direct consequence (DC)
And she lived on a island and ate parrots.	Reactions (R)
Multiple episodes	
Once there was this big dog on a farm.	Setting statements (S)
And he got hungry 'cause there wasn't enough food.	Initiating event$_1$ (IE$_1$)
The dog . . . his name was Max . . . was sad with no food, so his owner went to find some.	Internal response$_1$ (IR$_1$) Attempt$_1$ (A$_1$)
He met a witch, but she wouldn't give him food 'til he killed a yukky toad.	Initiating event$_2$ (IE$_2$) Internal response$_2$ (IR$_2$)
He was scared but he decided to build a trap.	Internal plan$_2$ (IP$_2$) Attempt$_2$ (A$_2$)
He dug a hole and filled it with frog food.	Direct consequences$_2$ (DC$_2$)
The frog wanted to eat the man but got caught.	Direct consequence$_1$ (DC$_1$)
The man went back to the witch and she got some hamburgers for the man and the dog.	
And the man and Max ate hamburgers and were happy.	Reaction$_1$ (R$_1$)

late in developing. The overall developmental sequence is as follows, although much individual variation exists:

- *Descriptive sequences* consist of descriptions of characters, surroundings, and habitual actions. There are no causal or temporal links. The entire story consists of setting statements.

   This is a story about my rabbit. He lives in a cage. He likes to hop around my yard. He eats carrots and grass. The end.

- *Action sequences* have a chronological order for actions but no causal relations. The story consists of a setting statement and various action attempts.

   I had a birthday party. (S) We played games and winned prizes. (A) I opened presents. (A) I got balloons. (A) I blew out the candles. (A) We ate cake and ice cream. (A) We had fun. (DC)

CHAPTER 7 LANGUAGE SAMPLE ANALYSIS

- *Reaction sequences* consist of a series of events in which changes cause other changes, with no goal-directed behaviors. The sequence consists of a setting, an initiating event, and action attempts.

    There was a lady petting her cow. (S) And the cow kicked the light. (IE) Then the police came. (A) Then a fire truck came. (A) Then a hook-and-ladder came. (A) And that's the end. (S)

- *Abbreviated episodes* contain an implicit or explicit goal. At this level, the story may contain either an event statement and a consequence or an internal response and a consequence. Although the characters' behavior is purposeful, it is usually not premeditated.

    There was a mommy and two kids. (S) And the kids baked a cake for the mommy's birthday. (S) They forgot to turn on . . . off the stove and burned the cake. (IE) The kids went to the store and buyed a cake. (C) The end. (S)

- *Complete episodes* contain an entire goal-oriented behavioral sequence consisting of a consequence statement and two of the following: initiating event, internal response, and attempt.

    This man was a doctor. (S) He made a monster. (IE) And it chase him around his house. (IE) He run in his bedroom. (A) He push the monster in the closet. (A) And the monster go away. (C) That's all. (S)

- *Complex episodes* are expansions of the complete episode or contain multiple episodes.

    Once there was this Luke Skywalker. (S) And he had to fight Darf Invader. (S/IE) They fought with swords. (A) And he killed him. (C) And he got in his rocket to blow up these kind of horse robots. (IE) And he shot them. (A) Then all the bad soldiers were killed. (C)

- *Interactive episodes* contain two characters who have separate goals and actions that influence each other's behavior.

    Sally never helped her mom with the dishes. (S) She got mad and said that Sally had to do it. (IE) So, Sally washed the dishes but she was mad. (IR) Then Sally dropped some dishes. (A) Then she dropped more. (A) And her mom said that she didn't have to do any more dishes. (C) And Sally watched TV every night after dinner. (S)

Specific structural properties associated with each structural pattern are listed in Table 7–31.

The SLP can note the setting and episodic structure for their completeness and relevance to the overall narrative. Another method of scoring is to award points or ratings based on setting complexity, characters, plot, and ending (Noel & Westby, 2014; Swanson et al., 2005).

Personal narratives differ from fictional narratives, so a strict story grammar analysis may not be a perfect fit. For example, personal stories usually include an indication of the purpose for relating the story or the point of the telling. In addition, personal narratives

Table 7–31. Structural Properties of Narratives

Structural Patterns	Structural Properties	Structural Patterns	Structural Properties

Descriptive sequence	Setting statements (S)(S)(S)	Complex episode	Multiple episodes
			  Setting statement (S)
			  Two of the following:
			    Initiating Event (IE$_1$)
			    Internal response (IR$_1$)
			  Attempt (A$_1$)
			  Direct consequence (DC$_1$)
			  Two of the following:
			    Initiating Event (IE$_2$)
			    Internal response (IR$_2$)
			  Attempt (A$_2$)
			  Direct consequence (DC$_2$)

Action sequence	Setting statement (S) Attempts (A)(A)(A)		
Reaction sequence	Setting statement (S) Initiating event (IE) Attempt (A)(A)(A)		
Abbreviated episode	Setting statement (S) Initiating event (IE) or internal response (IR) Direct consequence (DC)		

Complete episode	Setting statement (S)
	Two of the following:
	  Initiating event (IE)
	  Internal response (IR)
	Attempt (A)
	Direct consequence (DC)
			Expanded complete episode
			  Setting statement (S)
			  Initiating event (IE)
			  Internal response (IR)
			  Internal plan (IP)
			  Attempt (A)
			  Direct consequence (DC)
			  Reaction (R)

		Interactive episode	Two separate but parallel episodes that influence each other

often do not include an initiating event and hence no plan to overcome the problem. The teller is usually trying to make a point that the story supports, such as "It was the most terrible vacation ever."

Story grammar LSA alone may lack the sensitivity to differentiate children with language disorders from those without. Unfortunately, there is little normative data for clinical use. In general, children developing typically produce all of the elements of story grammar by age 10 years. Children's narratives can be used, however, to approximate their functioning level and to determine which structural elements are present. Table 7–32 contains several narratives analyzed by story grammar structural pattern and narrative level.

CHAPTER 7 LANGUAGE SAMPLE ANALYSIS

Table 7–32. Story Grammar Analysis

Narrative	Story Grammar Elements	Structural Pattern	Narrative Level
I.			
We went to a farm.	(S)		
I got to feed chickens.	(S)		
Then I saw cows in the barn.	(S)	Descriptive sequence	Unfocused temporal chain
Cows give milk.	(S)		
Cows stay in the field all day and eat grass.	(S)		
At night they come in.	(S)		
II.			
There was this boy who lived in a city.	(S)		
And one day a giant bug got out of this place where they keep bugs.	(IE)	Reaction sequence	Focused temporal chain
And the boy got in an airplane and shot it.	(A)		
III.			
Once there was two boys.	(S)		
One boy fell into a big hole with rats and he was scared.	(IE_1)		
His brother got a ladder but the rats ate it.	(IR_1)		
So, he threw his lunch in the hole.	(A_1)	Complex episodes	Narrative
The rats ate it, too, and the boy climbed up a rope and was safe.	(DC_1/IE_2) (A_2) (DC_2) (R)		

Note: Although the third narrative possesses advanced structural properties, it demonstrates some pronoun confusion. The relationship of the boys is not established until the third utterance.

Microstructure Analysis

Although much of this information, such as MLU_M, lexical density, and sentence types, was discussed previously, narratives offer different opportunities for exploration of a child's language. Let's discuss some measures appropriate for narratives.

Quantitative Measures

Several quantitative measures, mentioned previously, can be used with narratives. In addition, the longer extended language found in narratives may lend itself to analysis using T- and C-units. Other quantitative measures might include TNW, NDW, total number of T-units (LENGTH), mean length of T-units in words (MLT-W), total number of T-units that contain two or more clauses (COMPLEX), and the proportion of complex T-units (PROCOMPLEX) (Justice et al., 2006; Moore Channell et al., 2018). These values are presented in Table 7–33. Be cautioned that some of these data are from a pilot study, albeit a well-done one, and that there is wide variability among children with TDL, as seen in the standard deviation. Within 1 SD is where the normal population is considered to be.

The Grammaticality and Utterance Length Instrument (Castilla-Earls & Fulcher-Rood, 2018) is a valid tool designed to assess the grammaticality and average utterance length of a child's story retell. The child's prerecorded retell can be analyzed fairly quickly.

Table 7–33. Narrative Microstructure Measures

Age (Years)	TNW M ± SD	NDW M ± SD	Length M ± SD	MLT-W M ± SD	Complex M ± SD	Procomplex M ± SD
Oral narratives						
5	68 ± 47	39 ± 20	8.5 ± 5.4	6.8 ± 1.7	3.1 ± 3.2	0.33 ± 0.2
6	77 ± 54	43 ± 22	9.6 ± 6	7.5 ± 1.6	3.5 ± 2.8	0.37 ± 0.2
7	96 ± 74	52 ± 28	11.3 ± 9.1	8.5 ± 3.8	4.6 ± 4.3	0.38 ± 0.2
8	137 ± 77	69 ± 27	15.8 ± 8.9	8.1 ± 1.4	7.6 ± 5.2	0.45 ± 0.2
9	162 ± 96	79 ± 30	17.3 ± 9.6	8.4 ± 1.4	8.9 ± 6.1	0.51 ± 0.2
10	237 ± 196	101 ± 49	21.5 ± 14.5	8.9 ± 2.1	12.2 ± 9.8	0.55 ± 0.2
Written narratives						
11				9.14 ± 2.2		
14				11.19 ± 3.9		
17				11.27 ± 2.1		

Note: Columns include total number of words (TNW), number of different words (NDW), total number of T-units (Length), mean length of T-units in words (MLT-W), total number of T-units that contain two or more clauses (Complex), and the proportion of complex T-units (Procomplex).

Sources: Information from Justice et al. (2006) and Sun and Nippold (2012).

Moore Channell et al. (2018) offer somewhat different values.

Age (Years)	MLU_M of C-Units	NDW in 50 C-Units
5	6.8	88
10	9.0	107
15	10.6	118

CHAPTER 7 LANGUAGE SAMPLE ANALYSIS

Clausal density (CD) in a narrative task, measured by clauses per utterance, does not seem to have high sensitivity and specificity for children aged 4 to 9 years (Guo et al., 2021). This finding does not support the use of CD for identifying children with language disorders. If we change the measure slightly to CPS, we find that, at least for children aged 3;0 to 7;11 years, CPS demonstrates high sensitivity and specificity when paired with MLU_S (Pavelko & Owens, 2019).

In the narratives of teens, we find that both mean length, as measured in T-units, and CD increases with age. In addition, throughout adolescence, the use of abstract nouns, such as *accomplishment*, *loneliness*, and *mystery*, and metacognitive verbs, such as *assume*, *discover*, and *realize*, in narratives also increases (Sun & Nippold, 2012).

Episodic or episode structure and syntactic accuracy are good measures of language in children from CLD backgrounds (Muñoz et al., 2003). More semantically based quantitative measures, such as the number of different words, seem to vary with the method of elicitation (Uccelli & Páez, 2007).

Expressive Elaboration

Expressive elaboration occurs when the storyteller goes beyond information transmission and creates a pattern of theme, structure, story genre, and mood. The result is an interesting or well-crafted narrative. The skilled narrator selects words and sentence structure to attain the narrator's desired effect on the listener.

Literate Language. Although structural properties are essential for narratives, literate language contributes to development of narratives. **Literate language** contains abstract language features commonly used by teachers and included in the curriculum (Westby, 2005). Features of literate language related to narrative competence include

- metacognitive verbs (*think, know, remember, forget*);
- metalinguistic verbs (*say, talk, tell, ask*); and
- elaborated noun phrases (ENPs) (*the little girl in the car with her mom*).

These features appear in preschool and continue to develop into adulthood and are essential for relating the ordered relationships between events (Curenton & Justice, 2004; Nippold, 2007). Not surprisingly, these literate language features are used less frequently by children with language disorders (Greenhalgh & Strong, 2001).

Literal language features are used in expressive elaboration through appendages, orientation, and evaluation (Ukrainetz et al., 2005). Appendages alert the listener that a story is being told or ended and consist of five categories:

- Introducer or opening elements (*One morning last week . . .*)
- Abstracts, which provide summaries of events prior to the narrative (*This is about what happened when I . . .*)
- Themes, which provide summaries within the narrative (*This is why I'm so grouchy today*)

- Codas, which are general observations that show the effect on the narrator or characters (*So I learned not to run without looking*)
- Enders (*That's all*)

Orientations are setting statements that often consist of ENPs and include

- names (*Jill*);
- relations, which describe roles or jobs (*my teacher*); and
- personality attributes that persist throughout the narrative (*lazy*).

Finally, evaluation describes how the narrative and character perspectives are delivered. Evaluation consists of five categories:

- Modifiers, which consist of descriptive adjectives and adverbs in ENPs
- Expressions, which are multiword modifiers (*tired as a marathon runner*)
- Repetition of nouns, adjectives, or verbs (*walked and walked and walked*) for effect
- Metacognitive internal state words, which reflect thoughts (*remembered*), feelings (*depressed*), reactions (*surprised*), intentions, and physical states (*tired*)
- Metalinguistic dialogue words (*So she said . . .*)

By age 9 years, all children with TDL should exhibit some expressive elaboration in their narratives. Naturally, these vary by type of elaboration, so several narratives are required for a full picture of a child's abilities. Table 7–34 presents narratives with varying types of expressive elaboration.

> ***Food for Thought:*** **Given that by adolescence, written language is often more complex than spoken, might written narratives be of use in assessing literate language features?**

Cohesive Devices. We discussed cohesive devices previously, but in narratives they are especially important. Cohesion is the use of various linguistic means to link utterances together. In narratives, that linking forms a unitary text (Hickmann & Schneider, 2000). To tell an effective story, narrators must use cohesive devices that carry concepts across utterances. In narrative analysis, we're especially interested in

- referential cohesion, which maintains appropriate reference to the characters, objects, and locations;
- conjunctive cohesion, which sustains concepts across phrases and utterances; and
- lexical cohesion, which effectively uses vocabulary to link concepts across utterances.

CHAPTER 7 LANGUAGE SAMPLE ANALYSIS

Table 7–34. Types of Elaboration Found in Narratives by Age 9 Years

Evaluations—Most frequent; increase with age

Modifiers	Adjective, adverbs, and adverbial phrases*	*mighty, angry, shy, slowly, in between*
Expressions	Multiword modifiers	*as quietly as she could, wrong side of the tracks, all of a sudden*
Repetition	Repetition of a word for emphasis	*He ran and ran to get way, They were very, very happy*
Internal states	Words reflect intentions, thoughts, feelings, emotions, motivations, and reactions	*thought, sad, angry, tired, decided, planned*
Dialogue	Portions of narrative in which characters speak	*She shouted, "Stop that!"*

Orientations—Increase with age

Names	Characters identified specifically on first mention	*King Juan, Jack, Monica*
Relations	Relationships of jobs defined	*Monica's sister, teacher, pet*
Personality	Personal attributes that endure throughout the story	*always late, too young to, grumpy old woman*

Appendages—frequent; increase with age

Introducer	Beginning of narrative marked	*Once upon a time, One night, Yesterday*
Abstract	Summary prior to narrative or story title	*This is a story about why you shouldn't run away, This is called "My Best Day"*
Theme	Summary within narrative	*And this is why he was so scared*
Coda	Effect of narrative or lesson learned	*So they decided never to ride their bikes in the woods again*
Ender	Formal indication narrative is over	*That's it, The end, And they lived happily . . .*

Note: *Some occur so frequently that they should not be noted. These include *some, other, another, one, little, big, bad, on top, outside, behind,* and *after*.

Source: Information from Ukrainetz et al. (2005).

Reverential cohesion across utterances is controlled using noun phrases and pronouns and articles. As the name implies, conjunctive cohesion uses conjunctive words and phrases (*and, but, because, besides, in addition, finally, in contrast*). Lexical cohesion uses word variation to express cohesion, as in "She *grew* vegetables and when they had *grown fully*, she took them to the market to sell."

Children with language disorders and those with poor reading abilities exhibit some difficulty communicating well-organized, coherent narratives. The most common cohesive errors among children with language disorders are an incomplete tie, in which the child references an entity or event not introduced previously, and an ambiguous reference, in which the child does not identify to which of two or more referents they're referring.

Because there is little normative data on the development of these relations, descriptive LSA is the best diagnostic approach. In general, mature story grammar develops prior to mature use of cohesive devices. It is possible, therefore, to have good episodes but poor cohesion. The two are related but not dependent. The cohesion within and between episodes becomes important as children develop complex and interactive episodes. There is a metalinguistic quality about cohesion in that the speaker must pay attention to the text apart from the story itself.

Cohesion analysis describes the linguistic devices used to connect the elements of the text. Inappropriate or inadequate use of cohesive devices results in a disjointed text that is difficult to comprehend. As an SLP, you'll want to identify the linguistic means used to create a cohesive unit. These are clues to the sensitivity of the narrator to the perceived needs of their listener.

Reference. *Reference devices*, which refer to something else in the text for their interpretation, consist of pronouns, definite articles, demonstratives (*this*, *that*), and comparatives (*bigger*). The link with the referent should be clear and unambiguous. Referring expressions are adequate if they are appropriate for the listener's knowledge, shared physical context, and preceding linguistic context (Schneider & Hayward, 2010). Clarity is often a problem when a child changes the story narrator frequently, uses dialogue, or includes several characters.

Within the extended discourse of a narrative, the knowledge state of the listener needs to be constantly monitored. It takes some linguistic skill to bring a listener along as the narrative progresses. Children's ability to introduce and maintain referents in narratives develops gradually during the early school years.

Although children have some inadequate referencing in subsequent mention, preschool and young school-age children have more difficulty with first or initial mention of referents. When kindergartners must choose initial-mention referents based on listener knowledge, they tend to be less adept than older children at doing so. Even young school-age children have some difficulty with initial mention, although after age 9 years or so, in simple stories, children introduce characters similarly to adults. The ability to introduce referents in narratives continues to develop for some time after age 9 years (Schneider, 2008).

Difficulty in subsequent mention seems most related to story complexity. This is because in simple, short narratives, it may only be necessary to refer to characters once or twice after initial mention. Multiple characters, especially of the same gender, can also complicate subsequent reference.

Central nervous system abnormality associated with fetal alcohol spectrum disorder can be noted in the cohesive referencing errors of these children during narration and are a valuable diagnostic and research tool (Thorne & Coggins, 2016). Even when standardized testing fails to identify these children as having a language disorder, the increased demands of narratives find these same children failing to produce age-appropriate narratives (Coggins et al., 2007).

One way to measure cohesive referencing is to focus on a child's ability to establish and manage story elements using referential terms such as nouns and pronouns. Tallying Reference Errors in Narratives (Thorne, 2006) categorizes nouns and pronouns into error reference categories. These might include the following:

- Rate of noun reference errors (NREs) = NRE/total words
- Rate of noun reference errors by opportunity = NRE/opportunity
- Rate of pronoun reference errors (PREs) = PRE/total words
- Rate of pronoun reference errors by opportunity = PRE/opportunity
- Rate of all reference errors = (NRE + PRE)/total words
- Rate of all reference errors by opportunity = (NRE + PRE)/opportunity

A similar system can be adopted for any child exhibiting poor referential skills.

Semantic elaboration can also be used to assess referencing (Thorne et al., 2007). Semantic elaboration is measured by the use of nouns and pronouns to reduce ambiguity in the narrative, the specificity of the nouns and verbs used to introduce an entity (*thing* versus *hammer*) or action (*went* versus *drove*), and noun and verb elaborators (*large angry dog* and *ran quickly*, respectively). The Semantic Elaboration Coding System (Thorne, 2004) offers a convenient way to analyze these data.

Conjunction. Conjunctions link the underlying semantic concepts and thus represent the relationship of these units, which may be expressed by various syntactic units. The way episode parts are linked may reflect a child's underlying episodic organization.

We might expect, therefore, that conjunctive relationships between episodic elements would be more complex and difficult than those between sentences. This association seems to be true for both children with language disorders and those without. This may account for the fewer conjunctions found in the narratives of children with language disorders (Greenhalgh & Strong, 2001).

Lexical Items. Words themselves express relationships by the morphological endings used. The following example demonstrates this relationship:

He *had been writing* for several months. After the book was finally *written*, he celebrated for days. He swore never *to write* another novel.

Categorical relationships can be expressed and demonstrate convergent and divergent organizational patterns. Convergent thought goes from the members to the category, as in "She had petunias, dahlias, roses, and pansies in her garden, but she could never have enough flowers." Divergent thought goes from the category to the members, as in "She liked several kinds of sports but was best at soccer, rugby, and lacrosse."

Finally, words can express relationships that reveal underlying memory storage. In a narrative, the SLP can look for antonyms, synonyms, ordered series, and part–whole or part–part relationships. Ordered series include memorized sequences, such as the days of the week, or hierarchies, such as *instructor, assistant professor, associate professor*, and *full professor*. Part–whole relationships are expressed by entities that form a portion of the whole, as in *rudder–boat*, *pedal–bike*, and *January–year*. Finally, part–part relations contain parts of the same whole, as in *nose–chin*, *finger–thumb*, and *rudder–sail*.

Summary. Assessing children's use of cohesive ties has been attempted in several ways (Schneider & Hayward, 2010). Normative data are difficult to obtain given the influence of story complexity on these measures. In addition, not all cohesive ties are equal in the degree to which they contribute to cohesion, and focusing solely on certain linguistic forms may miss the overall cohesive abilities of a child.

Referential cohesion may be best considered in terms of function rather than particular linguistic forms. Although related, the ability to introduce and maintain referents successfully is different than mastery of individual linguistic forms.

Other researchers have suggested calculating *referential adequacy* (RA) by dividing the number of adequate referring expressions by the total number of referring expressions (Norbury & Bishop, 2003). Although this methodology overlooks different types of cohesion and degrees of inadequacy, RA measures have the advantage of focusing on the function of referring in context.

Unfortunately, for all these reasons, we are still searching for a normed narrative instrument of referential cohesion. The likely reason is the difficulty in specifying the rules for determining adequacy of subsequent mention, which depends on both the length of a story and the number and order of referents mentioned.

It might be more appropriate to focus, at least in part, on initial mention, which is more straightforward than subsequent mention (Schneider & Hayward, 2010). In addition, it's possible with initial mention to restrict analysis to the same set of referents by controlling for the number and type of referents through the use of picture cues, wordless books, and story retells.

Scoring based on the degree of adequacy of the initial mention can also be helpful. A total score for all referents could be divided by the number of referents mentioned initially. If you're interested in such a procedure, refer to the article by Schneider and Hayward (2010), who used this methodology with the Edmonton Narrative Norms Instrument (ENNI; Schneider et al., 2009). The authors were able to describe developmental changes with age and to distinguish between children with TDL and those with language disorders. The ENNI is available free of charge at http://www.rehabmed .ualberta.ca/spa/enni. A similar procedure could be used to establish local norms.

Reliability and Validity

Narrative LSA is not without its detractors. Naturally, reliability and validity will vary with the aspects of narratives measured.

Establishing developmental level by the number of story grammar components present appears to have very high inter- and intrajudge reliability. This developmental level and other quantitative measures, such as words per T-unit and words per clause, also correlate strongly with language test scores, suggesting that narrative LSA has strong construct validity.

One promising narrative assessment tool is the Narrative Scoring Scheme (NSS; Heilmann et al., 2010). NSS rates a range of microstructural and macrostructural narra-

CHAPTER 7 LANGUAGE SAMPLE ANALYSIS

tive skills required for school-age children to effectively tell a narrative. To do this, NSS incorporates multiple aspects of the narrative process into a single scoring system, combining both the basic components of story grammar approaches and higher inter-utterance text-level narrative skills.

The hybrid approach enables the SLP to examine each component of the narrative process while reflecting on a child's overall narrative skill. Each component is rated as proficient, emerging, or minimal/immature and contributes to a score of overall quality.

As an assessment tool, NSS appears to be both an efficient and an informative way to measure development of narrative macrostructure. NSS is significantly correlated with age and with each of the microstructural measures. In addition, there is a unique relationship between vocabulary and narrative macrostructure.

Summary

The near universal use of narratives in conversation suggests their importance in communication. Although there are few normative data on narrative development against which to compare a child's or adolescent's performance, an SLP can use the model described in this chapter as a basis for LSA and description of a child's narrative performance.

In general, the more mature the narrative, the more complete the structure and the story grammar. In addition to causal chains, more mature narratives contain

- greater cohesion to aid the listener in interpretation;
- more structural cohesion proceeding from one event to another in a logical fashion that demonstrates the narrator's attempt to guide the listener;
- more insight into the thoughts and feelings of the central characters; and
- greater use of devices for expressing time and place, leaving fewer extraneous details and loose ends.

An SLP should be cautious when evaluating children from cultures whose narratives do not closely follow the pattern described in this chapter. Narratives are extremely culturally based and will be discussed more in Chapter 8.

Computer-Assisted Language Sample Analysis (CLSA)

We cannot conclude the topic of LSA without considering the use of computers and computer software. Pavelko et al. (2016) reported that 78% of SLPs believe LSA takes too much time. However, few SLPs report taking advantage of formal LSA protocols.

CLSA can automate or shorten many LSA tasks, resulting in faster and more accurate analysis. In addition, a language sample analyzed with the aid of a computer program, such as Systematic Analysis of Language Transcripts (SALT; Miller & Iglesias, 2015), can provide broad information on a child's language abilities. Several language analysis methods are described in detail in Appendix C. I encourage you to read this appendix thoroughly as your introduction to CLSA.

Increasingly, SLPs are turning to CLSA as an aid (Benway et al, 2021; Finestack, Rohwer, et al., 2020). This is not a decision to take lightly, and you should take the time to research different computerized methods, coding requirements, costs, yields, and normative data.

Methods such as SALT (Miller & Iglesias, 2015) and SUGAR (Owens & Pavelko, 2021) were designed for use with computers. Others, such as Developmental Sentence Scoring (DSS; Lee, 1974) and Index of Productive Syntax (IPSyn; Scarborough, 1990), have been adapted to computer analysis. As one of the creators of SUGAR, along with Stacey Pavelko, PhD, I encourage you to investigate all these computer analysis methods and to visit both the SUGAR and SALT websites (http://www.SUGARlanguage.org; https://www.saltsoftware.com).

Adapting LSA from hand scoring to computer scoring can pose challenges (Benway et al., 2021). For example, Computerized Language Analysis (CLAN; MacWhinney, 2000; available at http://dali.talkbank.org/clan/) demonstrates poor reliability between hand and computer scoring on the IPSyn portion (Roberts et al., 2020). Differences can result from the differing formats, such as a computer program's inability to identify structures or errors.

SLPs need to remain current on evidence-based practice and new developments. I predict that researchers and clinicians will adapt procedures to lessen these difficulties.

See the thorough tutorials by Finestack et al. (Finestack, Engman, et al., 2020; Finestack, Rohwer, et al., 2020) and Pezold et al. (2020). Pezold and colleagues outline the differences between CLAN, SALT, and SUGAR. Within the tutorial, they address collecting language samples, analysis, time required, and the results for each program.

We can draw some conclusions from all these studies. First, although CLSA results can provide diagnostic information, they should be used as only one of several pieces of information to determine eligibility or diagnostic status.

Second, CLSA is almost exclusively morphosyntactic in nature. The exception is TTR, introduced on p. 263. Aspects of language that are omitted should be included via other methods in a thorough diagnostic assessment.

Third, CLSA results are largely quantitative (MLU_M, NDW) and don't translate into meaningful treatment goals. For example, increasing MLU is not a meaningful goal in and of itself and occurs as a result of increases in a child's language structure. Hand analysis will still be required. However, CLSA can streamline the process and highlight other areas for additional assessment or analysis.

SUGAR contains a subanalysis format based on age or MLU_S. Other methods include DSS, IPSyn, and Assigning Structural Stage (Miller, 1981). Analyses described previously in this chapter, such as PGU, may also be helpful.

The availability of a wide range of software and hardware technologies increases an SLP's opportunity to use CLSA. In general, the accuracy of computerized analyses is greater than or equal to the accuracy of analyses conducted by hand, and computerized analyses are more time efficient (Long, 2001). In addition, given the sensitivity of CLSA, it can be used efficiently to measure changes over time in response to intervention.

One danger in both testing and CLSA is having the method of testing or analyses dictate or heavily influence identification and intervention. The danger always exists that the method used to assess a child's progress directly affects the goals that an SLP

CHAPTER 7 LANGUAGE SAMPLE ANALYSIS

establishes for a child and the methods they use to achieve those goals. Once again, we must repeat the mantra to use multiple measures of a child's language.

Once mastered, CLSA is more efficient than LSA by hand. Although CLSA may quicken the analysis phase of sampling, it cannot replace the clinical intuition of a trained and experienced SLP. Nor can CLSAs fill the deficiency caused by a poorly collected sample. In a final analysis, only the SLP can use the data generated by LSA to make clinical decisions.

Conclusion

When standardized measures are used to assess a child's language, an SLP is more likely to focus on the discrete skills that are on those measures and to select these skills as goals for intervention. In other words, the very choice of a test can have serious consequences for a child's identification and subsequent intervention.

A language sample is a rich source of information on a child's language and the best example of a child's actual language use in context. LSA may be accomplished at the individual utterance level, across utterances and partners, and by conversational event. LSA should not be attempted until an SLP has a good understanding of the child's language and of the caregivers' concerns. Then a language sample can be collected and analyzed to examine the aspect of language that is a concern.

Utterance-level LSA is most appropriate for language form. Analysis of larger units, such as turns and topics, gives an SLP information on the use of language in context and answers questions about the efficacy of a child's use of language to communicate. A caregiver's style is also of interest if an SLP hopes to employ the caregiver as a language teacher and facilitator.

Although a conversational sample is a rich source of data, LSA is time-consuming. That was Amanda's concern at the opening of this chapter. Therefore, SLPs should focus on areas of suspected difficulty rather than attempt a blanket LSA.

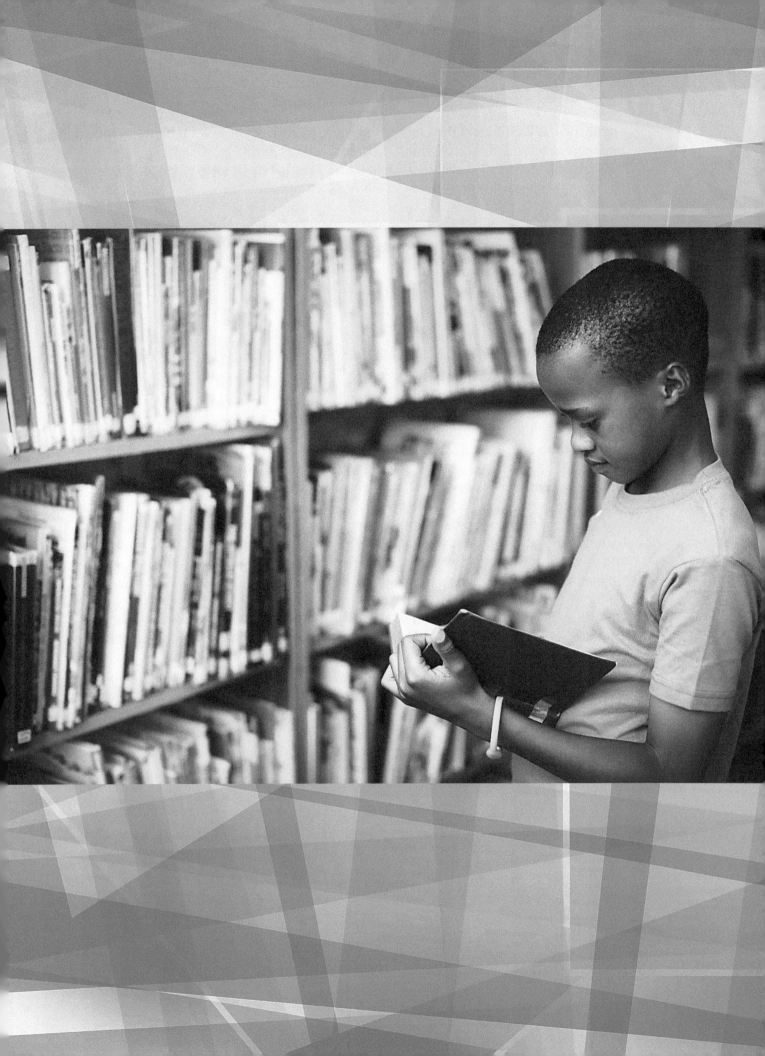

CHAPTER 8

ASSESSMENT OF CHILDREN FROM CULTURALLY AND LINGUISTICALLY DIVERSE BACKGROUNDS

Alejandro's parents came to the United States before he was born. Both parents worked until his mother had to quit because she was pregnant with Alejandro.

Alejandro spoke primarily Spanish when he went to Head Start at age 4 years. English came slowly, but it was sufficiently mature to pass his district's kindergarten screening. In school, he was very challenged by reading and writing and often did both with little comprehension or production of content. Instead of learning to read, he used a combination of memorized word shapes, pictures, or guessing to sound out words.

Multisyllabic words are especially difficult for him, and he confuses words that sound and look similar. Verb endings are also a deficit area. His teacher later learned that Alejandro had difficulty with Spanish as well.

Despite his district's English-only policy, Alejandro's speech-language pathologist (SLP), Ms. Catalina, who is fluent in her native Spanish, has been sending work home with him in Spanish. Otherwise, it would be difficult for his parents to instruct at home. Ms. Catalina has demonstrated how to use book-sharing as a tool for intervention. His parents read to him in Spanish, and he retells the narrative.

For Ms. Catalina, or "Cata" as she prefers, it was somewhat difficult to adapt her Spanish and her cultural expectations. Alejandro's parents speak a rural Guatemalan dialect. Cata was born in Bogota and was in high school when her college-educated parents immigrated to the United States. She went to college at UCLA. Her urban Colombian upbringing differs greatly from that of Alejandro's parents.

Language differences, such as dialects or the influence of a first or heritage language on English, are not disorders. This bears repeating. *Language differences are not disorders.*

Instead, such differences are valid rule-governed linguistic systems in and of themselves. However, children learning non-mainstream American English (NMAE) or learning American English as a second language can also exhibit language disorders, such as developmental language disorder (DLD), learning disability (LD), or any of the others discussed in Chapters 2 and 3. The task for you as an SLP is to separate these natural differences from disorders. Let's discuss the difference–disorder divide, then talk about children exposed to two or more languages, and follow this with a discussion of children speaking NMAE.

First, let me clarify terms. Multilingual children are described using a variety of terms. **English language learner** (ELL) is frequently used to refer to school-age children and **dual language learner** (DLL) to refer to preschool children (Weyer, 2018). The U.S. Department of Education (U.S. DOE, 2016) uses English learner (EL) for all ages. To simplify our discussion, we use ELL throughout this chapter.

Difference or Disorder?

Language differences are common and expected in the course of learning another language. There are differences in language form, content, and use. These differences can result in a child being misidentified as having a language disorder or having their language disorder thought to represent simply a language difference.

Just as with monolingual majority dialect American English-speaking (MAE) children, language disorder can affect the communication of second-language learners and NMAE speakers as well. Language disorders, because they often represent underlying cognitive processing problems, increase the difficulty inherent in learning another language or the majority dialect.

The rates of misdiagnosis in monolingual and ELL children differ, but underdiagnosis is more frequent than overdiagnosis across both groups (Grimm & Schulz, 2014). Diagnosis is especially challenging with ELLs, suggesting multiple measures should be used.

It is important that you, as an SLP, be able to distinguish between a disorder and difference that may be the result of interaction of the heritage language with English or of a NMAE use. As an SLP, you'll be faced with the dilemma of differentiating language difference based on cultural, linguistic, dialectal, and environmental characteristics from a possible underlying language disorder. This task is made all the more challenging for SLPs by the lack of appropriate assessment tools and methods, especially when an SLP is not proficient or even familiar with the child's heritage language or dialect.

Naturally, we'd expect a child who is an ELL to experience some challenges with English. American English is not an easy language to learn. Compared with peers from a similar cultural, linguistic, and socioeconomic background, however, an ELL with language disorder demonstrates several different behaviors that we'll mention later.

According to the Individuals with Disabilities Education Act (IDEA, 2006, Part B), assessment of children with special needs must yield accurate information on a child's

CHAPTER 8 ASSESSMENT OF CHILDREN FROM CULTURALLY & LINGUISTICALLY DIVERSE BACKGROUNDS **307**

functional, academic, and developmental knowledge. In addition, the assessment cannot be discriminatory based on language or culture (Dragoo, 2017).

For an SLP, the main goal in an assessment of a child who is an ELL is to determine if concerns about their English are related to

- being a multilingual language learner; and/or
- having a language disorder that underlies and influences all languages used by the child (American Speech-Language-Hearing Association [ASHA], 2004; Paul et al., 2018).

The results can impact a child's educational placement, future academic achievement, and participation in society (International Expert Panel on Multilingual Children's Speech, 2012; Johnson et al., 2010).

Language profiles of NMAE speakers and those with language disorders are not the same. In general, language disorder results in a more restricted range of language variation than does dialect (Oetting, 2019).

ELLs and children with dialectal differences are more likely to be identified as in need of special education services (de Valenzuela et al., 2006). In general, these children are overrepresented as having language disorder, whereas majority dialectal English-only speaking students are underrepresented.

Typically, SLPs make two common errors in evaluating the language of children with culturally linguistically diverse (CLD) backgrounds. Either children are identified incorrectly as having a language disorder, or those with a disorder are missed. For example, African American children from rural Alabama who speak the African American English dialect common to that area continue to delete final consonants beyond the age at which European American children do so. An SLP who is unaware of this difference might conclude, incorrectly, that these children exhibit a disorder.

The higher proportion of ELLs and children with dialectal differences in special education is most likely related to performance on standardized tests. ELLs score lower than monolingual children on tests administered only in English (Bialystok et al., 2010). Compared to monolingual children's performance on standardized language tests, however, ELLs perform below average, even in their heritage language.

State of Service Delivery

Although the demographics of the United States are changing, the overwhelming majority of SLPs will continue to belong to the majority culture for the foreseeable future. Approximately one in three SLPs has some bilingual clients, but more than 80% of these professionals do not feel confident in their abilities to serve these clients. It's estimated that only 6.5% of certified members of ASHA self-identify as providing services in languages other than English (ASHA, 2021). Inadequacies include a lack of academic preparation and unfamiliarity with different languages and/or cultures and a lack of appropriate assessment tools. Let's discuss these briefly.

Lack of Academic Preparation

Most academic programs offer little preparation for working with children from CLD backgrounds through either coursework or practicum. Until this deficiency changes, it is the responsibility of SLPs to educate themselves through online and in-person continuing education offered by ASHA and state and local professional organizations. Some colleges and universities, such as Columbia University, offer certification programs in working with CLD populations.

Unfamiliarity With Different Languages and Cultures

All aspects of our lives are overlaid by culture, a shared framework of meanings within which a population shapes its way of life. Thus, culture is what one needs to know or believe to function acceptably in a particular group.

Culture has been shaped by a population's history and evolves as individuals constantly rework it and add new ideas and behaviors. As such, culture includes, but is not limited to, history and the explanation of natural phenomena; societal roles; rules for interactions, decorum, and discipline; family structure; education; religious beliefs; standards of health, illness, hygiene, appearance, and dress; diet; perceptions of time and space; definitions of work and play; artistic and musical values, life expectations, and aspirations; and communication and language use. Culture interacts with language to influence cognitive and affective processes and the interpretation of behavior.

Each culture has a unique outlook. It is essential for you, as an SLP, to recognize that culture is pervasive and diffused throughout each of our lives. Therefore, culture influences our clients but also the way each SLP views other cultures.

SLPs from the majority culture in the United States typically have Euro-centered standards. These standards will influence each SLP's decisions about language disorder, although these standards may not apply within other cultures. For example, Vietnamese culture is much more tolerant of speech and language diversity than is U.S. majority culture. Likewise, the Navajo culture values a quiet, introspective persona, which may seem withdrawn by U.S. majority standards. Language differences affect much more than language form, including rules for appropriate interaction in specific contexts, awareness of content information required in different situations, appropriate structures for participation, and communication styles.

Words and concepts also are related culturally. For example, the word and the concept *crib* are not found in Korean. In contrast, the word is so familiar in the majority, English-speaking culture that one of my own children referred to the Lincoln Memorial with its many columns as "Lincoln's Crib." Table 8–1 offers other examples of cultural variants.

Although SLPs cannot know all cultures, they can become familiar with the cultural backgrounds of the children they serve. In addition, an SLP can become increasingly culture sensitive. It is important to respect other cultures and to recognize that no one culture is the standard. Many traditional notions of the U.S. majority culture are inappropriate in our global environment.

Learning about culture is ongoing and should result in constant reevaluation and revision of ideas and in greater sensitivity. Cultural competence and cultural humility

CHAPTER 8 ASSESSMENT OF CHILDREN FROM CULTURALLY & LINGUISTICALLY DIVERSE BACKGROUNDS

Table 8–1. Cultural Variants That May Influence Assessment

Concept	Other Cultures*	Majority U.S. Culture
Achievement	Cooperation and group spirit. Accept status quo. Manual labor respected.	Emphasis on competition and success. Define self by accomplishments. To the victor go the spoils.
Age	Elders are revered. Growing old is desirable.	Youth is valued.
Communication	Respectful, avoid eye contact, loudness for anger. Silence means boredom. Nonlinguistic and paralinguistic important.	Casual, direct eye contact, loud voice acceptable. Silence means attentiveness. Emphasize verbal.
Control	Fate.	Free will.
Education	Formal for few. Entrance into mainstream society. Elders, peers, and siblings are teachers. Active, physical learning. Spontaneous, intuitive. Testing not integral.	Universal, formal, verbal. Key to social mobility. Teacher is authority. Classroom passivity rewarded. Reflective, analytical. Tests are part of learning.
Family	Extended, kinship important, more varied, elder or parent centered. Male or female dominated.	Nuclear, small, contractual partnership, child centered.
Gender/role	Males independent, pampered. Females have many home responsibilities.	Relative equality.
Individuality	Humility, anonymity, deference to group.	Individual makes own life. Stress self-reliance.
Materialism	Excessive accumulation is bad, status ascribed.	Acquisition, symbol of success and power.
Social interaction	Contact, physical closeness. Kinship more important than friends.	Noncontact, large interpartner distance. Large group of friends desired.
Time	Enjoy the present, can't change future. Little concept of wasting time. Flexible.	Governed by clock and calendar, punctual, value speed, future oriented. Time is money. Scheduled.

Note: *No specific culture.

are not goals to be obtained but, rather, processes in which we can all progress. Cultural competence is the ability to interact effectively with people of different cultures in a way that acknowledges and respects these cultures and to offer clinical services that bridge differences and have a strong positive effect. It means being and interacting without judgment while acknowledging, respecting, and building upon diversity, seeing diversity as a potential strength. Finally, cultural competence is the understanding that equality is not equity.

Equality means all individuals are equal; each group or individual is given the same resources or opportunities. In contrast, **equity** recognizes different circumstances and allocates those resources and opportunities so that all have the potential for an equal outcome.

Cultural humility is other-oriented, an ability to maintain an interpersonal stance that is open to others in relation to aspects of their cultural identity that are most important to them. Such self-humility recognizes its own lack of cultural knowledge and stresses a commitment to collaborative lifelong learning focused on self-evaluation and self-critique. Through cultural humility, we decrease the barriers, differences, and power dynamics that can hinder true collaboration.

From the previous chapters, despite our best efforts, the inescapably subjective nature of the language assessment process should be obvious. You, the child, and the child's family each bring your own cultural assumptions. To make sense of all our behaviors, we must view them against the background of culture.

The following are guidelines for interacting with children and families from different cultures:

- Each dyad, SLP–child or SLP–family member, forms a unique cross-cultural interaction.
- Each encounter is subject to the cultural rules of both participants.
- Children perform differently because of their unique cultural and linguistic backgrounds.
- Different modes, channels, and functions of communication may evidence differing levels of linguistic and communicative performance.
- Cultural norms should be considered when evaluating behavior and making determinations of language disorder.
- Possible sources of conflict in assumptions and norms should be identified prior to an interaction and action taken to prevent them from occurring.

Becoming familiar with another culture and another language requires shedding many preconceived notions and becoming culturally aware. This requirement is followed by education about particular languages and cultures and about language development among children with CLD backgrounds. These can be accomplished by doing the following:

- Taking a foreign language course
- Taking a course in cultural diversity
- Joining local cultural organizations
- Attending cultural festivals and events
- Become a Big Brother or Big Sister
- Volunteering to work with culturally diverse youth, recent immigrants, or community organizations such as Habitat for Humanity

CHAPTER 8 ASSESSMENT OF CHILDREN FROM CULTURALLY & LINGUISTICALLY DIVERSE BACKGROUNDS **311**

- Joining organizations, such as National Coalition Builders Institute, that foster cooperation and understanding
- Joining church groups that foster interactions with religious institutions with different faith traditions
- Going out of your way to introduce yourself to individuals from other cultures
- Reading and traveling

Educating Yourself on Culture and Language Development

Cultural sensitivity and awareness are not enough. As an SLP, you must educate yourself about the dialects, languages, and cultures of the individuals you serve and about the process of dialect and second language learning.

> ***Food for Thought:*** **Did you imagine that you might need to make decisions about disorder and difference? Are they the same thing but disorder is a more severe form of difference? Or are they distinct?**

Cultures. The breadth of cultural diversity is beyond the scope of this text. Suffice it to say that each SLP should become familiar with the cultures of the children they serve. Reading and observation are both essential methods of learning. An SLP must remember that cultures are not monolithic and that there is much heterogeneity, especially in the Latino/Latina American population.

The need for professionals to understand and appreciate the beliefs and values of families with CLD backgrounds is critical. One study found that both parents/caregivers and Head Start staff were unaware of their differing assumptions about education, parenting, child learning, and disability (Hwa-Froelich & Westby, 2003). Of particular importance are differences in childrearing practices, family structure, attitudes toward language disorder and intervention, and communication style. Variants of communication style include nonlinguistic and paralinguistic characteristics, such as eye contact, facial expression, gestures, and intonation; intercommunicant space and the use of silence and laughter; pragmatic aspects, such as roles, politeness and forms of address, interruption rules, turn taking, greeting and salutations, the ordering of conversational events, and appropriate topics; and the use of humor. It is best if an SLP is somewhat cautious at first, until they have a sense of cultural expectations.

Cultures differ in their beliefs about health, disability, and causation. A great deal of discomfort may surround disorder and intervention. Families may be surprised by the extent of their expected role in functional intervention.

It's important, as an SLP, to consider a family's culture background in order to achieve the best child outcomes. Otherwise, recommendations you make may not be appropriate because they do not fit the family's pattern of interacting with young children. According to federal law and ASHA guidelines, intervention for language disorders must be responsive to the cultural and linguistic backgrounds of children and their families

(ASHA, 2008b, 2008c, 2008d, 2017; IDEA, 2004). For example, the Latino/Latina population in the United States is highly diverse. This variability is likely to impact the cultural validity of early language interventions for children and families from these backgrounds (Cycyk & Huerta, 2020).

Sociocultural norms inform a parent's views and approaches with their young children. **Cultural congruency** or the synchrony of intervention strategies and techniques with these norms—with the cultural values, beliefs, and behaviors of the community—is important for providing appropriate services. As discussed in Chapter 4, this is especially true in caregiver-implemented programs common with young children with language disorders. In summary, language interventions that match parents' or caregivers' beliefs, values, and practices will have more successful outcomes than those that do not (García Coll et al., 2002; Griner & Smith, 2006; Larson et al., 2020).

One example, the continuum of cultural orientation from individualism to collectivism, may be illustrative. Simply stated, individualism is oriented toward autonomy and personal success, whereas collectivism is oriented toward interdependence and group success. In childrearing, individualistic cultures tend to prioritize a child's independence and individuality, whereas collectivist cultures prioritize a child's compliance and responsibility to the group. This is not an either–or but, rather, a continuum. Although many parent-implemented programs represent individualistic cultures and foster child independence, many Latino/Latina communities hold more collectivist values (Caldera et al., 2015; Hofstede, 2001; Lynch & Hanson, 2004). In contrast, these communities may emphasize compliance and deference to adults (Guiberson & Ferris, 2019).

Some procedures, such as praising children and teaching pre-academics, may be acceptable to nearly all Latino/Latina parents and caregivers, but there is considerable disagreement beyond these techniques. For example, parents and caregivers may display considerably less acceptance for mothers as the sole intervention agents, homes as the intervention setting, following the child's lead, placing items out of reach to elicit requesting, and using only one language in intervention (Cycyk & Huerta, 2020). Some practices, such as the use of only one language, often English, violate good practice and are not supported by research.

The important message is that as a practitioner, you must truly collaborate with parents and caregivers, and you must research the communities you serve. Collaboration requires solicitation of ideas for goals and techniques and obtaining parental approval before implementation.

Second Language Learning. Children in the United States who are bilingual Spanish–English or who use Spanish only may perform very differently even from each other. These differences may reflect U.S. regional differences, country of origin, or dialectal or socioeconomic differences.

In general, second language learning is more difficult than first-language learning, which for most children is fairly effortless. A language assessment must distinguish between those errors that reflect this difficulty and those that represent a language disorder.

In sequential bilingual learning, the heritage language (L_1) reaches a certain level of maturity before acquisition of English, the second language (L_2), begins. Sequential learning may maximize the interference between the two languages. **Interference** is the influence of one language on the learning of another. For example, the English /p/ is difficult for Arabic speakers but not for Spanish speakers. Children who learn L_1 at home and are exposed to L_2 (English) in school usually move toward L_2 or English dominance in middle school, but the transition occurs earlier in comprehension than in production, suggesting interference in production (Kohnert & Bates, 2002).

The monolingual model of development is inappropriate when describing second language learning. Likewise, rate of learning is a poor index because of the many variables that affect second language learning.

Preschool children, because of their age, will have an immature L_1 when introduced to English. The result may be that a child fails to reach proficiency in either language. A child may be delayed in development of L_1 after exposure to L_2 if the second language is dominant in the culture. Although extremely important, this factor is rarely considered in language assessments. In general, competence in L_2 is related to the maturity of L_1. The more mature a child's use of L_1, the easier it is to learn L_2.

Initially, a child in preschool may be silent for a while after exposure to L_2 and appear to have a language disorder. It takes time for a child to decipher the new linguistic code. Although learning a second language is easier for younger children, older children possess metalinguistic skills that aid in this deciphering process.

School-age children exposed to L_2 may appear to have LD. The decontextualized language of the classroom may be especially difficult. If exposure to L_2 does not occur until after age 6 years, it may take 5 to 7 years to acquire age-appropriate cognitive and academic skills. The result is that in the United States, many children never fully develop L_1—often Spanish—and are deficient in academic use of English (L_2). L_1 may exhibit arrested development or be lost if it is not used, is not valued by the child, is discouraged by the parents and caregivers, or is considered less prestigious. As a preschooler, my godson refused to learn Spanish despite the family's daily use of Spanish in the home.

Factors that affect L_2 competency are individual characteristics, such as intelligence; learning style; positive attitude about one's self, one's own native language, and the target language; an extrovert personality and a feeling of control; a lack of anxiety about L_2 learning; and home and community characteristics, such as parental and community attitudes and the level of literacy in the home. Low socioeconomic status (SES) alone is not a negative factor but may be when paired with poor literacy or poor L_1 use in the home and/or little opportunity to converse one-on-one with mature L_2 users.

In general, the heritage language forms a foundation for the learning of L_2. What a child knows from one language is transferred to the other. This may be general knowledge about sentence construction and parts of speech or similar language processes if the languages are similar. For example, you know from your language development course that the progressive -*ing* verb ending is relatively easy to learn. It's similar to and consistent with the -*ando* verb ending in Spanish. It's reasonable to expect, therefore, that the progressive -*ing* would be easy for a Spanish-speaking child to learn. We might wonder if a child has a language disorder when they struggle with -*ing*.

Of course, interference also can occur, but its effects are usually minimal. A poor base in L_1 usually leads to difficulties in L_2.

Dialects and Language Learning. All language users are dialect users. We all speak and, to a lesser degree, we all write in a dialect of American English. Most dialects are close enough to the majority dialect or they may be the majority dialect of the area in which we live so that we are not disadvantaged by being a dialectal speaker. This is not true for everyone.

It is not possible to learn all of the dialects or languages one might encounter, especially in large metropolitan areas. Therefore, each SLP should attempt to learn the contrastive influences of other languages and dialects of children they serve. Common phonological, syntactic, and morphological contrasts are found in Appendix E. SLPs can also learn high-usage words and forms of greeting used in these language and dialect communities. Let's explore children using African American English (AAE) as an example of how dialects develop. We'll bring in other dialects and variations of AAE later.

Earlier language research in AAE focused not on the typical language development patterns of children speaking AAE but on how their development differed from those learning MAE. More recently, there has been a recognition of cultural and linguistic diversity and a shift in the study of child language acquisition from a deficit to a difference perspective (Stockman, 2007). This shift was aided by empirical evidence legitimized AAE as a linguistic system.

Not all children with different dialects of American English are the same. Each child's language will differ with the specific dialect spoken and the maturity of a child's language and dialect development. Although data are limited, we know that children learning AAE show only minimal evidences of their dialect by age 3 years. By age 5 years, however, most African American English forms are being used, at least in part.

Findings in the speaking and writing of third- and eighth-grade speakers of AAE suggest that during this period, speakers of AAE learn to dialect switch in their writing (Ivy & Masterson, 2011). Although third graders have comparable use of AAE in both spoken and written modalities, a difference in use between the modalities is found by eighth grade. In general, eighth graders use more AAE dialectal features in speaking than writing.

Although awareness of AAE appears to increase slowly throughout elementary school, actual production in speech gradually shifts to more MAE use (Isaacs, 1996). Interestingly, speaking NMAE does not seem to influence the ability to comprehend the majority dialect.

The challenge of accurate assessment is complicated by the large numbers of African American children with low-SES backgrounds. Low SES limits access to adequate health care and nutrition, early schooling, and other resources that can maximize developmental potential. As a result, children with low-SES backgrounds may be more prone to developmental delays than the general population.

One subgroup of families with low-SES backgrounds is those who are homeless. According to the U.S. Department of Housing and Urban Development (2021), 580,466 people experienced homelessness in the United States on a single night in 2020, an increase of 12,751 people, or 2.2%, from 2019. Approximately 30% to 40% of these are families with children. Nearly three-fourths of these families are headed by a single parent, usually a mother (Lowe et al., 2002; Weinreb et al., 2006). In addition to parental stressors, preschool children who are homeless are at risk for a combination of language, learning, or cognitive delays that later negatively impact school achievement (O'Neil-Pirozzi, 2003).

In general, AAE-speaking children reared in low-SES environments tend to use MAE morphological markers, such as past tense *-ed* (*walked*, *jumped*) and passive particle (*eaten*, *chased*), less frequently than African American children with mid-SES backgrounds (Pruitt et al., 2011). The weakness in morphological marking is related to the general vocabulary weakness of these children and may reflect their relatively impoverished language environment as a result of low SES.

Importantly, although children who speak AAE use morphological markers variably, none of their performance suggests language disorder (Pruitt & Oetting, 2009). In fact, their performance is distinctly different from that of children with language disorders.

Lack of Appropriate Assessment Tools

An SLP can expect the formal test performance of children with CLD backgrounds to be affected by cultural differences. Negative attitudes by the listener or tester also can affect children, causing poor performance. The result is lower expectations and inappropriate referral or classification.

Few nonbiased standardized language tests are available for evaluating children with CLD backgrounds. Tests are typically unique to one culture or language. Spanish versions of most tests fail to consider dialectal differences and are normed on monolingual Spanish-speaking children rather than on ELLs (Gutiérrez-Clellen & Simon-Cereijido, 2007). In two judicial decisions regarding placement of Mexican American and African American children in classes for children with intellectual developmental disorder (*Diana v. State Board of Education*, 1970; *Larry P. v. Riles*, 1979), the courts ruled that judgments made on the basis of responses to tests whose norming populations are inappropriate for these children are discriminatory.

Many of the English-based tests widely used by SLPs are normed on population samples with a disproportionately high number of monolingual English-only European American children with mid-SES backgrounds. Tests may yield lower scores for groups with low-SES backgrounds and for African American children. In addition, some test items may be culturally biased.

A critical need exists for nonbiased language measures for children of color, especially those from low-SES backgrounds. Having said all this, when we survey SLPs, we find that most use formal, standardized English tests to assess ELLs (Caesar & Kohler, 2007).

In general, poor performance leads to lower expectations. It is inappropriate to compare many ELLs to native speakers of English. The use of chronological norms is especially questionable, given the great variety in developmental rate among CLD populations. The child with limited English does not have language similar to an age-matched native speaker of English.

Clearly, there is a critical need to develop assessment measures appropriate for these children. Assessment in only one language underrates ELLs' overall language ability. Assessment and intervention with ELLs should be conducted in the native language as mandated by federal law (PL 94–142 and PL 95–561), legal decisions (*Diana v. Board of Education*, 1970; *Lau v. Nichols*, 1974; and *Larry P. v. Riles*, 1979), and state educational regulations.

Two promising tools for identifying language impairment in U.S. Spanish–English ELLs are the Bilingual English Spanish Assessment (BESA; Peña et al., 2018) and the Bilingual English Spanish Oral Screener (BESOS-2; Peña et al., 2015). Although ELLs score significantly lower than their functional monolingual peers, they are no more likely to fall in the at-risk range (Peña et al., 2011). In addition, the BESA sentence repetition task has strong internal validity that supports its use in clinical practice (Fitton et al., 2019).

Summary

SLPs must appreciate the rule-governed nature of native languages and dialects and know their contrastive features. It's also important for an SLP to remember that the use of an NMAE or use of a dialect of English influenced by a heritage language are not disorders.

Adequate service delivery by an SLP may require native or near-native fluency in both languages and the ability to describe speech and language acquisition in both languages, to administer and interpret formal and informal assessment procedures, to apply intervention strategies in both languages, and to recognize cultural factors that affect service delivery to a CLD community.

However, a language assessment should establish language dominance and the most appropriate language for intervention. One error often made by inexperienced SLPs is to assume that the heritage L_1 is dominant. My advice to you is that if you still have time in your college career to improve your use of another language, do so.

> ***Food for Thought:*** **Feeling somewhat abandoned? No tests. Imagine the challenge for an SLP who has just a few children whose heritage languages range from Karen to Pashto.**

Language Assessment of a Child Who Is an ELL

Languages other than English are devalued in the United States. This is the result of racial and ethnic discrimination and has resulted in a bilingual educational policy that sends a very clear message on the relative value of English.

It is important that an SLP understand the process of sequential bilingual acquisition. This is a dynamic process in which a child's language system is changing. Performance may vary widely within and across ELL children. Therefore, language assessments need to be tailored individually to each child.

In this section, we'll try to weave our way through current best practices in the assessment and treatment of children who are ELLs. I suggest that you read the excellent article on this topic by Pieretti and Roseberry-McKibbin (2016) in the *Communication Disorders Quarterly* that inspired much of this section of the text.

CHAPTER 8 ASSESSMENT OF CHILDREN FROM CULTURALLY & LINGUISTICALLY DIVERSE BACKGROUNDS **317**

A comprehensive assessment can reduce the potential misdiagnosis of language disorders in children who are ELL (Dragoo, 2017; Lewis et al., 2010; Peña & Halle, 2011; U.S. DOE, 2016; U.S. DOE, Office of English Language Acquisition [OELA], 2016). One of the primary difficulties you as an SLP will face is the paucity of appropriate assessment tools (Washington et al., 2019).

A thorough unbiased assessment might use a comprehensive biopsychosocial framework that considers not only a child's language abilities but also the child's developmental context. The World Health Organization's *International Classification of Functioning, Disability and Health–Children and Youth* (ICF-CY) enables SLPs to specifically address factors unique to each multilingual child. A comprehensive and holistic framework, the ICF-CY helps identify health conditions and related contextual factors that impact language functioning (ASHA, 2016; Threats, 2013; Washington, 2007). In addition, the ICF-CY provides a framework for functional intervention by examining language use in the context of a child's daily environment (ASHA, 2016; McLeod & Threats, 2008; Westby, 2007; Westby & Washington, 2017).

The ICF-CY has two parts:

- Functioning and Disability, including "Body Functions and Structures" or anatomy and physiology and "Activities and Participation" or a child's involvement in life situations
- Contextual Factors, including
  - Environmental Factors—the physical, social, and attitudinal environment
  - Personal Factors—background such as age, gender, and developmental history

Thus, a child's disorder is considered a dynamic interaction between health conditions and contextual factors. Although an exhaustive explanation of the ICF-YC is beyond the scope of this text, I encourage you to read the fine study of communication assessment tools and the ICF-TC by Wright Karem and colleagues (2019).

Who Are ELLs?

Although the most recent census data were not available at the time of writing, the U.S. Bureau of the Census (2011) had previously identified 207 different ancestral groups represented in the United States. In addition, more than 55 million people, 20% of the population older than age 5 years, spoke a language other than English at home (U.S. Bureau of the Census, 2011).

Currently, ELLs account for approximately 10.2% of the students enrolled in U.S. public schools, rising to 15.7%, 16.4%, and 22.1% in Texas, Nevada, and California, respectively (National Clearinghouse for English Language Acquisition, 2018). In Head Start programs for preschoolers, the percentage of preschool-age children who use a language other than English is approximately 30% (Office of Head Start, 2016). It's predicted that by 2025, 25% of all school-age children nationwide will be ELLs (Silverman & Doyle, 2013).

There is a strong link between language experience and language development in young children. Compared to monolinguals who receive concentrated input in one language, children simultaneously exposed to two or more languages receive less input and have less practice using each language and may be at increased risk for language delay (Kohnert, 2008; Kohnert et al., 2005; Paradis, 2007). On the other hand, possible developmental benefits may accrue from dual language use. Switching between two languages may possibly confer developmental advantages on some ELLs (Bialystok et al., 2008).

Most children in the United States who are exposed to two or more languages will do so sequentially, learning their heritage language or L_1 at home and subsequently learning English or L_2 in preschool or school. For these ELLs, accurate assessment of language skills is crucial to educational success (Bedore & Peña, 2008; U.S. DOE, OELA, 2021).

In the United States, a shift in language proficiency from the heritage language to English during the school years occurs regardless of whether the child receives an English-only or bilingual education (Castilla-Earls et al., 2019). In general, using percentage of grammatical utterances (PGU) as a measure, we find that initially PGU is higher in Spanish and lower in English. PGU in English improves over time, whereas PGU in Spanish declines in both instructional models mentioned previously. Improvement in English is steady with a small difference in the rate of growth among children in different programs.

The most common heritage languages among school-age children who are ELLs are Spanish, Chinese, Arabic, Vietnamese, Haitian Creole, Somali, Tagalog, Hmong, Portuguese, and Russian. Spanish-speaking ELLs are concentrated in a dozen states, with five—California, Texas, Florida, New York, and Illinois—having the highest numbers (National Clearinghouse for English Language Acquisition, 2018).

In the United States, the most important predictors of any child's academic success are race and SES. Unfortunately, many children who are ELLs also have low-SES backgrounds (Hammer, 2012). In addition, many individual children may have had no preschool experience as a bridge to school (Lopez, 2012). Thus, a child who is a second-language learner and speaks little English, is from a different culture, is poor, and has had no formal school preparation is likely to struggle in school.

English language proficiency is highly correlated with academic success. Although many children who are ELLs are academically successful and although being bi- or trilingual has linguistic, cognitive, social, and, later, employment benefits, many of these children have academic difficulty.

The problem is exacerbated by the paucity if bilingual classrooms in the United States. Most classes in American public schools are taught in English only, with few, if any, supports for students who are ELLs. Because they struggle with English as well as cultural differences, children who are ELLs are overrepresented in special education and on the caseloads of SLPs (Pieretti, 2011; Riquelme & Rosas, 2014; Wyatt, 2012).

It takes more than 3 years for children who are ELLs to approach the language norms of monolingual English speakers. Several factors affect second language learning, including a child's age, the heritage language, a child's aptitude for language learning, length of exposure to English in school, maternal education, and richness of the English environment outside school (Paradis, 2016). As might be expected, children with DLD who are also ELLs acquire English more slowly than peers with typically developing language (TDL).

Importance of Accurate Assessment

Among Latino/Latina American preschoolers with DLD, the child's Spanish language skills, level of English vocabulary development, and level of English are all important predictors of English acquisition (Gutiérrez-Clellen et al., 2012). In short, the better the child's skills in Spanish and the higher English vocabulary development and English use, the more likely a child with DLD is to develop English. It's easy to see from these data why accurate assessment is so important and the reason SLPs are required to deliver appropriate services to multilingual children (ASHA, 2004, 2017; Davison & Qi, 2017).

Any assessment of children with CLD backgrounds must recognize the relationship between the risk for language impairment and SES. For example, children in the United States who speak Spanish as their first or heritage language (L_1) are more likely to come from low-SES backgrounds (Krashen & Brown, 2005). SES and maternal education level influence language development in a number of ways. Higher maternal education is associated with better vocabulary development, language comprehension, and narration. In contrast, children from low-SES backgrounds with poorer maternal education have an increased incidence of language disorder (Schuele, 2001).

Overcoming Bias in Assessment of ELLs

The challenge in a communication assessment of ELLs is to differentiate difficulties that result from experiential and cultural factors from those that are related to language disorder. Both groups may have some language difficulties. However, ELL adolescents in need of language intervention exhibit greater difficulty expressing themselves, establishing greetings and opening and maintaining a conversation, listening to a speaker, and cueing a listener to a topic change.

Use of Interpreters

The accuracy of testing with ELLs may be increased by using interpreters who speak the child's heritage language. When an interpreter is not available, family members can aid the SLP.

All children perform significantly better with familiar examiners. This finding suggests the use of interpreters familiar with both the language and the culture of a child and their caregivers.

An SLP must recognize the limitations of the process and must select and train the interpreter carefully. They must work together as a team with mutual respect. Three factors seem critical in the use of interpreters: selection, training, and relationship to the family and community. Let's discuss these further.

Selection. Selection should be based on a potential interpreter's linguistic competencies, ethical and professional competencies, and general knowledge and personality. An interpreter should possess a high degree of proficiency in both the heritage language and English; be able to paraphrase well; be flexible; and have a working knowledge of developmental, educational, and communication terminology.

Ethical and professional competencies should include an ability to maintain confidentiality, a respect for the feelings and beliefs of others and for the roles of professionals, and an ability to maintain impartiality. Confidentiality is especially important if the interpreter is a resident of the immediate geographic area served.

Finally, it is very desirable for the potential interpreter to have a knowledge of child development and educational procedures. Personal attributes include flexibility, trustworthiness, patience, an eye for detail, and a good memory.

Training. Training must include the critical factors of assessment and intervention, including procedures and instruments. The interpreter must understand the importance of exact translation from L_1 to L_2 and the reverse.

Pre-assessment training must include the elements of a thorough assessment and the methods of specific test protocols, including technical language. Rapport-building strategies and questioning techniques also should be taught.

Prior to each evaluation of a child's language, the SLP and the interpreter should review each case and the assessment procedures; practice pronunciation of the child and family names, introductions, questioning, and nonlinguistic aspects of the interaction; and discuss the topics to be introduced. During the evaluation, the interpreter can interact with the child and caregiver(s) while the SLP records the data and directs the process. In the post-assessment interview with caregivers, the interpreter conveys the results of the evaluation as they are reported by the SLP.

Relationship With Family and Community. Prior to the assessment, the interpreter should try to get to know the caregiver(s) and child. It is very important that the interpreter convey the confidentiality of the proceedings, especially if the interpreter is from the community. During the assessment, the interpreter is to translate exactly. The SLP can aid this process by keeping interactional language simple and use of professional jargon to a minimum. It is the interpreter's responsibility to ensure that the caregivers thoroughly understand the process and the results and recommendations.

Summary. Working through interpreters can be difficult and does not address some of the other problems in assessment of ELLs. The following list contains suggestions for working successfully with an interpreter. The SLP should do the following:

- Meet regularly and keep communication open and the goals understood.
- Have the interpreter meet with the child and caregiver(s) prior to an interview to establish rapport and to determine their educational level, attitudes, and feelings.
- Learn proper protocols and forms of address in the native language.
- Introduce themselves to the family, describe roles, and explain the purpose and process of the assessment.
- Speak more slowly and in short units, but not more loudly.
- Avoid colloquialisms, abstractions, idiomatic expressions, metaphors, slang, and professional jargon.

CHAPTER 8 ASSESSMENT OF CHILDREN FROM CULTURALLY & LINGUISTICALLY DIVERSE BACKGROUNDS 321

- Look directly at the child and caregiver(s), not at the interpreter. Address remarks to the caregiver(s).
- Listen to the child and caregivers to glean nonlinguistic and paralinguistic information. What is not said may be as important as what is said.
- Avoid body language or gestures that may be misunderstood.
- Use a positive tone that conveys respect and interest.
- Avoid oversimplification and condescension.
- Give simple clear instructions and periodically check the family's and child's understanding.
- Instruct the interpreter to translate the client's words without paraphrasing.
- Instruct the interpreter to avoid inserting their own words or ideas in the translation or omitting information.
- Be patient with the longer process inherent in translation.

Although these suggestions will not ensure success, they may lessen some friction that potentially could disrupt effective delivery of services.

Testing in Both Languages

Grammatical ability of ELL preschoolers seems to be related to lexical or vocabulary variables in the same language. For example, among preschool Spanish–English ELLs, lexical–semantic knowledge in one language has an impact on the grammatical skills in that language (Simon-Cereijido & Méndez, 2018). Interestingly, there does not seem to be a relation between vocabulary and grammar skills across languages. These data would lend support to testing in both languages.

Testing in both English and Spanish is difficult for many monolingual English-speaking SLPs. It has been shown, however, that SLPs can accurately identify language disorder in a Spanish–English ELL once the child uses English at least 40% of the time (Bedore et al., 2018). For children using a lower percentage of English or speaking a different heritage language, more research is needed into how to positively identify language disorder.

Summary

None of the ideas for decreasing bias is as important as a thorough language assessment that actively explores a child's language and communication system. As I've stressed in the past several chapters, a thorough language assessment has many components and requires planning and consultation.

> ***Food for Thought:*** **Although I have no doubt that you will assess a child in as nonbiased a way as possible, will you be able to say the same for the methods you used? Do testing measures seem adequate?**

An Integrated Model for Assessment for ELLs

In an assessment, language may be treated as an autonomous cognitive ability divided into many components. In this approach, language is not viewed as holistic.

It's more appropriate to use an integrated approach for all children, especially those with CLD backgrounds. Such a model of assessment uses the child's natural environment and depends on descriptive analysis rather than on normative test scores. An SLP focuses on the functional aspects of language and on flexibility of use.

The overall question would be: "Is this child an effective communicator in their communication environment?" It follows then that the criterion would not be norm referenced but, rather, communication success referenced. Data could be collected in natural settings as the child converses with their natural conversational partners, parents, caregivers, teachers, and peers.

It's critical that an SLP recognize language diversity. Among Spanish–English ELL preschoolers, diversity is related to several factors, including home and classroom environments and experiences. This difference underscores the importance of a thorough evaluation, including highlighting a child's relative strengths in both languages and considering the best intervention approach to support the child (Halpin et al., 2021). Such an approach also supports the notion throughout this book that language assessment and intervention is not "one-size-fits-all."

Components

When we're assessing the language of children who are ELLs, our most powerful weapon is information (Riquelme & Rosas, 2014). The more data an SLP collects from multiple sources, the more likely it will be that the diagnosis is accurate. The models for gaining that information with children for whom English is not their heritage language vary naturally but follow a systematic process not unlike what we've discussed previously in this text. For example, Pieretti and Roseberry-McKibbin (2016) recommend the following steps:

- Pre-evaluation process, including
  - A comprehensive teacher evaluation of the child's classroom performance
  - A case history collected from the child's parents/caregivers
  - Screening of kindergarten and first-grade students
  - Response to intervention
  - A review of the results of previous language proficiency testing
- Preparation for assessment
- Assessing
  - Formal tests and measures
  - Informal measures
    - Dynamic assessment
    - Language sampling

Pre-Evaluation Process

The evaluation of the child's classroom performance should be as unbiased as possible. Subjective teacher ratings using the Bilingual Language Assessment Battery: Preschool Teacher Report (Pua et al., 2013) have been shown to be an effective method of screening bilingual preschoolers for language difficulty (Pua et al., 2017).

Parent reports are another valid and valuable tool that helps differentiate language difference from language disorder (Goldstein et al., 2010; Grech & McLeod, 2012; Hammer et al., 2012; Kuder, 2013; Simon-Cerejido, 2013). Parental questionnaires have been shown to be highly accurate in identifying ELLs with language disorder (Paradis et al., 2013). In addition to being asked to describe and to compare a child's language to that of other children in the school, neighborhood, and family, informants can also be asked about behaviors that may indicate language disorder.

As mentioned throughout this text, respondents will give more valid responses if given a list of behaviors rather than if they are asked a general question about behavior. A comprehensive list of behaviors is presented in Table 8–2 (Pieretti & Roseberry-McKibbin, 2016).

Although we all would agree that a heritage language may influence learning of a second, it's not as simple as this statement implies, Prior to assessing a child's language, it's important to learn the following from parent and teacher interviews (Pieretti & Roseberry-McKibbin, 2016):

- The primary language: Language learned first and used most frequently in the early stages of language learning.
- The proficiency levels: Level of skill in the use of a language. This data is often available through proficiency testing accomplished periodically within the school. Of interest are the level of proficiency and the developmental trend.
- The dominant language: The language spoken most proficiently by the student in different language environments. Language dominance can vary with the task and with the aspect of language being measured.

The Language Exposure Assessment Tool (LEAT) is a valid and reliable cross-linguistic assessment tool for characterizing early language exposure of young children across cultural settings (DeAnda et al., 2016). A computerized interview-style assessment, the LEAT is a format that enables parents and caregivers to estimate dual language exposure of their children.

Parents can be a valuable source of information. Not surprisingly, Spanish-speaking parents and caregivers are as accurate in reporting the expressive vocabulary and grammar of their toddlers as monolingual English-speaking parents and caregivers (Thal et al., 2000). Parental reports of ELLs' vocabulary and word combinations are consistent with sampling findings (Patterson, 2000).

The data collection stage is particularly important for ELLs. Many variables affect second-language development and are of interest. In addition, seemingly simple information such as age—Is the child age 1 at birth or a year later?—is culturally dependent and can greatly affect determinations of impairment.

Table 8–2. Characteristics of Children With Language Disorders Who Are ELLs

Compared to children with TDL who are ELLs, those with language disorder have . . .

- Slower development than siblings or peers raised in a similar cultural/linguistic environment, including delayed language acquisition in the primary language
- Communication difficulties at home and school
- Need for a more structured academic program of instruction
- Communication difficulties when interacting with peers from a similar background
- Slow academic achievement even when academic English proficiency is adequate
- Information-processing problems, such as poor memory
- Difficulty attending
- Family history of communication disorder, special education, or learning difficulties
- General disorganization and confusion, including a lack of organization, structure, and sequencing in spoken and written language; difficulty conveying thoughts
- Poor sequencing skills, resulting in communication that is disorganized and incoherent, and leaves the listener confused
- Reliance on gestures to communicate
- Inordinate slowness when responding to questions
- Need for frequent repetition and prompts during instruction and communication
- Syntactic problems such as short mean length of utterance and overly simple sentence structure; specific difficulty with morphology in both the primary language and English
- Deficits in vocabulary, including difficulties in the use of precise vocabulary and overuse of empty words such as *stuff*, *things*, and *that*
- Inappropriate social use of language, such as digressing from topic or being insensitive to the needs or communication goals of conversational partners
- Difficulty with narratives

Sources: Hammer and Rodriguez (2012), Kohnert (2013), Paradis et al. (2011), Riquelme and Rosas (2014), Rosa-Lugo et al. (2012), and Roseberry-McKibbin (2014). Edited list compiled by Pieretti and Roseberry-McKibbin (2016).

Considerations for ELLs include the degree of exposure to English-speaking peers, self-esteem, personality (introverted vs. extraverted), motivation to learn English, family attitude toward English, ethnic community's view of education, the SES of the family and of English-speaking peers, and the process of learning a second language. The same child may appear very different depending on the stage of English development.

Maintenance of the heritage language is related to migrant status, such as first or second generation, and to type of early childhood care (Verdon et al. 2014). Although longitudinal analyses demonstrate a decline in heritage language use across early childhood, patterns of loss are varied. Environmental and personal factors include parental language use, the presence of a grandparent in the home, type of early childhood care, first- and second-generation immigrant status, and parental perception of support from the educational environment.

CHAPTER 8 ASSESSMENT OF CHILDREN FROM CULTURALLY & LINGUISTICALLY DIVERSE BACKGROUNDS **325**

Although SLPs routinely screen all kindergarten and first-grade students, monolingual English-language screening tests may be of little value with an ELL child. An experimental version of BESOS (Peña et al., 2015) has been reported to be useful for predicting risk for language disorder in ELLs in first grade. The combined semantics and morphosyntax scores in the best language resulted in predictive sensitivity of 95.2% and predictive specificity of 71.4%, with an overall accuracy of 81% for predicting risk for language disorder.

Response to Intervention. We'll talk more about response to intervention (RTI) in Chapter 12 when we discuss classroom and curricular language intervention. For now, just know that RTI is a classroom-based assessment and intervention approach that occurs within a three-tiered process by providing services and interventions to struggling students through small-group instruction and side-by-side teaching (Long, 2012; McGill-Franzen & Smith, 2013; Roth et al., 2013). In addition, RTI is a method for evaluating in a dynamic manner a student's ability to learn over time when provided with instruction.

The SLP can check with the teacher(s) to find out how the ELL student is responding. The child who is an ELL and has been given extra supportive learning opportunities through RTI but continues to have problems beyond those of his peers most likely will need the SLP to provide language intervention. Later in the assessment, the SLP may try additional teaching strategies to determine if a child can use these to help them learn.

Preparing to Assess

Based on the information so far, an SLP should consider the best, most valid, and most reliable assessment methods and materials. Guidelines from IDEA (2004) and from ASHA (2017) recommend that when feasible, assessment should be in both the child's heritage language or best mode of communication and in English. This will necessitate the use of multiple sources of information and possibly the use of trained translators.

A child's language proficiency in each language may help an SLP determine which language is best to use in an assessment. For many children, testing in both languages will be best. It's likely that a child is still in the process of learning both languages, so use of the combined data from both the heritage language and English can be useful in making clinical decisions (Brice et al., 2010; Hammer & Rodriguez, 2012; Patterson & Pearson, 2012; Peña et al., 2012).

Each child's language skills must be compared to sociolinguistic factors such as the following:

- Age at exposure to each language
- Extent of exposure to each language
- Ability to use each language
- Comparative linguistic structure of the two languages
- Individual child differences (Goldstein, 2006)

Assessment in both languages is especially important for preschool and kindergarten children in order to evaluate development in each (Hammer et al., 2007).

A child's phonological repertoire can be an important determiner of morphological use. It is important, therefore, in an assessment to know the phonological properties of both languages of an ELL child.

Language assessments should occur where a child and their caregivers are most comfortable, such as the home. Parents, especially recent immigrants, may speak little or no English. A properly trained interpreter can be very helpful in obtaining needed information. Occasionally, older siblings have sufficient English skills to answer questions or to translate for their parents or family members. Table 8–3 contains possible questions to be asked in an interview for both ELLs and children with dialectal difference, discussed later.

When possible, the SLP can observe the child in several settings with different activities, partners, and topics. These data will give the SLP an idea of the extent of a child's bilingualism and possible language and communication difficulties. Of additional interest are the child's language use, academic strengths and weaknesses, and learning style.

Assessing

It's very common for SLPs to use formal standardized tests with ELLs to distinguish a language difference from a language disorder (Kimble, 2013; Wyatt, 2012). Unfortunately, although federal law (IDEA, 2004) does not require the use of formal, standardized measures in assessment, many SLPs rely almost entirely on these measures. With most ELLs, informal assessment is more appropriate.

Note that children who are ELLs, whether or not they have a language disorder, have better receptive language than expressive language. Children with language disorder have a significantly larger gap than their ELL peers with TDL (Gibson et al., 2014).

Formal Tests and Measures. Data collection and observation are often followed by testing and language sampling. According to SLPs, the primary problem in assessment of children who are ELLs is the lack of appropriate, nonbiased assessment instruments (Roseberry-McKibbin et al., 2005). However, when standardized formal measures are used, it's important for an SLP to remember that tests are static procedures in which scores may be obtained in one or two testing sessions, thus representing a child's performance at one point in time. In addition, static measures can be affected by environmental factors such as poverty, lack of preschool experience, and lack of familiarity with English.

Test scores should not be taken at face value. For example, the omission of some morphological endings by ELLs is similar to the error pattern of children with DLD, leading to possible misdiagnosis (Paradis, 2005). Although differences do exist, they are often subtle and require great care when examining assessment results. Given Alejandro's difficulty with verb endings, mentioned in the introduction, the SLP will want to probe this aspect of language well in both languages.

When Spanish–English ELL children with TDL and those with language disorders are compared on use of English past tense, different error patterns emerge (Jacobson &

CHAPTER 8 ASSESSMENT OF CHILDREN FROM CULTURALLY & LINGUISTICALLY DIVERSE BACKGROUNDS **327**

Table 8–3. Possible Interview Questions for Children With CLD Backgrounds

Demographic

How long has the family been in the United States?

In which country were the parents/caregivers born? From which country did the family emigrate?

How much contact does the family have with their native country? Is there any plan to return?

*How long has the family been in this community?

Is the family connected to a large community from their native country?

Family and Childrearing

*How old is the child? What is the child's general health?

*Which family members live in the household? Number of siblings? Other individuals?

In what cultural activities does the family participate?

*Who is primarily responsible for the child? *Who else participates in caregiving?

*Approximately how much time do the child and caregiver spend together on a typical day?

*With whom does the child play at home?

*How much education do family members have? In what language?

*Does the child misbehave? How? How is the child disciplined? Who disciplines?

Please describe any media the family use. Are any in the native language? If so, how often does the child watch such shows?

*Are stories read or told to the child? If so, in what language? How often?

*Are there books, magazines, or newspapers in the home? In what language?

*At what age did the child begin school? *Has the child attended school regularly? *How many schools has the child attended? What language was used in the classroom?

*Please describe a typical day for the child.

Attitudes and Perceptions

*Please explain your concern for the child's communication. Is blame assigned? If so, to whom or what?

*How does the family view intervention? Is there a feeling of helplessness?

How does the family view Western medical practices and practitioners?

Who is the primary provider of medical assistance and information?

*From whom does the family seek assistance (organizations and individuals)?

*What are the general feelings of the family when seeking assistance?

*Does one family member act as the family spokesperson when seeking assistance?

*How is the child expected to act toward parents, teachers, or other adults? Adults toward the child? Are there any restrictions or prohibitions, such as the child not making eye contact or not asking questions?

*How important are English language skills? How much English is used at home?

continues

Table 8–3. *continued*

Language and Communication

What language is spoken in the home? Between adults? Between caregivers and the child? Between the children? When playing with neighborhood friends? Other caregivers and the child?

What language is used in community activities, such as church, Scouts, and team sports?

At what age did the child begin to learn English? Where and how?

*At what age did the child say the first word? Use two-word utterances?

Note: *Applicable to children who are ELLs or speak NMAE.

Schwartz, 2005). For example, in addition to scoring lower with regular past tense -*ed* on real and nonsense verbs and with irregular past tense verbs, ELLs with language disorder make significantly more omission errors, whereas ELLs with TDL make overgeneralization errors (*eated, sitted*).

All is not lost. American English standardized tests can be used with modified procedures to enhance a child's performance. Modifications may aid an SLP in describing a child's language and communication skills. Obviously, the scores from such testing would be invalid, although the descriptive information may be invaluable. If reported, the scores must be qualified by a description of the modified procedures.

Some tests have been normed on population samples from different languages, such as children speaking English and Spanish, by using English and a Spanish translation. Results of translated tests must be used very cautiously because they assess structures important for speakers of English and ignore those of the other language. Although development of the possessive -*'s* morpheme (*Mother's keys*) is important in English, the translation (*las llaves **de la madre***) has no equivalent morphological ending.

The standardized norms from such translated tests could be used to identify children with language differences. Children who exhibit language disorders relative to their peer group could be identified by use of the peer group norms. Even this peer procedure may bias results, given the diversity of some populations, such as Latino/Latinas. Norms for all speakers of a language fail to consider dialectal variations. Other variables, such as SES, family grouping, length of time exposed to English, and quality of the heritage language used at home, affect the child's performance.

ELLs are at increased risk of being misclassified for having a language disorder (Grimm & Schulz, 2014; Kraemer & Fabiano-Smith, 2017; Sullivan & Bal, 2013). As might be expected, children who use English more do well on test items such as morphological markers for plural or the third person -*s*. More complex forms, such as question noun–verb inversion (transforming *He is happy* to *he happy?*) and relative clauses (*A girl **who's in my class** is here*), place a higher demand on memory and are more difficult (Bedore et al., 2018).

In semantics, often assessed through single-word vocabulary measures, ELLs with DLD and those with TDL have similar performance if tested in only one language (Anaya et al., 2018; Peña et al., 2015). Language experience, based on current use or age of acquisition, accounts for up to 61.9% of the variance in semantics test scores and 64.4% in morphosyntactic scores in ELLs (Bedore et al., 2012). Variation in language input reduces exposures to words in either languages, resulting in less semantic knowledge than that of monolingual children (Hoff et al., 2012; Peña et al., 2002). Greater exposure in either language is reflected in semantic test score (Sheng et al., 2013).

Data from semantic testing with Spanish–English ELL children with and without DLD indicate that children do significantly better if items are adjusted for the language experience of the child (Jasso et al., 2020). For example, selecting items specifically for children with high Spanish experience improves diagnostic accuracy. These results suggest that SLPs need to refine semantic test items to more accurately represent the continuum of exposure. By doing so, fewer ELLs may be diagnosed as having a language disorder.

The Morphosyntax and Semantics subtests of the Bilingual English–Spanish Assessment (Peña et al., 2018) have a reported sensitivity of 93.3% and a specificity of 86.7% in distinguishing Spanish–English-speaking 4- and 5-year-olds with language disorder and without (Lazewnik et al., 2019). These values are far better than those of the translated/adapted Spanish and/or English versions of standardized assessments. If we combine these subtests with mean length of utterance in words from the child's better language sample (English or Spanish), Lazewnik and colleagues (2019) suggest that confidence in the findings can be above 90%.

Difficulty with Spanish morphology can be a potential indicator of DLD in Spanish-speaking ELLs. Spanish morphological markers with good diagnostic accuracy include both noun and verb markers, especially subjunctive mood, and clitics (Bedore & Leonard, 2001, 2005; Castilla-Earls et al., 2016, 2021). Without going into great detail, subjective mood indicates a speaker's attitude, often in an unreal or imagined state, as in "If I were you . . . " or "It's important that she hold my hand . . . ." Notice that the speaker uses "were" when we are in the present and that the verb *hold* does not have the usual third person *-s* even though it is following *she*. Clitics are unstressed words, often occurring in contractions, such as *-m* in "I'm" or *-ve* in "we've." My examples are in English, of course, and not in Spanish.

The languages used in testing and the manner of their presentation differ with each child and the purpose of the evaluation. It is important to establish the primary language, language dominance, and language proficiency in both languages. Testing in both the heritage language and English seems essential for assessment of disorder. Successive testing in the stronger language, followed by the weaker, results in the best performance, especially for young children with monolingual L_1 homes, although simultaneous testing may be best for children who exhibit poor competence in both languages or who speak a combined L_1 and L_2 language, such as "Spanglish" (Spanish–English) or "Konglish" (Korean–English).

Mode of Administration and Scoring. The mode of administration and scoring can greatly change the reported responses of ELLs on vocabulary assessment. Many vocabulary tests ask children to supply words used to name entities and actions. In a monolingual test, a child with two languages may be at a disadvantage.

The number of correct responses increases as SLPs move from monolingual to bilingual administration and from monolingual scoring to conceptual scoring in which the child is credited for different aspects of meaning (Bedore et al., 2005). For example, in conceptual scoring, although a child may not have the name of something in English, they may be credited for the name in the heritage language. In other words, the child has the concept, as evidenced by the word in Mandarin, but not the English word equivalent.

> ***Food for Thought:*** **There might be two ways to think about testing results. With conceptual scoring, we might get a truer picture of a child's language system(s). But some might say, "It's an English test, so how you do in English should be the criterion."**

If, for example, a Spanish–English-speaking child is shown a picture of a house cat, they might respond with "cat" or "gato" or with both words. That is one aspect of the definition, the entity's name. If the child adds, "It's like *leon* [lion] in jungle," they have added a new aspect to the definition and demonstrated conceptual knowledge. This example is very simplistic. Conceptual knowledge can be assessed using questions such as the following in response to objects and pictures:

Tell me three things about . . .

Describe what an X looks like.

This is Rosa. Tell me what she looks like.

What shape is X?

What do you do with X?

What is the difference between X and Y?

What are they going to do?

If we compare simultaneous and sequential ELLs, both score significantly below monolingual children from similar SES backgrounds on English receptive and expressive vocabulary measures. Conceptual scoring removes some of this difference in receptive vocabulary and increases the proportion of children with vocabulary scores within the average range (Gross et al., 2014). Conceptual scoring doesn't fully ameliorate the inherent bias in single-language standardized vocabulary measures, but it can help in reducing vocabulary deficits that may be used to determine language disorder in ELLs.

Although conceptual scoring, or giving a child credit for correct responses in either language without counting the correct responses twice if present in both languages, can potentially decrease the differences between monolingual and ELLs (Bedore et al., 2005), it's not the only adjustment an SLP can make.

Another aspect of vocabulary development is taxonomic awareness, sensitivity to the hierarchical organization of words. Taxonomic awareness can be assessed by category membership and similarity and dissimilarity measures. As an SLP, you can also be alert for children who may misname an item but give a response that is related taxonomi-

CHAPTER 8 ASSESSMENT OF CHILDREN FROM CULTURALLY & LINGUISTICALLY DIVERSE BACKGROUNDS **331**

cally, as in saying "Gato" (Spanish for *cat*) when the target is *kitten* or saying "Yánsè" (Mandarin for *color*) when the target is *yellow*. Although there is still much research to be accomplished, data indicate that use of conceptual scoring and taxonomic exploration can reduce the test score differences between monolingual English-speaking children and ELLs with heritage languages as different as Spanish and Mandarin (Lam & Sheng, 2016).

The overwhelming majority of studies of language assessment with multilingual preschool children focus on semantic skills (73%), but few measure use and participation (5%). There is a critical need for development and use of evaluative measures that assess all aspects of language, especially pragmatics (Wright Karem et al., 2019).

Informal Assessment Measures. Informal assessment is an ideal measure of the language of ELLs, whether used alone or along with more formal standardized procedures (Grech & McLeod, 2012; Riquelme & Rosas, 2014; Wyatt, 2012). As noted throughout this text, informal measures can be more ecologically valid assessments that consider the environment, home, and culture of the child and family. In addition, informal measures can assess language in real-life contexts (Haynes & Pindzola, 2012). The only real criteria are that these measures be valid and nondiscriminatory and that they be used in an equitable manner. Informal methods may include language and narrative sampling, dynamic assessment, and measurement of information-processing skills (Pieretti & Roseberry-McKibbin, 2016).

Language Sampling. Language sampling in both English and the child's heritage language, collected in familiar contexts with various conversational partners, offers the best opportunity to evaluate a child's language as it is used in everyday situations (Jacobson & Walden, 2013; Paul & Norbury, 2012; Peña et al., 2012; Rosa-Lugo et al., 2012; Wyatt, 2012). Code switching and different language use in different contexts are extremely important information for determining the effectiveness of a child as a communicator.

Sampling should occur in monologue and dialogue situations in both languages. Monologue activities might include static, dynamic, and abstract tasks. Static tasks describe relationships among objects in a context and might include directing others to perform a task or describing entities by location, size, shape, or color. Dynamic tasks describe changes over time as in narration. Finally, abstract tasks might include opinion-expressing tasks, such as stating or justifying a position.

Dialogue situations can include a variety of partners because of the special constraints that each imposes on a child with a CLD background. At least a portion of the sample should include a parent, caregiver, sibling, or peer as a partner. The classroom is especially important because of the academic difficulties these children may encounter.

In each context, different conversational partners can pose communication problems for a child. Change and problem-solving encourage communication and enable an SLP to determine the effectiveness of the child as a communicator. In addition, such situations can offer clues to the learning style of the child. Guidelines for collecting a language sample from children with CLD backgrounds are presented in Table 8–4.

With ELLs, it is important to establish patterns of language use both in L_1 and L_2. Two possible patterns to be mindful of are interlanguage and code switching. **Interlanguage**

LANGUAGE DISORDERS: A FUNCTIONAL APPROACH TO ASSESSMENT AND INTERVENTION IN CHILDREN

Table 8–4. Guidelines for Collecting Language Samples From Children With CLD Backgrounds

Observe the child in various communication contexts, especially low-anxiety, natural communication environments.

Observe the child with speakers of both languages or dialects. Language mixing during collecting may confuse the child.

Record conversations with the child's family for comparison.

Explore with the family the child's communication in the home and community environment.

Use culturally relevant objects to stimulate conversation. Pictures should contain members of the child's racial/ethnic group.

Avoid the tendency to "fill in" for the child's communication gaps. Observe the child's strategies for getting the message through.

Note:

Language uses and purposes. How flexible is the child's system?

Success at communicating. Are certain content and situations more successful?

Communication breakdowns. Where do they occur? With whom?

Strengths and weaknesses. What strategies are used to compensate for weakness?

Anxiety and frustration

---

is an individualistic combination of the L_1 and L_2 rules, plus ad hoc rules from neither or both languages. This "hybrid" language may vary among children and within an individual child across situations. Usually, interlanguages are transitional in nature, but some features may stabilize as a permanent form, especially if there is little motivation to change. Of interest are the rules used by the child and any situational variables.

Linguistic **code switching** is more formal and is the shifting from one language to another within and/or across different utterances. A complicated, rule-governed behavior, code switching does not signal poor or immature language emergence, although it may be used by children when they have inadequate English skills. As with interlanguage, code switching is influenced heavily by contextual and situational variables. For example, the Spanish-speaking storyteller might use English when referring to Anglos and Spanish when referring to Latinos/Latinas. Code switching follows agreed-upon community rules and usually occurs to enhance meaning; emphasize a change of topic; and convey humor, ethnic solidarity, and attitudes toward the listener.

The SLP should note specific uses of interlanguage and code switching in different contexts with various partners. It is especially important to identify patterns that may impede the transmission of meaning or interrupt communication.

Sampling should be based on the realistic demands of a child's communication contexts, such as the classroom. In this setting, a sample should reflect the contextual, performance, and instructional constraints of the situation. A child can then be

CHAPTER 8 ASSESSMENT OF CHILDREN FROM CULTURALLY & LINGUISTICALLY DIVERSE BACKGROUNDS **333**

measured against the minimal competency needed to function within that context. That's a functional assessment.

Ideally, testing and language sample analysis (LSA) complement each other. For Spanish–English ELLs, the synthesis may vary with age and the methods used in sampling. For example, among younger school-age children, ages 5;6 to 8;11 years, positive correlations can be found between the two measures in both languages (Danahy Ebert & Pham, 2017). Among older children, ages 9;0 to 11;2 years, there are fewer correlations. These mixed results may reflect the method of sample elicitation. This study used wordless picture books, which may be inappropriate for older ELLs.

You'll notice as you read further that the factors to consider in LSA with a child who is an ELL are similar to the factors discussed in Chapter 6 for sampling with children who are not ELLs. For example, it's even more important to collect the sample in a variety of familiar contexts or settings with the child engaged in communication with a conversational partner with whom the child feels comfortable (Peña et al., 2012).

As is frequently the case, you as an SLP may not speak the heritage language and yet, as discussed, need to collect and analyze both languages. Now you can appreciate why we need multiple partners to help. If you speak no Mandarin and you are the child's conversational partner when you collect your sample, how will you elicit Mandarin speech?

If possible, a bilingual SLP can be asked to help by collecting and analyzing a sample in the child's heritage language. Although not as ideal, a trained interpreter can also assist.

Most children with language disorders have difficulty with the morphosyntactic or grammatical aspect of language. Children who are ELLs with language disorders are no different, and this challenge should be evident in both languages. English grammatical errors can be expected among those with little exposure to English.

The most frequent morphological errors of ELLs are presented in Table 8–5. Morphological markers often are omitted or overgeneralized. Some Spanish speakers lump English syllables together, decreasing intelligibility. A Cuban American friend calls me "Bobowens." This chunking may cause small units such as morphemes to be deemphasized or omitted.

Examples of grammatical errors common to ELLs with language disorder include the following:

- Difficulties with verb tense morphology in both English and, more important, the primary language. Spanish-, Danish-, and Afrikaans-speaking children with language disorders who are learning English use fewer tense markers than similar children with no language disorder (Christensen & Hansson, 2012; Grinstead et al., 2013; Southwood & van Hout, 2010).
- Less use of the past tense marker in English (Blom & Paradis, 2013). As mentioned in Chapter 6, narratives are a good way to elicit past tense verbs.

Although we still need much more study on language differences and the errors ELL children with language disorders make in both languages, we have enough research and clinical data to demonstrate that an SLP shouldn't diagnose a child as having language disorder based solely on the grammatical errors the child makes in English. As with more

Table 8–5. Most Frequent English Morphological Errors of ELLs

Morpheme	Type of Error	Possible Explanation
Articles	Omission or overgeneralization of *the*	Articles are used infrequently in many languages.
Auxiliaries and modals	Omission	Many languages do not have auxiliary verbs and rely on verb markers.
Contractions	Omission	Unstressed forms often omitted; a phonological error.
Copula	Omission	Unstressed forms often omitted.
Gerund	Omission of *-ing* ending	Many languages do not have this form.
Plural *-s*	Omission or error in agreement, as in *many tree*	Unstressed forms often omitted; used when other languages mark by adjective.
Possessive *-'s*	Omission or overgeneralization	Many languages use the possession of possessor form.
Prepositions	Substitution errors	Very complex system in English; multiple meanings of words.
Pronouns	Substitution errors, noun–pronoun agreement errors	Most languages do not have as many pronouns as English.
Regular past *-ed*	Omission or overgeneralization	Unstressed forms often omitted.
Third-person *-s*	Omission or overgeneralization	Exception to English rule of no person or number markers.

formal testing, language samples should be collected and analyzed in both English and a child's heritage language (Jacobson & Walden, 2013; Paul & Norbury, 2012; Rosa-Lugo et al., 2012; Wyatt, 2012).

Number of errors per T-unit has been found to be a significant value for predominately Spanish-speaking children (Restrepo, 1998). Five- to 7-year-old Spanish-speaking children developing typically made only .09 (SD = .05) errors, whereas those with language disorder made .39 (SD = .21) errors.

Narrative Analysis. Although there do not appear to be any significant differences between ethnic groups in narrative organizational style or use of paralinguistic devices, there are some differences of which SLPs should be aware (Gorman et al., 2011). In the narratives of first and second graders, African American children include more fantasy, Latino/Latina children name the characters more often, and Caucasian children make more references to the nature of character relationships. Although these changes do not significantly change the character of the stories, they give us added insight when soliciting narratives from these children.

The effect of English exposure on Spanish–English-speaking children varies by age of exposure and by language feature. Comparing children with simultaneous Spanish and English exposure from birth to those with Spanish in the home and English exposure in preschool, a longitudinal study reported that although children with preschool exposure had fewer English narrative structures initially, they demonstrated faster rates of growth during the preschool years (Bitetti & Scheffner Hammer, 2021). Although macrostructure features differ in content, each makes a unique contribution to narrative quality. Children such as Alejandro at the beginning of this chapter may have considerable challenges with reading and writing.

In early stages of learning English, ELLs with language disorder have a receptive–expressive gap in narrative comprehension and production (Gibson et al., 2018). Although this gap is present in kindergarten, it seems to dissipate by first grade. Interestingly, the use of single pictures during narrative generation compared to multiple pictures or no pictures during narrative retells seems to minimize the receptive–expressive gap.

ELLs with TDL make more efficient use of English input compared to ELLs with DLD. Thus, English exposure and richness predict narrative abilities for ELL kindergarten children with TDL but not ELLs with DLD. The takeaway is that exposure alone is not enough.

Children from some Spanish-speaking and some Native American cultures may have less experience with story narratives. To varying degrees, these cultures make extensive use of more descriptive narratives. Thus, the use of pictures and elicitation techniques, such as "Tell me a story about this picture," may evoke a very different narrative from what is sought.

ELLs with DLD do more poorly in story grammar ratings than their ELL peers with TDL (Govindarajan & Paradis, 2019). Narrative microstructure components such as grammar are similar. This data suggests that story grammar might differentiate between children with TDL and those with DLD better than microstructure. For example, in storytelling tasks Cantonese–English ELL preschool and kindergarten children use more story grammar elements when speaking in English (Rezzonico et al., 2016).

The narratives of Japanese children may be succinct collections of experiences rather than single detailed sequential events. Children from Latino/Latina cultures often do not relate sequential events. Furthermore, story grammar elements in one language predict elements present in the other.

Narrative retells are relevant tools in predicting performance of ELLs on a standardized English vocabulary assessment. Specifically, the number of different words (NDW) in narratives is related to performance on standardized vocabulary assessments (Wood et al., 2018).

The classification accuracy of LSA is greater in story retelling than in storytelling tasks for 4- and 5-year-old Spanish–English-speaking children. Grammatical errors per communication unit (C-unit) and lexical diversity or the number of different words are the most useful indicators of language abilities in story retelling.

In general, preschool Spanish–English ELLs from socioeconomically disadvantaged backgrounds have lower mean length of utterances in words (MLU_W), total number of words, average hourly vocalizations, and conversational turns compared to their monolingual English-speaking peers (Wood et al., 2016). Interestingly, MLU_W does not seem to be related to either average hourly vocalizations or average hourly conversational turns.

ELL children may use English words in either very restricted or overextended ways. Restricted use may be limited to specific features of a word or to word-for-word transfer in which the word has only the meaning of its L_1 equivalent. In the latter, for example, the English *for*, which is *para* in Spanish and has slightly different syntactic uses, might be used only where *para* would be used.

ELLs may also exhibit confusion with noun phrase element order and pronoun use. For example, bilingual Russian–Hebrew-speaking children with DLD use a smaller set of pronouns but use them to introduce characters in a narrative, thus threatening the referential cohesion or connection (Fichman & Altman, 2019).

Dynamic Assessment. Dynamic assessment (DA) examines a child's capacity to learn rather than assessing the child's knowledge at one point in time as tests do. DA is based on the educational notion of zone of proximal development (Vygotsky, 1978), or the difference between a child's current performance on a task and the amount of guided assistance needed by the child to be successful. Thus, in DA, an SLP is interested not only in a child's performance but also in the best way to facilitate learning and in the child's ability to respond to learning.

The three primary DA methods are "testing the limits," graduated prompting, and test–teach–retest (Gutierrez-Clellan & Peña, 2001). In testing the limits, an SLP probes behind a child's response using elaborative feedback and verbal explanations by a child to determine their understanding of the task and the way in which they arrived at the response. For example, a child may have interpreted the word *buoyancy* as boy-in-seat (Peña, 2002).

Graduated prompting is a method of probing a child's readiness for learning. By subtly manipulating the prompts given to a child, the SLP determines the level of support needed by a child in order to be successful. In essence, the SLP is trying to bridge the gap between what a child knows and the requirements of the task.

The most common method is test–teach–retest (Haynes & Pindzola, 2012; Kuder, 2013; Long, 2012). Succinctly, in the test–teach–retest method, a child is initially tested to determine a level of performance, followed by intervention to teach what a child is lacking, and then the child is retested to determine if they have acquired this newly taught information.

The method of teaching called mediated learning experience (MLE) is an individualized approach to the response and strategies used by a child and includes explaining the importance of the learning and giving evaluative feedback (Peña, 2002). Several types of mediation are possible, including the following:

- Informing a child of the purpose for the interaction and attempting to maintain a child's involvement

- Focusing a child's attention on important features and helping a child understand their importance and relevance

- Bridging concepts and learning beyond the immediate context by relating specifics of the task to other experiences

- Encouraging a strategic, deliberate approach to problem-solving and manipulating a task to help a child be successful

The focus is not simply on what a child learns but also on how a child learns. An example of MLE is presented in Table 8–6. In retesting, or posttesting, children with language disorders usually demonstrate little change, indicating their difficulty learning (Peña et al., 2001).

Several studies have supported the use of DA in determining language differences versus language disorder in children from CLD backgrounds (Hasson et al., 2013; Peña et al., 2006, 2014). The SLP can use a child's ease or difficulty of learning to determine if language disorder is present and to provide some guidance for the direction of intervention.

DA has excellent potential for assessing the language of children from CLD backgrounds. The very open-ended and individualized nature of DA, however, may be a challenge for some SLPs. The lack of definitive methods reflects the individualization necessary in assessment when seeking the best adult mediation for a particular child who may or may not have language disorder. Although an SLP may like DA in the abstract and use it on occasion, without a standard against which to compare children, this same SLP may feel that they can't use DA to make clinical decisions.

The following are of interest to an SLP, relative to peers from similar linguistic, cultural, and SES backgrounds (Pieretti & Roseberry-McKibbin, 2016):

- How much structure and individual attention is needed for the child to acquire new language skills? More prompts, modeling, and repetition than needed by peers could indicate language disorder.

- During instructional activities, how often does the child exhibit off-task behaviors or inappropriate responses?

- Does the child require instructional strategies that differ from those used effectively with peers?

Narrative assessment of school-age Spanish–English ELLs offers a good example of the use of DA. A DA of narrations might consist of collection and analysis, mediated instruction, and a second collection and analysis (Peña, 2002). With school-age children, the SLP first can collect narratives in response to wordless picture books and analyze each for the number of words, C-units, clauses, clauses/C-unit, episodic structure, story components, and story idea and language. Possible wordless picture books include *Bird and His Ring* (Miller, 1999b); *Frog, Where Are You?* (Mayer, 1969); *One Frog Too Many* (Mayer & Mayer, 1975); and *Two Friends* (Miller, 1999a). Other wordless picture books can be found by typing those words into a search engine.

In the second step, the SLP can choose one or two areas of the narrative for an MLE. The SLP helps the child explore the goals of a story, the importance of these goals, the consequences of omitting these goals, plans for using this information, and developing strategies.

Table 8–6. Example of Mediated Learning Experience

Introduction

Today we're going to play with some special toys and use them in special ways. While we're using the toys, we'll think about the actions we do with each and the different names we use. Now, what are we going to be talking about? [Child response]

Um-hm, and why do you think it would be important to be able to name the different actions that we can do? [Child response]

Good, so we can explain our actions to other people. Can you think of anything else? [No response]

Do you ever ask for some help from your mother? [Child response]

And . . . [Child response]

Yes, of course, we can use actions to ask others to help us. Suppose I called your mother and said, "Dad!" [Child response]

You're right, it would be the wrong name. To help people understand us, we call things by their right name. I know that you have a dog. What's his name? [Child response]

Okay, if I called him something else, would he answer? [Child response]

No. So names are important. We call actions by their right name too. I have a whole box full of different objects. Some tell us what we do with them. Here's one your mother uses. It's called an iron. And what do we do with it? [Child response]

Right, we iron, we iron clothes. That was a hard one. How should we name the actions that go with each object? [No response] Would it help to name the object? [Child response]

Okay, let's begin that way. Suppose that you know the name of the object but not the name of the action? [Child response]

Well, I could tell you but can you think of a way to show me what you know? [Child response]

Good, you could show me by doing the action. Then together we can figure out the name of the action, maybe from the object used or there might be other ways to remember. [Lesson continues]

Within Lesson

Now we've named all the actions. Some objects have more than one. Let's try something else. You name the action and I'll name the object. Only one rule, you cannot repeat an action. If you can't think of the action, act it out and I'll try to help. [Continues]

Do you know how to play Simon Says? [No response] Well, in this game you get to be the queen and you tell me what to do. Let's use your name: "Catalina says, 'Eat!'" [SLP pretends to eat in a very sloppy manner. Child laughs.] Now you try one. [Continues]

Wow, that was fun. What a busy queen you are! Look at this. I have a book full of actions. Let's see if we can describe what's happening in the book. [Continues]

Conclusion

You worked really hard today. Do you remember what we learned? [Child response]

Why are action names important? [Child response]

And what did you do when you couldn't think of the action word? [Child response]

The second collection and analysis is similar to the first but attempts to answer five questions (Peña, 2002):

- Was the child able to form a more complete and coherent narrative?
- How difficult was it for the SLP to achieve positive change?
- Did the child pay attention and include more elements in the second narrative?
- Was the child able to transfer the learning without SLP support?
- Was learning quick and efficient?

Children developing typically usually make rapid changes and are very responsive.

For more mature children and adolescents, several narratives can be collected in various contexts and analyzed as above and for the "rules" appropriate for each type of narration. It must be remembered that not all cultures tell the same types of narratives.

> ***Food for Thought:*** **Dynamic assessment seems more prominent than discussed in other assessment chapters. Why is that? Does DA have a crucial role with children who are ELLs?**

The characteristics of each type of narration based on temporal, referential, causal, and spatial coherence are included in Table 8–7. The SLP must remember that the "rules" for certain types of narration may be unfamiliar to some children, and the result may reflect a difference rather than a deficit. The types of cohesion used by the child should reveal their narrative style.

In the second step, the different types of narratives are explained to the child by using cues, such as "Talk like a book in school" or "Talk like you would to a friend," and examples. Within the training, the child is given different types of narratives to produce. Feedback is used by the SLP to seek clarification, additional information, relevant comments, and reference. After some intervention, the SLP attempts to determine whether the child can learn different types of narration, can transfer the types of cohesion across contexts, and can tell narratives without cueing and feedback.

Two measures that seem particularly important are the length of causal sequences and the number of unrelated statements. Among children speaking Spanish, an increase in the length of causal sequences and a decrease in the number of unrelated statements are indicators of greater causal cohesion.

Dynamic procedures work well with children from different sociocultural backgrounds. The procedures require that the task be explained, that the reasons for certain responses be stated adequately, and that the child respond differentially to the SLP's cues.

Researchers in one promising study targeted missing story grammar elements and subordination within two 25-minute test–teach–retest sessions and found overall results to have very high sensitivity and specificity (Petersen et al., 2017). Let's look a little closer. Although implementation requires precise methods, we discuss the process in a generalized fashion. I suggest you read the Petersen et al. (2017) article for the specifics.

Table 8–7. Types of Narration and Cohesion

Temporal Coherence

Is there a temporal order of events?

Are temporal connectives necessary? If so, are they used?

Are shifts in time marked?

Causal Coherence

Are physical and mental states used to interconnect actions? (He was very tired, so he went to sleep.)

If not, can connectives be inferred easily?

Are causal connectives necessary? If so, are they used?

Referential Coherence

Participants

Is adequate reference to the participants made?

Are new characters introduced clearly? If not, are they referred to as if introduced elsewhere in the text?

Are characters reintroduced in an unambiguous manner?

Can the referent be inferred from general world knowledge?

Props

Is identification of specific objects necessary? If so, are props mentioned adequately? If not, are props introduced by gestures or deictics, such as "that thing"?

Can the identity of props be inferred from descriptions or functions?

Spatial Coherence

Is information about location necessary? If so, are locations identified?

Are shifts in location clearly marked?

An SLP could use a wordless children's book, such as *Frog, Where Are You?* (Mayer, 1969), to collect a narrative retell sample from the child. The SLP tells the narrative in either English or the heritage language as the child is shown the appropriate pictures from the book. After the SLP's story, the child is given the book and asked to retell the story in that same language. This procedure is then repeated in the other language. The SLP should use a script to ensure that the stories contain the same elements.

Each cycle in a four-step teaching model begins with the SLP reading an unfamiliar story aloud in English. The story should have clear story grammar elements and adverbial subordinate clauses.

Adverbial subordinate clauses serve the same function as adverbs or adverbial phrases. For example, temporal subordinate clauses tell when something happened, as in

He was sad and went home *after his team lost the game.*

CHAPTER 8 ASSESSMENT OF CHILDREN FROM CULTURALLY & LINGUISTICALLY DIVERSE BACKGROUNDS **341**

The SLP then helps the child retell the story using verbal prompts, illustrations, and colored icons representing the main story grammar elements. In instruction, the SLP targets story grammar elements and adverbial subordinate clauses that were omitted or poorly presented in the child's narrative. In each successive step, prompts and supports are systematically removed to foster independent retelling.

The entire four-step model can be completed in less than 30 minutes. In the study by Peterson et al. (2017), the instruction took place on two successive days. The retest phase follows instruction. Finally, the pre- and posttest performances are compared to assess learning. Continuing research will attempt to shortened the DA process even further and provide more easily accessible norms.

Measures of syntactic complexity, such as increased use of subordinate clauses with increased age in monolingual English-speaking children, may not be appropriate for all ELLs, such as those speaking both Vietnamese and English (Dam et al., 2020). Although Vietnamese–English-speaking children may subordinate clauses in both Vietnamese and English, the number has been found to differ by language.

DA of narrative ability in children who are Ells indicates that a combination of examiner ratings can accurately identify children with language disorders. Composite scores include

- modifiability, characterized by compliance, metacognition, and task orientation;
- DA story scores, based on setting, dialogue, and complexity of vocabulary; and
- ungrammaticality, derived from a posttest narrative sample.

Please read the original research by Peña and collaborators (2014) for scoring specifics. DA conducted in English provides a systematic method for measuring learning processes and learning outcomes.

Assessment of Information-Processing Skills. As mentioned in Chapter 2, children with language disorders have difficulty with information processing (Chiat & Roy, 2007; Haynes & Pindzola, 2012; Kohnert, 2013; Leonard et al., 2007; Munson et al., 2005; Rispens & Baker, 2012). Although not guaranteed, assessment of information-processing skills can be a way to circumvent a child's formal language assessment difficulties that are due to lack of the background linguistic knowledge assumed by standardized tests (Kohnert, 2013; Paradis et al., 2011; Wyatt, 2012).

Verbal working memory tasks combined with other more robust linguistic measures seem useful in assessing preschool-age dual-language children with DLD (Guiberson & Rodríguez, 2020). The same is not true for nonverbal working memory measures.

The validity of information processing-based measures has been demonstrated for ELL children from diverse linguistic and cultural backgrounds (Guiberson & Rodriguez, 2013; Hwa-Froelich & Matsuo, 2005; Restrepo & Gutiérrez-Clellen, 2012; Thordardottir et al., 2011). Among children with TDL who are also ELLs, vocabulary may be affected and influenced by first-language exposure, but nonword and sentence repetition is not (Engel de Abreu et al., 2013; Fortunato-Tavares et al., 2012; Thordardottir & Brandeker, 2013). Second language learners with language disorder may have difficulty with both tasks.

Although children who are ELLs can be compared to their peers with TDL, SLPs must use some judgment when selecting materials. For example, nonwords selected for a repetition task should be phonologically familiar to the child and consistent with the child's articulatory abilities. Nonsense words should be checked to make sure that they're not words in the heritage language or risk invalidating the results (Wagner et al., 2005).

Language Assessment of Children Speaking NMAE

African American children, as the second largest racial group in the United States, make up approximately 17% of children enrolled in public schools (Fry, 2007). The reported academic underachievement of many of these children, who are from families with low SES backgrounds, has been attributed by some professionals to the AAE dialect that many of these children bring to school, which differs from the MAE dialects used for instruction. Those AAE-speaking children who are bi-dialectal are better able to navigate the language of the classroom when they attend elementary school.

It's good to remind ourselves that variation due to a dialect difference represents a typical sociolinguistic process and large groups of children contribute. In contrast, variation due to language disorder represents atypical language learning mechanisms by a relatively small group of children (Oetting et al., 2016).

It's important to consider a child's dialect use when assessing language ability, especially with language features that are variable in NMAE dialects. For example, when assessing the morphosyntactic features of past tense -*ed*, third-person singular -*s*, and plural -*s*, children with TDL who speak NMAE dialects may overtly mark past tense and third-person singular less often compared to their MAE peers (Eisel Hendricks & Adlof, 2020). In turn, these same NMAE speakers may overtly mark these morphosyntactic markers more often compared to peers with developmental language disorder.

Careful Use of Standardized Tests

The research on African American children's language has helped in developing more culturally sensitive clinical procedures. As a result, SLPs have recognized the need for more options in assessing children's spoken language. Some considerations are not dissimilar from those we discussed with ELLs.

In the past, the norm-referenced standardized tests used to identify children with language disorders often did not include African American children in their normative samples or included them in such small numbers as to be inconsequential. Compared to norming samples that were overwhelmingly majority dialectal speakers, AAE speakers performed poorly. It's important to remember that not all African American children use AAE and not all AAE speakers are African American.

Even when African American children are included in tests' normative samples, some groups of children continue to obtain below-average scores, whereas others do not (Champion et al., 2003; Qi et al., 2003, 2006; Thomas-Tate et al., 2006). This fact is a reminder that African American children are a heterogeneous group.

The challenge in an assessment is to distinguish differences that are due to normal dialect use from those that are due to language disorder. Most standardized tests were not designed to make such a distinction.

Measures to counter negative bias in existing standardized tests may include the following (Stockman, 2010):

- Creating local norms for evaluating African American children's test responses
- Comparing the performances of a child and their parent on the same test
- Embedding test items in more familiar tasks or thematic contexts
- Using community judgments of typical use

As mentioned previously, local norms can be used along with those from the test. Although these dual norms can be used to compare the performance of children to that of the standard group and of their peer group, it must be remembered that most likely the test uses MAE. It seems more appropriate to compare a child's performance to that of other children also using the same dialect. Unfortunately, we have very little data on the validity of this procedure.

A recent example of adaptation is for Jamaican Creole English-speaking children. Standardized language assessment scoring procedures can be adapted using adult models. This is an ecologically valid approach that supports a more accurate assessment (Wright Karem & Washington, 2021). Adults from the same linguistic community can aid in developing an adapted scoring procedure that considers the influences of linguistic features on responses. The responses of adults inform this scoring adaptation and, in turn, increase the diagnostic accuracy of the standardized measure.

Although more research is needed, **dialectal scoring** for children who speak AAE and Southern White English (SWE) shows promise as an alternative scoring method for verb tense and agreement (Oetting et al., 2019). For example, dialectal scoring might count as correct three types of nonmainstream responses: *is* for *are*, *was* for *were*, and zero verbal *-s* (*he run*) versus MAE (*he runs*). All three variations are found in both AAE and SWE. This type of scoring does not appear to affect diagnostic distinctions between children with DLD and TDL, but it does decrease the number of dialectal speakers who may be misdiagnosed as having a language disorder (Cleveland & Oetting, 2013; Oetting & Garrity, 2006).

An alternative measure is the Diagnostic Evaluation of Language Variation, Norm Referenced (DELV-NR; Seymour et al., 2018), a norm-referenced standardized test designed to assess both those who speak AAE and those who speak MAE. Designed for children ages 4;0 to 9;11 years, the DELV yields performance profiles in syntax, pragmatics, semantics, and phonology.

Variations exist in dialects. Within AAE, for example, the Fluharty Speech and Language Screening Test, Second Edition (Fluharty, 2001), accepts an /f/ for /θ/ substitution on the word *teeth* as a dialectal response, but in New Orleans, African Americans substitute /t/ to produce *teet* (/tit/).

Finally, test procedures that ask children to repeat what the SLP says may go against the cultural norm. Some African American children are not expected to imitate adults.

Alternative Assessment Approaches

Alternative assessment approaches may include spontaneous oral LSA and procedures that measure learning potential. Spontaneous speech is natural, authentic, readily accessible to observation, and implicitly sensitive to linguistic differences because speakers choose their own words and how they are said.

An SLP can use analysis techniques that have been adapted to take AAE grammatical patterns into account or those that look for development of phonologic, morphosyntactic, semantic, and pragmatic performances that are noncontrastive in AAE and the majority dialect (Stockman, 2008; Stockman et al., 2008). Some measures of spontaneous speech performance, such as length of communication units, can help identify language disorder.

Similar to standardized tests, samples attempt to describe a child's existing language status, which reflects past learning. An SLP is left with the question of whether a child's performance reflects limitations on the child's language experiences in the environment or the child's inadequate ability to learn from those language experiences.

An SLP's use of DA and fast-mapping strategies can minimize the effect of past learning experiences on current performance by evaluating a child's ability to learn from new linguistic input. DA has been described previously.

Fast-mapping assessments are based on a child's quick incidental learning of words seen during typical development. Children with TDL learn most words without deliberate instruction from caregivers, and this learning can occur with very little input. Novel word learning is less dependent on prior experience than typical vocabulary testing. For example, mid- and low-SES 2-year-old African American children with TDL do not differ significantly on fast-mapping novel word tasks, although they differ significantly in their responses on norm-referenced standardized tests of receptive and expressive vocabulary (Horton-Ikard & Weismer, 2007). Similar results are reported when African American children's performance is compared with that of other racial and ethnic groups (Rodekohr & Haynes, 2001).

Although discussed with regard to speech production, this notion of variation within a dialect may be a novel one for you. Let's take a moment to demonstrate morphosyntactic difference across speakers of five dialects: AAE, AAE-speaking children from the Gullah/Geechee (GG) corridor of South Carolina whose AAE is influenced by their GG heritage (Berry & Oetting, 2017), Cajun English, SWE, and MAE. I'm borrowing heavily from Oetting (2019).

Seven forms are considered unique to some dialects and/or some speakers within a dialect. Six have been identified in children speaking AAE and SWE, including use of *ain't*; *I'ma*; *fitna/finna*; some past tense forms, such as *brung* and *fount*; some reflexive forms, such as *hisself*; and some pronoun forms, such as *ya'll* and *allya'll*. The remaining form—copula and auxiliary BE—is found in GG-influenced AAE. These differences are explained in the following paragraphs.

These unique forms are a small subset of linguistic rules that are not produced at particularly high frequencies. In fact, dialectal differences are most pronounced when we examine the rates at which these forms are produced. Even within dialects, there is considerable individual variability. Nonetheless, an SLP must consider these differences when evaluating a child's language.

CHAPTER 8 ASSESSMENT OF CHILDREN FROM CULTURALLY & LINGUISTICALLY DIVERSE BACKGROUNDS 345

Some forms likely reflect dialect-universal processes of contraction and analogy:

Contraction

fixing to → fitna/finna

I'm going to → I'ma

Analogy

drink – drank so *bring – brang*

Rates of use affect some forms but not others. For example, among AAE-speaking preschoolers, rate of use affects children's marking of auxiliary BE and DO but not modals (Newkirk-Turner et al., 2014).

Similar to adults, children who speak AAE, SWE, and other dialects of English do not produce nonmainstream forms randomly (Oetting, 2019). Linguistic context can influence when a nonmainstream form is produced. For example, BE contexts, such as the form of BE (i.e., *am, are, is, was/were*), contractibility (contractible *I'm* versus uncontactable *I am*), and grammatical function (copula versus auxiliary), may have differing rates of use.

All three variables affect AAE-speaking children, whereas only the type of BE and grammatical function affect SWE speakers (Roy et al., 2013). AAE-speaking children produce high rates of marking for *am* and *was/were*, lower rates for *is*, and even lower rates for *are*. By comparison, SWE-speaking children produce high rates of marking for all forms except *are*. In contrast, GG-influenced AAE-speaking children have lower rates of marking for all forms (Berry & Oetting, 2017).

In general, children with DLD do not produce a different set of unique forms, effects for linguistic context, or functions than have been produced by their AAE and SWE dialect-speaking peers with TDL (Oetting & McDonald, 2001). Children with DLD produce lower rates of marking (i.e., *She bes busy*) and higher rates of zero marking (i.e., *She be busy*) for several substructures, such as infinitives, compared to their dialect-speaking typical peers (Oetting & Garrity, 2006; Oetting & Newkirk, 2008; Pruitt & Oetting, 2009). For example, AAE- and SWE-speaking kindergartners with DLD overtly mark tense and agreement at lower rates compared to children with TDL who speak the same dialect (Oetting et al., 2019).

In addition, children with DLD produce dialect-specific unique forms or dialect-specific rates, contexts, and functions of grammatical structures. They learn the dialects of their communities. Children with DLD do not seem to contribute additional language variation to their communities by producing unique forms or by using grammatical structures in differing ways.

> ***Food for Thought:*** **Will there be some methods discussed in evaluation of children who are ELLs that will be appropriate with dialectal speakers of American English?**

Model of Language Assessment of a Child Who Speaks NMAE

Many of the assessment practices in Chapters 4 through 7 and those in our discussion of ELLs are appropriate when assessing children who are NMAE speakers. For this reason, I won't repeat what was said previously but, rather, highlight additional considerations. Much of the research has been conducted with children who speak AAE rather than other nonmainstream dialects, and this section reflects that emphasis.

When assessing a child who uses AAE, the SLP must be aware of multiple layers of dialectal use that can affect pronunciation, grammatical rules, and word usage. A child may be erroneously judged as having delayed or disordered language. This outcome is likely to occur when the child exhibits a high density or rate of AAE use (Stockman, 2010). As a consequence, children who speak AAE are either overdiagnosed with speech-language disorders or underdiagnosed because observed differences are attributed to dialect use.

Components

As with any diagnostic assessment, you, as an SLP, will want to collect the best, most nonbiased data possible. You'll want to be as accurate as possible so that those children who need intervention qualify and those with TDL do not.

Pre-Evaluation

Assessment begins as mentioned in Chapter 4 with data gathering. This collection process might include screening all children who are ELL or NMAE speakers. The Expressive Vocabulary Test, Third Edition (Williams, 2018) is a screening measure. Earlier editions have been reported to be culturally fair and appropriate for use with African American children (Thomas-Tate et al., 2006).

Among other options available, two quickly completed dialectal density measures are the Diagnostic Evaluation of Language Variation–Screener Test (DELV-ST; Seymour et al., 2003), Part I, and a dialect variation score (DVAR; Terry et al., 2010) obtained from the DELV-ST.

A DVAR score is the percentage of scorable items on Part 1 of the DELV-ST that vary from the MAE dialect. Using the elicited responses from a standardized test such as the DELV allows easier comparisons across children. A DVAR score is calculated by dividing the number of items that varied from MAE by the total number of scoreable items and multiplying this value by 100. The resulting score is the percentage of use of AAE features. The mean or average DVAR scores and the standard deviations (in parentheses) are as follows (Horton & Apel, 2014):

Kindergarten	67.95 (± 26.06)
First grade	49.30 (± 28.54)
Second grade	33.90 (± 20.30)

Pre-Assessment Planning

An SLP must choose assessment measures carefully. This means researching individual tools online and considering evidence-based practice to obtain the most unbiased tools possible. As an SLP, you'll also want to considered alternative scoring methods, such as dialectal scoring, and the use of informal measures.

Assessment

As in any good assessment, an SLP should use a combination of formal and informal assessment techniques and measures.

Formal Tests and Measures. The following five guidelines should be considered prior to using standardized tests with children from CLD backgrounds:

1. What is the relationship of the norming population and the client? Are enough NMAE children included to give a fair representation? Are separate norms used for different groups of children?

2. What is the relationship of the child's experience and the content areas of the test? Items using farm content, for example, may have little relevance for children in the inner city.

3. What is the relationship of the language being tested and the child's dialect dominance? This issue is critical in determining language disorder. The determining factor should be the child's ability to function within their own dialectal community.

4. Will the language of the test penalize a nonstandard child by use of idiomatic or metaphoric language?

5. Is the child penalized for a particular pattern of learning or style of problem-solving?

Parents, who presumably speak the same dialect, may be used as referents when very little normative data are available. A language test can be given to both the parent and the child. Once enough data have been gathered, the SLP can compare the child's performance with that of the adult. Assuming the adult has no language disorder, child use that reflects parent use but that differs from MAE would represent a dialectal difference, not a disorder. For example, zero-marking of final plosives found in AAE would result in omission of the regular past tense *-ed*. Just testing the child, an SLP might assume that the child does not have past tense. Parental use would confirm a dialectal difference.

Dual sets of norms—those from the test and locally prepared ones—can also be used to compare the performance of children with CLD backgrounds to that of the standard group and of their peer group, but they must be used cautiously because most likely the test will still be in MAE. It seems more appropriate to measure a child's performance in their dialect and compare this performance to that of other children also using that dialect.

Unfortunately, we have very little data on dialectal development and even fewer tests. However, scoring modifications for children who speak AAE can result in measurement that more accurately reflects a child's language knowledge and abilities while somewhat negating the influence of NMAE use (Eisel Hendricks & Adlof, 2017).

When measuring dialectal use in children speaking AAE, SLPs have limited valid and reliable measures of nonmainstream dialect use from which to choose. For example, scores of African American children with low-SES backgrounds on an older version of the Preschool Language Scale, Fifth Edition (Zimmerman et al., 2011) suggest that although the test was generally nonbiased, some items should be interpreted with caution because they were problematic for these children (Qi et al., 2003). This is a lesson for all of us to use standardized tests with caution.

Although tests may not be inherently bias, they may overlook dialectal differences or cultural norms. If SLPs are sensitive to dialectal differences, more open-ended tasks, such as sentence recall, can yield moderate-to-high levels of diagnostic accuracy in identifying DLD among speakers of nonmainstream dialects of English, such as AAE (Oetting et al., 2016).

Semantic knowledge, the underlying concepts, may be a better framework than language form for speakers of some dialects, including AAE and Appalachian English. The adequacy of the semantic knowledge of these children is often questioned on the basis of the form of their language. It is assumed, incorrectly, that children using NMAE dialects acquire concepts later than do speakers of dialects closer to MAE.

Both Latino/Latina and African American children's standardized vocabulary test scores increase significantly from pre- to posttest after they are exposed to test-taking strategies (Peña et al., 2001). As you might suspect, children with TDL obtain significantly higher posttest scores than children with language disorders. These outcomes suggest that learning mechanisms are more likely intact for children with TDL but not for those with language disorders.

Informal Assessment Measures. Normative testing should be supplemented by probing. Children with CLD backgrounds score lower on knowledge-based testing, such as that found in many normative procedures, but score the same on process-based assessments, such as comprehension and production in real conversations.

Sampling. Although samples of 50 to 100 utterances are often recommended, longer samples are needed when children speak NMAE. Across nonmainstream dialects, some grammatical structures are expressed in a variety of ways rather than categorically. For example, the plural -*s* may be omitted by children speaking AAE when a number precedes the noun but not on other occasions.

Children who speak NMAE demonstrate dialect-specific and dialect-universal patterns in their early acquisition of auxiliaries. For example, auxiliary verb use by 3-year-olds who speak AAE varies by auxiliary type and the amount of nonmainstream dialect characteristics, called *dialect density*, in a child's speech. In general, among AAE-speaking preschoolers, dialect density is related to a child's marking of BE and DO but not modal auxiliaries (Newkirk-Turner et al., 2014). Marking of BE is influenced by its surface

CHAPTER 8 ASSESSMENT OF CHILDREN FROM CULTURALLY & LINGUISTICALLY DIVERSE BACKGROUNDS **349**

form, which varies considerably with *am*, *is*, *are*, *was*, and *were*, and the following verbal element. Marking of BE and DO is also influenced by the specific syntactic construction. These findings suggest that in an evaluation, the SLP should carefully analyze the use of auxiliary verbs within their linguistic context.

Young AAE speakers begin producing auxiliary verbs between 19 and 24 months. As would be expected, initial forms are restricted and occur in syntactically simple constructions. Subsequent rates of use vary by auxiliary verb type (Newkirk-Turner et al., 2016). For example, rates of BE and DO marking vary with the syntactic construction. BE occurs most frequently in declaratives. DO first appears in the negative as *don't* and, not surprisingly, is used most in negative sentences throughout the preschool years. Modal auxiliaries also appear first as negatives in the *-n't* form (*can't*, *won't*) and have only limited use by AAE-speaking preschool children.

The rate of BE marking is further affected by the form of the verb (*am*, *is*, *are*) and what follows in the sentence. First appearing as *I'm*, the *am* form occurs most frequently through the preschool years, followed by *is*, which exceeds use of *are*. In addition, the BE auxiliary is used more frequently in the present progressive tense than preceding *go* or *gonna*, an early way to mark future tense (*I go tomorrow*). Addition information plus a developmental chart can be found in the study by Newkirk-Turner et al. (2016).

Children's use of the infinitive TO is also affected by their dialect, linguistic context, and the presence or absence of DLD (Rivière et al., 2018). Among children speaking AAE, SWE, and Cajun, contexts including verbs of motion especially affect use of infinitives. This suggests that an SLP must consider both dialect and linguistic context when assessing use of infinitives.

When evaluating AAE–speaking children, the SLP should be mindful that dialectal variations exist. For example, children speaking Creole variations, such as Gullah/Geechee, have been found to have variation in their use of the verb BE, including unique forms, such as /də/; unique uses of forms such as BEEN; and varying rates of use of forms of BE used by other speakers of AAE (Berry & Oetting, 2017). Gullah/Geechee speakers traditionally resided in the coastal areas and the sea islands of North Carolina, South Carolina, Georgia, and Florida and are descendants of Central and West Africans enslaved on these isolate islands. If you are working with children speaking Gullah/Geechee, I suggest reading the excellent article by Berry and Oetting (2017).

A final consideration is communicative functions (CFs) or the reasons for communicating. These differ by SES, race/ethnicity, or gender among preschoolers and their mothers (Kasambira Fannin et al., 2018). In addition, CF production may be influenced more by maternal demographic characteristics at the time of children's school entry than by child demographics, such as SES.

Although children differ little on the rates of CF use, those from low-SES homes produce fewer utterances and less reasoning. Boys use less self-maintaining utterances and more predicting.

Mothers exhibit more sociocultural differences in CFs compared to children. African American mothers use more directing and less responding compared to European American and Latino/Latina American mothers. Mothers from low-SES backgrounds also do more directing and less responding.

Narratives. Narrative performance among various cultural, ethnic, and linguistic groups may differ greatly. These differences reflect both cultural and individual differences in storytelling.

> ***Food for Thought:*** **Every aspect of narration is culturally based. How will you decide if a child's narrative is culturally appropriate or disordered?**

Storytelling is never context or culture free. Rather, it is the product of the contextual interaction of the narrator and the audience and of the sociocultural norms of each, which shape each person's presuppositions and expectations. Even the purpose and context for narratives vary across cultures.

Telling narratives is a social event governed by cultural norms and values. Not every culture expects the narrative monologues seen in MAE. Among some Latino/Latinas, Native Americans, African Americans, Jewish Americans, and Hawaiian Americans, stories are produced conversationally with audience cooperation. The story is built by the storyteller acting out the parts as the audience challenges and contradicts.

Listeners, both African American and White, tend to rate narratives in similar fashion, allowing more leeway for variation from MAE in personal narratives and less in fictional ones (Mills et al., 2021). In general, teachers rate narratives that differ more from MAE lower than parents and caregivers do.

Planning ecologically valid narrative collection requires an SLP to be mindful of the many functions narratives can serve in various cultures, such as informing and entertaining. An SLP should attempt to reflect and later foster narrative skills valued by children's culture (Bliss et al., 2001).

SLPs must be alert to possible bias in interpretation of children's narratives. For example, with little guidance in the professional literature, SLPs may have their own preference for what constitutes a good narrative. African American children often tell topic-associating narratives in which events that happened at different times and places may be combined around a central theme. Current literature focuses almost exclusively on story structure over the performative aspects of storytelling, although there are potential sociocultural influences on children's use of stylistic and creative features in their narratives.

Interestingly, the features of narratives by elementary school African American children differ depending on the elicitation task (Mills, 2015). For example, syntactic elaboration and MLU_W are higher when no visual cues are used, whereas NDW is higher with both no visual cues and picture sequences. Single picture cueing is the least effective method.

African American children from low-SES backgrounds in both gifted and general education classrooms produce fictional narratives of similar length, lexical diversity, and syntactic complexity. In general, children in gifted classrooms produce lower rates of AAE and perform better on standard vocabulary measures compared to children in general education classrooms (Mills, 2015).

Summary. Despite the incredible difficulties inherent in accurately assessing children with CLD backgrounds, there is hope. The same integrated, functional methodology proposed for native speakers of English can be used with some modifications with these children as well. With sensitivity, unbiased administration of testing, and sampling within the everyday context of a child, a fair and meaningful assessment can be accomplished.

The differences between majority and minority children on knowledge-based tests are not found on process-based evaluations. It may be possible to reduce bias in language testing of children with CLD backgrounds by using methods and tools that emphasize processing abilities, such as memory and perception, rather than language experience and knowledge. Process-based tests can be useful in distinguishing language disorder from experiential difference. Processes are the mental operations required to manipulate linguistic material. Testing might include such tasks as nonword vocal repetition, completion of two language tasks simultaneously, and following directions. To ensure that past learning is minimized, tasks should be completely novel, and task-related vocabulary and grammar should be familiar or, if not, reviewed prior to testing.

Conclusion

Unfortunately, sometimes a battery of readily available tests is given to every child regardless of possible language disorder or CLD background. For some professionals, this passes for an individualistic and thorough assessment. As with intervention, assessment procedures must be designed for the individual child. Standardized tests are only a portion of this process. Language tests are only aids to an SLP and cannot substitute for the informed and sensitive clinician.

Both cultural and linguistic factors influence performance in an assessment. These may lead to misinterpretations and miscommunication. An SLP must be careful not to stereotype behavior and draw incorrect and unfair conclusions. For example, Latino/Latina American children may seem uncooperative and inattentive when, in fact, their behavior signifies different concepts of time, body language, and achievement.

An SLP can avoid biasing data interpretation by asking the following questions:

- Are there other variables, such as limited exposure to English or contextual factors, that might explain the child's difficulties with English?
- Are the problems related to English language learning or dialectal differences?
- Are similar problems exhibited in L_1, the heritage language?
- Can the problems be explained by cultural difference?
- Is there any consistency in linguistic problems that might suggest an underlying rule?
- Can the problems be explained by any bias related to materials or procedures?

An SLP should interpret the child's performance in light of the intrinsic and extrinsic biases inherent in the assessment process.

Intrinsic biases, such as knowledge needed and normative samples, are part of the test, whereas extrinsic biases, such as sociocultural values and attitude toward testing, reside in the child. When different groups of children score similarly to the norming population—as on the Communication and Symbolic Behavior Scales (Wetherby & Prizant, 2003)—it suggests a less biased assessment device.

Language use patterns of both a child and an SLP and the language-learning history of that child also may influence the assessment. Communication and interactive style are culture bound.

Bias can be overcome by

- identifying variables that might affect the assessment;
- analyzing tests and procedures for content and style;
- taking variables into account and changing assessment procedures; and
- using dynamic assessment techniques.

Each child's level of acculturation will differ with the age of the child and the extent of exposure to both cultures.

Assessment of ELLs and NMAE-speaking children is an important but often less-than-accurate process. Unfortunately, ELLs and NMAE-speaking children are often diagnosed with language disorder although they may simply have had fewer opportunities to learn English or MAE compared to their English-speaking monolingual or MAE peers. Dynamic assessment shows promise as an effective method for identifying ELLs and NMAE-speaking children with language disorders.

Dynamic assessment tasks are appropriate and deemphasize grammar in favor of ability to communicate and learn. Tasks are interactive, focused on learning, and yield information on learner responsiveness.

A thorough assessment includes a variety of flexible procedures designed to heighten awareness of a potential language problem and to enable an SLP to delineate more clearly the language abilities and specific disorder of a child with a CLD background. For training to be truly functional, a thorough description of a child and that child's language or languages must be made.

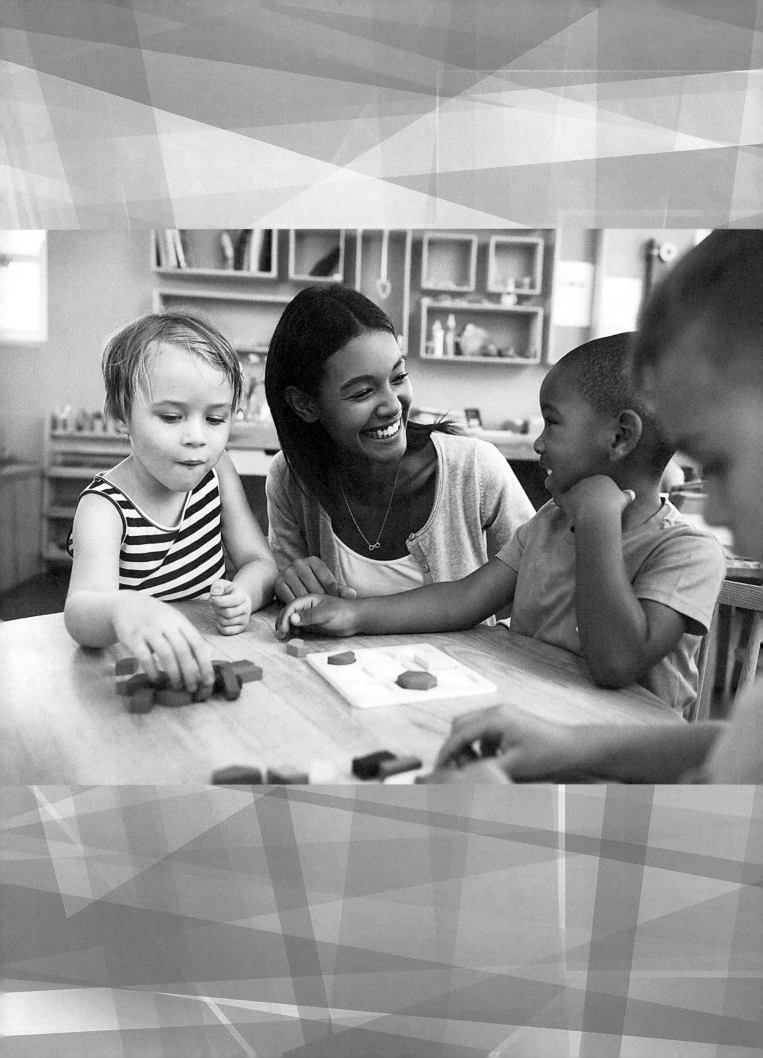

CHAPTER 9
A FUNCTIONAL INTERVENTION MODEL

As a new speech-language pathologist (SLP), Kendra is frustrated, not with her job or with the children in her caseload, but with the results of her intervention rarely evidenced beyond the therapy room door. It feels like an uphill battle.

She's explored multiple approaches, read journal articles, and attended conferences. Most research addressed specific language targets. She's looking for an overall approach that can inform her intervention but leave room for her own creative touch.

Her graduate program stressed rigid, behavior methods that don't hold much interest or show much promise for Kendra. Her school is in a rural district, and she's unsure how much support she'll have for trying something radically different.

Just what the "something" is has yet to be determined.

Often, language intervention does not consider either the integrated nature of language or the context of language use. Language is viewed as a set of rules, rather than as a holistic social tool. Although the focus may include form, content, and use, the overall design may be additive, rather than integrative. Often, the stated goal is to learn specific language units, not to enhance overall communication.

Language methods that emphasize very specific skills run the risk of obtaining very specific effects. When taught without a thought to context and use, newly acquired forms may fail to generalize to everyday conversational use.

It need not be this way. Clinical intervention can be a well-integrated whole in which the various aspects of language combine to enhance communication. The purposes of intervention can be

- to teach a generative repertoire of linguistic features that can be used to communicate in socially appropriate ways in various contexts; and
- to stimulate overall language development (Duchan, 1997).

But it takes work and thought on your part as the SLP.

Dr. Alan Kamhi (2014) has done a fine job of summarizing much of what we know about language and literacy intervention (Fey et al., 2003; Nelson, 2010; Paul & Norbury, 2011; Reed, 2012), and I encourage you to read his article. Let's borrow some of what he said and save some for the following chapters. We can begin with the understanding that *more is not always better* when it comes to language intervention, *nor is increased feedback always better*. Both are especially true with regard to mass learning, often characterized by drill. **Mass learning** is learning that occurs all at once instead of spaced over time.

It's also important to recognize that learning plateaus are more likely with repetitive intervention, such as language drills. Learning seems to stall. In this situation, simply increasing the frequency of intervention may not result in better language and literacy outcomes (Denton et al., 2011; Fey et al., 2013; Ukrainetz et al., 2009).

Practice that's distributed and has intervals between learning episodes is more effective. In addition, distributed practice results in better retention. Although true for many types of learners, this guidance seems to be especially true for children with language disorders (Riches et al., 2005; Yoder et al., 2012).

All this discussion suggests that determination of language targets and the type of intervention may be our keys to success. It also leads me to believe that a more natural, non-drill intervention that spreads intervention throughout the day may be a better approach.

Because many of the principles in Kamhi's (2014) article are distributed throughout this text, we'll only mention one more here. We can summarize this as *focus on a child's knowledge or language deficits rather than on cognitive processing*, such as sequencing and prioritizing, and on cognitive abilities, such as attention and memory (Kamhi, 2011). In other words, it's better to teach sequencing through narration rather than as a separate skill. This notion is addressed further in Chapter 11.

A functional language intervention model discussed throughout this text attempts to target language features that a child uses in the everyday context, such as the home or the classroom, and to adapt that context so that it facilitates the learning of language. This contrasts with the more traditional model's targeting of smaller units of behavior, sometimes taught in isolation and devoid of context.

Table 1–1 contrasts the traditional and functional models of intervention. Take a quick look back just to refresh your memory.

I don't want to leave the impression that some professionals are uninformed or that older methods were detrimental. We learn as we go. That's what evidence-based practice (EBP) is all about. For example, when I began in the field, I worked with children who were not talking. There were few of us back then.

We would teach a child to say a word and then teach the child how to use it. That was backwards. Without a use for the word, the child had no reason to learn it. We now realize that a gestural means of communication can establish an intention, such as requesting, and also provide the vehicle for teaching words used in requesting. Teaching language devoid of purpose is counterintuitive.

That realization and change is called *evolution*. Similarly, we realize that more traditional methods of language intervention may be limited and we try new ones, such as functional intervention. We don't throw out older methods; rather, we change and modify them based on new knowledge.

The functional approach recognizes a need to orient language teaching toward the inclusion of family members and teachers and toward the use of everyday activities for encouraging functional communication. Therefore, routines within the home, school,

CHAPTER 9 A FUNCTIONAL INTERVENTION MODEL

and community are used with an array of language teachers. In this way, aspects of language can be taught as they relate to one another within the context of a meaningful experience. As a result, the intervention experience more closely approximates patterns of typically developing language (TDL). Content is based on common experiences.

A functional approach, with its integrative and interactive aspects, changes the nature of the clinical interaction and the role of an SLP. The SLP as teacher also becomes a consultant for other language teachers, who interact more frequently with the child, teaching them to modify the contexts within which language can occur and to elicit and modify the child's language. The SLP and caregivers collaborate in the child's language intervention.

Concern for generalization is foremost and governs the overall intervention approach. Planning by an SLP, along with the other language teachers, is essential. Implementation and generalization may be hampered or impeded by any number of factors, such as the targets selected, the intervention setting, the teaching methods used, and caseload and scheduling considerations.

Intervention should begin with a generalization plan that identifies features of a child's communication environment relevant to generalization. Often, generalization is the last step in the intervention planning process, rather than the overall organizing aspect I'll suggest.

> ***Food for Thought:*** **Does it seem odd or natural to identify the variables that affect generalization for a child before you even begin intervention?**

Once the appropriate generalization variables have been identified, you, the SLP, can begin to design intervention strategies. The relevant features of the communication environment that have been identified can now be enlisted. Ideally, such intervention enables an SLP to

- develop linguistic constructs at a child's developmental functioning level, taking into account the strategies children normally use when acquiring language;
- integrate all linguistic areas within the communication framework; and
- provide meaningful and age-appropriate contexts.

In this chapter, we discuss principles of intervention in a functional approach and an overall model for intervention, focusing on the variables that affect generalization.

Guidelines

Use of a functional approach to language intervention requires you to be mindful of certain guidelines that aid communication with and learning by a child. It is important to engage a child in meaningful dialogue or in some other communication event, and this event becomes the vehicle for learning and generalization.

LANGUAGE DISORDERS: A FUNCTIONAL APPROACH TO ASSESSMENT AND INTERVENTION IN CHILDREN

This section includes some of the most important guidelines for a functional approach. Undoubtedly, some important ones have been omitted that you'll want to include in your repertoire.

Be a Reinforcer

As communicators, all of us continue to interact with individuals who provide positive feedback and reinforcement. As much as possible, we avoid communicating with certain individuals who are nonresponsive, caustic, or overly critical. Children avoid certain potential conversational partners for many of the same reasons. If you want children to communicate with you, then *you must be someone with whom children want to communicate*. Kendra, the SLP at the beginning of the chapter, learned in graduate school how to use reinforcement but never thought of herself as a reinforcer.

Children respond most readily to adults who convey genuine caring and respect for them. These attitudes are conveyed by meeting a child halfway. Adults who desire to be effective conversational partners must appreciate the world from a child's perspective. It may help to recall that for children, the world is full of wonder and delight, full of things that cannot be explained, and full of magic. One of my sons burst into tears after being shown how to do a magic trick, protesting, "But I wanted real magic."

Adults demonstrate concern for children and adolescents when they are willing to attend to a child, to listen, and to accept their topics. As much as possible, intervention should be nonintrusive, with teachers providing supportive, evaluative feedback. By reducing your authority-figure persona, demonstrating an attentiveness and a willingness to adopt a child's topics, and remaining accepting, you, as an SLP, can send a message of acceptance of the child as your partner.

Few child responses are totally linguistically wrong. Hopefully, even seemingly incorrect utterances can demonstrate the child's understanding of the situation and of the underlying relationships. Acceptance of a child includes acceptance of these utterances. Usually, some portion of the utterance can be reinforced.

> *Child:* I need help with ear-gloves.
>
> *SLP:* That's right, they are like little gloves for your ears. We call them *earmuffs*. Here, let me help you put on your *earmuffs*.

The partner has accepted the child's utterance, recognized the child's understanding of the situation, corrected the utterance, and left the child's ego intact. What a marvelous teacher!

The intervention setting itself should "create and sustain an atmosphere containing fun, surprise, interest, ease, invitation, laughter, and spontaneity" (Cochrane, 1983, p. 160). In such an atmosphere, children will be eager to participate.

One of my best lessons on verbal sequencing within narration used mime, complete with white face paint. The children enacted familiar everyday event sequences, such as making breakfast, while other students tried to guess the name of the sequence. After the correct guess was given, the actor stated each event in the sequence while performing it.

CHAPTER 9 A FUNCTIONAL INTERVENTION MODEL

Finally, each actor attempted to reconstruct the sequence verbally. The lesson was messy, fun, enjoyable, and thoroughly successful.

Children also respond favorably if you, as the SLP, occasionally play the clown or buffoon. I may wear a cooking pot on my head in order to evoke a response. On other occasions, I purposely may make incorrect verbalizations or actions. I've even conducted intervention dressed as a chicken. These behaviors add to the magic of the communication situation and encourage children to communicate.

Closely Approximate Natural Learning

Language intervention strategies should approximate closely the natural process of language acquisition. The teaching event should be communicative in nature and use language as it naturally occurs. Teaching language devoid of its communicative function deprives a child of intrinsic motivation and of one essential element of generalization.

Natural language models—parents, teachers, aides, and others—should be the principal resources for implementation of language intervention. These individuals serve as language models with or without the SLP's input. Their potential as language teachers can be exploited best, however, when they are guided by the SLP in content selection and taught in facilitative techniques. When using these language teachers within the child's everyday situations, the role of the SLP changes to that of collaborator.

Follow Developmental Guidelines

The language development of children with TDL can guide the selection of teaching targets. As a group, these children develop language in a similar, albeit individualistic, manner. Generally, language form is preceded by function, with easier, less complex structures being learned first. Children use the language they possess to accomplish their language goals. These uses are the framework within which new forms develop. The overall result is a hierarchy that suggests steps for teaching language.

Of course, no SLP would ever adopt a language intervention hierarchy without adaptations for a child and the contexts in which they function. Rigid adherence to a developmental hierarchy is inappropriate. Good teaching may suggest alternative hierarchical teaching patterns.

As an SLP, you should be aware of the prerequisites for successful communicative behaviors at the functioning level of a child. The child learning plurals need not be able to count but must have a notion of *one* and *more than one*. Likewise, successful use of *why* questions and answers requires an ability to reconstruct events in reverse. These cognitive skills may need to be taught prior to attempting the linguistic means noting this knowledge.

Similarly, the child needs to understand the requirements and demands of different communication situations to communicate effectively within them. For example, the requirements of classroom give-and-take are very different from having a face-to-face conversation or from talking on your smartphone.

As with much learning, simple rules are combined and modified or enlarged to form higher order rules. By carefully analyzing each new teaching target and monitoring progress, an SLP can ensure that a child possesses the appropriate skills for new learning.

Language development and disorders can be very individualistic and may not follow the dictates of a developmental hierarchy. Aspects of language will develop at rates influenced by perception and cognition, opportunity, needs, and teaching. Of more importance for intervention is the selection of teaching targets that help a child function more effectively within the everyday environment.

The language rules of most children, whether correct or not, are valid for those children at that time. For example, young children say things such as "Mommy eat" and "More juice," which demonstrate adherence to simple word sequencing rules. The rules are appropriate to the child's level of linguistic competence.

At various levels of intervention, it may be appropriate to target child rules rather than the correct but more difficult adult ones. To require children with language disorders to use adult sentence forms seems unfair, especially when we do not require such behavior from young children with TDL.

Even the expectation that a child will use a new language feature following a brief period of intervention may be unrealistic. Children with TDL learn and extend or retract their language gradually after many encounters and trials over time. Eventually, these rules come to resemble those of adults. Therefore, it is inappropriate to expect near-perfect performance from children with language disorders shortly after a target is introduced.

Rule learning is complicated and time-consuming. As a child progresses, the language targets can be modified accordingly.

Follow the Child's Lead

Often, the expectation that a child will not communicate effectively becomes self-fulfilling. If an SLP expects a child to communicate and plans for that communication, the child will meet this expectation.

It is important, therefore, that an SLP or other language teacher attend to the content and intent of each child utterance and respond appropriately. In this way, teaching occurs when a child is paying attention and the language being used has positive consequences.

Language teachers can choose either to direct and maintain a child's attention or attend to what interests the child. Although the former is an adult-oriented or -centered approach that gives the adult virtual control of the entire interaction, it may not be the most effective approach. Children with intellectual developmental disorder (IDD) are less likely to follow such teacher attempts to redirect attention. In contrast, these children learn some things more easily when the teacher follows the child's attentional lead and builds on the focus of the child's attention.

A more child-centered approach guarantees joint or shared reference, enhances semantic contingency, and reduces noncompliance by a child. With **semantic contingency**, an adult comments on a child's topic or previous utterance, thus facilitating processing by the child. Children appear to attend most and be able to comprehend best speech that occurs during joint-attention activities.

Child actions or utterances provide contextual support within which to comprehend language. Such support aids the processing of children with IDD who have memory storage and retrieval problems.

CHAPTER 9 A FUNCTIONAL INTERVENTION MODEL

A child's verbal behavior should be interpreted by others in terms of its possible intention, rather than viewed as inappropriate or incorrect. In other words, a request is still a request even though the form may be wrong, the item desired misnamed, and so on.

Children signal those things in which they are most interested by their actions or through verbalizations. This gauge can be used to keep child interest and motivation high in the intervention setting. Often, I will say to a child, "What toy do you want to play with?" Although the topic is open-ended, the technique is very specific—as we discuss later—permitting a flexible choice of topic within certain limits I've set.

Although more functional, naturalistic intervention is not the only approach possible, indications are that following a child's lead while prompting for language is likely to elicit speech production in both children with autism spectrum disorder (ASD) and those with TDL (Walton & Ingersoll, 2014). Furthermore, for children with ASD, a parent's use of orienting cues helps a child verbally respond.

We can draw from this discussion that following a child's lead, setting the context with language and then asking follow-on questions is valuable. In other words, the child looks at a dog, and the parent talks about the dog briefly and then asks a question ("Do you want to pet the doggie?") or sets the expectation that the child will respond ("I wonder what he wants").

When a child initiates an interaction and is responded to accordingly, the value for learning is greater than when a child's initiation is ignored or penalized. Ignoring or penalizing a child will result in a decrease in future initiations.

While observing a lesson in a training apartment in preparation for an older teen's move to his own apartment, I overheard the following exchange:

SLP:	What are you doing?
Adolescent:	(Matter-of-factly) Dusting furniture.
SLP:	Good. What else are you dusting?
Adolescent:	You live in apartment?
SLP:	You didn't answer my question. What else are you doing?

The client obviously was interested in living arrangements and would have joined such a conversation willingly if the SLP had followed his lead.

> ***Food for Thought:*** **Is a child or are you more likely to be involved in a conversational exchange when your topic has been adopted?**

As an SLP, you can follow the child's lead and manipulate the conversation to encourage the desired language features. Continued use of directive responses by the SLP mentioned in the example will diminish the child's initiating behavior. Who wants to talk about dusting anyway?

Actively Involve the Child

Language acquisition occurs with the active participation of the learner. Language learning is not a passive process. In like fashion, more rapid learning occurs when a child with a language disorder is participating actively in some event.

Children's active participation is a significant aspect to effective language therapy. The level of their active engagement is significantly, positively related to their language gain regardless of the amount of intervention (Schmitt, 2020). In addition, the more actively involved the child, the greater and more stable the generalization. Ideally, intervention should consist of motivating participatory activities with the potential for a variety of language use contexts.

Remember the Influence of Context on Language

Context can be a major determiner of what is said and how it is said. Language is a socially based cultural form. Its use reflects an individual's linguistic, interpersonal, and contextual competence within a given situation. An individual's knowledge of the event or situation influences the way they use language in that situation.

Language intervention should occur within the contexts of everyday events and conversational give-and-take or that of other communication events. The language teacher needs to create a rich context in which a child with a language disorder can experience a variety of linguistic and nonlinguistic stimuli and be supported in their linguistic attempts.

The content for these dialogues is the common experience of the intervention setting. The skillful SLP or other language teacher can manipulate both the linguistic and nonlinguistic context to attain desired targets from the child.

So can you! We'll discuss how in Chapter 10.

Use the Scripts Found in Familiar Events

As noted previously, a script is an internalized set of expectations about routine or repeated events organized in a temporal–causal sequence. As such, scripts contain shared event knowledge based on common experiences that aid and enhance memory, comprehension, and participation.

Routinized events for which children have scripts provide specific situations in which children can learn appropriate language. Familiar activities of high interest, such as making popcorn, pudding, or cake, can be used as the contexts for language intervention. The event sequences contained in scripts can be used to teach language expression and comprehension and can aid recall.

Naturally, scripts will differ with a child's maturational level and, to some extent, with the individual. Even very young preschoolers remember events in an organized manner similar to adults in general structure and content. As children mature, their scripts become longer, more detailed, and contain more options ("Sometimes . . ."), alternatives ("You either . . . or . . . "), and conditions ("If . . . , then you . . . ").

CHAPTER 9 A FUNCTIONAL INTERVENTION MODEL **363**

Design a Generalization Plan First

Considerations of generalization are essential to treatment program design and should be identified prior to beginning training. Table 9–1 is a suggested generalization plan format. In designing such a plan, an SLP considers the individual needs of the child and environment and the relevant variables that will affect generalization.

Generalization Variables

To ensure generalization to the everyday environment of a child, the SLP must manipulate the generalization variables most likely to result in that outcome. As you may recall from Chapter 1, the variables that affect generalization can be grouped by content and context (see Table 1–2). Content variables include the teaching targets and teaching items. Context variables include the method of teaching, language teachers, cues, contingencies, and location of teaching. Each of these variables and considerations of their use for intervention within a functional model are discussed, expanding on the brief introduction in Chapter 1.

As a student, Kendra, the SLP introduced previously, had thought of generalization as work sent home after each session. She never imagined that concern for generalization could drive everything she does.

Table 9–1. Possible Generalization Plan Format

Intervention targets:

Identify settings, situations, and persons across which training can occur.

					Settings			
		Situation:	Situation:	Situation:	Situation:	Situation:	Situation:	Situation:	Situation:
P e r s o n s									

Cues:

Consequences:

Teaching Targets

Intervention can be conceptualized as a two-step process (Kamhi, 2014). A *short-term* context-specific appearance of a language feature is a child's performance. But a long-term context-independent appearance or generalization of a language feature is called *learning*.

Lack of generalization can be attributed to poor performance by the child but can also reflect the methods used by the SLP. One way an SLP limits learning is by choosing narrow restricted targets. Broad-based language rules, in contrast, have a much less narrow scope. The challenge, therefore, is to design language intervention that facilitates the acquisition of broad-based language rules.

Language intervention needs to be relevant to the child's communication within the environment and to target the language process, rather than language products or units. The SLP should consider two questions:

- What is the function of the forms and content I'm teaching?
- Are the forms and content being taught within communication events in which the intended function can actually be accomplished?

In general, more frequently required language forms and content are more relevant to a child's world and, therefore, are more likely to generalize. For example, if a child is expected in class to relate past events through oral narration, that child is likely to encounter past tense frequently. Similarly, communicative needs in the home can be introduced into intervention.

Well-chosen language targets can increase the effectiveness of a child as a communication partner. Within a functional approach, the first goal of intervention is successful communication by a child at their present level of functioning.

As mentioned previously, developmental guidelines can aid target selection. Goals approximating a developmental sequence are more successful than those that do not. Stated simply, earlier emerging forms are easier to learn, which is why they appear early. In intervention, they can be learned in fewer attempts and are a step toward later emerging forms. For example,

Mommy eat cookie is a step toward

Mommy eating cookie, which in turn moves a child closer to

*Mommy **is** eating a cookie.*

In addition, earlier emerging forms generalize more readily into a child's use system and move the child to a higher level of use.

In addition to data from development, research literature is critical in selecting appropriate treatment goals. This is especially true with complex syntax.

Please don't interpret my words to mean always target what's easy to teach and learn. In general, what shows rapid improvement in performance doesn't always result in long-term retention and transfer. Selecting difficult targets can create hurdles for a learner and

CHAPTER 9 A FUNCTIONAL INTERVENTION MODEL

slow the rate of apparent learning, but these same targets can also optimize long-term retention and transfer (E. Bjork, 2004; R. Bjork, 2011; Diemand-Vauman et al., 2011).

A functional model would suggest teaching forms useful in the natural setting while attending to the developmental order of these forms. The overriding criterion for target selection should be to aid the child in communicating what is necessary in the contexts in which they most frequently communicate. This practical approach is especially important for children who experience pragmatic difficulties, such as those seen in children with traumatic brain injury (TBI) and social communication disorder.

The best way to determine need is through environmental observation. If, for example, a child frequently requests items in the environment but is generally ineffective, then requesting might be chosen as a target. When there is very little opportunity for a possible language target to occur, it might be best to identify other content for teaching or find ways to increase opportunities.

Infrequent opportunity for possible teaching targets to occur may be the result of low environmental expectations or few requirements for a child to produce these forms or functions. For example, there may be few opportunities for a child to ask questions when there is little expectation that they will do so. In such cases, low expectations can become self-fulfilling. The communication environment may need to be restructured to facilitate use of newly acquired communication skills.

An SLP can identify both targets and everyday situations in which each target is likely to occur and in which its use will be affected by and, in turn, affect the context. For example, questions should be taught in situations in which they make sense and in which they perform their intended function of gaining information. SLP instructions such as "I'm coloring a picture; ask me what I'm doing" violate the function of questions. Usually, we do not ask questions for which we already have the answer or can determine it easily.

Instead, we can modify both the situation and the cue to elicit a question more appropriately. For example, the SLP might talk on a smartphone and state, "How can you find out what I'm doing?"

Teaching Items

The teaching items are the linguistic locations where the target will be taught. For example, if the target is past tense -*ed*, then the teaching items are the verbs that will be used for this teaching.

As an SLP, you should plan to teach enough examples of the language feature being targeted to enable a child to generalize to untrained members. For example, it is neither desirable nor possible to teach all possible noun–verb combinations. The goal should be to teach enough examples from the noun class in combination with sufficient examples of the verb class so that the child will generalize the rule *noun + verb* to all members of these two classes. Obviously, this process is being simplified in this introductory discussion, and more planning and thought are required.

In addition, a sufficient number of items must be taught so that a child can determine both the relevant and irrelevant aspects of the communication context. For example, words or phrases such as *yesterday*, *last week*, and *in the past* are relevant for use of the past tense. The child forms a hypothesis that states, "In the presence of *yesterday*, *last week*, or *in the past*, use the past tense." Other aspects may be irrelevant, such as the specific nouns or pronouns preceding the verb. For example, the pronoun *I* is irrelevant and can be used with any tense. If the child is taught to use the form *Yesterday, I . . .* , *Last week, I . . .* , and *In the past, I . . .* , the resultant incorrect hypothesis might be "In the presence of *I*, use the past tense."

Knowledge of both the relevant and irrelevant aspects of the context is essential for learning. A child needs to learn those cases in which the target language feature is required and those in which it is not.

Initially, teaching should limit irrelevant dimensions so as not to confuse the child. For example, the child first may learn to use regular past tense with *yesterday*. Such words as *today* do not signal the tense as clearly and should be introduced later. Gradually, more irrelevant dimensions, such as longer sentences, can be introduced.

When a particular syntactic form or function is being targeted, it is especially important to select content words or utterances already in the child's repertoire. In this way, the SLP is changing only one thing at a time, past tense *-ed*. With the targeting and introduction of new words, an SLP should also select familiar structures. In the reverse, new language structures, such as question verb–noun reversals as in *can he*, should be taught with familiar words. This principle stated succinctly is "new forms–old content/old forms–new content."

Processing constraints are the limited capacity of the brain to process information. When these boundaries are reached, trade-offs occur. For example, children omit more grammatical markers in longer, more complex sentences than in shorter, less complex ones. Children with language disorders are particularly susceptible to these constraints because linguistic processing uses more capacity than it does for children with TDL. Teaching items that exceed the information-processing constraints of these children may result in inadequate learning and poor generalization.

Often, a language feature fails to generalize because a child has not learned the conditions that govern its use. For example, if a child learns only by imitation, they internalize the variables that affect imitation, not the variables found in conversation. In order for a behavior to generalize to another context, such as conversation, teaching should include variables found in that context.

Because some children with language disorders may lack metalinguistic awareness or the ability to consider language out of context, rule explanation is not a viable clinical tool for their learning. As a result, an SLP must structure the environment so that linguistic regularities are obvious.

Contrast teaching is one method of overcoming generalization problems. In **contrast teaching**, a child learns those structures and situations that obligate use from those that do not. For example, use of the third-person *-s* marker is required with singular nouns and third-person singular pronouns. A child must recognize also that plural nouns and other pronouns do not require this marker.

Conversational use requires recognition of contexts within which the target does or does not appear. Using several different contexts, both linguistic and nonlinguistic, ensures that a child does not misidentify linguistic variables nor assume that the SLP and the therapy setting are the only contexts in which the target is to be used.

CHAPTER 9 A FUNCTIONAL INTERVENTION MODEL

Ideally, functional teaching uses multiple examples, such as the several categories of linguistic responses or teaching items, several teachers, and several settings. These features are essential for generalization.

Method of Teaching

Language is a set of rules that allow a person to use language features in different communication contexts to express varied intentions. A rule is an abstraction that describes language similarities. If language is a rule-governed social tool, then the goal of intervention should be to use these rules to participate in social communication.

> **Food for Thought:** If language is a social tool, how does that affect ways in which an SLP might teach it?

The most effective intervention approach for older school-age children and adolescents with deficits in language form is an integrated one in which naturalistic stimulation approaches are supplemented by deductive teaching procedures. In a deductive method, children are presented with a rule guiding the use of a morphological inflection or marker along with models of use (Finestack & Fey, 2009). Although this statement would seem to fly in the face of functional approaches outlined in this text, this is not the case.

Strict stimulation-only approaches occur in natural contexts all the time, but a child is usually unaware of the language feature and is not required to respond. Stimulation is much more open-ended than the functional intervention we'll be discussing in which an SLP can engage a school-age child's metacognitive abilities in the learning process by helping the child become conscious of the intervention target and informing them of the principles and patterns underlying the target. Rules can then be deduced from the SLP's specific examples and from actual use by the child.

It is not practical for most children and most intervention targets for the SLP simply to explain the language rule being taught. Instead, teaching consists of the rule being applied within situations that contrast the critical conditions that apply to the rule. For example, try to imagine teaching regular past tense to a child as follows:

When a verb is used in the past tense, an *-ed*, pronounced as /t/, /d/, or /əd/, is added to it to produce a past tense verb, as in *walk/walked*.

Instead, we might teach regular past tense in the following manner:

Every day I *walk*, yesterday I *walked*.

Every day we *talk*, yesterday we *talked*.

The word *yesterday* tells us to add the /t/ sound. Now you try it. I'll start.

Every day I walk, yesterday I _____..

Good. Let's try again. Every day they rake, yesterday they _____.

I know you walk to school every day. Tell me about yesterday.

An SLP can provide organized language data to a child as an illustration of rule use. Thus, the child would be presented with paired minimally different situations that do and do not invoke the rule. Then the child can be asked to apply the rule. For example, pronoun use might be contrasted with noun use.

SLP: We're going to play imagination. Try to find the picture. I'm thinking about a ghost. Which ghost? He has a big nose. Wow, you found that really fast. Okay, you think of something else.

Child: Blue eyes.

SLP: I don't know what you're talking about. What's the name of it?

Child: A doll.

SLP: Um-hm. What about the doll?

Child: It has blue eyes.

SLP: I found the doll and it has blue eyes. It's easy when I know what you're talking about. Try another. I'm thinking . . . .

Child: Thinking of a dinosaur. He's got sharp teeth.

SLP: Oh, I know which dinosaur has the sharp teeth. This one. I know that you have a new pet. Tell me about your pet.

By presenting these contrasting situations and encouraging the child to practice, the SLP helps the child assemble the data necessary to identify the critical elements of the rule. Once the child is aware of the critical elements, the SLP has the flexibility to present these elements in any communication situation, such as talking about a pet.

The strength of the rule-teaching approach is in the way it simplifies the learning task by condensing relevant input and highlighting critical conditions. Abstract grammatical rules are difficult for children with language disorders to learn directly.

Functional techniques are more effective than stimulation alone because they incorporate behavioral principles and also use the context of naturally occurring conversations that can be modified systematically by the language teacher. In addition, functional techniques are not simply presenting a stimulus and reinforcing the correct answer. For example, the following exchange might occur with a child for whom we have targeted future tense:

SLP: That sounded like fun. What about tomorrow?

Child: Zoo?

SLP: What about the zoo?

Child:	Go zoo.
SLP:	Now?
Child:	Go zoo tomorrow?
SLP:	You will? Maybe I can go. Sure, I WILL. What about you? Tomorrow you . . .
Child:	**Will** go zoo.
SLP:	Yeah. Tomorrow you **will** go to the zoo. I love the zoo. I wonder what **will** happen there.

Generalization is more likely than with more structured drill-like approaches because the cues used resemble the varied ones found in real communication events. In addition, the child's attention is focused on a topic while receiving linguistic input about that topic.

A functional model provides a dynamic context for teaching language. Language teaching that works for a child in real communication events should generalize to those events. The focus should not be merely the correctness of a child's language but also its communicative potential.

In general, functional intervention in combination with more structured remediation facilitates both acquisition and generalization of language targets to usage within natural environments. The functional approach involves

- selecting appropriate language targets for a child and environment;
- arranging the environment to increase the likelihood that a child will initiate;
- responding to a child's initiations with requests for elaboration of the target forms;
- reinforcing a child's attempts with attention and access to objects in which the child has expressed interest; and
- attempting to have the child respond in a similar manner.

Interactions between adults and children arise naturally in situations, such as play, and can be manipulated systematically by the adult to give the child practice in communication.

A child signals a potential topic by demonstrating interest or requesting assistance. The child's topic provides an opportunity for the adult to teach the language target. The child is more likely to talk and be more interested in the content of this talk if the topic has been established by the child.

Within these communication contexts, an SLP models the responses that fulfill a child's communication goals. Because the purpose of language is established in the environment, form and content may be learned more easily. In short, the child is taught a more effective way to communicate within a particular context. The SLP also models behaviors for the caregivers in order to facilitate teaching and increase the likelihood that natural situations will occur in which the child is successful.

When the desired interactions do not occur, the SLP can manipulate the environment to enhance its language-teaching potential. Both linguistic and nonlinguistic aspects of the context can be altered to elicit the desired communication. We'll discuss how to do that in Chapter 10.

Activities can be planned around communication contexts that are highly likely to occur for the child. Teaching for the child's typical environment and tasks should be as close to that environment in materials, situations, and persons as possible. Activities can include a child's usual reasons for talking and typical topics, can rely on previous experiences and introduce new ones, can use familiar focuses of communication, and, when possible, can include the child's natural communication partners.

Each child's individual learning or cognitive style also must be considered by an SLP. Children are most comfortable with new experiences and information presented in a manner consistent with that style.

By considering why and how children use words and gestures, you can increase your ability to provide the most natural and optimal situations for eliciting and teaching communication. The combination of appropriate context and specifically targeted language features facilitates maximum carryover and generalization outside the clinical environment.

There's a general consensus that generalization is less difficult than initial learning. An SLP can aid this process by following another principle cited by Kamhi (2014), which states that *varied learning and practice conditions are more efficient than constant and predictable instruction*. In other words, the more we consciously try to bring in the variable real world, the easier generalization becomes—something we established in Chapter 1.

Conversation, by its nature, is variable and unpredictable. A language skill learned in this environment should transfer well to different conversational contexts (E. Bjork, 2004). Succinctly stated, changes in the instructional context enhance learning. In this way, newly learned skills are linking to a range of contextual cues (R. Bjork, 2011). Thus, long-term learning and transfer to novel contexts is enhanced when the conditions of instruction and practice are varied.

Language Teachers

If the goal is language use within a child's everyday contexts, then a lone SLP working only in a clinical setting is limited as to what they can accomplish. The brevity of child–SLP contact necessitates the use of a wider variety of social contexts, including various communication partners. These partners supply a strong social base for intervention, providing a reason for language use.

The appropriate partners to be used in teaching will vary with the age and circumstance of the child. Whereas parents may be appropriate for preschool children, they may have more limited interaction with their school-age children, for whom teachers and peers may be more effectual. Successful use of the language taught in intervention programs depends, in part, on the expectations of these significant others in the child's environment.

Among aided augmentative and alternative communication (AAC) users, intervention can focus on using their device within peer interactions. For children with complex communication needs, the most frequently reported intervention components are the use of AAC within social interactions with peers who've been taught to promote interaction (Therrien et al., 2016).

Peer intervention, including peer mediation and direct instruction, can be an effective way to focus on social interaction with kindergarten and first-grade children with ASD (Kamps et al., 2015). Children with ASD display significantly more initiations to peers, have significant growth for total communications, and show more growth in language and adaptive communication compared to children not in peer-mediated interactions. In addition, teachers' ratings of children's prosocial skills reveal significant improvements.

Peer social groups can be used to teach social and communication skills through games and table play activities, such as card and board games. Intervention interactions with typical peers can provide multiple practice opportunities to improve reciprocal social communication.

Specific skills taught in these groups could include (Kamps et al., 2015)

- requests and shares ("Ask and share");
- comments about one's own play activities or actions ("Tell about my toys");
- comments about peers' play activities or actions ("Tell about friends' toys");
- social niceties, such as *please*, *thank-you*, and giving compliments ("Talk nice"); and
- play organizers, such as giving ideas about setting up games and rules ("Ways to play").

Peer group sessions might last for 25 to 30 minutes three times per week. Within these peer sessions, children's language can be prompted by adults.

Parents can be successful language teachers with their children. Most success has been reported for children in early stages of language and cognitive development. For example, parents of children with ASD have been taught to provide intervention services within the daily routines of their preschool children at home (Kashinath et al., 2006).

Without intervention, it is often difficult for toddlers with language disorders and their parents to establish mutually rewarding interactional patterns. Such children are less likely to succeed in a preschool setting. Their experience level and their success in communicative interaction are often minimal, and they may exhibit poor listening skills. Children who are not successful in communication often become resistant or negative and develop attention-getting behaviors.

A child must have the opportunity to communicate; thus, a teacher must be attentive and responsive. A teacher must consistently recognize a child's attempts to communicate and provide appropriate responses. Parents need to be taught more than just modeling language, and their progress as teachers should be monitored.

Communication partners, such as teachers and parents, can be an effective part of an intervention team if they are trained and monitored thoroughly. An adult must be trained in both

- the how, or the best teaching techniques; and
- the what, or the goals and materials for intervention.

Training of adults can be accomplished in a combination of ways, including direct teaching and modeling, in-service teaching, and the use of telephoned and written/illustrated instructions.

To provide effective intervention services at home, parents and caregivers need realistic input from you as the SLP. For example, teaching might include user-friendly written handouts explaining the teaching strategy and/or target, videorecorded and live demonstrations, practice and critique, and discussion.

Caregiver Conversational Style

The difficulties experienced by children with language disorders reflect their everyday contexts as much as their so-called disorder. If this is so, then conversational partners must assume some of the responsibility for the communication of these children. For example, although adult interaction-promoting strategies, such as extended conversations and questions to promote turn taking, are positively related to language productivity in preschool children, adults in child care centers are more responsive to the context of interactions than to the language abilities of a child (Girolametto & Weitzman, 2002).

If we want change to occur, we need to change these adult behaviors. The quality and quantity of spontaneous conversational behavior of children with language disorders are negatively related to the number of verbal initiations and directives by their adult conversational partners.

In response to children's language deficits, adults modify their own language. Mothers of children with language disorders repeat more than do mothers of children with TDL. Most of these maternal repetitions are imperatives (demands) or directives (commands). The frequency of these parental directions and self-imitations is negatively correlated with the rate of a child's language growth. In a highly directive interaction style, there is often no connection between the directive and any utterance of the child.

Adult verbal control of interactions also seems to adversely affect the verbal output of children. For example, although the question–answer style of adult communication may help children maintain a conversational topic, it can discourage children from commenting outside the topics initiated by the adults and is counterproductive to the goal of spontaneous conversational behavior by the child.

Adult directive style includes verbal conversational behaviors that

- control and initiate conversational topics;
- lead the conversation; and
- structure the nature of the child's contribution.

These behaviors ensure a cohesive and fluent conversation at the expense of the child's spontaneous initiations.

Food for Thought: Do you like being told what to do all the time? That's a directive style. How about a child? What might a child prefer?

CHAPTER 9 A FUNCTIONAL INTERVENTION MODEL

In contrast, the use of an adult facilitative style of conversation can increase the use of topic initiations, questions, and topic comments by children with language disorders. Adult facilitative style

- allows a child to control and initiate conversational topics;
- follows a child's conversational lead; and
- encourages a child to participate in various ways.

A facilitative adult is less interested in conversational flow than in providing an opportunity for a child to participate and to assume control of the conversation. Specific behaviors that define each style are given in Table 9–2.

As has been mentioned several times throughout this text, following the child's attentional and conversational lead is an effective clinical tool. For example, parental utterances that follow a child's current focus of attention or respond to a child's verbal communication facilitate the process of vocabulary acquisition. For children with ASD, following the child's lead mitigates the need to use attention-following of others as a word-learning strategy (McDuffie & Yoder, 2010).

Mothers who receive training in facilitative techniques are more responsive to and less directive of their children's behavior than are untrained mothers. These changes in parental behavior are related to child language changes, such as increased mean length of utterance in morphemes (MLU_M), increased number of utterances, increased lexicon, and improved standardized test scores. Children whose parents receive training initiate more topics, are more responsive, use more verbal turns, and have a more diverse vocabulary. For example, in a twice-weekly 1-hour social interaction–based intervention for

Table 9–2. Characteristics of the Directive and Facilitative Styles

Directive	Facilitative
Initiate at least half of the topics of conversation.	Initiate fewer than half of the topics of conversation.
Use direct questions to initiate most topics.	Use indirect questions or embedded imperatives to initiate most topics.
Use primarily direct questions and occasional imitations or expansions to maintain topics.	Use primarily direct statements, encouragements, imitations, expansions, or expansion questions and occasional direct questions to maintain topics.
Do not ask for clarification directly, relying instead on encouragement, imitation, and expansion strategies.	Use direct clarification questions or statements when necessary and appropriate.
Do not allow lapses in turn taking to occur, but use direct questions to require the child to respond.	Allow lapses between turns to occur, and after a short wait, initiate topics as noted above.

children with ASD, preschool children made significantly greater gains in social interaction skills compared to children in more traditional models of intervention (Casenhiser et al., 2015).

Following a 12-week Developmental Reciprocity Treatment parent-teaching program, including introduction to developmental approaches, imitation and building nonverbal communication, functional language development, and turn taking, parents reported improved social quality of life (Gengoux et al., 2019). Their children with ASD improved in core autism symptoms and in number of words produced.

An increase in the percentage of semantically related or contingent utterances can, in turn, provide greater opportunity for topic maintenance and turn taking. With more opportunity to participate, the child gains more control over both the adult's behavior and the exchange process.

Children's spontaneous verbalizations can be enhanced when adult teachers provide a high level of verbal feedback coupled with little verbal directing. Examples are given in Table 9–3. Data from several studies suggest that children's conversational abilities can be increased by adult behaviors that are highly responsive to a children's spontaneous communicative behaviors. Best results seem to occur when teachers receive frequent, regular, structured training, including role-playing and critiques.

Shared or dialogic reading can also improve children's language. Similarly, dialogic book reading can be an effective way to elicit some language structures, such as bound morphemes (see Appendix D) (Maul & Ambler, 2014). The fundamental reading technique in dialogic reading can be summarized by the acronym PEER:

- Prompt the child to say something about the story.
- Evaluate the child's response.
- Expand the child's response by rephrasing and/or adding new information.
- Repeat the prompt to ensure the child has learned from the expansion.

Table 9–3. Examples of Minimally Directive Verbal Feedback to Children
Child: I went to the zoo, yesterday. *Partner:* Oh, that's one of my favorite spots. I love the monkeys best.
Child: I have a birthday party, tomorrow. *Partner:* Oh, that should be fun. What do you want for your birthday?
Child: We went whale watching on vacation. *Partner:* I've always wanted to do that. Bet it was exciting. Tell me about it.
Child: My picture is a cowboy. *Partner:* A big cowboy on a spotted horse.
Child: I'm gonna be a ghost for Halloween. *Partner:* Don't come to my house; I'm afraid of ghosts. I think I'll be a witch and scare your ghost.

Note: In each of these five exchanges, the adult followed the child's lead by commenting on the child's topic and then cueing the child to provide more information or waiting for a reply.

Imagine that the parent and the child are looking at the page of a book:

The parent says, "What happened?" (Prompt) while pointing to the book.

The child says, "Boy falled," and the parent might follow with "Boy falled? That doesn't sound right." (Evaluation)

The parent replies, "The boy fell off his bike." (Expansion)

The parent follows, "What did he do?" (Repetition)

It is feasible even for parents in dire economic situations to participate in and benefit from language-based group intervention with their children while residing in family homeless shelters. Despite the many demands made on and restrictions faced by mothers and children who are homeless, parents—even those with limited language skills—can be taught to use facilitating language strategies during interactions with their preschool children in shelters (O'Neil-Pirozzi, 2009).

Children living in shelters can show positive language growth when parents received as little as four 90-minute small-group program sessions, held weekly over the course of 4 weeks (O'Neil-Pirozzi, 2009). Attendance by parents can be increased if teaching sessions are offered at a convenient time and place and by providing child care and light refreshments.

Intervention may empower homeless parents' sense of self-worth and foster strong, positive parent–child bonds during a time of family instability. Given the temporary nature of shelter living, intervention should be as brief and convenient as possible, while maximizing effectiveness by teaching across multiple contexts (Dickinson & Tabors, 2001; Tabors et al., 2001).

Among families with low-SES backgrounds, promising language improvements have been reported for parental shared book reading (Colmar, 2014). Parents are taught easy-to-learn strategies for reading and talking in everyday conversations, such as pausing and encouraging the child to talk more and following a child's conversational lead. These simple changes in the way parents had previously interacted with their kindergarten children positively affect the children's language.

The results of a meta-analysis of 18 studies of parent-implemented language interventions with preschool children found all these approaches to be effective (Roberts & Kaiser, 2011). Parent-implemented language interventions have a significant, positive impact on both receptive language and expressive syntactic skills. Parent teaching has a positive effect on parent–child interaction style in terms of responsiveness, use of language models, and rate of communication. Parents who receive parent training are significantly more responsive than those who do not. Unfortunately, without specifics on parent teaching and its actual implementation, it is difficult to determine what specific parent teaching works best.

Families and Children From Culturally Linguistically Diverse Backgrounds

Although families within the same culture differ, recognition of cultural contributions by an SLP increases the likelihood of appropriate and effective intervention. Table 9–4 presents guidelines for SLPs to follow when interacting with culturally diverse families.

Table 9–4. Guidelines for Interacting With Culturally Diverse Families

Do not make assumptions based on cultural stereotypes.
Cultural rules govern each encounter for both the family/child and the speech-language pathologist. Be aware that responses to stimuli, such as a clinic room, may be very different across cultures.
Learn about the cultures of the families and the children you serve.
Use cultural mediators or interpreters when necessary.
Learn to use words, phrases, and greetings from the culture of the family/child.
Be patient; allow more time for interactions. Use as few written instructions as possible, unless a family member has good English reading comprehension. Allow time for questions.
Recognize that the family may not be prepared for the amount of professional–family collaboration found in functional approaches.
Encourage family input without embarrassing family members. Involve the family to the extent that they wish to be involved.
Ensure that goals and objectives of the professionals and the family match.
Involve the cultural community when possible.

Source: Information from Lynch and Hanson (2004) and Wayman et al. (1990).

As an SLP, you should be mindful of the differing expectations and perceptions of various ethnic and racial identities. The role of parents and caregivers, the expectations for children, and the attitudes toward disability, medicine, healing, self-help, and professional intervention within a minority population should be understood thoroughly prior to intervention. For example, mothers from Puerto Rico who live on the mainland seem to hold beliefs about early education and literacy that reflect both their original culture and also more North American notions (Hammer, Rodriguez, et al., 2007). Children and professional intervention services are viewed quite differently across Asian, Latino, and African American cultures.

Likewise, an SLP's conversational style may have a great effect on future involvement with members of that community. Successful SLP–family collaboration should be characterized by mutual respect, trust, and open communication.

Although I have tried to make the teaching techniques mentioned in Chapter 11 culture-free, the model of intervention proposed in this text is based primarily on North American psycholinguistic research of White, middle-class families and, therefore, contains an implicit, if unintended, cultural bias. When we ask mothers to use these techniques at home, we need to be very sensitive to cultural differences that define how parent–child interactions occur (Johnston & Wong, 2002).

An SLP must determine these cultural belief systems and modify intervention techniques accordingly. Otherwise, intervention may be less effective, or worse, parents may actively resist intervention efforts.

Information can be gleaned from reading research studies, talking with community representatives, and working closely with parents. Nothing beats getting involved with the cultural community, attending religious services, clubs, and festivals, and talking with and listening to parents, caregivers, and community members.

Once you enter someone else's culture, many of your assumptions must be set aside. Even when things seem similar, they may not be. Let's use Chinese culture as an example and explore the implications for intervention (Johnston & Wong, 2002). Based on research literature, we can make the following broad characterizations of Chinese cultural beliefs:

- The ideal self is embedded in interdependent social relations, requiring obedience and respect of others over self-fulfillment and independence.

- Human behavior is very malleable rather than biologically based.

- When a child goes to school, they pass from a period of nonunderstanding to one of understanding in which the child can be expected to succeed.

As a result, caregivers are less likely to join preschool children in play or to engage them in social communication. Instead, parents are more directive, focusing or refocusing a child's attention.

These beliefs impact intervention in myriad ways. For example, a parent may not understand our insistence on the importance of early intervention. Any discussion of this topic must include the importance of early intervention for later success in school, a Chinese cultural value.

Similarly, the notion of following a child's lead does not flow naturally from beliefs in interdependence and respect for elders. It might be better to help Chinese mothers construct more formal teaching lessons to be used several times each day within the home (Johnston & Wong, 2002). Note that the use of the home environment still retains the basic functional nature of intervention.

Given differences in cultural beliefs, there are likely to be occasions when well-intentioned intervention recommendations run counter to cultural expectations of the family you serve. To be successful, an SLP must find "functional equivalents" that achieve the same ends (Johnston & Wong, 2002). For example, parents of a young child with a language disorder are often encouraged to engage in book-sharing activities. The goal of social communication rather than book reading per se may be unfamiliar to some families. Other methods can be found that attain the same goal while being more culturally appropriate to the child and family, such as oral storytelling.

Language is one of the primary modes of socialization and acculturation for children. When a child learns English in an English-intensive educational program, they are in danger of losing their heritage language. This may be especially true for children with language disorders who receive remedial intervention for English but no help with their initial language. Given the interdependence of emotional, cognitive, and communication development in young children and the needs these children have for family support, it is important that SLPs also support the home language of these children (Kohnert et al., 2005). This does not necessitate intervention in both languages.

Potentially, well-trained parents can be as effective as SLPs in administering intervention in the heritage language (Law et al., 2004). As mentioned previously, an SLP can directly teach a parent to become the primary intervention agent for their child. Successful caregiver teaching requires the following:

- Specific language facilitation strategies versus general stimulation
- Use of multiple sessions and instructional methods with parents
- Systematic progression of skills
- Activities tailored for the individual child

Rather than suggest that parents cease using one language at home—a huge imposition, especially for families that freely mix languages—it seems best to target activities, such as book reading, in which one language would be used exclusively. Where necessary, it may be helpful to use paraprofessionals from the language community or siblings as in-home teachers.

Preschool Teachers

The language of preschool children exposed to early deprivation and trauma improves with high-quality early care and education programs, such as preschool and Head Start, compared to similar maltreated children who are not enrolled in these types of programs (Merritt & Klein, 2015). In addition, there is a positive correlation between these programs and lower caregiver neglect.

High-quality preschool language experiences are especially important for children from disadvantaged backgrounds and those at risk for language disorders (Dickinson & Tabors, 2001; Hubbs-Tait et al., 2002). Unfortunately, many preschool classrooms, especially those serving children from low-SES backgrounds, do not provide an optimum environment for facilitating children's language skills (Dickinson et al., 2008; Justice et al., 2008). Teachers may provide little explicit facilitation of children's language skills through use of questioning, modeling, and recasting. In turn, young children may have limited opportunity for multi-turn conversations with their teachers (Justice et al., 2008).

Unfortunately, EBP provides little guidance on how to achieve higher quality language instruction in preschools short of intensity-sustained levels of interaction that may lack feasibility for real-world settings. One promising approach, teaching preschool educators to be more conversationally responsive to children within the classroom setting, benefits children's language, especially vocabulary, and literacy development, especially print-concept knowledge, but requires further study (Cabell et al., 2011). It is not surprising, given their better overall language skills, that children of high and high-average language ability seem to benefit most.

Responsivity education attempts to increase adults' capacity to be conversationally responsive partners with children and to promote reciprocal interactions that support children's active participation in an exchange. Adults promote reciprocity by smiling and maintaining eye contact, consistently responding to children's communication efforts

CHAPTER 9 A FUNCTIONAL INTERVENTION MODEL

and recasting or expanding a child's productions, cueing a child to take another turn, using a slow pace so as to not dominate, and asking open-ended questions (Girolametto & Weitzman, 2002; Yoder & Warren, 2002).

Teaching Cues

If you accept the premise that pragmatics is the governing aspect of language, then as an SLP, you should be concerned with the context within which teaching occurs. Certain linguistic and nonlinguistic contexts require or provide an expectation of certain linguistic units.

In part, the problem of lack of success in generalization is due to response programs in which children are taught specific responses to specific cues. A child's everyday world lacks this careful control. The everyday context contains many irrelevant stimuli that do not and cannot elicit communication behaviors taught with specific cues.

At the same time, without training, caregivers and teachers may be presenting cues and prompts in such a diverse manner as to inhibit learning. They can be taught to focus their attention and to manipulate the environment to elicit the behaviors desired and then to broaden the communication prompts.

Often, traditional approaches rely on very narrow and somewhat stilted cues unlike those found in conversation. The use of these traditional cues, such as "Tell me the whole thing," may result in teaching characterized as "apragmatic pseudoconversational drills" (Cochrane, 1983). Pragmatically, the cues may not make sense. As a result, the conversations within which teaching occurs are little more than drill with a conversational veneer.

Verbal and nonverbal cues can be varied to ensure that the child does not become dependent on one stereotypic stimulus. A **system of least prompts** can be used, in which an SLP rates each type of prompt from least to most intrusive and supportive (Timler et al., 2007). Through the course of intervention, the SLP works to minimize prompting whenever possible and to allow the context to prompt the targeted language features. For example, children with ASD can be taught to initiate requests and to make comments through a system of decreasing prompts, moving from sentence completion ("Can I . . . ") through answering ("What could you ask your friend?") (Thiemann & Goldstein, 2004).

Relevant, common stimuli within the everyday communication context can serve to elicit a child's new language targets if these stimuli are included in the teaching. Targets can be taught across several behaviors, teachers, and settings to ensure generalization. The overall goals are for the newly trained behavior to be emitted in response to a variety of stimuli and for a single stimulus to result in a variety of responses. These goals can be achieved by using contrast teaching, response variations, and linguistic and nonlinguistic cue variations. With *contrast teaching*, mentioned previously, relevant and irrelevant stimuli are presented together so that a child learns which ones affect the newly learned behavior.

Response variation teaches a child that several responses can be used to achieve the same communication goal. For example, a drink can be attained by saying "Want drink," "Drink please," "May I have a drink?" "I'm thirsty," and "Are you as thirsty as I am?"

Contingencies

Once a child has produced language, the adult teacher can begin to modify that language if necessary. In short, the child's utterance is the stimulus to which the adult responds. These responses or contingencies help form the context for the child's utterance.

You may recall from your language development course that maternal responsivity, characterized by positive responses to child communication initiations, is important for early communication and language development (Owens, 2020). For children with fragile X syndrome, caregiver responsivity continues to have a significant effect on receptive vocabulary, expressive vocabulary, and the rate of different words children produce through age 9 years (Brady et al., 2014). Thus, maternal responsivity remains a potential target for language intervention beyond preschool.

Natural maintaining consequences should be identified prior to beginning teaching. As much as possible, these consequences should be related directly to the response. Such consequences as "Very good" and "Good talking" should be avoided. When a child message ("I saw monkeys") and the consequence ("Good talking") are unrelated both semantically and pragmatically, the child's language fails to retain its communicative value. Communication behaviors can be maintained by conversational responses ("Oh, I think monkeys are funny. What did they do?"). Often, simply attending to a child is sufficient to maintain the child's participation.

Conversational replies as reinforcers? Who knew? Kendra, the SLP from the beginning of this chapter, had learned in her classes that saying "Good talking" told a child what they did correctly. But over time, it sounded empty and meaningless.

In addition, use of phrases such as "Good talking" to evaluate every language production disrupts the flow of the conversational interaction. The repetitive nature of theses phrases also may cause a child to stop paying attention to the feedback.

> ***Food for Thought:*** Do you sometimes get tired of the ways things are said. Watch any TV cop show and you'll hear "We're so sorry for your loss." Every drop of sincerity has been drained. What about our old favorite, "Good talking"?

As much as possible, conversational consequences should be semantically and pragmatically contingent and should serve to acknowledge a child's utterance. Semantic contingency, the relatedness of a parent's or teacher's response to the content or topic of a child's previous utterance, has a positive effect on the rate of language development. In the previous example, "I think monkeys are funny," the adult response is semantically contingent.

Adult speech that is semantically contingent decreases the amount of processing a child has to do to understand and analyze the structure and meaning of an adult's utter-

CHAPTER 9 A FUNCTIONAL INTERVENTION MODEL

ances. The sharing of a conversational topic and common vocabulary decreases a child's memory load. The adult's utterance provides a prop or scaffolding for the child's own analysis and subsequent production. For children with expressive vocabulary delays, the semantic contingency of adult responses has more effect on a child's language than does the structure of the adult response. In contrast, frequent topic changing or refocusing of a child's attention by an adult impedes the child's language acquisition.

It is not enough, however, just to comment on a child's topic. In the following example, the teacher's response is semantically contingent but lacks pragmatic contingency:

Child: I want cookie, please.

Teacher: Johnny wants a cookie.

The teacher's response should make pragmatic sense within the conversational framework. In this example, more appropriate responses might be "What kind of cookie do you want?" "Okay, but just one," "Help yourself," and "No cookies until after lunch." This example shows why contingencies such as "Good talking" violate **pragmatic contingency** and do not help continue the interchange. A child's language is reinforced more naturally when its purpose and intention are met.

The SLP can recast a sentence containing the target structure or can recast a sentence that does not contain the structure so that the recast will do so. In the first instance, the child says "Boy eating cookie," and the adult recasts "He is eating." In the second example, the child says "Boy cookie," and the adult recasts "The boy is eating the cookie." This can then be followed by a conversational reply that continues the exchange. Children with developmental language disorder (DLD) and low MLU_M benefit more from recasts following utterances in which the child is prompted to attempt the structure prior to the adult's recast (Yoder et al., 2011).

In brief, behaviors that attempt to increase a child's participation in the interaction —that is, a child-centered interactional style—enhance a child's language skills. By relinquishing some control and adopting the child's topics, language teachers can ensure more child participation and interest.

Overall, in the clinical setting it is important that adults accept a child's utterance as representative of the child's understanding of the world and of the requirements being asked. Answers considered wrong by the adult may, in fact, represent a child's somewhat different perspective. A child's meaning can be negotiated by the partner and child as the exchange continues.

Such child-centered language interventions are correlated with greater generalization gains in grammar for children with DLD than are therapist-directed methods (Yoder & McDuffie, 2002). Chapter 10 discusses both linguistic and nonlinguistic cues and responses in more detail.

Location

As noted in Chapter 1, location of teaching includes both the physical location in which teaching occurs and the conversational context formed by a child and an adult. In many ways, the conversational context is more important for generalization because it does

Physical Location

When possible, language teaching should occur wherever a child is likely to use the newly taught language feature or skill. Most communication takes place within familiar events that influence the way the participants communicate. Storytelling at home, conversation in the car, and classroom interactions all have different rules for participation. Therefore, language intervention should take place within these types of discourse events and others that occur in a child's everyday physical locations.

The everyday environment provides natural and familiar stimuli for intervention and for generalization. Children with lingering pragmatic deficits, such as those with TBI, are particularly in need of environmentally based intervention.

Obviously, adults will need to be taught their new roles as language teachers. Parents or caregivers may come to a clinic or school to be trained. If this is not possible, evening group sessions or written guidelines can be helpful. Even if caregivers only modify their expectations for their child, this change will help with the generalization.

Conversational Context

Language should be evaluated and taught within a dynamic context in order to make sense to the child. Language and communication are influenced heavily by the context of what precedes and follows both linguistically and nonlinguistically and by the expectations for participation within that context. Ordering at a fast-food restaurant presents different expectations from chatting with a friend on the phone. Each event follows certain scripts.

Sentences taught out of context are, therefore, more difficult for a child to learn. Ideally, SLPs are not teaching static forms but a generative, versatile system. The contextual expectations and scripts must be examined prior to beginning intervention within each context. Teaching approaches can be adapted to this setting to approximate more closely conversational exchange.

Conclusion

By carefully considering the variables that affect generalization, an SLP can modify teaching to maximize carryover. Targets and design decisions can be made on the basis of the likely effect on generalization and on ultimate use within the events and situations of a child's everyday environment. Language can be elicited and modified by using techniques that mirror the conversational style used by a child's usual partners within these contexts. Motivation is provided by a child's desire to participate in enjoyable activities with responsive and attentive adults.

The language context is crucial. For example, meta-analyses demonstrate that teaching working memory and controlled attention directly does not seem to have long-term effects, nor to generalize to other areas (Melby-Lervåg & Hulme, 2013; Randall & Tyldesley, 2016; Schwaighofer et al., 2015; Shipstead et al., 2016). A more beneficial approach is to use language in context to help a child with DLD acquire new ways to process language and organize long-term memory. Narrative recall may help a child "chunk" and organize information to aid comprehension (Gillam et al., 2018).

Within a conversational context, adults can adhere to the following guidelines:

- Expect the child to communicate.
- Respond to the child's topics and initiations.
- Respond conversationally and build the child's utterances into longer, more acceptable ones.
- Facilitate communication within the everyday activities of the child.
- Cue the child in a conversational manner to elicit the language desired.

All of these principles are discussed in Chapter 10.

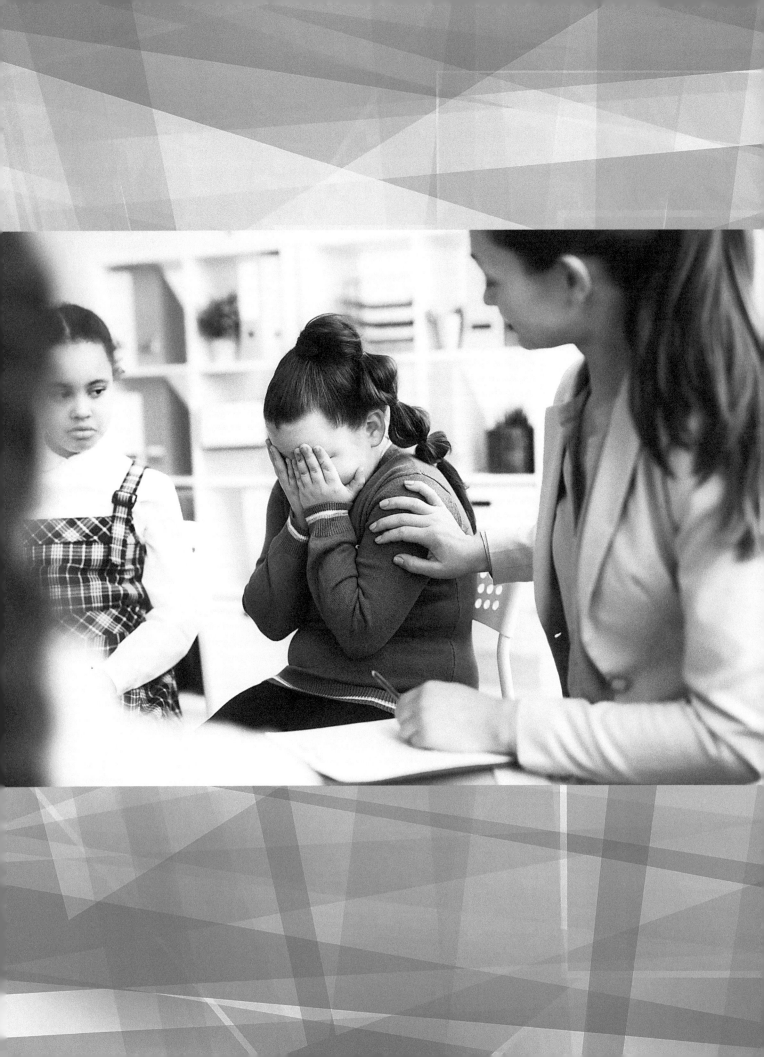

CHAPTER 10

MANIPULATING CONTEXT

According to his parents, Tad's language was appropriate for his age until about age 4 years. Up to that point, he had seemed quiet but his parents believed him to be at least as advanced as his sister. He deferred to her when in a communication situation. His grandmother even referred to him as "Tongue-tied Tad."

In a preschool classroom environment away from his sister, Tad's language was on center stage and his lack of language skill was in full view. His teacher recommended a language evaluation and with the parents' permission scheduled an assessment by a district speech-language pathologist (SLP), Ms. Ramirez.

After some observation and administering the Preschool Language Scale and selected subtests of the Clinical Evaluation of Language Fundamentals, Ms. Ramirez collected a language sample while Tad responded to a picture book. Ms. Ramirez reported that Tad was a very social child with several deficits in language form. His sentences were basic with little elaboration. Often, the form of his utterances mirrored what Ms. Ramirez had just said.

Ms. Ramirez recommended intervention and proposed a functional model that will include both his parents and the preschool teacher. She will teach them simple techniques for responding in a way that maximizes his chances to communicate and to hear targeted language structures being used. For now, caregivers will not require Tad to use the more complex syntax of the adults.

In contrast, Ms. Ramirez will provide models and require Tad to respond in a similar manner. Although she was initially concerned about his mirroring her language, she believes that this habit can be used to help him produce more mature complex language.

The demands of both the nonlinguistic and linguistic context give rise to both the form and content of the language we express. It would seem to follow, therefore, that a primary goal of language intervention would be for a child to learn the appropriate language skills to function effectively within everyday nonlinguistic and linguistic communication contexts.

Within each activity, an SLP or other language teacher can strive to provide an active experience along with language use. If the SLP and other language teachers learn to manipulate these experiential contexts, they can provide a child the maximum learning possible.

When language can be used to achieve goals within everyday communication contexts, the chances of generalization to these contexts increase. Language acquires a purpose or function, and thus, teaching becomes functional in nature.

386 LANGUAGE DISORDERS: A FUNCTIONAL APPROACH TO ASSESSMENT AND INTERVENTION IN CHILDREN

In this chapter, we explore various strategies that can be used to manipulate the nonlinguistic and linguistic contexts in which language occurs. These strategies can be used within the everyday activities of a child and, thus, can become a part of that natural environment. As much as possible, natural and conversational strategies can be used.

Nonlinguistic Contexts

The nonlinguistic context—what is happening in the environment—offers a rich source for eliciting language. As an SLP, you can manipulate the nonlinguistic contextual cues to elicit desired language and to ensure that a child initiates language.

Often, the teaching paradigm allows the child with a language disorder little control. Therefore, the child assumes a passive, responsive role that can inhibit learning.

Certain nonlinguistic contexts naturally elicit more language than do others. For most adults, cocktail parties are more likely to elicit language than are theater engagements. Some situations also dictate the type of language used. Most adults do not question and challenge sermons—at least not while the sermon is being delivered. In contrast, learning situations, such as in your classroom, are supposed to encourage questioning.

If targets have been selected to help a child communicate better, then, hopefully, the SLP already has identified the contexts in which the child attempts these targets. In other words, the nonlinguistic contexts that are highly likely to elicit the target are known.

Ideally, once the nonlinguistic context elicits the target language behavior, the SLP can help the child modify the target into a correct form for that situation. In theory—and this is key to our success—a child who makes a meaningful response in context will be interested in that response, will attend, and will be motivated to change it in the way desired by the SLP. This corrected response should generalize more easily to everyday use because it is being taught within the context of everyday events and conversations.

Table 10–1 contains a sample of nonlinguistic contexts and the type of language each may elicit. Small group projects or tasks usually elicit lots of language from children. For younger children, role-play and dress-up are good contexts for language. Routines, either current or newly learned, can be contexts for interaction within the home or the classroom.

Within these nonlinguistic contexts, language may be elicited through the use of delays, introduction of novel elements, oversight, and sabotage. Delaying or waiting for a child to initiate communication is often a very effective nonlinguistic strategy, especially after a child has demonstrated use of a language feature, even when incorrect.

Food for Thought: **Think of different child activities and opportunities in each for specific language targets. For example, game playing elicits turn taking.**

Let's assume that the language teacher is waiting for a child to initiate the interaction. The adult may sit near the child and look questioningly or display some interesting item while looking at the child. When the child looks at the adult, the adult does not speak

CHAPTER 10 MANIPULATING CONTEXT 387

Table 10–1. Nonlinguistic Contexts and Language Elicitation

Turn Taking and Requesting Objects

Provide only one plastic knife for children to share as they make a fruit salad.

Provide one highly desirable outfit in the dress-up corner of the class.

Provide only enough art supplies for half of the children and request that children share equipment.

Following Directions and Directing Others

While working in a group, re-create the teacher's construction-paper collage. The teacher should be careful not to supply precut paper or to help children with the color tints. The goal is to get the children to ask for help and to direct others and themselves.

In groups of two, duplicate a cake decoration previously completed by the teacher.

As a group, plant seeds in cups as the teacher has done previously. A more involved project might involve planting a garden, keeping the different crops straight, and making signs.

Bake while following a written or pictured recipe.

Put together a model by following written or oral directions.

Play dumb. By making lots of mistakes, the teacher can have children direct or correct the behavior.

Have a child explain how to do something known by only that child.

Have children direct each other through activities blindfolded.

Have the child be the teacher.

Requesting Information

Give only partial directions for completing a task.

Put objects that the children need for a task in an unusual location so that they will need to ask for the location.

Introduce visually interesting items but do not name them or explain their function to the children.

Giving Information

Have children explain class projects to children from another class.

Have children explain class projects to parents at a special event or Parents' Night.

Have children tell about events they experienced—for example, summer vacation, a weekend trip, a birthday party. This task and explaining how something is accomplished are excellent vehicles for sequencing.

Have children request information from children who need to improve their ability to give information.

Have children tell make-believe stories.

Reasoning

Have children try to float or submerge objects in water. Include objects that float and those that do not so that the children must find various combinations.

Build a suspension bridge from straws, string, toothpicks, and tongue depressors.

Design a city with transportation, schools, recreation facilities, and residential, industrial, and business areas.

continues

Table 10–1. *continued*

Reasoning *continued*

Play initiative games in which groups of children must solve a common problem.

Make large projects in connection with class projects. For example, children might design the "perfect" world; make montages that demonstrate male and female roles; or design a board game, such as On the Way to Your Birthday, that illustrates stages of fetal development.

Requesting Help

Pose problems that children cannot solve themselves.

Sabotage activities, such as holes in paper cups, dried markers and paints, glue bottles glued shut, not enough chairs, missing gloves and hats, and so on. The list is endless.

Imagining and Projecting

Set up a drama or dress-up center. Set up a puppet stage with a variety of characters.

Set up simulated shops and stores or a housekeeping center.

Role-play. (Role-play can elicit a variety of intentions.)

Protesting

Play dumb, as in forgetting to give children peanut butter and jelly with which to make sandwiches.

Miss a child's turn or withhold needed objects.

Violate a routine or an object function by using objects in novel or nonsensical ways.

Give a child too much of something or more than is needed.

Put away objects before the child is finished using them.

Ask a child to do something that is not physically possible (but safe).

Initiations

Pose problems and wait for children to initiate communication.

Ask children to talk to lonely animals for you.

---

for a specified period of time unless the child does. If the child does not verbalize, the adult may use a linguistic model or prompt to get the desired verbalization.

Novel or unexpected events can be introduced into a situation to evoke communication. Most individuals will notice and remark on such events. For example, a kitten, guinea pig, or bright toy might be found in an unexpected spot. Even children functioning at the single-word level will comment on elements in a situation that are novel, different, or changing.

Oversight or forgetting by an adult will elicit language from a child who's eager to become the teacher themself. I often play dumb, forgetting object locations or children's turns. Needed objects, such as glue or scissors, can be omitted or used by the teacher in unusual ways to prompt a reaction by the child.

Finally, sabotage of activities or routines involves taking actions or introducing elements that will not permit the activity to continue or to be completed. My favorite example is the classroom teacher and aide who would buckle the children's boots together and turn their coats inside out sometime during the day. One can imagine the chaos at the end of the day and all of the language elicited as children requested assistance.

Linguistic Contexts

In the following sections of this chapter, we explore myriad approaches to eliciting and modifying children's language. Although this text stresses a functional approach, that model of intervention has several aspects. Nor is it always appropriate to rely exclusively on only a single intervention approach. At times, a child needs more direct instruction. Let's briefly explore explicit instruction before moving to other strategies.

Exposure to Grammatical Targets

The professional literature identifies three approaches to the exposure of grammatical targets to children with language disorders. Let's briefly investigate each approach and see what it has to offer to a conversational approach. For a more detailed discussion, see the fine in-depth article by Leonard and Deevy (2017), from which much of the following discussion has been taken.

The Input Informativeness Approach

Development of children with typically developing language (TDL) can be gauged across languages by the degree to which overt forms are available in the input heard by children. For example, in English, children hear not only forms with overt markers (e.g., *He walks the dog twice a day*) but also unmarked forms (e.g., *I/you/we/they walk the dog twice a day*; *Can he walk*) and irregular forms. In general, the more overtly marked forms in parents' speech, the earlier a child with TDL will develop productive use of these forms (Hadley et al., 2011). The feasibility of this procedure in intervention has been demonstrated in a procedure called *toy talk*, in which overtly marked forms are used repeatedly within a play situation (i.e., *The doll eats ice cream*; *The puppy jumps on the sofa*) (Hadley & Walsh, 2014). Toy talk is easy to implement. Parents and others are encouraged to comment about the actions of toys that are the focus of play, emphasizing the overt forms used.

The informativeness of overt marking through procedures such as toy talk can provide optimal input for children with language disorders. In addition, the procedure is readily transferred to other contexts, making it very functional. Ideally, because this methodology can be used within real conversations, children receiving this overt input will gain knowledge not only of the individual morphemes but also of the concept behind each form.

The Competing Sources of Input Approach

When English-speaking children make morphological errors, the most frequent errors are omissions. These omissions may not be as simple as this statement implies. For example, *he/she/it* requires the third person *-s* marker. In contrast, *him/her* does not. In a child's defense, adult input may include *Help her make cookies* or *We saw her make cookies* from which a child might be easily confused. Thus, a child's omission may occur in the form of *Her make cookies*.

In studies with novel or invented verbs, children produced the novel verb in a way that was highly consistent with how they heard the verb being produced by the adults (Finneran & Leonard, 2010; Theakston et al., 2003). In addition, there is a correlation between the proportion of young children's errors, such as *Me make it*, and the proportion of sentences in the input with the same sequence (e.g., *Let me make it*) (Kirjavainen et al., 2009).

With the past tense *-ed* marker, use is also inconsistent. Irregular past tense forms are common, and in negatives and questions the past tense marker is often subsumed in the auxiliary verb, as in *He didn't jump on the trampoline yesterday* or *Didn't you play with her yesterday?*

Children with DLD/SLI are more likely than younger and older peers with TDL to use a novel verb consistent with how they heard it presented by adults (Leonard & Deevy, 2011; Leonard et al., 2015). Sentence comprehension difficulties of children with DLD may pose a special problem when sentences require integration of new information. The SLP can simplify sentences that contain the new structure.

These data suggest that an SLP needs to be concerned not only with the frequent presentation of morphemes but also with avoidance of certain input utterances. Such an approach may work initially, but at some point, a child with a language disorder also needs to be able to interpret utterances that seem counter to the language rule. An alternative would be to explain the inconsistency and demonstrate the meaning using the targeted form (Fey et al., 2017). Unresolved learning issues suggest that some inconsistency problems may need to be taught one morpheme application at a time until a child generalizes its use.

A competing source of input approach would place emphasis on relative frequency and on actively avoiding certain exceptions. In the question, *Does she like ice cream?* the phrase *she like* is in direct contrast to *She likes ice cream* and thus potentially confusing. Other combinations, such as *I/we/you like ice cream*, while possibly confusing, do present the basic premise that *I, we*, and *you* do not take the third person *-s* and would thus be acceptable in intervention as illustrating the underlying concept.

The High Variability Approach

Young children and adults who have language disorders and those who don't are able to learn morpheme use when input is variable (different words) but consistent (presence of target morpheme) (Gerken et al., 2005; Gomez, 2002; Grunow et al., 2006; Torkildsen et al., 2013). Individuals are able to learn rules of grammar from disparate examples. Failure to do so occurs when a child cannot distinguish new examples that conform to the rule from those that are "ungrammatical."

The emphasis in the high variability approach differs from that in either of the other input approaches. Emphasis in the high variability approach is on the way in which morpheme use is influenced by other details in the sentence.

CHAPTER 10 MANIPULATING CONTEXT

In general, children who learn target forms in a high variability condition make greater gains than those who learn the same forms in a low variability condition (Alt et al., 2012; Plante et al., 2014). If we consider children with TDL, they learn language in just such a variable context.

The SLP will need to select the target words and phrases carefully. For example, teaching the third person *-s* within the context *he walks* (*talks, jumps, plays*, etc.) may inadvertently teach the child that the third person *-s* appears only in conjunction with the pronoun *he* (Plante et al., 2014). Similar learning may unintentionally occur if the same word order is used repeatedly (Plante et al., 2013).

> ***Food for Thought:*** **Is there some basic logic in the notion that variability fosters independence and generalization? Why? If not, why?**

The context is also important. For example, in a book-sharing activity, several verbs may offer an opportunity to use a target morpheme. In recast sentences, however, the SLP is constrained by the verbs used by the child.

Common Ground

Although our discussion has been limited to morphological learning, each approach has wider application and offers unique contributions. I hope you can see that high-frequency input is important.

According to the high variability approach, however, it's not sufficient simply to present target morphemes frequently. These morphemes should appear with a wide variety of target words and in differing linguistic contexts. In order to have variability in a child's utterances, the SLP may need to plan their own linguistic input to the child. The SLP should be mindful to place the input example in the final sentence position as much as possible because of the salience or importance of this position and the tendency for speakers to elongate and emphasize final morpheme production in this location (e.g., *Every day she walks*).

In summary, the three approaches each provide increased frequency but go beyond that to define a different role for input. For example, the first or input informativeness approach increases the frequency by focusing on specific details of the input. In a contrastive approach, a child experiences the language feature in contexts in which other words may or may not influence its use. Finally, high variability offers some variety while avoiding non-use contexts to prevent inappropriate extraction of non-use forms.

Each of these strategies can be easily incorporated into input-oriented intervention procedures. More research data are needed to determine if these approaches, used singly or in combination, can provide a coherent intervention approach.

Explicit Instruction

Explicit instruction tries to make a child consciously aware of the underlying language pattern. In a study with 5- to 8-year-old children with developmental language disorder

(DLD), Finestack (2018) compared the efficacy of an explicit approach to an **implicit approach** targeting three grammatical forms of varying linguistic complexity. Novel forms were used so the children had no prior experience with the targets, although the novel targets resembled true English grammatical forms, such as a marker for gender which in English is reflected in the pronouns *he* and *she*.

Methods from Finestack's (2018) study can be adapted for teaching real English structures to children with language disorders. Each session began with a learning check, followed by the teaching task and another probe at the end. Note that learning is checked once to record carryover from the last session and again to measure new learning. Pictorial cues and sentence models were presented via a computer. After several models, a rule was presented guiding use of the linguistic form. This was followed by a cloze or fill-in-the-blank procedure in which the child attempted to finish a sentence using the targeted structure. The procedure, modified for more interaction, is diagrammed as follows:

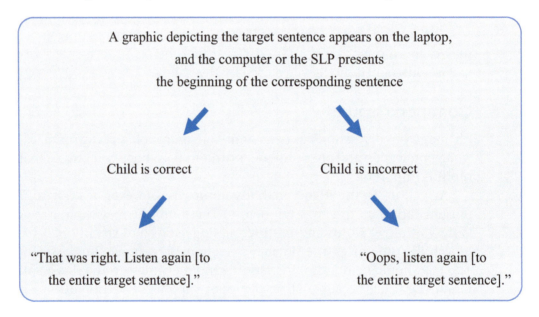

Periodically, the child was reminded of the underlying rule.

Study findings indicate that compared to implicit instruction with no rule explanation, children are more likely to acquire, maintain, and generalize novel grammatical forms when taught with explicit instruction (Finestack, 2018). This methodology does not preclude using the more conversational approaches mentioned later in this chapter and instead presents some techniques that are just good teaching, such as probing, modeling, and the use of multimodality input. In addition, occasional reminders of the rule or why we're learning a language target enhance learning.

Failure to follow principles such as these leave the SLP with the hope that a child will deduce the underlying rule on their own. Such hope may be inappropriate given that a child has already failed to generalize a language rule from previous exposure.

Research indicates that combining implicit language teaching approaches with explicit approaches is beneficial when teaching grammatical forms to children with significant weaknesses in language (Bolderson et al., 2011; Calder et al., 2018; Kulkarni et al., 2014; Smith-Lock et al., 2013). In contrast to implicit approaches, explicit instructional approaches aim to make the child conscious of the target and the underlying pattern or rule that guides the language structure. This is done by directly teaching the child the linguistic context in which a target structure is obligatory—for example, explaining that when we talk about what a person or a thing does habitually, we put a /z/ (or /s/ and /Iz/) at the end of the verb (e.g., "He runs").

Intervention that includes explicit instruction is more beneficial than implicit techniques alone (Bangert et al., 2019; Finestack, 2018; Finestack & Fey, 2009; Motsch & Riehemann, 2008). In general, intervention research indicates that with as few as 10 sessions, some children, including those with DLD and autism spectrum disorder (ASD), achieve high levels of accuracy with explicit teaching, although long-term effects are not robust.

One type of explicit instruction that investigators have examined is the Shape Coding system (Ebbels, 2007), which involves visual cues (Kulkarni et al., 2014). The Shape Coding system uses a variety of shapes, colors, and arrows to indicate parts of speech and morphology in combination with explicit discussion of grammatical rules.

Conversational Milieu

As the previous discussion and the results of several studies mentioned throughout this text highlight, varied linguistic and nonlinguistic contexts can enhance both learning and generalization. Simple exposure to language is not enough. Manipulating these contexts to enhance a child's language learning requires skill.

The goal of language use within a conversational context necessitates a thorough evaluation of the linguistic cues used with children in the teaching situation. Cues such as "What do we say?" and "Now, tell me the whole thing" are examples of pseudo-conversational cues mentioned previously. Both cues have their place but tend to be overused in intervention while rarely occurring in the real world.

Eliciting language through constant prodding or interrogation can be unpleasant and actually result in less talking by a child. The interaction is one-sided, with the child assuming the role of passive receiver or occasional reluctant speaker.

Linguistic contexts can be divided into those that model language with or without a child's response and those that directly and indirectly cue certain responses. Contingencies are strategies used following a child's utterance that attempt to confirm the utterance or, if necessary, modify it in some way. Several language teaching techniques are presented in Table 10–2. Most, but not all, are discussed.

Modeling

The efficacy of the modeling approach has been demonstrated repeatedly. *Modeling* is a procedure in which an SLP produces a rule-governed utterance at appropriate junctures in conversation or activities but initially does not ask the child to imitate. The technique compares favorably with more active techniques, such as question–answer, that require responses by a child.

Table 10–2. Language Teaching Techniques

Type	When	Purpose	Examples

Focused stimulation
  Self-talk
  Parallel talk
	Beginning of intervention	Model	Yesterday, I *walked*, my brother *rode* his bike, mommy *drove*.
			
			Yesterday, I *went* to the store.
			
			Yesterday, you *made* a cookie.

Imitation
  Immediate
  Delayed
	After child is familiar with language target	Model and familiarize child with production	Say "He rode a bike."

Expansion	When child produces target error	Model child's utterance in more mature or more correct form	*Child:* Yesterday he will eat ice cream. *SLP:* Yes, yesterday he ate ice cream.
Expansion with imitation	When child produces target error	Repeat child's utterance in more mature or more correct form and require production	*Child:* Yesterday he will eat ice cream. *SLP:* Yes, yesterday he ate ice cream. Now, you tell me.
Modeling and parallel sentence production	After child is able to imitate	Offer examples and child forms their own response	*SLP:* I measured the sugar. I added the flour. I poured the milk. Tell me what you did? *Child:* I mixed the dough.
Direct rule learning	Best with older children; teaches language rule	Explicit instruction	When we talk about something that happened before, we . . .
Classification	When child is beginning to produce the target	Contrast structures	Now and yesterday. I am running. Is that "now" or "yesterday"?
Paraphrase or change structure	When child is beginning to produce the target	Independent production with structure	He is running. Tell me what he did yesterday.
Completion	When child is beginning to produce the target	Independent production with structure	*SLP:* Look at the picture. Yesterday, . . . *Child:* Yesterday he ran.

CHAPTER 10 MANIPULATING CONTEXT

395

Table 10–2. *continued*

Type	When	Purpose	Examples
Buildup	When child is able to produce the target	Give child the elements to build a longer utterance	Yesterday he rode. On his bike. Now he is riding his bike. Tell me what happened yesterday.
Question–answer	When child is able to produce target	Elicit target	What did the boy do yesterday? [May or may not model answer]
Choice-making	When child produces the target inconsistently	Provide a possible model	Ride or rode?
Judging correctness	When child is producing the target inconsistently	Help child self-monitor	Yesterday, he will ride his bike. Is that correct?
Making obvious errors	When child is producing the target inconsistently	Help child self-monitor	Yesterday, we will swim. What should I say?
Reformulation	When child is producing the target inconsistently	Additional practice	Rode yesterday bike he. Make a sentence from those words.
Identification	When child is producing the target inconsistently	Find the target in speech	I'm going to tell a story. Raise your hand whenever you hear me use past tense.
Correction model	When child makes an error	Production and correction with maximum assistance	*Child:* Yesterday I see a puppy. *SLP:* Yesterday I saw a puppy.
Correction model/request (imitation)	When child makes an error	Production and correction with maximum assistance	*Child:* Yesterday I see a puppy. *SLP:* Yesterday I saw a puppy. Now you tell me.
Incomplete model/request	When child makes an error	Production and correction with maximum assistance	*Child:* Yesterday I see a puppy. *SLP:* Saw. Now you tell me.
Reduced error repetition request	When child makes an error	Production and correction with some assistance	*Child:* Yesterday I see a puppy. *SLP:* See? *Child:* Saw. *SLP:* Tell me again.

continues

Table 10–2. *continued*

Type	When	Purpose	Examples
Error repetition request	When child makes an error	Production and correction with some assistance	*Child:* Yesterday I see a puppy. *SLP:* Yesterday I see a puppy? *Child:* Saw. Saw a puppy. *SLP:* Tell me again.
Self-correction request	When child does or does not make an error	Self-monitoring and correction with minimal assistance	*Child:* Yesterday I see a puppy. *SLP:* Was that right? [Was that correct?]
Request for clarification	When child does or does not make an error	Independent production and correction with minimal assistance	*Child:* Yesterday I see a puppy. *SLP:* I don't understand.
Repetition request	When child says the target correctly	Independent production	*Child:* Yesterday I saw a puppy. *SLP:* Yesterday I saw a puppy. Tell me again.
Expansion request	When child says the error correctly	Independent production	*Child:* Yesterday I saw a puppy. *SLP:* Tell me more.
Turnabout or reply	When child says the error correctly	Independent production	*Child:* Yesterday I saw a puppy. *SLP:* A puppy? What color was he? [That sounds like fun. Tell me about him.]

Modeling can be used in any of the following ways:

- As a high-frequency response in very structured situations
- As a specific language stimulation technique
- As an element in comprehension teaching

In general, modeling closely approximates the language-learning environment of children with TDL and is an effective language-learning strategy for a child with a language disorder. You may recall from the beginning of the chapter that Ms. Ramirez planned to use a stimulation technique via other people in Tad's world.

CHAPTER 10 MANIPULATING CONTEXT

One issue is how much to model. Providing a telegraphic or simplified prompt, such as "Mommy eat," for a child to imitate does not appear to offer any advantage in intervention. Children are just as likely to attempt to imitate a grammatically complete prompt. In addition, including bound morphemes and function words, such as articles, encourages a child who is ready developmentally to imitate them (Bredin-Oja & Fey, 2014).

It is expected that the child will acquire some aspect of the language behavior of the language teacher and use it in a similar context later. Interactive modeling considers the child to be an active learner who abstracts the rules used in forming utterances and associates these utterances with events and stimuli in the environment. Use of modeling should be considered in light of the previous discussion on variable contexts and explicit–implicit teaching.

Focused Stimulation. It's best to model the teaching target for a child prior to attempting to elicit the target. Within such focused stimulation, an SLP produces a high density of the targets in meaningful contexts without requiring the child to respond. Two varieties of this stimulation are *self-talk* and *parallel talk* (see Table 10–2). Obviously, activities will need to be chosen carefully to provide sufficient opportunities for the target to occur.

Focused stimulation should be semantically and pragmatically appropriate. The target feature is presented frequently while, at the same time, placing little pressure on the child. The following is an example of focused stimulation within a conversational context:

Child: Mommy make hamburgers. Mommy make 'tator salad.

SLP: *She* must be a good cook. *She* made hamburgers and potato salad. And what else. *She* made . . .

Child: Cake.

SLP: *She* did? *She* made a cake. Yummy. Maybe *she* also made hot dogs?

Child: Uh-huh.

SLP: *She* made a very nice picnic for the family. Did *she* get to play any games or did *she* just work?

The language feature being targeted—the pronoun *she*—appears in the initial part of the sentence or in elliptical utterances in which shared information is omitted. Such frequent modeling plus recasts of the child's utterances, explained later, can be used effectively in facilitating use of several language structures.

Although a grammatical feature can be made more salient or conspicuous by emphasizing it, this can change the basic meaning of a sentence. Say the following sentences out loud, emphasizing the boldfaced word:

I'll see you next week.

I **will** see you next week

Whereas the first is probable, the second is definite. Or the following:

I do my homework every day.

I **do** my homework every day.

In the first, we have a statement of fact. The second, however, seems like a defensive response that has a different meaning. An SLP must be careful, therefore, that added emphasis does not change the meaning of the utterance.

Targets can also be placed at the end of a sentence to aid working memory and enhance learning (Fey et al., 2003). This can occur in syntax ("The girl is running to school. *She really is*"), morphology ("He rides to work. He doesn't walk; *he rides*"), or semantics ("Don't put the block on the box. *Put it in*"). Here's an example of how it might work (Fey et al., 2003):

Child: I do it.

Adult: What about me?

Child: You too.

Adult: Great. You won't do it alone. We **will**. We **will** do it together.

Child: We do it.

Adult: Yes. We **will** do it together. We **will**!

Once a target has been modeled thoroughly, the SLP can ask the child to respond in a manner similar to the model. Note this change. Children who are young, low-functioning, or delayed may need imitation teaching, with a complete model presented immediately before their response.

Imitation. Imitation is a procedure in which the child repeats the language behavior of an adult, with the expectation that the child will acquire some aspect of the language teacher's language. Imitation by a child enables them to become accustomed to the language feature being taught and its phonological patterns. This is especially important if the feature is difficult to produce.

Imitation can be used as a first step in programs to teach specific language targets or as a correction procedure when the child fails to respond or responds incorrectly. The procedure has been used successfully with several types of language disorder.

Imitation can be a useful tool in language intervention as long as we recognize its limitations (Eisenberg et al., 2020). Use of imitation can result in rapidly achieving production of grammatical targets. The technique is not recommended as the sole or long-term method of intervention for working on grammar.

Several studies have demonstrated that although imitation can increase performance and generalize to untaught items, the results have only limited generalization to conversational speech. Conversely, conversation-based therapy results in faster or higher usage in conversational speech.

Priming. By monitoring a child's progress, an SLP can provide varied cues, including partial models and/or delayed imitation. This methodology, called **priming**, occurs when the utterance of one person influences the structure, vocabulary selection, or sounds used by a second speaker.

Structural priming occurs when a sentence produced by one speaker influences the structure of the sentences of a second speaker. This influence occurs even when the second speaker's productions do not contain the same words or thematic relations as the preceding sentence. For example, after hearing *The woman sent presents to her friends*, a speaker is more likely to produce a sentence such as *The girl gave cookies to her parents*. The sentence heard by the second speaker is referred to as the prime sentence, and the sentence produced by this speaker is the target sentence.

The effects of priming are not fleeting or limited to the effects on the next sentence. Priming effects persist even when there is intervening information or sentences (Bock & Griffin, 2000; Hartsuiker et al., 2008; Konopka & Bock, 2005). Although our discussion will of necessity be short, I suggest that you read the excellent tutorial by Leonard (2011), from which much of this discussion is taken.

In a more structured approach, priming is called **parallel sentence production**. The SLP provides a model of the type of utterance desired. The child is not expected to imitate the model but, rather, to provide a similar type of sentence. For example, I might describe a picture with "The girl is throwing the ball" and then ask the child to describe a second picture of a boy catching a ball. You might recall from the beginning of the chapter that Ms. Ramirez was going to use a similar technique with Tad.

Structural priming has it limits and appears to work best at the phrase level (Pickering & Ferreira, 2008). In other words, priming for the present progressive (*is catching*) would work best if the child already has the structure of the basic sentence into which it fits (subject + verb + object).

As you might imagine, the effects of priming on a child vary with the child's age. In general, parallel sentence production occurs with 3-year-olds only when

- there is considerable lexical overlap between the priming sentence and the child's target sentence (Bencini & Valian, 2008); and
- the child is able to repeat or imitate the priming sentences.

In contrast, 4-year-olds show the effects of priming after only hearing the priming sentences (Savage et al., 2003; Shimpi et al., 2007). Not surprisingly, we find more parallel sentence production among 3-year-olds with TDL than among those with DLD (Leonard et al., 2000; Miller & Deevy, 2006; Thothathiri & Snedeker, 2008).

Summary. Both strategies that require a child response, such as questions, imitation, and parallel sentence production, and those that do not, such as focused stimulation, can result in improved language but not for all children. Given that priming works best at the phrase or the less-than-a-sentence level, it does have relevance for elaborated noun and verb phrases and other phrasal structures such as prepositional phrases.

A child may be asked to respond to questions for which an SLP has modeled the answers previously. Initially, the modeled answer may follow the question, but this format can be altered so that the answer precedes the question, is given partially, models a similar answer, or precedes the question by increasingly longer periods of time.

Although the modeling procedure seems stilted in writing, it can be applied very flexibly and works well with groups of children. In small groups, children who have acquired a certain target can serve as models for those who have not. By varying turns, an SLP can ensure that sufficient models are provided for different children. In a reversal of roles, the SLP can serve as a model for a child, while the child cues the SLP.

Modeling alone may be less effective than other, more structured methods. Although modeling is effective in changing the behavior of children with TDL, it is less effective than imitation with children with language disorders who may benefit more from other approaches.

Direct Linguistic Cues

Linguistic cues for certain targets can be direct or indirect. Direct elicitation techniques might include those in Table 10–3.

Substitution. Substitution requests also can be used. For example, pronouns can be substituted for nouns that have become old information. The language teacher might make a statement, such as giving one descriptor ("The dog is little"), and then ask the

Table 10–3. Direct Linguistic Cues

To Elicit . . .	Use . . .
Verbs	"What is he doing (are you doing)?" Use any tense. A benefit is that the question contains the target tense.
Noun subjects	"Who/what is verbing?" Again, the tense can be altered for the situation.
Noun objects	"What is he/she verbing?" Tense can be altered for the situation. Obviously, verbs that do not take objects should not be used.
Adverbs or adverbial phrases	"When/where/how is he/she verbing?" Tense can be altered. "How" questions can be used also to elicit process answers, as in "How did you make the airplane?"
Adjectives or adjectival phrases	"Which one . . . ?" Tense can be altered. There should be an obvious contrast between choices for the response, such as *big* and *little*. These differences might be noted prior to questioning. Responses of a particular type can be modeled, as in "Which one ate the cookie, the littlest bear, the middle-size bear, or the biggest bear?" To keep the child from responding "That one," the SLP may want to cover the child's eyes or use some barrier.
Specific words	Completion sentences, as in "She is playing in the _____." Rising intonation after the last spoken word will signal the child to respond. If the SLP plays dumb or acts forgetful, the child's behavior makes more sense conversationally.

CHAPTER 10 MANIPULATING CONTEXT

child to make a comment ("What can you tell me about the dog?"). This procedure also can take the form of a guessing game, as in "Is the dog little? Well, if the dog isn't little, what can we say?" Of course, our goal is "He is . . . ."

Tad, mentioned at the beginning, will repeat an utterance using a similar form. Given this behavior, the SLP or other adult can use this behavior for the frame of the utterance but ask Tad to substitute a pronoun for a noun.

Although these linguistic cues are conversational in nature, they will seem very nonconversational if used in contexts in which they make no sense pragmatically. An SLP can model a response prior to asking the child a question, as mentioned previously. For example, "I think I want the yellow one. What about you?" This type of cue is more likely to elicit a longer utterance and is more conversational in tone. The goal is a sentence of similar construction. Contrast this with asking, "Which one do you want?" which may result in "Red."

Mand Model. One variation of the direct linguistic cue is a **mand model**. This technique has been used effectively with preschoolers and with children with DLD. This procedure follows a routine that is established prior to beginning any activity. The routine serves as a chain in which one stimulus cues the next. The mand model approach typically is used for teaching new language features.

In the four-step mand model teaching sequence, an adult first attracts a child's attention by providing a variety of attractive materials. This inducement may not be necessary if the child already displays an interest. Thus, the adult establishes joint attention with the child. In the second step, after the child has expressed interest, the adult (de)mands, "Tell me about this" or "Tell me what you want," requesting a behavior taught previously. If there is no response, the adult moves to step 3 and prompts a response or provides a model to be imitated. In step 4, the adult praises the child for an appropriate response and gives the child the desired item.

Even preschool peers can be taught to use the mand model technique effectively. In these situations, production by children with language disorders generalizes to unprompted productions.

Indirect Linguistic Cues

Indirect linguistic cues are more conversational and situational in nature. For example, when attempting to elicit questions, the SLP might use unfamiliar objects hidden in boxes to set the nonlinguistic context. Beginning with "Boy, is this neat," the SLP peeks into the box. An exchange might continue as follows:

Child: What's in there?

SLP: This. (Takes the object out. Waits.)

Child: What is it?

SLP: A flibbity-jibbit. It does everything.

Child: What it do?

Notice the elicitation of questions. It is easy to see the interplay of nonlinguistic and linguistic cueing.

Another indirect linguistic technique requires the SLP or language teacher to make purposefully wrong statements. For example, to obtain a negative statement, the SLP can focus on a child's clothing, a technique I have dubbed "the emperor's new clothes":

SLP: (Touching child's red sweater) What nice blue pants.

Child: Not blue pants.

In both examples, the child has given a final response that may be something less than what is desired. The SLP now can respond and begin to shape the child's previous utterance into an acceptable form, as in *It's not blue pants*. We'll use contingencies to correct the utterance. Right now, we're just eliciting it.

> *Food for Thought:* **Check out Appendix F. Can you think of other indirect ways of getting specific language features.**

These examples are only a very few of many indirect techniques. Others examples are listed in Appendix F. Take a look. The possibilities are only limited by your imagination.

Contingencies

Conversational consequences can be divided roughly into those that do not require a child's response and those that do. Each type provides some feedback to the child, and each differs with the functioning level and degree of learning exhibited by the child.

Contingencies Requiring No Response. Although it's best if SLPs provide well-formed language models (Bredin-Oja & Fey, 2014), it's also important not to respond negatively to a child's language. Instead, an SLP's response can provide an evaluation of the attempt and/or reflect a corrective response. Contingencies that require no response from a child are nonevaluative or accepting in nature and can be used to increase correct production or highlight incorrect production for self-correction.

When a child initiates or responds to some cue, the SLP or other language teacher focuses full attention on the child, creating joint reference on the child's topic. Because the child has established the topic, it now acts as a motivator for the child and can be used to modify the child's language. Modifying techniques that do not require the child's response include fulfilling the intention, use of a continuant, imitation, expansion, extension and expiation, breakdowns and buildups, and recast sentences.

By fulfilling the intention of a child's utterance, such as handing the child a requested item, the adult signals the child that the message was acceptable as received. No verbal response is required.

CHAPTER 10 MANIPULATING CONTEXT

A continuant is a signal that a message has been received and acknowledged. These signals usually consist of head nods or verbalizations, such as "uh-huh" and "okay." Continuants fill a speaker's turn by agreeing with the previous utterance.

Imitation. In imitation, the adult repeats a child's utterance in whole or in part but makes no evaluative remarks. Rising intonation, signifying a question, is not present. Again, this behavior primarily acknowledges the child's previous utterance. Imitation is especially helpful to the child when correctly produced features of interest are emphasized ("She **is** riding the bike"). Imitations might be preceded also by phrases such as **That's right** ("That's right, she **is** riding the bike").

Expansion. In contrast to imitation, expansion or recast/expansion is a more mature, or more correct, version of the child's utterance that maintains the child's word order—for example:

> *Child:* It got stolen by the crook.
>
> *SLP:* Uh-huh, it *was* stolen by the crook.

The use of expansion as a teaching tool is very limited for children functioning above about 30 months of age.

In a variation of expansion, the SLP can prompt the child to imitate the expansion, although such requests disrupt the flow of conversation. A more appropriate variety of expansion for older children is a reformulation in which two or more child utterances are combined into one utterance that includes the concepts of each, as in the following:

> *Child:* The dog bited the man. The man runned away.
>
> *SLP:* Oh, the dog bit the man, who then ran away.

The use of expansion and of a cloze, or fill-in-the-blank, procedure by adults produces more responses, more interpretations, and more syntactically complex utterances by children than does a question-and-answer procedure (Bradshaw et al., 1998).

Extension. For older children, extension is a more appropriate response. Extension is a reply to the content of the child's utterance that provides additional information on the topic, as in the following:

> *Child:* It got stolen by the crook.
>
> *SLP:* Oh, I wonder if the crook stole anything else.

Much of our behavior in conversations consists of replies to the content of the other speaker, and these comments can be used effectively regardless of the age or functioning level of the child. Extensions signal the child that the adult is attentive and interested.

404 LANGUAGE DISORDERS: A FUNCTIONAL APPROACH TO ASSESSMENT AND INTERVENTION IN CHILDREN

Breakdowns and Buildups. In combination, **breakdowns and buildups** consist of dividing the child's utterances into shorter units and then combining them and expanding on the child's original utterance. The purpose is to help the child understand intrasentential relationships. I use this strategy as my great-great-uncle used to do to aid the processing of information, mulling it over before commenting:

Child: It got stolen by the crook.

SLP: (Emotional, disbelieving) It was? (Hmmm) It was stolen. Stolen by the crook. (Disgusted) By the crook. (Finally) It was stolen by the crook.

This strategy works well, especially if the SLP or teacher plays dumb or uses a silly puppet who just does not seem to get things right. The child may shake his head or say, "Uh-huh," in agreement between the adult's utterances.

Recasts. **Recast sentences** maintain the child's meaning or the relations while modifying the structure, and they immediately follow the child's utterance. Recasts repeat at least one of the major lexical elements while modifying other parts of the utterance. For example,

Child: He not eat.

Adult: The dog is not eating his food. Is he hungry?

Child: Not hungry.

Adult: The dog is not eating his food. He is not hungry. Is the cat eating?

Child: Uh-huh.

Adult: The cat is eating his food. The dog is not eating his food.

We may be splitting hairs in this example because these types of recasts are very close to expansions. Recasts can also be in another syntactic form:

Child: It got stolen by the crook.

SLP: Was it stolen by the crook?

OR

It was stolen by the crook?

OR

The crook stole it.

OR

Did the crook steal it?

Sentences can be recast in whatever form the SLP has targeted, although adult comments are easier for children to process than question forms. Note that even though the form

CHAPTER 10 MANIPULATING CONTEXT

has changed, the relations have not: *crook-steal-it.* Although children with DLD can benefit from the use of recasts, this consequence must be produced in much greater quantity than found in typical conversation to be of value (Proctor-Williams et al., 2001).

The adult's additional information may be syntactic, semantic, and/or phonological depending on the target of intervention. Extensions, in contrast, are conversational replies in which adult responses continue a child's topic and add new information but do not necessarily contain any of the child's words. A meta-analysis of 35 research studies concluded that although the available evidence was limited, it supports the use of recasts in grammatical intervention (Cleave et al., 2015).

Most recasts are corrective in nature and range from simple to complex depending on the amount of information. Ideally, a recast expands or corrects the child's utterance in a way that supplies the child with an example of their specific language goal(s). Often, the child is not required or prompted to imitate the adult.

Recasts support intervention by presenting feedback to the child in a way that highlights language features the child has not mastered (Camarata & Nelson, 2006). Because the adult's recast immediately follows the child's utterance, it's assumed that the child notes the difference between their production and that of the adult.

The immediacy and shared focus of both the child's initial utterance and the adult's recast increase the likelihood that the child will attend to the adult utterance. The proximity and similarity of the two utterances can reduce linguistic processing demands on the child and allow for the child to make a critical comparison.

Recasts are provided within the interactional context of child–adult communication. Because of this context, the child's attention to the adult's language should increase, motivation to communicate should be enhanced, and generalization to conversation should be strengthened (Camarata & Nelson, 2006). In other words, the increased frequency of meaningful language input changes the child's language.

The effectiveness of recasts is based on four assumptions (Fey et al., 2003):

- It is easy for the child to attend, because the recast sentence is based on the child's utterance.

- It is easy for the child to comprehend, because the recast sentence is similar to the child's sentence.

- It is easy for the child to notice the change, because the recast sentence differs from the child's sentence primarily in the use of the targeted feature.

- It is easy for the child to understand underlying relationships, because the recast sentence occurs in context.

Although recasts may be an effective way to respond to a linguistic error, they are not as effective as structured cueing to elicit the correct response (Smith-Lock et al., 2015). Compared to direct cueing, recasts that require no child response are not as effective. Cueing requires a child to be actively involved, whereas recasts without a child response enable the child to be passive.

A word of caution is needed. Although both modeling and response strategies have led to reported gains in children's language abilities, children with DLD will most likely require more input (Proctor-Williams et al., 2001). In addition, merely providing more frequent input may not achieve the therapy goal, especially if the variability of the input is not considered (Ambridge et al., 2015). This leads us inevitably to our final group of techniques.

Contingencies Requiring a Response. Contingencies that require a response are used when a child is able to produce the target reliably but has failed to do so or has produced the target inaccurately. A skilled use of both nonlinguistic and linguistic contextual cues should set the stage for production of the target, hopefully in a situation in which it makes good pragmatic sense.

In a conversation, the child has an interest in the interaction and in their own utterance. Thus, the child is motivated to modify production in order to maintain the conversation and receive the adult's attention.

Most of the contingencies discussed here note the child's error or require the child to find the error and request that the child produce the target more correctly. A second contingency type requests repetition or a correct or expanded utterance to strengthen correct production. A hierarchy of both types, ranging from contingencies that provide maximum input to the child to those that provide the minimal, would be *correction model/request, incomplete correction model/request, choice-making, reduced error repetition/ request, error repetition/request, self-correction request, contingent query, repetition request, expansion request,* and *turnabouts.* These techniques are shown in Table 10–2.

Correction Model/Request. In a correction model/request, the language teacher repeats the child's entire utterance, adding or correcting the target that was omitted or produced incorrectly, for example:

> *Child:* I *builded* a big tower out of blocks.
>
> *SLP:* I *built* a big tower out of blocks. Now you say it. (or "Tell me that again.")

The child is requested gently to repeat the SLP's model. Note that the error has been corrected for the child.

Initially, the target may be emphasized to aid the child in locating the corrected unit. Later teaching might restate the child's utterance as a question, as in, "You *built* a big tower out of blocks?"

Because the entire utterance is desired in the child's response, the SLP can act confused to maintain the conversational nature of the interaction rather than saying "Tell me the whole thing."

> *SLP:* You *builded* a tower out of big blocks? I thought you *built* a big tower out of blocks. I'm confused, tell me again.

In a correction model/request, the child is provided with a complete or only slightly altered model of the correct utterance.

CHAPTER 10 MANIPULATING CONTEXT

The SLP should require the child to produce correctly only those units that are currently targeted for intervention. It may be difficult to reinforce utterances even when they contain errors, as in the following example:

Child: I *builted* the most biggest tower out of blocks.

SLP: You *built* the biggest tower out of blocks?

Child: Yeah, I *built* the most biggest tower out of blocks.

SLP: Uh-huh, how big was it?

OR

Yeah? What kind of blocks did you use?

OR

Oh! Where is the tower now?

Note that the SLP ignored "most biggest." Instead, the SLP remained focused on the target and on the hierarchy of teaching strategies being used.

Incomplete Correction Model/Request. In contrast to a correction model/request, an incomplete correction model/request provides only the corrected target. Thus, the child has less support. The child must provide the rest of the utterance, as follows:

Child: I *builded* a big tower with blocks.

SLP: *Built.*

Child: I *built* a big tower with blocks.

Initially, the child will need a cue to repeat the utterance with the corrected target.

Choice-Making. As the child begins to exhibit some success at self-correcting, the SLP can offer choice-making: "Is it *builded* or *built*?" The SLP must be careful to use this form occasionally when the child's initial utterance is correct as well as when it is incorrect. Otherwise, the child will recognize that the question is only used when they make an error. In addition, the location of the correct answer should vary so that the child does not develop a strategy of always picking the first or second of the pair choice.

If the child fails to make a correct choice, the SLP can provide a corrected model by using an incomplete correction model/request. That's how a hierarchy works. The SLP moves up or down depending on the amount of support required by the child.

Reduced Error Repetition/Request. Once the child has learned the target reliably within more structured situations, the SLP can use other techniques that require the child to supply the missing or correct target. With reduced error repetition/request, the SLP repeats only the incorrect structure with rising intonation, thus forming a question.

This contingency informs the child that the language unit in question is incorrect and must be corrected—for example:

> *Child:* I *builded* a big tower with blocks.
>
> *SLP:* *Builded?*
>
> *Child:* Built.

The SLP's question is more conversational than the cue found in correction model/requests and is less disruptive to the flow of conversation. If the child fails to recognize the error, the SLP can provide a choice.

Error Repetition/Request. With error repetition/request, the SLP repeats the entire utterance with rising intonation. The child must locate the error or omission and correct it, as in the following:

> *Child:* I *builded* a big tower with blocks.
>
> *SLP:* I *builded* a big tower with blocks?

The emphasis on the error can be increased or decreased as needed. For example, increased emphasis might be used to aid the child in finding the error. If this technique is unsuccessful, the SLP might provide a reduced error repetition/request.

Ideally, the SLP will place the rising intonation at the end of the sentence, not after the error. If increasing independence comes from locating the error in context, then not signaling the error with intonation seems essential.

Once the child's target knowledge is reasonably stable, the SLP can use the error repetition/request even when the child is correct. This procedure helps children scan their productions spontaneously and to self-correct.

Self-Correction Request. A self-correction request does not provide the child with a repetition of the previous utterance. Instead, the SLP asks the child to consider the correctness of that utterance from memory—for example, "Is [was] that right [correct]?" and "Did you say that correctly?" If the child is unsure, the SLP can provide an error repetition/request.

Contingent Query. In contrast to the somewhat stilted tone of the self-correction request, the contingent query is more conversational. A contingent query is a request for clarification.

In general, contingent queries are concerned more with comprehension of the message being sent than with specific targets. For example, if I miss something, I might say "What?" Nevertheless, this technique can be used effectively to signal the child that something may be amiss with the production. The child is left to scan recent memory to determine where communication breakdown occurred.

Use of contingent queries should be limited because they can disrupt communication and frustrate the speaker who is continually asked to repeat. Young school-age children dislike having to repeat more than once or twice.

Contingent queries may be specific or general, depending on the abilities of the child. In response to the sentence, "I built a big tower with blocks," the SLP might respond, "What did you do with blocks?" "What did you do?" or simply, "What?" If the child falsely assumes that their production was correct and merely repeats the error or omission, the SLP might use a self-correction request.

Repetition Request. Correct productions of the target can be strengthened by asking the child to repeat. With a repetition request, the SLP simply says, "Tell me that again," or, "Could you say that again?" This technique also can be used conversationally, implying that the listener missed some portion of the transmission, not that the transmission was in error.

Expansion Request. If the child produces the target correctly but in a smaller unit than desired, such as a one-word response following a reduced error repetition/request, the SLP can use an expansion request. The typical cue, "Tell me the whole thing" is not conversational in tone. It is better for the SLP to fake confusion and ask for a total restatement, as in the following example:

> *SLP:*   Built? Built what? I get so confused. You better tell me again.

Turnabout. Turnabouts may be more effective than repetition requests and are more conversational in nature. In a turnabout, the SLP acknowledges the child's utterance or comments and then asks for more, as in "Uh-huh, and then what did you do?" or "Wow, what will you do next?" or "That sounds like fun; what happened then?" The corrected form can also be placed in the comment to provide yet another model.

The turnabout technique has been taught successfully to high school peers and parents and has been used effectively in conversational intervention with children with language disorders. This partner-as-SLP strategy reportedly can improve conversation skills significantly. The parents of Tad, the child mentioned previously, can engage him in open-ended turnabouts to increase his use of sentences.

Questions used in turnabouts should be of a topic-continuing nature and thus support the child's efforts to maintain the topic. This style of responding is especially helpful to preschool children and children with language disorders.

Several relational terms also may be used in open-ended utterances to aid the child in providing more information of a specific nature. For example, the SLP might repeat the child's utterance with the addition of *but* to elicit contrary or adversative information, or *and* to elicit complementary information:

> *Child:*   We played games at the party.
>
> *SLP:*   What fun. You played games at the party *and* . . .
>
> *Child:*   And we had cake and ice cream.

410 LANGUAGE DISORDERS: A FUNCTIONAL APPROACH TO ASSESSMENT AND INTERVENTION IN CHILDREN

Hierarchy. The conversational contingencies discussed in this section can be arranged in a hierarchy similar to that in Table 10–4. This arrangement and the specific techniques will differ with the language unit being targeted and with the child.

The SLP who is familiar with this hierarchy can respond to the child's utterances in a top-down manner that enhances language stimulation and facilitates language learning. In the next section, we'll put the techniques together in a conversational milieu.

> *Food for Thought:* Can you see why as an SLP, you don't need to cave in and give the answer to the child? There are many steps between independent use and imitation.

Table 10–4. Hierarchy of Conversational Contingencies

For the examples, the child's utterance is "I sawed two puppies." The SLP should use the contingency farthest down on the list that ensures the child's success with minimal input.

Facilitator Input	Conversational Contingency	Example
Maximum	Correction model/request	I saw two puppies. Can you tell me again? (The cue to say it again is optional, unless the child does not repeat spontaneously.)
	Incomplete correction model/request	*Saw.* Can you tell me again? (Again the cue is optional.)
	Choice-making	Is it *saw* or *sawed*?
	Reduced error repetition/request	*Sawed?*
	Error repetition/request	I sawed two puppies?
	Self-correction/request	Was that right?
	Contingent query	I didn't understand you. Say it again, please. (Other options include *Huh?* and *What?* or, in this example, *What did you do?*)
	Expansion request	Tell me the whole thing again.
	*Repetition request	Tell me again.
Minimum	*Turnabout	You did? I love puppies. What did they look like?

Note: *Used with complete, correct responses.

Conversations: Top-Down Teaching

The methods presented so far are helpful no matter what method of intervention is used by an SLP. It is in the arrangement of these techniques that everything can change.

A functional approach is one that uses conversation whenever possible as the milieu for instruction. Employing a top-down intervention model, an SLP helps a child repair conversational errors as they occur within context. In other words, both the teaching and the target have a communication purpose. You may recall that Ms. Ramirez, Tad's SLP, was considering a functional conversational approach.

Initially, the SLP selects targets based on the child's needs and activities. Topics of conversation are based on the child's interests and experience. Placing intervention within everyday routines or play is ideal. By manipulating both the nonlinguistic and linguistic context, the SLP can elicit the targeted language feature and then provide just enough input to aid the child's production. The amount of input needed by the child depends on the child's ability and will differ across children.

The SLP provides just enough input to help the child be successful. In other words, the child is given the least amount of help necessary. Over time, as a child gains more independence, this level of input can be decreased further. For example, a system of least prompts, sometimes called a least-to-most prompting procedure (Ault & Griffen, 2013; MacDuff et al., 2001; Neitzel & Wolery, 2009), can be used even with minimally verbal children. For example, it's been used effectively to help children with ASD compose multisymbol messages using augmentative and alternative communication (Finke et al., 2016).

Let's assume that a child is working on irregular past tense and the SLP is inquiring about the past weekend, specifically what the child saw, ate, drank, and so on. In this example, the child can self-repair but requires that the error be highlighted in order to do so. Note in the following exchange how the child needs more assistance than first assumed by the SLP. It is also important to note that the SLP does not correct the error for the child. Supplying the correct response builds dependence on this type of help and does not foster independence.

Child:	I sawed two puppies.
Partner:	Was that right? (Self-correction request)
Child:	Uh-huh.
Partner:	I sawed two puppies? (Error repetition/request)
Child:	Yeah.
Partner:	Sawed? (Reduced error repetition request)
Child:	Saw. I saw two puppies.
Partner:	What was that? (Repetition request to strengthen correct production)
Child:	I saw two puppies.

Partner:	Oh, I think I love puppies more than kittens. What did they do? (Turnabout)

When the child gives the correct response, the SLP does not respond with that tired old "Good talking!" Instead, the SLP strengthens the correct response by asking for a repetition, then replies conversationally and uses a turnabout to elicit the next response. Let's eavesdrop some more.

Child:	At the pet store.
Partner:	I'm confused. What happened?
Child:	I saw the puppies at the pet store?
Partner:	Umhm, you saw them at the pet store. Pet stores are fun. When did you go?
Child:	I goed on Saturday.
Partner:	Was that right?
Child:	I went on Saturday.
Partner:	Oh, you went to the pet store on Saturday and saw the two puppies. Did you go alone?

Each response by the SLP tries to elicit another that includes use of the target, the irregular past tense, but not just any irregular past tense verb. The specific verbs were chosen well in advance and taught using a variety of methods.

The functional approach to intervention can be challenging for an SLP at first. Once you begin to think in a new way, and with practice, functional teaching becomes second nature—just the way the SLP talks with children. The intervention approach can be used in almost any interaction with a child, thus giving an SLP ultimate flexibility.

> ***Food for Thought:*** Imagine having a therapeutic conversation—one in which a child participates in a meaningful exchange of information and learns language at the same time.

Conclusion

Within functional communication, an SLP's role becomes one of accepting the child's spontaneously occurring verbal or nonverbal behavior and treating it as meaningful communication. The SLP or other language teacher interprets the behavior in a manner that is contextually appropriate and collaborates with the child in communicating the message in a more effective way.

CHAPTER 10 MANIPULATING CONTEXT

As an SLP, you are a teacher. Not a classroom teacher, although you may do that on occasion too, but a teacher nonetheless. What does that mean? One of the best explanations is provided by Melanie Schuele and Donna Boudreau (2008). In fact, it's so good, I'm quoting it for you:

> Teaching involves helping a child do something that he or she was not able to do previously, or helping a child do something better or more independently (Vigil & van Kleeck, 1996). Thus, a teacher . . . explains, models, highlights critical concepts, carefully sequences teaching, provides sufficient practice, and scaffolds, contingent on the child's current level of performance. At the outset of learning, the adult literally carries the child through the task. . . . Over time, the adult gradually yields control; the adult guides the child to successfully complete the pieces of the task, providing support when needed. As the child gains skill and independence, the adult provides less and less support (Vigil & van Kleeck, 1996). Learning is best characterized . . . by moving a child from successful performance with maximal support to successful performance with little or no support. At each step along the way, the teacher or clinician must be proficient at providing the appropriate amount and type of support. (pp. 10–11)

Commit this to memory!

Throwing out questions or cues haphazardly and hoping for the right response or providing the answer when the child is incorrect is not teaching. Teaching is a systematic analysis of what the child is lacking that results in their non-success.

It's essential for an SLP to break any learning task into the sequential steps required to move from where the child is now to where we want the child to be, which is successfully learning the task, whether it's using plural -s or initiating a topic. To be an effective teacher, the SLP must now plan how intervention will proceed within and between each step of the sequence.

Decisions on sequencing should be determined by the complexity of the task. It goes without saying that simple tasks are targeted before complex tasks. Success in earlier tasks should lead to success on later ones. Earlier tasks need to target emergence and initial establishment of a skill and provide enough support that there is a high probability of a child being successful.

To teach effectively, the SLP must plan how intervention will proceed at each step. This requires consideration of the task but also necessitates paying attention to the learning characteristics of the individual child and the cognitive and linguistic requirements of the task.

The SLP must consider the way in which they cue or prompt a child's response. Framing the question is essential to success.

As a child becomes more successful, the SLP can provide less scaffolding or structure. You can enhance teaching by anticipating the types of support that a child is likely to need and the types of error the child is likely to make. Both should be used to plan intervention strategies.

In addition, effective intervention depends on the ways in which the adult responds to the child's attempts. Both cueing and responding should be designed to facilitate growth toward more independent and more complex performance. The nature of the child's errors and successes indicates the amount of scaffolding or support a child needs. Guidelines include the following precepts:

- Formulate a response based on the reason for a child's error.
- The manner of responding will depend on where the child is in the learning process.
- The SLP's response should be designed to facilitate achievement of the teaching goal while still preserving the goal of maximum independence with minimal support.
- Responses to correct an inadequate response may be similar to the child's because they both highlight the problem-solving task for the child.

Both the nonlinguistic and linguistic contexts can be manipulated by an SLP and other language teachers to teach language to a child and to encourage use of structures recently acquired. By using the various techniques described in this chapter, you as the SLP can maximize interactions with the child with a language disorder.

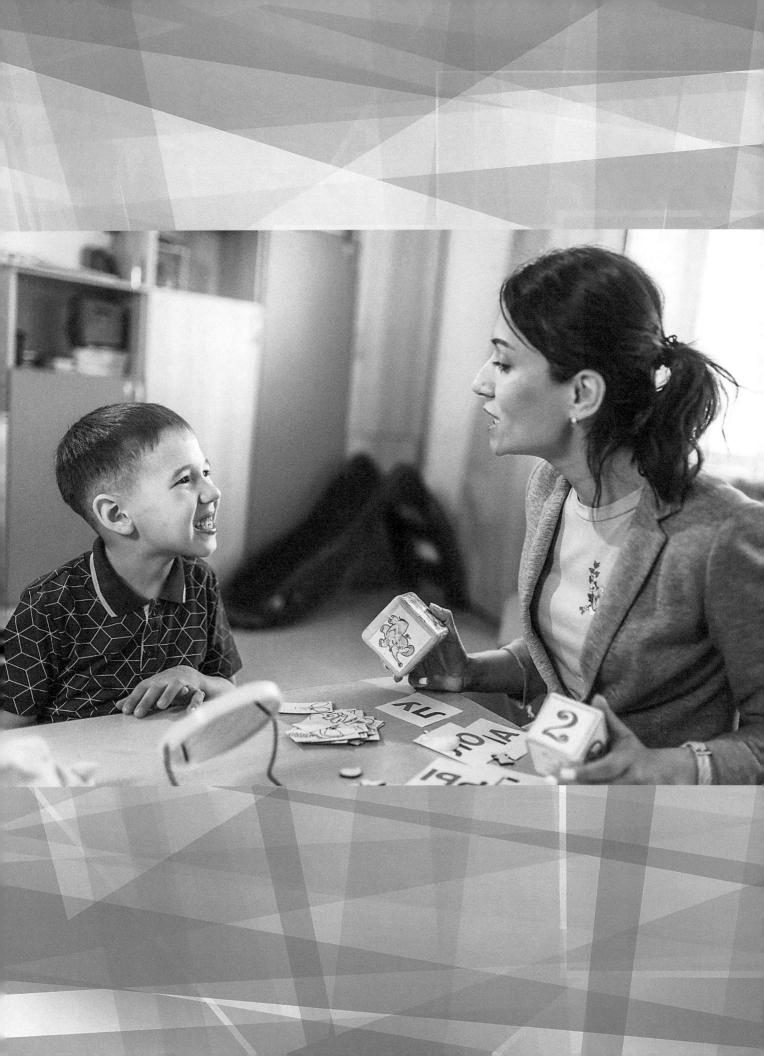

CHAPTER 11

SPECIFIC INTERVENTION TECHNIQUES

Carrie seemed to be constantly in trouble, fighting with other girls and being inappropriate in her remarks to teachers. Her parents said she was "impossible" at home. She didn't follow directions or even simple hints to do one thing or another.

In her own communication, Carrie is imprecise, often using words such as "thing" or "one." She doesn't seem to understand what her listener needs. It seems as if she expects others to know what is in her mind.

In class, she had difficulty following directions and asking questions. In conversations, she was often off-topic and misinterpreted the comments of others as criticism or belligerent behavior. She responded in kind.

She had few friends that anyone could recall and was a loner both at school and at her church. Many neighbors and parishioners spoke of her as being mentally ill.

Her parents wondered if her behavior was the result of a blow to the head as a child when she fell from a jungle gym onto concrete and was unconscious for almost an hour until she was seen in a local hospital. "She was never the same after that," her father explained.

His loving child seemed to change, unable to control her emotions, impulsive, rigid in her behavior. In conversations, she blurts out whatever she's thinking, interrupting other children and adults.

The success of intervention varies with the particular linguistic feature trained, the manner and duration of the training, and the characteristics of the individual child. Prior to beginning intervention, you, as a speech-language pathologist (SLP), will want to examine all deficit areas for a child and apply a "so what?" criterion that considers the importance of individual deficits for a child's overall communication.

It is also important to consider generalization before beginning intervention and to make critical teaching decisions on the basis of generalization to the everyday environment. Even if using a more traditional approach, at least a portion of each lesson should involve use in a conversational milieu. Intervention that focuses solely on linguistic form while ignoring use can result in limited progress and lack of generalization.

A functional approach will be my overall model for intervention. At all levels of instruction, some elements of the functional intervention model can be used even within more traditional teaching.

Intervention should be fun and challenging, using real conversational exchanges between the child and caregivers wherever possible. Thus, both partners are involved actively in the process.

In this chapter, we explore some proven and some promising techniques for language intervention. I have attempted to include the best evidence-based practices (EBPs). We'll introduce cognitive considerations first because they'll be referred to throughout the chapter.

For clarity, I have divided the chapter into four aspects of language: pragmatics, semantics, syntax, and morphology. We'll discuss hierarchies for teaching and techniques that lend themselves well to each area. The final portions of the chapter deal with the special needs of children from culturally linguistically diverse (CLD) backgrounds and with the clinical application of computers.

Despite gaps in the literature, a general consensus on the basic principles and procedures of language therapy exists (Fey et al., 2003; Nelson, 2010; Paul & Norbury, 2011; Reed, 2012). One disconnection is between our current learning and language development knowledge and our clinical practice. The following are things we do know (Kamhi, 2014):

- Learning is more difficult than generalization.
- Instruction that varies the conditions of learning and practice is more efficient than instruction that is constant and predictable.
- Varied stimulation (distributed practice) is a more effective teaching strategy than focused stimulation (massed practice).
- The more feedback is not necessarily the better.
- More therapy is not always better.
- Telegraphic utterances (e.g., *push ball, mommy sock*) should not be provided as input for children with limited language.
- Increasing levels of mean length of utterance (MLU) and targeting Brown's (1973) 14 grammatical morphemes are not appropriate language goals. Complex syntax is more difficult to teach, especially with preschool children, but more beneficial.
- Sequencing is not as important a skill for narrative competence as conceptual understanding of the topic and cohesion and coherence.

The best intervention addresses language holistically so that a child can experience newly acquired language as it is used in communication. Some SLPs accomplish this goal by targeting skills in more than one area of language or by using a stage approach in which a few teaching targets from a stage of development are targeted simultaneously. Suggested activities are presented in Appendix G.

Cognitive Considerations

SLPs can intervene with cognitive deficits affecting communication, such as those found in children with traumatic brain injury (TBI), through basic principles of cognitive rehabilitation that can be embedded in a functional context (Sohlberg & Turkstra, 2011). This means that if you choose to work with individuals with cognitive communication disorders (CCDs; American Speech-Language-Hearing Association [ASHA], 2004), you'll need special advanced teaching beyond the scope of this introductory text. The principles of cognitive rehabilitation include

- collaboration with the child and caregivers to determine needs and goals that are functional in nature;
- practice to directly target the child's needs within functional contexts;
- sufficient practice so that skills can be learned; and
- a generalization plan built into intervention (Sohlberg & Mateer, 2001).

Taken together, these principles translate into cognitive rehabilitation for children that includes individualized, contextualized goals to support generalization for their academic and social participation (Ciccia et al., 2021). The most functional and natural treatment settings are school and home.

Given the nature of CCDs, services in schools should rely heavily on a coordinated team-based approach. In interdisciplinary teams, each member can contribute their expertise and integrate care through regular meetings in which they synthesize both knowledge and treatment practices (Hardin & Kelly, 2019).

Information Processing

As discussed in Chapter 3, differences in information processing help us understand some disorders further. These differences can suggest certain intervention techniques to be used when working with children. For example, children with intellectual developmental disorder (IDD) process information differently from those who do not have IDD. Possible techniques to use with these children are represented in Table 11–1 and reflect the characteristics of children with IDD in general.

In addition, as an SLP, you must be mindful of individual learning styles as well as the characteristics of certain identifiable groups of children. Group characteristics do not represent any one individual. That said, accommodations must be made in intervention for the special learning needs of boys with fragile X syndrome (FXS). In short, with these boys, an SLP can take advantage of their more visual learning style while stressing listening and comprehension. Intervention sessions must also accommodate to these boys' short attention spans, difficulty with transitions to new activities or topics, other sensory deficits, and low tolerance of stress (Mirrett et al., 2003).

Some children with FXS have nonverbal learning disability (NLD), which is characterized by deficits in visual and tactile perception, psychomotor skills, and learning novel information. Although language form is relatively unaffected in children with NLD, subtle pragmatic and semantic disorders exist. Individual differences will be even more varied.

Table 11–1. Techniques to Use With Individuals With Intellectual Developmental Disorder

Attention

- Aid attending by visually or auditorily highlighting stimulus cues. Likewise, gestures used to highlight important information can enhance the auditory message. Cues should be gradually decreased.
- Teach child to scan stimuli for relevant cues.

Discrimination

- Highlight and explain similarities and differences that will aid discrimination. Preschoolers do not understand terms such as same and different. Teachers must demonstrate likenesses and differences, such as hair/no-hair. Meaningful sorting tasks with real objects can be helpful. Overall size and shape (not *circle*, *square*, or *triangle*) and function are relevant characteristics for preschoolers.

Organization

- "Pre-organize" information for easier processing and storage. No "winging it" here. Visual and spatial cues may be helpful.
- Train associate strategies. What things go together? Why?
- Use short-term memory tasks, such as repetition of important information, to aid simultaneous and successive processing. Repetition and interpretation are helpful.

Memory

- Train rehearsal strategies, such as physical imitation. Gradually shift to more symbolic rehearsal tasks.
- Use overlearning and lots of examples.
- Train both signal (sounds, smells, tastes, and sights) and symbol recall of events. Signals, which are easier to recall, can be gradually reduced.
- Word associations for new words will improve recall of the words. Likewise, sentential and narrative associations will improve recall.
- Highlight important information to be remembered, thus enhancing selective attending.
- Use visual memory to enhance auditory memory.

Transfer

- Training situations should be very similar or identical to the generalization context. Use real items in training, at least initially.
- Highlight similarities between situations, especially if training and generalization contexts differ. Help child recall similarities.
- Help child recall previous tasks when approaching new problems.
- Use people in child's everyday contexts for training.

CHAPTER 11 SPECIFIC INTERVENTION TECHNIQUES

Pragmatics

Traditional language intervention goals are product oriented. In addition to learning a language form, it's essential that children understand the functional qualities or uses of these structures. Thus, when appropriate, linguistic forms should be targeted within a functional context.

Through role-play, videotaped interactions, and meaningful interactions, an SLP can teach a child to identify when communication is inadequate, inaccurate, or inappropriate. An SLP may directly target a number of pragmatic skills within a single lesson and can use many everyday events and play activities to teach pragmatic skills. For example, telephone conversations can teach several pragmatic skills, such as acknowledgment of the interaction, conversational opening and closing, topic maintenance, and referential communication. The use of different situations can help a child adapt to differing scenarios. For example, by pretending that they are lost, a child can learn requesting and gaining assistance and information, along with following directions.

Construction toys, such as Legos, can teach requesting assistance, referential communication, giving and following directions, and topic maintenance. More difficult tasks will require requesting assistance.

Several children's books can be enacted to help a child learn roles. The use of puppets or dolls or different costumes also will aid the learning of role taking. It should be remembered that the goal is to take roles in communication. This is not theatrical practice.

Finally, an SLP can use any number of activities for referential communication. Children can describe objects seen in books, on computers, or even through toy periscopes. Such activities as I Spy and Twenty Questions also aid referential communication growth and foster requesting and giving information. In addition, object descriptions can be a part of requesting similar objects, as in "I want the fuzzy bear."

Effective intervention should enhance language and social skills while generalizing to authentic interactions (Timler et al., 2007). Although more structured clinician-centered intervention methods may be required for some children and targets, generalization to a child's everyday environment is key to success.

Social Skills and Autism Spectrum Disorder

Social communication and self-regulation are areas of struggle for children with both ASD and TBI. Deficits in social communication can negatively affect academic performance (Welsh et al., 2001), be associated with anxiety and depression (Barnhill, 2001), and affect friendship and employment outcomes in adults (Howlin et al., 2013). Self-regulation deficits negatively impact academic and social interactions for children (Jahromi et al., 2013) and are correlated with young adults' self-reports of lower quality of life compared to non-ASD peers (Dijkhuis et al., 2016).

Although group interventions are common practice for targeting social communication goals in children with high-functioning ASD, evidence for the efficacy is mixed (Rao et al., 2008). Both social communication and self-regulation are skill areas that predict outcomes for children, but there's little research on interventions addressing both of these skill areas in school-age children with high-functioning ASD.

It's generally believed that social cognitive interventions are more effective than behavioral approaches for children with high-functioning ASD. These methods teach social problem-solving skills to be used to change behavior flexibly across contexts as opposed to teaching fixed social rules (Crooke et al., 2016). I'm reminded of Carrie at the onset of this chapter and her rigid social behavior.

A parent-assisted blended intervention combining components of Structured TEACCHing and Social Thinking has been shown to be effective in teaching social communication and self-regulation concept knowledge to children with ASD and their parents (Nowell et al., 2019). Both parents and children demonstrate an increase in social communication and self-regulation knowledge.

The essential elements of Structured TEACCHing are

- an environment structured to make activities understandable;
- use of child's strengths in visual skills to supplement weaker skills;
- use of special interests to promote engagement; and
- support for self-initiated meaningful communication (Mesibov & Shea, 2010).

The TEACCH model encourages parent-assisted intervention in support clinic–taught communication; therefore, parents are active participants.

Social Thinking is a cognitive-based methodology focused on building social concepts and social knowledge to aid understanding and using of social behaviors (Crooke et al., 2016; Winner, 2013). The purpose is to establish awareness needed to adapt behavior and flexibly meet social expectations across communication contexts and partners (Crooke et al., 2016).

Intentions

Children select and acquire utterances that are communicatively most useful. As an SLP, you'll be concerned with the breadth of intentions that a child is able to express. The following sections address the teaching of several intentions. Appendix F also provides several indirect linguistic cues useful for eliciting different functions.

Calling for Attention

Children seek attention from adults. The form of attention-requesting is usually a child calling a person by name or gaining attention by some other means, such as tapping the listener's shoulder, moving into the visual field of the listener, leaning in the direction of the listener, or using eye contact. The child also may specify how the adult should respond by making a request. These sequences are easy to teach within a variety of activities.

Within the classroom, teachers might give a child an object and ask the child to take it to an adult who, for the purpose of teaching, initially ignores the child. The child also might be asked to relay a message to someone else.

Adults should attend to a child as soon as the child requests attention. If the child continually demands attention or uses inappropriate behavior to get attention, the adult

CHAPTER 11 SPECIFIC INTERVENTION TECHNIQUES

will have to set some limits, such as only responding in certain situations and never responding to inappropriate behavior.

> **Food for Thought:** It may seem very basic to call for attention, but it does take some social skill. It's importance can be seen in the tantrums that follow a child being ignored.

Requests for Action or Assistance

Requests for action can be taught at mealtime, within small group projects, or during almost any physically challenging task. An SLP needs to design situations in which children require assistance to complete a task. To encourage requesting, a language teacher can use games in which children must solve problems. Tasks also may be sabotaged (see Table 10–1). In requests for actions or assistance, attention is gained first, and the form of the utterance is interrogative (*Can you . . . ?*) or imperative (*Hold my . . .*).

SLPs can modify a child's behavior by ceasing reinforcement for a less desirable form while providing reinforcement for a second, more acceptable one. It is important to establish well-generalized use of the acceptable communicative act in situations previously associated with the less desirable alternative.

Although young children with ASD can learn new communicative behavior, they may fail to use that behavior conditionally (Sigafoos et al., 2002). *Conditional use* means using the behavior that best matches a particular context. In some cases, individuals with significant developmental disorders (DDs) find a socially unacceptable response option more reinforcing than a more conventional one. Screams may get more attention than politely asking and may require less effort (Sigafoos et al., 2002).

An SLP cannot assume that a child's obligatory use of a communicative behavior, such as requesting assistance, will result in correct conditional use. Conditional use requires a child to use one communicative behavior when it is needed but refrain from using it when it is not. For example, when items are nearby or easy to manipulate, a child can be taught to help themselves, and when items are distant or difficult to manipulate, the child can produce a request. This can be accomplished in graduated steps in which a child attempts a desired task and is initially successful. As the task becomes increasingly more difficult, the child must request assistance. In this way, conditional use can be established even with children with ASD (Reichle et al., 2008; Reichle & McComas, 2004).

Requests for Information

Children with language disorders often do not see other persons as sources of information and may produce few such requests of this type. Although the environment can be manipulated to encourage requests for objects and actions, it is not as easy to encourage or increase a child's need and desire to seek information.

Requests for information require that a language teacher omit essential information for some novel or unfamiliar task, such as an art project, a new game, or some challenging academic task. Objects unknown to a child may be introduced without being named or their purpose explained. A child can be prodded gently to ask questions if asking does not occur spontaneously.

A child must recognize both the need for this information and that another person possesses the knowledge. Recognition of need is often the most difficult aspect of this teaching. Confrontational naming tasks, such as labeling objects pulled from a bag, some known and others unknown, may encourage initial requesting for information. The form of requests for information is either a *wh-* or *yes/no* interrogative with rising intonation, as in "What's that?" or "Is that a marker?"

An SLP or other adult also might encourage the child to ask questions by questioning them about another person's feelings or actions of which the child has little knowledge. The child then can be cued with "Why don't you ask (name)?" This tactic can be used with naming tasks as well, as in "See if Juan knows what this is."

A child should be expected to ask questions that reflect the forms they are capable of producing. The SLP's verbal responses discussed in Chapter 10 can be used to help the child modify incorrect, inappropriate, or immature responses or learn new ones.

Requests for Objects

An adult can easily teach requests for objects within art tasks, group projects, snack time, job training, or daily living skills training, such as dressing and hygiene. It is essential that a child actually desire the object they are to request and that the language teacher can actually provide it.

An SLP or other teacher can modify the environment to increase both the opportunities for requesting and the behaviors that direct a child's attention to these opportunities. Many situations, especially those with groups of children, provide an opportunity for overlooking a child's turn, thus encouraging requesting. Of particular importance is a coordinated program designed to teach requesting for use in the everyday environment by approximating that environment and by teaching those within that to model and elicit requests. Table 11–2 includes general guidelines for caregiver elicitation techniques.

Expression of this intention usually begins with eye contact or some attention-getting behavior, such as calling a name. The form, usually accompanied by a reaching gesture, is interrogative (*Can I have . . . ?*) or imperative (*Give me . . .*) and specifies the desired object.

An SLP can elicit denials by giving the child something other than what they requested or by giving the child something undesirable. The child can reject either an action or a proposal. The speaker uses emphatic stress, and the utterance is in a negative form.

Responding to Requests

Responses may take the form of an answer to a question or a reply to a remark. These forms are very different and require different skills and syntactic forms.

In responding to questions, children must recognize that they possess the answer and that they are required to reply. Initial teaching might disregard the correctness of the answer in favor of reinforcing answering in general. Responding with an incorrect answer is preferred over no answer at all. Some children with language disorders have

CHAPTER 11 SPECIFIC INTERVENTION TECHNIQUES

Table 11–2. Guidelines for Caregiver Elicitation of Requests for Objects

Make statements throughout the day about objects that the child might prefer. Wait for a response.

Use elicitation behaviors to accompany high-interest activities and play. These behaviors include the following:

Modeling with an imitative prompt. Facilitator provides a model of a request and asks the child to imitate.

Direct questioning. Facilitator asks, "What do you want?" or "What do you need?"

Indirect modeling. Facilitator provides a partial model followed by an indirect elicitation request, such as "If you want more X, let me know" (or "ask me for it") or "Would you like to X or Y?"

Obstacle presentation. Facilitator requests that the child accomplish some task but provides an obstacle to accomplishment.

"Please get me the chalk over there." (There is no chalk.)

"Pour everyone some juice." (The container is empty.)

General statement. Facilitator makes a verbal comment about some activity or object that the child might want to request. The facilitator entices the child.

"We could play Candyland if you want to."

"I have some Play-Doh on that high shelf."

Set up specific situations to elicit requesting.

Provide direct and indirect models as often as possible without requiring the child to imitate.

Provide a model at appropriate times when the child appears to need assistance or is looking quizzical.

Have the child attempt difficult tasks in which help is occasionally needed.

Respond *immediately* and *naturally* to any verbal request.

---

difficulty identifying the emotions of others and of themselves and placing these in a form of expression. We can teach awareness and expression through a three-step intervention model (Way et al., 2007):

1. Connecting physical experience and emotions
2. Increasing awareness of own emotional state
3. Connecting emotion to expression

Activities within each step are presented in Table 11–3.

Replies

Replying is more difficult to teach than answering because a response is expected from the child but not required. A child can be helped to recognize the need to reply by

Table 11–3. Teaching Emotional Awareness and Expression

Connecting physical experience and emotions

- Bodywork, such as recognizing one's heartbeat, sweating, flushing, or a stomachache, can help a child turn their attention internally.
- Connecting physical states to specific feelings and learning methods to calm oneself when feeling anxious or upset.

Increasing awareness of own emotional state

- Drawing the child's attention to the important features of expression, then modeling language to express those feelings. SLPs might observe and comment on facial expressions, body expressions, vocal affect, and labels or words in affective experiences.
- Role-playing various feelings.
- Identifying feelings of characters in stories, videos, or photos; or using art therapy.
- Using *feelings strips* on which is the unfinished sentence, "I feel . . . ," into which children can insert feelings/faces to describe their feelings. In this way, children are taught physical cues for different feelings at the same time as they learn to become aware of their own.
- Identify single feelings and then learn to recognize multiple feelings at a particular moment. Begin with *primary* emotions such as joy, sadness, anger, fear, disgust, and interest, and then progress to more sophisticated *complex* emotions that require self-reflection, such as empathy, sympathy, guilt, envy, shame, regret, and pride.

Connecting emotion to expression

- Drawing pictures to express feelings nonverbally in preparation for addressing them verbally.
- Expressing emotion through role-playing, pretend play, and acting out dramas.
- Creating a skit from an index card listing multiple feelings, and then having other children guess the feelings being portrayed.
- Acting out stories from books, TV shows, and movies.
- Reading and listening to narratives and making sense of character perspectives in the context of story events. SLPs can use questions that probe linguistic and socioemotional awareness and questions that guide students to reflect on feelings and organize these ideas using language to describe, report, predict, and interpret feelings and motivations.
- Oral and written storytelling to share personal narratives while developing integrated language skills and expressiveness.

Sources: Information from Denham and Burton (1996) and Hyter et al. (2006).

physical signs from the SLP, such as a head nod, or the passing of an object to signal "It's your turn."

A child's ability to reply may be hindered by an inability to determine the topic or to formulate a response. An adult may enhance linguistic processing by having the child repeat the previous speaker's comment. Over time, the adult can modify this procedure to teach the child to whisper the speaker's comment; mouth it; and, finally, silently repeat until the process is internalized by the child. In this way, children can be helped to identify important information in comments and in formulating replies.

Statements

Show-and-tell, discussions, and current-event activities help children state information. During discussions of high-interest topics, such as holidays, pets, and family events for children or dating, friends, and competitive games for adolescents, a caregiver can encourage offering of opinions.

A teacher also can use mock radio and television broadcasts. With a little cutting and some paint, they can convert a large appliance box into a television from within which children can deliver daily newscasts of information.

Partners have different informational needs, and knowing the correct amount requires some presuppositional skill. Children can be taught how much information to include (see the section titled Presupposition later in this chapter).

Initially, the child must secure the listener's attention and state the discussion topic. Later, statements can be expanded into narratives whose purpose is also to convey information.

Conversational Abilities

More than other areas of language intervention, the teaching of conversational abilities requires the use of actual conversational situations. Ritualized communication that interferes with interpersonal communication, such as echolalia, can be modified gradually into acceptable and conventional routines, such as greetings, conversational initiations, and requests for repair. For children with Asperger's syndrome, high-functioning autism, or other social interactional difficulties, the following conversational goals seem appropriate (Kline & Volkmar, 2000):

- Conventions of verbal and nonverbal communication, including initiating a conversation and selecting appropriate topics
- Social awareness and social problem-solving, including perceiving verbal and nonverbal cues and making inferences
- Self-evaluation and management, including ability to participate in diverse communication activities and to control one's own behavior

Children with high-functioning ASD need support to improve their communication skills and interactions with peers (Kelly et al., 2018). It would be appropriate to form a mentor system with peers with typically developing language (TDL), including opportunities to practice social communication skills.

These children may also benefit from comprehensive instruction in the basic components required for successful conversation, including explanations for why these components are necessary (Müller et al., 2016). Intervention outcomes may be enhanced through a variety of strategies, including peer-directed interactions, questions, use of *wh-* words in topic introduction, extending conversation through topic maintenance, and use of conversational repair.

Social routines can be memorized and practiced in different situations that help a child become more flexible. Variations can be taught through different adults and situations. For example, one does not offer to shake hands when the potential partner has their arms full.

In a study of adolescents with TDL, several behaviors that may or may not be present in teens with language disorders occur frequently (Turkstra et al., 2003). These include

- looking at a conversational partner, especially when listening;
- nodding and showing neutral and positive facial expression;
- responding verbally to acknowledge understanding (*uh-huh*, *yeah*); and
- giving contingent responses.

These behaviors suggest targets for helping children with language disorders interact more appropriately. You may recall that contingent responses may be semantically contingent (on-topic) and/or pragmatically contingent (appropriate).

Although limited, research data suggest intervention methods that may work for some teens (Brinton et al., 2004). A two-step intervention program could target

- helping youth with language disorder think of conversation as a reciprocal endeavor that requires adjustment for one's partner; and
- providing interactive strategies to solicit and act on conversational contributions by others.

Intervention can occur within structured, conversation-focused, small-group activities (Nippold, 2000). The atmosphere should be positive with plenty of opportunity for success. Within this context, the SLP models appropriate responses, and this modeling is followed by teen practice, then peer analysis and feedback with the use of video recordings and small-group discussion. Scripted sequences and role-play can be very helpful.

Video clips and guided observation and comment can be used to aid an adolescent to comment on the nature of exchanges, feelings and thoughts of participants, and interpretation of reactions. The bulk of the time, however, should focus on interactive strategies, moving from highly structured situations in which turns and topics are controlled to more free-flowing conversations. Carrie, mentioned at the beginning, will need a supportive environment to learn to exchange information and to discuss feelings.

Children can be taught in variations of comment–question, in which they make a contingent comment on their partner's utterance and then ask a related question, as in turnabouts. Listening and comprehension skills can also be enhanced. From here, additional interactional techniques, such as how to ask someone's opinion or how to draw listeners into the conversation, can be taught.

> ***Food for Thought:*** Although it may seem easy to enter a play situation, we should keep conversational entry in perspective. Each of us has been in a situation in which conversational entry seems awkward or strained.

Entering a Conversation

Although entering an interaction can be a formidable challenge to children with language disorders, they can be taught play-entry strategies through modeling and prompting by an adult (Selber Beilinson & Olswang, 2003). Four nonverbal "low-risk" strategies can be taught initially through modeling and visual picture prompts:

- Walk over to your friend.
- Watch your friend.
- Get a toy like the one your friend is using.
- Do the same thing as your friend.

A fifth, "high-risk" strategy includes verbal initiation.

Verbal Initiation. In modeling verbal initiation, the classroom teacher, aide, or SLP helps a child select a toy similar to that of another child and says to the second child, "We're building with blocks just like you." This can be an opening for the other child to respond by asking the child to join. A more direct model might include telling a child what to say.

When a child can successfully imitate the opening behavior, the adult gradually reduces the model and tries to prompt it through toys and picture and verbal cues. These are also reduced until a child can initiate spontaneously. Other strategies might include interpreting (*I think Mohammed wants you to play with him*), giving suggestions (*Maybe Kwanzi would like to see what you made*), referring to a peer (*Maybe Alex can help you hold the paper while you glue it*), and commenting on similarities (*Jin is making a costume too. Tell him about yours.*) (Weitzman & Greenberg, 2002).

Although we have to be cautious with small research studies, one promising approach with social initiations among children with ASD targets involved initiating questions during social interactions. Using the motivational procedures of pivotal response treatment (PRT), researchers were able to increase social question-asking of both targeted and untargeted questions (Koegel et al., 2014). Gains were also made in overall communication and in adaptive behavior.

PRT procedures included child choice, interspersal of maintenance and acquisition tasks, rewarding attempts, and the use of direct and natural reinforcers (Koegel & Koegel, 2006, 2012). The components are as follows (Koegel et al., 2014):

- Child choice: Begin with highly desired items and provide an opportunity for the child to *initiate* a question about the item.
  - *"What is it?"* The SLP places a variety of highly desired objects in an opaque bag and verbally prompts the child to initiate "What is it?" or an approximation. After the child asks the question, the SLP opens the bag, labels the object, and waits for the child to repeat the label. The child's repeated label is followed by a natural and direct reinforcer. The prompt is gradually faded or reduced.

- *"Where is it?"* The SLP hides the desired item and verbally prompts the child to ask the question or an approximation. Natural and immediate reinforcement involves responding with the location of the desired item to enable the child to find it. Again, the prompt is faded upon repeated success by the child.

- *"Who is it?"* Children are taught this question using their preferred miniature characters and pretend-play activities. When a new, unknown, character is incorporated into play, the SLP prompts the child to ask, "Who is it?" In response, the SLP names the character and gives it to the child. Prompts are faded as before.

- *"What happened?"* Motivation is increased by indicating that something surprising or exciting had just happened. The child is prompted to ask, "What happened?" The SLP immediately and naturally reinforces the child by answering. Prompts are faded.

- Intersperse maintenance and acquisition tasks: Gradually introduce neutral or less desired items and fade prompts.

- Reinforcement of attempts: Adult answers *child* approximation of a question about stimulus item or action.

- Natural reinforcer: Child is provided with a natural reinforcer, such as an opportunity to interact or play with the item.

The SLP and/or parent participate in an activity with the child. The adults scaffold or structure the activity until the child begins to anticipate the routine and the reward. The scaffold is gradually reduced.

Presupposition

A speaker's semantic decisions are based on their knowledge of the referents (the thing to which words refer) and the situation and on *presuppositions*, or social knowledge a listener needs. A speaker provides information that is as unambiguous as possible. In other words, the speaker and the listener share the same linguistic context.

Often, children with language disorders are unaware of their audience's needs. Carrie, mentioned at the start of the chapter, is ambiguous in her identifying of topics of comment. Two aspects of teaching might be (a) what information to relay and (b) how much.

What to State. "What" can be taught with descriptive or directive tasks in which a child is the speaker. A listener tries to guess or draw the described object or to follow the directions. The adult can use barrier games, in which they place an opaque barrier between the speaker and the listener. Because the speaker and the listener do not share the same nonlinguistic context, the bulk of the information must be carried by the linguistic element in an unambiguous manner if the listener is to comprehend. The list of fun activities in which a child directs an adult in how to do something is endless.

CHAPTER 11 SPECIFIC INTERVENTION TECHNIQUES

431

When the child is the listener, the SLP can send ambiguous or incomplete messages or directions to give the child an opportunity to identify the missing semantic elements. Obstacle courses are a good vehicle through which the child can be directed or direct others.

How Much to State. Teaching the correct amount of information to transmit may be more difficult. Of course, giving insufficient information in the tasks previously mentioned would make the directions difficult to follow. The SLP can teach children to give more, as well as more accurate, information.

For a child who gives too much information, these tasks may be taught initially one descriptor (color, size, etc.) or one step in a task at a time. The relating of very discrete or limited events, such as combing your hair or washing your face, also can control the amount of information to be relayed.

The SLP can help the child monitor their own production to know when redundancy occurs. This is accomplished by gently reminding the child that certain information was relayed previously. In subsequent teaching, the SLP can quiz the child about the novelty or the lack of information presented. This will help the child identify the correct amount of information.

Referential Skills

Referential skills include identifying novel content and describing this content for a listener. Children with learning disability have been taught successfully to use referential skills through the use of barrier or guessing games. The description of physical attributes (*It's big and white and furry*) is somewhat easier to teach than are relational terms, such as location (*He's in front of the computer*). Guessing games can be lots of fun and very instructive.

Topic. Topic offers an encompassing framework for considering other language skills. Unlike greetings, which vary only slightly across situations, topics and methods of topic introduction and identification are context-dependent.

Topic Initiation. *Initiation* is the verbal introduction of a topic not currently being discussed. Children with language disorders often do not understand the purpose of conversations or are reluctant to introduce topics for discussion. Topic initiation implies an active conversational strategy. A child with a language disorder may not be adept at introducing topics clearly or may have very limited topics to discuss. Children with ASD or TBI may introduce unusual or inappropriate topics.

The SLP might first teach the child to gain a listener's attention. Topic initiation has been taught through the use of an SLP or language teacher waiting and through teaching the purpose of conversation. In the first step, a language teacher maintains eye contact for 10 seconds but does not speak. Delay can be an effective strategy for prompting children to initiate.

If the child does not initiate the conversation during this wait, the adult can explain the purpose of conversation and the enjoyment that can result. They also can describe the roles of speaker and listener. Then the adult returns to the waiting strategy. If the child still does not respond, the adult can suggest that the child find something of interest to discuss by looking on the internet at pictures from the child's life. The adult then returns to the waiting strategy. If the child fails to initiate again, the adult can model a topic initiation.

It is important that the adult focus fully on the child when they initiate and follow the child's lead. The adult should try not to interrupt the child. If the child inadequately introduces a topic, the adult can request further information to identify the topic.

The SLP initially can tolerate inappropriate topics to give the child some success. Gradually, the SLP can discuss the inappropriateness of some topics and gently steer the conversation to more appropriate ground. They can suggest topics ("Maybe you'll tell me about . . . ") and leave it for the child to initiate. The SLP also can teach the child to ask other people about their likes and dislikes, favorite foods, sports, TV shows, or exciting trips or vacations in order to include other-oriented topics in the child's repertoire.

To increase the frequency of memory-related topics, you as the SLP can encourage the child to talk about feelings or activities. Elicitation can be direct ("What did you do yesterday?") or indirect ("I wonder what you did yesterday").

The SLP can encourage the child to ask the same information in turn. In addition, you can engage the child in activities and then ask the child to discuss what was done. The SLP can provide feedback. Future-related topic initiations are similar, such as discussing what the child will do next. The use of such conversationally based strategies can increase nonimmediate topic initiations, as well as the general level of syntactic performance.

Topic Maintenance. An SLP can continue the conversation by commenting on the topic a child initiates and by cueing the child to respond. The SLP can use turnabouts—usually a comment followed by a cue for the child to respond, such as a question—to keep the conversation flowing and on-topic. Questions should make pragmatic sense; that is, the adult should not know the answer prior to asking. Table 11–4 is a list of various turnabouts.

Off-topic responding may indicate that a child is inattentive or cannot identify the referent or topic presented. Children who are inattentive may need help determining how to focus their attention.

An SLP can help a child who cannot sort through the information to identify the referent or topic through the use of questions and prompts that highlight those semantic cues of importance to the child. Practice conversations with various partners and topics can provide an opportunity to learn and generalize. The adult can keep the child on-topic with such cues as "Anything else you can tell me about (topic)?" and "Tell me more about (topic)."

When an adult and a child have shared the same experience, the adult can act as a guide to keep the child on-topic. The adult also can help the child sequence events through the use of questions ("Then what happened?") or probes ("Are you sure that happened next?").

As the SLP, try to avoid dead-end conversational turns. Dead-end comments result in a short response, such as "yes" or "no," that ends the interaction.

CHAPTER 11 SPECIFIC INTERVENTION TECHNIQUES

Table 11–4. Variety of Turnabouts

Type	Example
Tag	*Child:* Baby's panties. *Mother:* It's the baby's diaper, isn't it?
Clarification (contingent query)	*Huh?* *What?*
Specific request	*What's that?*
Confirmation	*Horse?* *Is that a hippopotamus?* (Hand object to partner and give quizzical glance)

Expansions
    Suggestions
    Corrections
    Behavior comment
	
	I want one.
	No, it's a zebra! (Expectant tone)
	You can't sit on that.

Expansive question for sustaining conversation	*What would the police officer do then?*

Duration of Topic. An SLP or an adult can help an incessant talker by using very limited topics with definite boundaries, such as "What animals did you see at the zoo?" If the child strays beyond the topic, the adult can interrupt. They then can remind the child of the topic and gently bring them back to it.

The adult also should alert the child when they have provided enough information or are redundant. Such phrases as "You've already told me about X" or "I'll only answer that question one more time" help the child establish boundaries.

Children who provide too little information can be encouraged to provide more with "Tell me more." An SLP also can play dumb with such utterances as "Well, I guess it was pretty boring if that's all that happened." In general, children remain on-topic longer when they are enacting scenarios, describing, or problem-solving.

Turn Taking

It is important not to initiate turn-taking teaching while also attempting to teach topic maintenance. Too many new teaching targets may confuse the child. An SLP may have to tolerate off-topic comments initially to correct inappropriate turn taking.

Turn taking can begin at a nonverbal, physical level. An SLP and a child can pass items back and forth as they use them. The item then becomes the symbol for talking when you hold it. Many structured games also require turn taking.

The SLP can provide a turn-taking model by imitating the child's spontaneous speech or using verbal games and motion songs with groups of children. Later, the SLP can use turnabouts or a question–answer technique to help a child take verbal turns.

Nonlinguistic cues, such as eye contact and nodding, can also signal the child to take a turn. The SLP can decrease questioning gradually in favor of these nonlinguistic cues and wait for the child to take a turn. Children can be taught attention-getting devices, such as increased speaking volume, to gain a turn. Games in which the child directs other people are highly motivating turn-taking activities.

Turn taking is appropriate if it does not interrupt others. Our friend Carrie seems unable to turn take, impulsively saying things that pop into her mind. A child such as Carrie who is overly assertive and who continually interrupts may need to be reminded not to do so.

The SLP might focus instruction on identifying when speakers have completed their turns. They also should explain appropriate interruptions, as in emergencies. Structured exchanges through use of a smartphone or mock police radio may help children understand the importance of turn allocation through play. Structured games, such as Twenty Questions, also foster turn-allocation learning. In fact, there are many games that require turn-taking skills and can be adapted for conversational teaching.

> ***Food for Thought:*** **Are these conversational behaviors evident in your daily interactions? Sit back and notice.**

Conversational Repair

Children with language disorders often seem unaware of the distinction between understanding and failure to understand and rarely act when they do not. Males with ASD respond less to clarification requests compared to those with TDL, Down syndrome (DS), or FXS both with and without ASD. In contrast, those with FXS with ASD respond more inappropriately that those with ASD, DS, or TDL (Barstein et al., 2018).

Communication breakdown goes beyond the five traditional domains of language (syntax, morphology, phonology, semantics, and pragmatics) and can reflect problems of cognition. This means that both assessment and intervention should target underlying cognitive processes that impact communication. For example, cognitive deficits, such as those seen in children with TBI, can manifest as difficulties in many areas, including recall of newly learned information, attending, and direction following (Ciccia et al., 2021).

An SLP may modify comprehension monitoring through the use of recorded language samples. Recorded samples can be replayed throughout teaching.

Steps in Teaching Requests for Repair. The child can be taught first to identify, label, and demonstrate active listening behaviors, such as sitting, looking at the speaker, and thinking about what the speaker says. After learning to distinguish successful and unsuccessful performance of the three behaviors, the child labels and demonstrates each. The child also might repeat the previous speaker's utterance or reply to such questions

CHAPTER 11 SPECIFIC INTERVENTION TECHNIQUES

as "What did (name) just say?" This can be worked into many play situations, such as playing store or restaurant.

Next, the child can be taught to detect and react to signal inadequacies, such as insufficient loudness, excessive rate, or competing noise. These obstructions are relatively easy to identify and enable a child to learn the difference between understanding and not understanding.

Within everyday activities, the adult can encourage clarification requests from the child by mumbling or talking too fast. This technique works especially well when giving directions needed to complete some fun task. The SLP or adult occasionally can ask the child, "What did I say? How can we find out?"

Once able to identify signal inadequacies, a child can be taught a variety of responses for requesting clarification. Requests may include general appeals, such as "Pardon?" (or "What?"), "I can't hear you," and "Wait. . . . Now say it again" (or "Again please"), or more specific requests, such as "Talk louder please" (or "Louder"), "Could you talk more slowly?" (or "Slow down"), and "Did you say *X*?" It is best to begin with more general requests and then move to more specific ones. The request form should reflect the child's overall syntactic level.

Next, a child can be taught to detect and react to content inadequacies, such as inexplicit, ambiguous, and physically impossible commands. For example, because inadequate content may not always be obvious, the SLP can ask the child to repeat the message to themself and/or to the speaker and to attempt the task demanded. Again, the child is taught various methods for requesting clarification of inadequate content.

This part of the teaching can be great fun, with the adult making outrageous statements and ridiculous demands of the child as in a game of "Simon says." I still remember the expression on the face of a small child with DS whom I had asked to get into his lunch box. The SLP can insert intentional content inadequacies into any number of daily activities.

Finally, the SLP can teach the child to identify and react to messages that exceed their comprehension capacity by the presence of unfamiliar words, excessive length, and excessive syntactic complexity. This level of comprehension breakdown may be the most difficult to detect.

Steps in Teaching Identification and Reaction. A child can practice identification and reaction in the form of clarification requests in real-life situations in which these difficulties are likely to occur. Most novel activities include unusual jargon that the adult can use to confuse the message. For example, cooking offers such words as *ladle, simmer,* and *skillet.*

As teaching progresses, the child should learn to identify the point of actual breakdown for the speaker. The child can be aided in identifying where the breakdown occurred through questions from the SLP.

Although this sequence is taught easily in an audio-recorded mode, generalization to actual conversational use should not be neglected. The introduction of puppets, dolls, or role-playing at each step can facilitate this generalization. Written scripts may be used with older children, targeting frequent conversational contexts.

Narration

Narrative intervention may focus on the organization of, cohesion within, or comprehension of the narrative. Modeling and practice are especially important. Specific targets will vary.

Whether the teaching target is comprehension or narrative retelling, or story production, it is important to control for the many variables that can affect a child's performance, including the following (Boudreau & Larsen, 2004):

- Number of characters
- Plot line clarity
- Number of episodes
- Number and complexity of utterances
- Clear resolution
- Age appropriateness
- Interest level

It is also important to manage the external prompts needed by a child, such as the use of sequential pictures and verbal prompts. Prompts can range from those needed to craft the narrative, such as "In the beginning . . . " and "How did the story end?" to more open-ended prompts, such as "What happened next?"

Narrative Structure

Knowledge of episode structure forms a narrative frame within which the child can interpret complex events and unfamiliar content. An SLP can facilitate development of internalized narrative organization through the following:

- Involving children in organized activities, such as daily routines, to help them organize their own real-life scripts. Go over each event in a routine with children.
- Using scripted play in which children enact everyday activities that gradually become more variable and less bound to the immediate context.
- Reading and telling real-life stories with clear scripts. The narratives can be based on the child's experience.
- Helping children transfer from event-based to linguistic organization by telling them narratives with clearly structured story grammars and then having them dramatize the stories.

These exercises may be performed orally with young children or in writing with older.

Scripted play is especially useful with preschool and early school-age children and is discussed in detail in Chapter 12. Initially, it is very important that the scripts describe familiar motivating events, such as going to the market or getting ready for school. The script should be introduced and discussed prior to play. The script is played and discussed afterward.

CHAPTER 11 SPECIFIC INTERVENTION TECHNIQUES

With each replaying, the children change roles, modify the events, and use fewer concrete objects. As children become more adept at recounting the script, the SLP encourages telling of the narrative without an enactment.

The SLP or teacher can facilitate production of event descriptions by having children describe familiar events as they occur or as recalled from pictures or videotapes. Children can role-play and describe familiar events as they occur.

Familiar events depicted in child drawings can be used for sequencing. An SLP can help the child identify the setting and characters by asking them to describe the picture; for example:

Adult: Well, what do we have here?

Child: This is me in the kitchen, and I'm making breakfast.

Adult: So, we might say, "This morning, I was in the kitchen making breakfast." What did you do first? (or Then what happened? or What's this next picture?)

After completing a step-by-step description, the child can be encouraged to tell the entire narrative.

Recalling a sequence of events requires attention and memory processes. More important for narratives is conceptual knowledge or the logical temporal order of events, the how and why one thing relates to another.

Focusing only on recitation of the order of events misses the logical connections that relate one thing to another and aid narrative recall or creation. Rather than focusing on sequencing ability, SLPs can target the specific concepts and language of the narrative discourse (Kamhi, 2014).

Guidelines. In an excellent tutorial, Spencer and Petersen (2019) set out narrative intervention guidelines that reflect EBP. Their principles are as follows:

- **Build story structure before vocabulary and complex language.** As a child becomes more familiar with the narrative frame, the SLP can require increasingly more complex language. The SLP can model, prompt, and encourage the use of correct syntactical forms, first in oral and later in written narratives.

- **Use multiple exemplars to promote metalinguistics and generalization.** Narratives differ; thus, their use promotes learning rather than memorization. A child's telling of a more mature narrative demonstrates both generalization and metalinguistic development. Strategically designed stories can contain intense and targeted narrative practice (Brown et al., 2014; Favot et al., 2018; Petersen et al., 2014; Spencer Kelley et al., 2020; Spencer et al., 2015; Spencer & Slocum, 2010).

- **Promote active participation.** Active involvement leads to increased learning. Children prefer interactive instruction in which they have a prominent role (Knapp & Desrochers, 2009).

- **Contextualize, unpack, and reconstruct stories.** A minimally complete episode consists of a problem, an attempt, and a consequence. The SLP can tell the entire story in its complete and complex form first to provide a context and ensure that a child sees it as a whole. Once the whole narrative is modeled, it can be broken into smaller, more manageable chunks with multiple opportunities for the children to practice each part. Corrective feedback, modeling, and prompting can aid the child's recall. After supportive telling/retelling of each part, the narrative can be reconstructed into its whole.

- **Use visuals to make abstract concepts concrete.** Storytelling is a demanding task for children with language disorders. Visual supports can be an effective teaching tool for making abstract concepts, such as story grammar and clausal subordination, more concrete. Visuals can correspond to story grammar elements, less common vocabulary, and complex language features (Gardner & Spencer, 2016). In addition, visuals, such as graphic organizers and concept maps, can support retellings (S. Gillam et al., 2015; Petersen et al., 2014; Spencer et al., 2013). As a child gains more independents, visuals can be faded or reduced.

- **Deliver immediate corrective feedback.** Effective feedback is immediate and specific and focuses on what the child should have said, with minimum attention to the child's incorrect response (Archer & Hughes, 2011; Watkins & Slocum, 2004).

- **Use efficient and effective prompts.** The SLP can select appropriate prompts and use them efficiently and effectively. Spencer and Petersen (2019) recommend a two-step prompting sequence in which the SLP asks a question about what the child missed, such as "How did Judy feel?" followed by a model of an appropriate response if the child is unable to answer the question.

- **Individualize and extend.** For school-age children, the SLP can extend intervention to include grade-appropriate academic and social skills. Materials such as *Story Champs* (Spencer & Petersen, 2016), *Story Grammar Marker* (Moreau & Fidrych, 2008), and *SKILL* (S. Gillam et al., 2018) offer suggestions for how to extend narrative intervention into academic skill areas.

- **Arrange for generalization opportunities.** Throughout this text, we've stressed generalization. An SLP can intentionally plan for generalization by involving classroom teachers. Within classroom activities, the SLP can model presentation and feedback techniques for the teacher. Family narrative activities can also be encouraged through suggestions sent home to parents or caregivers.

- **Make it fun.** Narratives are the perfect context for practicing language. As an SLP, you can make narrative intervention fun by being animated when listening, using exaggerated facial expressions and comments, and reflecting the narrative back to the child. Peers can be taught to paraphrase another student's narrative similarly. Games and other activities, such as art, can increase children's enjoyment and aid learning. For example, combining movement wand storytelling enhances intervention outcomes (Brinton & Fujiki, 2017; Culatta et al., 2010; Duncan et al., 2019).

Reminiscing. Two effective strategies for teaching personal narratives are reminiscing and making parallels between a child's personal experiences and those in other people's stories (Westby & Culatta, 2016). *Reminiscing* or recalling memories leads to better autobi-

CHAPTER 11 SPECIFIC INTERVENTION TECHNIQUES

ographical memory (Cleveland & Morris, 2014). It's best not to use a question-answering task but to be more collaboration in remembering.

In a clinical setting, it is best to reminisce about therapy or classroom activities that the SLP shares with the child. Parents share many more experiences with their child and can also be enlisted. Photos or videos of a shared experience can be used to help children recall and/or write the story that goes with the pictures. The photos provide support. The SLP and child may also reminisce about shared movies or videos.

Clinicians can also model the telling of a narrative about an event and ask children to relate their own similar experience. Some fictional narratives can evoke event narratives and model construction of similar real-life stories (Westby & Culatta, 2016).

Once a child with a language disorder is able to produce complete and coherent personal event narratives, an SLP might begin to assist with generating coherent life stories. Books and discussions about emotions, character traits, and threads in themes can highlight these aspects of life stories. Character traits often lead to actions that have consequences for the character. Books should be chosen carefully to reflect a child's cultural and linguistic background as well as life experiences.

To help a child think about significant turning points in their life, the SLP might ask about the following (Calkins, 2006, p. 21):

- First or last time you did something hard to do
- First or last time you did something you now do every day
- First or last time with a person, an animal, a place, or an activity
- A time you realized something important about yourself or someone else
- A time you realized that a huge change in your life almost happened

Graphic organizers may be a helpful way to arrange events to chart significant events.

Once a simple structure is mastered, additional details and events can be added to elaborate the narrative. These might include descriptions, causal factors, emotions, and dialogue. Teachers and parents can be enlisted to elaborate a child's personal narratives (Boland et al., 2003).

Teaching fictional narratives does not result in increased functional communication (Cannizzaro & Coelho, 2002). In contrast, personal narratives are used in a variety of natural contexts. Another aspect of generalization is the frequency of target's use, and personal narratives occur more frequently than fictional ones.

Episode Knowledge. Episode knowledge, mentioned previously, can be taught through the use of children's books. Book selection should be based on the following criteria (Naremore, 2001):

- Familiar event scripts
- Pictures that support the episodes
- Clearly sequenced episodes
- Appropriate length and language level
- Stories "pretested" for retelling by the SLP

The SLP should select stories that contain all episodic elements. Intervention can begin with a mediated approach by discussing with the child the importance of stories for communication.

After reading a book together, the SLP can help the child analyze the story following a "problem–solution–result" format. The SLP helps the child break the story into pieces, identify the parts, and recombine them again into a cohesive narrative.

For children who may not relate to books, the SLP can construct one-episode narratives of experiences familiar to the child. Pictures and real objects may aid the child's participation.

Narrative Retells. Preliminary data suggest that we can improve some young school-age children's functional use of both the macrostructure (story grammar) and microstructure (causality) in their narratives through books (Petersen et al., 2010). More sophisticated oral narratives share a variety of microstructural features with written language, including the use of causal and temporal subordinating conjunctions, coordinating conjunctions, adverbs, elaborated noun phrases, mental and linguistic verbs, and specific nouns with clearly referenced pronouns (R. Gillam & Ukrainetz, 2006; Greenhalgh & Strong, 2001; Nippold et al., 2005). Steps in literate narrative intervention are presented in Table 11–5.

Narratives can be retold, although retelling is not the overall goal. Ideally, the child will internalize knowledge to use composing and comprehending conversational and book-based narratives (Naremore, 2001). Both narrative length and structure can be improved if children have a model on which to base their narrative and a structure inherent in the model, such as story retelling using pictures (Tönsing & Tesner, 1999).

Retelling can begin with short stories of a few minutes' length. If the story is longer, the SLP may choose only a segment for retelling. Generalization can be enhanced if the narrative is related to classroom content or to events in the child's life. Pictures can be used to depict elements of the story grammar. With older children, an SLP can explicitly teach the elements of story grammar and use graphic story organizers to help children produce complete episodes. Stories retold many times can be modified by one element that will change the outcome.

Narrative telling can be extended in both speech and writing. If a child is able to retell a story with two or three complete episodes, they are probably ready to begin composing original narratives (Naremore, 2001). This can be accomplished within a story context with the SLP supplying the supporting structure initially. Gradually, the SLP supplies fewer episode portions. In each narrative, the child completes the story by supplying the final elements until they can compose an entire narrative. The teaching of longer written narratives is discussed in Chapter 13.

Children then can progress to fictional narratives or their own original stories. The adult can use questions to move children to more sophisticated ways of organizing and expressing concepts and relationships. Chapter 12 includes a discussion of replica play and narratives in the classroom.

Narrative use is the next logical step. Children should have the opportunity to practice forms of narration within a variety of role-playing situations.

CHAPTER 11 SPECIFIC INTERVENTION TECHNIQUES

Table 11–5. Possible Steps for Narration Teaching

1. The SLP models storytelling from pictures in a book.

2. The SLP and child co-tell the story in the same format with story grammar icons as prompts.

3. The child retells the narrative with SLP verbal prompts and pictures in a book but no story grammar icon prompts.

4. The SLP and child co-tell a story from a single complex scene picture and story grammar icon prompts.

5. The child retells the story from a single complex-scene picture while the SLP uses verbal prompts but no story grammar icon prompts.

6. The SLP and child listen to the child's recorded narrative while looking at the single complex-scene picture. The SLP places an icon on the table when each story grammar element is heard. After listening, the SLP and child identify missing story grammar elements and co-tell the story using the same single simple-scene picture and story grammar icon and verbal prompts.

7. The child retells the story from a single simple-scene picture while the SLP only uses verbal prompts as needed.

8. The child tells an original narrative using story grammar icon prompts and SLP verbal prompts as needed. Simultaneously, the SLP draws pictures illustrating the narrative.

9. The child retells the story using these pictures but without story grammar icon prompts and only minimal verbal prompts.

10. The child retells the narrative without using any visual prompts and only minimal SLP verbal prompts as needed.

Source: Information from Petersen et al. (2010).

SKILL. Sandi and Ron Gillam, who have contributed mightily to the field of communication sciences and disorders, have pulled together many of the elements of narrative intervention and teaching we've discussed plus EBP and a healthy dose of innovation to produce an approach to narrative intervention called Supporting Knowledge in Language and Literacy (SKILL) (S. Gillam & Gillam, 2018).

Let's explore SKILL as a means for summarizing much of what's been discussed so far. Although we don't have room for a discussion of the entire SKILL program, I'll outline the program for you as a possible intervention model. The program is divided into three sequential phases:

Phase 1: Teaching story structure, including story grammar elements (SGEs) and the causal framework. Understanding of the main story elements is taught in the context of wordless picture stories and then written narratives. Each story element is associated with an icon on a sequenced storyboard that serves as a graphic organizer.

The amount a child must recall is reduced by working in small groups and using key words and phrases to cue SGEs. SKILL uses story modeling, story retelling, and story generation.

To aid recall, SKILL uses a *whole-to-part-to-whole model*, enabling children to use world knowledge for overall recall, then specifics of the story that relate to the whole story. For example, the story may be about a man chopping wood. Using world knowledge, each child's expectations are explored. These elements are related back to the overall narrative. Students practice answering questions and generating stories. Teaching strategies can include co-telling, parallel story development, and retelling practice through the use of storyboards.

Phase 2: Stabilization of story structure and explicit instruction on multiple linguistic targets includes linguistic structures, concepts, and vocabulary in more elaborate, complex stories. Grammatical targets include elaborated noun phrases, adverbs, mental verbs, linguistic verbs, subordinated and coordinated clauses, and causal language. Students are taught to add dialogue and complications to their stories to increase linguistic complexity.

Phase 3: Metacognitive instruction targets internalizing story structure and linguistic structure by providing students with multiple opportunities to retell, create, tell, edit, and revise their own spontaneously generated stories with and without supports. For example, story prompts may go from story construction with multiple sequential pictures to a single picture and then to no picture. A child might progress as follows:

- Retell a narrative with assistance
- Create stories with assistance
- Retell a narrative without assistance
- Create stories without assistance
- Retell, sequenced pictures, single scenes, verbal prompts

The SKILL approach, which teaches children the critical cognitive and linguistic skills needed to support narration, has reported positive effects on children's narration (S. Gillam & Gillam, 2016).

Cohesion

Cohesion comes in many forms. Conjunctive cohesion is the easiest form to teach. Children's oral narratives can be collected and transcribed into a "book." Use of conjunctions and the relationships expressed can be analyzed. Simple stories containing various clausal relationships also can be read to children. In a retelling, a child usually will not express relationships and conjunctions that they don't use in everyday speech.

Once a child's narrative relationships and conjunctions have been analyzed, the SLP can begin to introduce other conjunctions. A developmental order of introduction may be helpful, although the first priority should be conjunctions omitted or

CHAPTER 11 SPECIFIC INTERVENTION TECHNIQUES

used incorrectly in the relationships expressed. Other types of relationships and terms are as follows:

Temporal	*and then, first, next, before, after, when, while*
Causal	*because, so, so that, in order to*
Adversative	*but, except, however, except that*
Conditional	*if, unless, or, in case*
Spatial	*in, on, next to, between, etc.*

The SLP can introduce narrative relationships with or without a conjunction and then, using a question–answer technique, prompt a child to produce the desired conjunction. If the child responds incorrectly, the SLP can reread or retell the relevant portion of the narrative, model a response including the conjunction, discuss the meaning, and prompt the child to respond again. The important aspect of the teaching is understanding the relationship expressed. The final stages of teaching include original narratives produced by the child.

Referential cohesion uses nouns, pronouns, and articles to designate old and new information in the narrative. Questions and answers can be used to direct the child as a narrative is told. Pronouns and articles are discussed in more detail later in the section on syntax.

Retellings by the SLP might use a fill-in-the-blank technique, in which the child provides the appropriate word. Gradually, emphasis on narrative-structured can be reduced.

Comprehension

Narrative comprehension can be improved by beginning with predictable narratives concerning everyday events or routines familiar to a child. A child's internalized script aids both comprehension and recall. Variations in the narrative are introduced gradually, moving to more unfamiliar and fictionalized events. Comprehension and recall can be facilitated by having children draw or write common event sequences.

Before using a narrative, an SLP should review it with the child. Help the child bring their knowledge to the task. This prenarration task is discussed in detail in Chapter 12.

Data suggest that the use of subjectivity or the character's thoughts and feelings can enhance comprehension of fictional narratives. Children can be taught to focus on a character's reactions as a way of making sense of the events in the narrative. There are no right or wrong answers; rather, the child's responses explain events in a manner comprehensible to the child.

Success has been reported with SKILL, mentioned previously. SKILL is based on the construction–integration (C-I) model of text comprehension (Kintsch, 2013). According to the C-I model, the reader or listener uses knowledge of words and language structures to create the microstructure of the text (Perfetti & Stafura, 2014). The SLP helps a child associate word meaning with its syntactic role in the sentence. With each successive sentence, the listener or the reader forms links, and a microstructure is constructed. Storytellers, listeners, and readers construct a mental model of the narrative called a macrostructure that represents the relationship among key ideas.

> *Food for Thought:* Are the conversations of your friends and family and of yourself filled with narratives, even short one-sentence ones? Notice the talk around you and you may be surprised.

Semantics

Meaning is the relationship of a symbol to the underlying concept. Different strategies are used by different children and by the same child at different developmental times to construct meanings.

Children with language disorders often use one strategy exclusively or predominantly. For example, the meanings expressed by some children with ASD seem to be unanalyzed, situationally related "chunks." A word is exemplified by the context in which it's learned; thus, the meaning of *gift* is *birthday*.

Vocabulary acquisition is associated with early reading skills and with improved writing quality (Graham et al., 2015; Olinghouse & Wilson, 2013). Early measures of vocabulary predict reading comprehension from preschool to adolescence (Ouellette, 2006; Quinn et al., 2015; Tannenbaum et al., 2006). For school-age children, individual differences in vocabulary development are related to differences in the amount of reading a child experiences.

Children with language disorders, who have smaller and less diverse vocabularies, are at risk for poor academic performance (Catts et al., 2006; McGregor et al., 2013). In general, children with language disorders and reading difficulties have fewer words in their vocabularies, have fewer and more sparse networks connecting words, and learn words more slowly compared to their peers (Cain et al., 2004b; Kan & Windsor, 2010; McGregor et al., 2013). However, the relationship between vocabulary and reading is not causal. They tend to change together.

The experiential or world knowledge base is also important, especially for the child younger than age 7 years. The child needs an opportunity to have meaningful, real experiences. In intervention, play in the snow can precede a lesson on the words used in that activity.

Early word meanings are acquired within event-related experiences, especially predictable, everyday routines and their accompanying scripts. As with all of us, children experience the world through their senses by touching, smelling, and tasting and then describing the sensation. Adults can help children encode features of these events and the entities to which children attend. Older elementary school children can learn from the experiences of others, much as adults do.

Vocabulary and Word Meaning

Vocabulary is more than a list of words and their meanings. Word knowledge is a rich variety of information about each word that supports our literacy and academic learning. Words are not isolated but exist within a network of concepts or mental representations. In addition, words are grouped into relationships, categories, synonyms, antonyms, and

CHAPTER 11 SPECIFIC INTERVENTION TECHNIQUES

the like that are important for storage and access or retrieval. These connections are called semantic networks. Finally, and this is important for intervention, words are not learned in one sitting. Meanings and word use emerge gradually from multiple exposures to a word. Deeper understanding is built with each successive encounter.

Early vocabulary growth occurs through exposure to oral language. In school, vocabulary development is fostered primarily through exposures to words in textbooks and other written venues, such as social media. Children learn approximately 2,000 to 3,000 words per year. Explicit teaching of vocabulary accounts for only approximately 300 to 400 words per year. The majority of new words learned by school-age children are the result of exposure to written text and other media.

Several factors may influence new word learning for both children with TDL and those with language disorders. For example, children acquire new words more readily if they consist of frequently occurring phonemes in common word locations and if the novel word is presented before the meaning (Bedore & Leonard, 2000; Storkel, 2001; Storkel & Morrisette, 2002). In general, access paths to words for all children are strengthened with successful use.

McKeown (2019) and Elleman et al. (2019) offer excellent tutorials on vocabulary intervention that I highlight with additions from other authors. I encourage you to read both tutorials. According to McKeown, effective vocabulary instruction promotes more than just knowing word meanings. An SLP can help children with language disorders understand how words work and how to use word knowledge effectively.

Semantic intervention consists of several different but related levels of intervention involving a variety of interrelated intervention strategies that are much more complex than simply teaching vocabulary words. At its core, word meaning consists of concepts or knowledge of the world. Semantic teaching must recognize the importance of these underlying concepts and include cognitive aspects of concept formation. Let's begin our discussion with word selection and progress through other factors important for teaching and learning.

Word Selection

If we conceptualize words as falling into three tiers, it helps us decide which words to teach (Beck et al., 2013). Tier 1 words form a large group characterized by everyday oral language, and children learn these readily when hearing them in context. In contrast, Tier 3 words tend to be limited to specific domains (e.g., *genome*, *integers*) or are extremely rare (e.g., *septuagenarian*). These words are best learned within their particular domains when needed.

In the middle, Tier 2 words are characteristic of written language but are not so common in everyday conversation. These words have high utility for literate language users and are general academic words common across various domains of academic texts. Good databases of academic words are available in print and online (Beck et al., 2008; Coxhead, 2000; Gardner & Davies, 2013; Stahl & Nagy, 2006). In general, these words are good candidates for instruction (McKeown, 2019).

Unfortunately, there's no definitive list of words that every student must know. The best advice is to select from texts students are reading and experiences they are having within the classroom curriculum. Collaboration with teachers is essential.

In general, it is easier to learn words for known concepts than to learn both words and concepts at the same time. The choice of which words to teach should be based on the likely frequency of use, typical development, need within the classroom and use in textbooks, and likelihood of the child learning the word from context alone. Even slang expressions might be taught to aid socialization, especially among adolescents.

Typically, children have a small repertoire of Tier 2 words when they enter school, but these increase as children become readers. Tier 2 words are beneficial because they are found in a variety of texts and contexts. Because deeper understanding of words takes time to teach effectively, SLPs and teachers need to be judicious in word selection.

Words are often learned in a specific context and with one of many possible meanings. Students provided with varied contexts and supportive interactions begin to understand a word's shades of meaning.

Preschool children's learning of academic vocabulary words is enhanced in a school learning plus home review condition in which families review words frequently at home (Soto et al., 2020). The primary hurdle is motivating parents.

Home review can be enhanced by promoting parent involvement and buy-in through in-person teaching, video modeling, and daily text message reminders. Even with these aids, some families, especially those in high-stress homes, will find it difficult to practice vocabulary words at home. More research is needed to identify effective strategies to help parents overcome barriers to home intervention.

Two factors that can affect word learning include lexical similarity and semantic similarity (Storkel & Adlof, 2009). **Lexical similarity** is neighborhood density, which is the number of words that differ by one phoneme from a given word. Preschool children with TDL tend to learn high-probability/high-density novel words more rapidly than low-probability/low-density novel words (Storkel, 2003, 2004; Storkel & Maekawa, 2005).

Semantic Similarity. **Semantic similarity** involves the closeness of semantic representations or meanings. Known words that are similar compete with each other. This can lead to poorer performance in recognition or recall (D. Nelson & Zhang, 2000).

Many Tier 2 academic terms—the ones children need to succeed in school—have low probability and low neighborhood density but few semantic similarities. Morphological approaches can strengthen understanding of word formation. It is also helpful to teach morphological variations, such as *evolution, evolve,* and *evolving.*

Direct vocabulary instruction should focus on high-frequency words used in the classroom. Words can be taught through a variety of methods and across several situations, relating them to other words and building on the initial knowledge a child may possess. Multisensory approaches in which the child both listens to and produces the word will help form a phonological representation. SLPs can provide examples from other contexts and encourage the child to do likewise.

Morphological Awareness

Morphological awareness is implicit knowledge of meaning units or morphemes within words. As we encounter words, we learn to use morphemes to help us infer the meaning. Morphological awareness, discussed in more detail in Chapter 13, is related to both

CHAPTER 11 SPECIFIC INTERVENTION TECHNIQUES

vocabulary development and reading comprehension (Nagy et al., 2006) and is impaired in some children with language disorders (Gilbert et al., 2014; Kieffer, 2014).

Root words can be expanded in a number of ways with morphological affixes (e.g., *un-*, *im-*, *-ly*, *-ish*). Thus, knowledge of morphological markers can expand the size of one's vocabulary. This does not mean teaching morphological markers in isolation. This rarely translates to learning and understanding of new words (Bowers et al., 2010; Curtis, 2006).

Flexibility must be introduced along with root word instruction. This can be accomplished through problem–solution tasks in which a child attempts to ascertain the meaning of a word given its linguistic context. Be aware that root word instruction has the potential to be boring. Be creative.

Intervention can be combined with spelling instruction, dividing words to discover their meaning, and sorting words by morphological affixes. Word segmentation abilities have been associated with word learning in school-aged children with TDL and also those with ASD, but not those with developmental language disorder (DLD). When initially given exposure to the phonology found in subsequent word-learning tasks, however, the performance of children with DLD improves (Haebig et al., 2017).

Suffixes are easier to learn than prefixes and should be introduced first (see the section titled Morphology). Prefix teaching should begin with concrete, easy-to-define prefixes, such as *un-*, and proceed to more abstract ones. The most frequently used prefixes in American English are *un-*, *in-*, *dis-*, and *non-*.

Contextual Cues

Context is one way that we ascertain a word's meaning and is most likely the primary way we learn new words and word meanings. Full meanings are slowly revealed through experiences in multiple contexts. This process suggests that word instruction be incremental and in context. As a word's meaning broadens, it loses its connection to a specific context, allowing the word to be used flexibly.

Most likely, a child will not need a full adult definition when the word is first introduced. As an SLP, you should not expect dictionary definitions from children younger than age 12 years. By that age, however, a child with TDL can define words, draw conclusions, and make inferences.

The SLP can expose a child to multiple examples of events and things in familiar contexts in order to help the child perceive features of words being used. In class and at home language teachers can act as mediators, framing, focusing, and providing salient features of experiences for the child.

Within activities, children can be encouraged to describe word features. Descriptors then can be used to determine similarities and differences and to label the world. For example, instead of naming unfamiliar entities such as the names for types of trees, children can be encouraged to stretch their existing language and give descriptive names, such as *five-pointed leaf tree*. These self-made descriptions then become the vehicle for learning and remembering tree names.

Contextual analysis teaches children to use context to determine an unknown word's meaning. Unfortunately, context alone can be unreliable. Therefore, in instruction, an SLP needs to ensure that the context supports the word meaning being taught. It's best to take advantage of related words in reading and to point out similarities and differences of meaning rather than to specifically target root words and morphological markers in isolation.

Children and adolescents with language disorder need to learn how to use the context to establish word meaning. Contexts provide a number of cues that can be classified as temporal (time), spatial (location), value (relative worth), stative descriptive (physical description), functional descriptive (use), causal (cause and effect), class membership (type), and equivalence (similarity/difference). Class membership and functional descriptive are the easiest for children, whereas stative descriptive seems to be the most difficult.

Context should be established for the child prior to introducing the word numerous times. A child will need help in determining what they know. This can be followed by repeated exposures in a variety of play or interactive contexts. Narratives can provide a context for introducing novel words.

Word learning is enhanced when words receive emphatic stress while being presented within stimulus sentences (Ellis Weismer & Hesketh, 1998). Stress is important given the difficulty children with DLD have in using syntax to acquire vocabulary (Rice et al., 2000).

Teaching also proceeds from more contextual meanings, as in "hit the ball," to less contextual, more figurative meanings, such as "hit the roof," and multiple meanings, such as "a hit musical." Obviously, these multiple meanings and uses would be introduced gradually, not all at once.

The adult can help the child understand that meaning varies with context. Varying contexts provide for maximum usage and exposure. Storytelling in which a novel word must be used is also a good strategy and uses context to facilitate use.

Semantic Networks

As mentioned previously, words do not exist in a vacuum but, rather, as part of a semantic network of related concepts (Borovsky et al., 2016; Ford-Connors & Paratore, 2015). These networks facilitate both comprehension and production and foster retention and word finding and retrieval. It's important for a child to understand how concepts are related. This can be fostered using graphic organizers, discussion surrounding relationships, and work in small groups (Ebbers & Denton, 2008).

Teaching can include words that mean the same (synonyms), sound the same (homonyms), or are opposites (antonyms). This teaching will help a child organize language for easy storage and retrieval. Common prefixes and suffixes are also important, as is syllabication. A child's meanings can be consolidated by building on the child's current vocabulary while correcting errors and misconceptions of meaning.

The semantic features of words can be analyzed to expand the characteristics associated with words and to aid categorization. Words can be classified according to their semantic features, as in Figure 11–1. Sorting tasks perform a similar function, and children can be encouraged to make their own associations.

Effective Instruction

Effective instruction means focusing on words in ways that promote word meanings but also understanding how words work and how to utilize word knowledge effec-

CHAPTER 11 SPECIFIC INTERVENTION TECHNIQUES

Figure 11–1. Analyzing semantic feature similarities.

	Transportation	Four-Wheel	Two-Wheel	Engine-Powered	Pedal-Powered	Runs on Rails
Motorcycle	X		X	X		
Bicycle	X		X		X	
Car	X	X		X		
Bus	X	X		X		
Train	X			X		X

	Animals	Bird	On Farm	Wild or Zoo Animal	Gives Milk	Four-Legged
Chicken		X	X			
Duck		X	X			
Cow	X		X		X	X
Elephant	X			X	X	X
Goat	X		X		X	X

tively. Thus, effective techniques might include the following (Elleman et al., 2019; McKeown, 2019):

- Present definitional and contextual information
- Provide words in multiple contexts
- Encourage active processing of word meanings

These recommendations flow from the nature of word understanding. Teaching a single definition devoid of context will foster little comprehension or use. Rather, we help a child "own" a word.

As mentioned throughout this text, learning is not passive. Children must engage with words, manipulating concepts, using words, and making connections to other words and concepts. Passive activities have poorer results than tasks that require students to respond using a target word, such as writing a story containing the target word (Wright & Cervetti, 2017).

Active processing requires students to deliberately attend to, engage with, and use word meanings to enhance learning. The more a word is used meaningfully, the easier it is to access. For example, the SLP can offer contrasting word choices, as in "Tell me if you'd be *eager* to do what I say or *reluctant* to do it." This can be followed with a list of activities under each choice (McKeown, 2019). Choice-making can be fun if you're creative with the options. When we make choices, we reflect on the features of a word.

Open-ended questions using a target word, such as "How could we *offer* to help a person who seems lost?" can also help students consider the features of a word's meaning. Feedback can be used to help a child refine their answer or think more deeply about the meaning, as in "Yes, and what else?" or "Why did you decide on *X*?"

Elleman et al. (2019) reviewed several studies conducted with older elementary school children. Recommendations from this research include the following:

- Use multiple activities, such as discussion, collaboration, morphological word solving, writing, and games and manipulative activities.
- Semantic mapping can be used to relate one word to another and explain underlying connections.
- Use root word and morpheme instruction plus problem-solving tasks related to word meaning.
- Teach and use words in a variety of tasks across content area.
- Use multiple teaching strategies.
- Promote use of high-utility words and academic language.

In addition to engaging children's morphological knowledge, an SLP can teach by (Alderete et al., 2004)

- using interactive book reading;
- direct vocabulary instruction; and
- fostering word consciousness through "playing with language."

The Vocabulary Acquisition and Usage for Late Talkers methodology offers promise as an effective method to teach single words (Alt et al., 2021). Within a given session, a child may hear four to eight words modeled in various sentences multiple times and be given opportunities to produce the words. During modeling, a target word can appear in varying locations within an adult sentence and be modified, as in *talk*, *talked*, *talks*, and *talking*.

Many commercially available games can be used as is or modified for vocabulary teaching, including Boggle, Pictionary, and Scrabble. Semantic organizers, such as spidergrams, can be used to build associations. Children can use semantic organizers to "brainstorm" or to tell all they know about a word. Figure 11–2 is a typical spidergram.

Multimodality Instruction. Some children benefit from multimodal input. For example, 4-year-old children with DLD learn vocabulary words better if the verbal word is accompanied by an iconic gesture illustrating a property of the referent, such as a specific action being used to illustrate the meaning of a verb being taught (Vogt & Kauschke, 2017). Another method to improve vocabulary learning among school-age children with TDL and those with ASD and with DLD is the use of orthography or written words along with oral presentation (Ricketts et al., 2015). Signing in support of speech has also shown promise for children with DLD, even with children in late elementary school (van Berkel-van Hoof et al., 2019).

Interactive Book Sharing. Exposure to storybook reading has been shown to be an effective way for kindergarten children to learn new words, especially those with poor

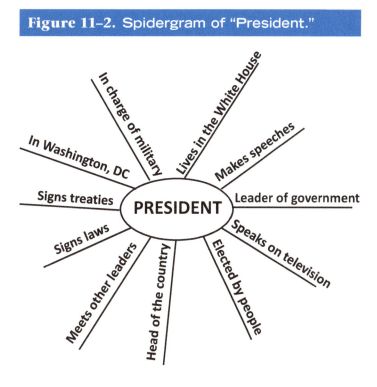

Figure 11–2. Spidergram of "President."

vocabularies (Justice et al., 2005). To be effective, reading should be paired with other word-teaching strategies, such as explaining an unfamiliar word when it occurs in the story, offering synonyms, acting out the word, and pointing to the referent.

Although interactive book reading has shown promise as an effective word-learning technique for children with DLD, we still do not know the most effective way to use this approach. The ideal number of exposures to a word during book sharing has yet to be determined. Children with DLD are able to learn a significant number of words during treatment, regardless of the number of exposures and the frequency format (Storkel et al., 2019).

Word Retrieval. Word learners benefit from retrieval practice of the newly taught words (Chapman et al., 2006). Repeated spaced retrieval (RSR) practice or spaced interval retrieval promotes learning of both word form and meaning information. Compared to retrieval immediately after learning, RSR seems to be more efficient for children's word processing (Haebig et al., 2021).

In interactive reading, children can be encouraged to talk about objects, characters, and events and also to expand to more nonimmediate talk that goes beyond the text. The child can be taught via levels of abstraction to progress away from the immediate text. Immediate prompts ask children to point to, name, and describe by physical traits. To reorder their perceptual skills, children can be asked the meanings of words used in the text, identifying characters and events by less perceptually based descriptions. Finally, children reason in response to questions about why events occurred or why emotions developed. After-reading activities can focus on discussion of words from the text and their meaning in context.

For children with DLD, different teaching cues seem to affect learning in differing ways (Gray, 2005). For example, semantic cues (*It's made of wood*) foster comprehension, whereas phonological cues (*It begins with /s/*) aid expression. Because children with poor vocabularies can have difficulty with both phonological and semantic aspects of words, intervention with both should be explored (Nash & Donaldson, 2005). Overlearning of new words in both expressive and receptive mode also seems warranted, especially for children with DLD (Gray, 2003).

Expressive use and retrieval among 7- to 12-year-olds is positively influenced by a child's greater familiarity with the word. Other factors include greater familiarity with the word's lexical neighbors and lower neighborhood density (R. Newman & German, 2002). The latter is surprising given the beneficial learning effects of high density.

Perhaps the most fun involves word play, matching synonyms, riddles, art, drama, and poetry. Children also enjoy creating words that do not exist in the dictionary or giving existing words new definitions. Such original words can be used along with real words to try to encourage children to make educated guesses about word meaning. In a recent conversation, a group of English language learning children used the word *skinship*, which they defined as the relationship between family members who touched frequently. Creative!

Although computers alone are inadequate for teaching vocabulary, computers can act as a supplement to classroom instruction. For example, in schools serving children with low socioeconomic (SES) backgrounds, 6- to 9-year-olds made large gains in word recognition, receptive identification, expressive labeling, and decontextualized definitions, in part through computer adjuncts to reading instruction (Goldstein et al., 2017). More research is needed to identify specific techniques that are the most effective.

Explicit Instruction

Ideally, intervention would lead to rapid access to word meanings in academic tasks and in literacy. Although most children and adults learn meanings gradually through multiple exposures, explicit vocabulary instruction can also be an efficient way to expand the vocabularies of both children with language disorders and their peers with TDL. However, multiple exposures in contexts and through a variety of activities are still essential (Ford-Connors & Paratore, 2015; Kamil et al., 2008; Wright & Cervetti, 2017).

Explicit instruction is effective in increasing vocabulary learning and reading comprehension of the words taught (Wright & Cervetti, 2017). Children with reading difficulties benefit much more from explicit vocabulary instruction compared to their peers with TDL (Elleman et al., 2009).

Although learned vocabulary may decrease over time without repeated input and use, an explicit vocabulary intervention can produce significant immediate gains in children's vocabulary knowledge. For example, the Story Friends program is effective in teaching challenging vocabulary to preschoolers with limited vocabularies (Spencer Kelley et al., 2020). In Story Friends, explicit vocabulary instruction is embedded in prerecorded storybooks. Learning can be enhanced further by integrating review and practice of target vocabulary into classroom and home practice activities.

Considerations With English Language Learners and/or Children From Low-SES Backgrounds

As you may recall from foreign language classes, vocabulary is an essential part of learning another language. Initially, vocabulary instruction with children who are English language learners (ELLs) should link American English vocabulary to the heritage language. Crosson and colleagues (2019) argue for instruction that not only makes this connection for children but also is "robust," occurring in both classroom and clinical settings, focusing on high-utility academic words and morphological analysis. This is the gist of English Learners' Robust Academic Vocabulary Encounters, a program that adheres to five recommended principles (Crosson et al., 2019):

- Make cross-linguistic connections to other languages whenever possible. Connection to words in the heritage language may help a child learn and remember root meaning when the roots are similar to English.

- Teach semantic networks connecting words that carry the same root. Students can be guided to notice word relations through roots—that is, *able, ability, enable, disable, inability.*

- Explicitly teach orthographic and phonological changes. Discerning the meaning of words that carry roots might be tricky because of the orthographic and phonological variations; hence, the connection may be difficult to decipher, especially if the variations occur infrequently. Students may need assistance to notice connections.

- Teach for fluent access to root meanings. The goal is to emphasize roots and strengthen connections between orthographic and semantic representations.

- Emphasize a flexible, problem-solving orientation using roots for learning academic word meanings.

As an SLP, you can focus on high-utility academic words and teach morphological problem-solving to foster word learning, as mentioned previously.

Preschool Spanish–English-speaking ELLs from low-SES backgrounds have benefitted from intensive vocabulary intervention embedded in e-books (Wood et al., 2018). It's especially effective when e-book experiences are supplemented with vocabulary instruction, including explanations in Spanish, repetition in English, checks for understanding, and highlighted morphology.

A word gap in vocabulary size and experience typically exists for children in low-SES communities when beginning school compared with their mid-SES peers. Although many children from low-SES backgrounds would benefit from instruction to enrich vocabulary and language, explicit instruction occurs infrequently in preschool settings. Children's learning of academic vocabulary can be enhanced by a combination of small-group intervention and teacher- or SLP-led class-wide instruction (Seven et al., 2020).

Semantic Categories and Relational Webs

Words fulfill different semantic roles, such as *agent* and *action*, that specify the relationships among those referents. Thus, a child forming a sentence must keep in mind both the referent and the semantic role.

Words and phrases also modify the meaning of basic sentence elements by indicating qualities, such as perceptual attributes (*big, old*), manner (*quickly*), and temporal aspects (*first, later*), and relationships between larger sentential units, such as additive (*and*) or causal (*because*). As a listener, the child can only comprehend other people to the extent that they understand the various relationships underlying other's utterances.

Semantic Classes

Semantic classes govern word use. A portion of word definition is the semantic class into which a word can be placed. Let's just use one class as an example.

The *agent* is usually found in the subject position of a sentence. English is a subject-prominent language in which a large number of elements are associated with the subject of the sentence. These elements include subject–verb agreement, as with variations of the verb BE (*am, is, are*) and the third person singular, present tense -*s* ending; pronouns; and auxiliary verb–subject inversions in questions. These elements are important syntactically.

An SLP can teach the concept of subjecthood using a functional approach in which they teach the child the purpose of a subject. The function of a sentence's subject, represented by a noun, pronoun, or a noun phrase, is to designate the perspective used in the sentence. If the sentence contains action, the agent designates the actor. Subjects can also be identified by the pronouns used with them.

The SLP can teach children to identify the subject by using the following forms:

- Subjective: ***He** is running.*
- Objective: ***Him**, he is running.*

The first is taught in conversational response to a "Which one is . . . ?" type of question, and the second in response to a "What is the man doing?" or "Who is . . . ?" type of question. Children can deduce the function of the subject and its separateness from the topic by the varying contexts in which they are used. There are endless possibilities for teaching subjecthood within play and conversation.

Children can learn each sentence form in response to questions within ongoing activities. Teaching should begin with the first sentence type because it is included within the second. Once children have learned the formats, the questions can be alternated. Later, the habitual or simple present form of the verb, such as *eat* or *drink*, can be introduced to teach children subject–verb agreement within the same subject-highlighted format.

Other semantic classes may be taught in a similar manner. Table 11–6 presents suggestions for teaching. Question cues can help children identity the semantic class of different words within a variety of activities.

CHAPTER 11 SPECIFIC INTERVENTION TECHNIQUES

Table 11–6. Suggestions for Teaching Semantic Classes

Instrument

Initially, this class can be trained in the final position of the sentence, preceded by the word *by*, as in "The wood was split *by his axe*." Position and the preposition *by* act as signals for this class. This class can also be signaled by the verb *use*, as in "John *used the rake* to gather the leaves." This sentence type can be prompted by questions such as "How did . . . ?" and "What did John use to . . . ?"

Patient/Object

This class may be taught initially by using the final position in the sentence as a direct object to transitive verbs. Question prompts such as "What did Carol throw?" may be used to elicit this class.

It is somewhat more difficult to teach this class in the subject position because that position is usually occupied by an agent. If agents are taught in response to a who type of question, patients might use *what*, as in "What grew in the park?"

Dative

The dative class is most frequently and obviously used as an indirect object. This function can be clearly signaled initially by use of the prepositions *to* and *for*. Question prompts can include these cues and the word *whom*, as in "For whom did Mary buy the flowers?"

Temporal, Locative, and Manner

These classes are relatively easy to teach because each has specific questions that prompt usage.

Prepositions, such as *in*, *on*, and *at*, are used with these functions, as are *to*, *with*, and *by*, which are used to mark other semantic class use.

Accompaniment

The final position in the sentence and the preposition *with* should be used in training to signal this class.

A *with whom* question prompt can be used to elicit response.

Relational Words

Relational words fulfill many functions in language. Relationships may be based on quantity or quality and may be general or specific. Other relational words are used to mark location and time. Conjunctions relate one clause or thought to another. Each type of relational word requires specific intervention considerations.

In general, relational terms can be acquired through descriptive tasks, in which a child must differentiate between one entity and another, or through narrative tasks, in which a child must aid the listener to differentiate characters. An SLP can help the child initially by keeping the task context-bound and by controlling the number of items or characters. By playing dumb or acting confused, the adult can help the child provide

456 LANGUAGE DISORDERS: A FUNCTIONAL APPROACH TO ASSESSMENT AND INTERVENTION IN CHILDREN

additional or essential information. Narratives are also effective vehicles for acquiring conjunctions, especially when the adult synthesizes larger, more conceptually complex sentences based on those of the child.

Quantitative Terms. A child does not need to be able to count to learn quantitative terms. Initial teaching can begin with the concepts of *one* and *more than one*. The second concept can be marked variously by *many, much, some,* and *more*. Such terms as *these* and *those* should be introduced with some caution because of deixis, or interpretation from the perspective of the speaker.

The distinction between *many* and *much* is complex and should not be introduced with children functioning at a preschool level. In general, *many* is used with regular and irregular plural nouns, such as *cats, shoes,* and *women*. In contrast, *much* is used with mass nouns—nouns that refer to homogeneous, nonindividual substances, such as *water, sand,* and *sugar*.

Later quantifiers can include words such as *few* and *couple*. These can be followed by other quantifiers, such as *nearly, almost as much as,* and *half*. Table 11–7 presents common quantitative words. The ordering of these words in the noun phrase is very important and

Table 11–7. Common Quantitative and Qualitative Terms	
Quantitative	**Qualitative**
One, two, three, four . . .	Big, little, long, short
Many, much, lots of	Large, small, fat, thin
Some, few, couple	Soft, hard, heavy, light
More, another	Same, different, alike
Nearly, almost all	Old, young, pretty, ugly
As much/little as	Blue, green, red . . .
Plenty	Hot, cold, warm, chilly
Half, one-fourth, two-fifths	Wide, narrow
10%, 75%	Sweet, sour
Units of measure: inch, foot, mile, cup, pint, quart, gallon, centimeter, meter, kilometer, liter, ounce, pound, gram, kilogram, acre	Nice, mean, funny, sad
	Fast, slow
	Smooth, rough
	Clean, dirty
	Empty, full
	Angry, afraid
	Comparative and superlative relationships: *-er, -est, as x as, x-er* than

is discussed in the syntax section of this chapter. The use of numerical terms and fractions and percentages must wait until school age and requires some mathematical skill.

Quantitative terms can be taught within many naturally occurring situations using anything from counting blocks and Legos to candy and treats. Books and many finger-plays also contain counting.

Narratives can contain several characters or objects that can be grouped in various ways throughout the story, using words such as *both*, *only one*, and *all three*. It is also easy to create situations in which children request a number of objects, as in response to "How many do you want?" Quantitative terms also naturally occur within any play that replicates commerce, such as a fast-food restaurant or market.

Qualitative Terms. Qualitative terms include such words as *big* and *tall*, plus *bigger* and *tallest*, which use the *-er* and *-est* morphological markers, and such phrases as *as big as*, *not as wet as*, *smaller than*, and the like. Table 11–7 presents common qualitative terms. In general, children learn to use the comparative *-er* before the superlative *-est*, and teaching should follow that pattern. It is best to begin with the regular use of these two markers before introducing exceptions, such as *better* and *best*. Words can be expanded into phrases, as in going from *bigger* to *bigger than*.

Children seem to acquire concepts one semantic feature at a time. A corollary to this hypothesis is that broad, nonspecific concepts (e.g., *big*) are learned before more specific concepts (e.g., *long*). In this example, *big* refers to overall size, whereas *long* refers to size only in the horizontal plane.

The SLP should introduce terms and relationships in the order in which comparative terms develop. Table 11–8 includes common pairs of comparative terms and the approximate age at which most children can use them correctly.

In general, conceptual word pairs are acquired asymmetrically. Children ages 3 to 7 years appear to learn the positive member of conceptual pairs, the one that represents more of the dimension characterizing the pair, prior to learning the negative member (Bracken, 1988). For example, *big* and *little* are opposite poles of the dimension size. *Big* represents more size and is, therefore, the positive member. These data suggest that positive members should be taught first to children with language disorders.

Many play situations and narratives include qualitative terms. It is also easy to devise conversations in which children must contrast one thing with another. By acting confused and asking "Which one?" an SLP can elicit responses such as "The big one" or "The green fuzzy one." Within several situations, such as play or snack, children can be offered choices based on some contrasting feature, such as size or color.

Spatial and Temporal Terms. Several words are used to mark both space or location and time and, thus, are potentially confusing. Among the most commonly used words in English are prepositions, such as *in*, *on*, *at*, and *by*. In the syntax section of this chapter, we discuss prepositional phrase teaching. Other terms, such as *first* and *last*, also note place and time.

Spatial concepts are best taught first in relation to the child and then with "featured" or fronted objects, such as a video screen, and finally with nonfeatured objects, such as

Table 11–8. Common Comparative Word-Pairs

Positive–Negative (Age)	Positive–Negative (Age)	Positive–Negative (Age)
same–different (36–60 months)	inside–outside	high–low (42–60 months)
in front of–behind (48–54 months)	over–under (42–48 months)	forward–backward
into–out of	front–back (48–52 months)	happy–sad
top–bottom (48–54 months)	above–below (66–72 months)	old–young
rising–falling	right–wrong	large–small (78–84 months)
healthy–sick	heavy–light (30–48 months)	long–short (horizontal) (54–60 months)
big–little (30–48 months)	tall–short (30–84 months)	hot–cold
deep–shallow	loud–quiet	dark–light
thick–thin	sharp–dull	tight–loose
hard–soft (30–42 months)	solid–liquid	a lot–a little
smooth–rough	full–empty (36–48 months)	fast–slow
more–less (42–72 months)	with–without (48–54 months)	early–late
all–none	arriving–leaving	always–never
old–new	first–last (60–66 months)	
before–after (66–72 months)	on–off (24–36 months)	
open–close	up–down (36–60 months)	

Note: The order represents when each member is learned respectively—that is, high at 42 months and low at 60 months.

Sources: Information from Bracken (1988), Edmonston and Thane (1990), and Wiig and Semel (1984).

a wastebasket or a ball. The latter is more difficult to learn because it involves deixis, or interpretation based on the speaker.

In general, vertical dimensions (*on top*) are learned before horizontal. Horizontal front and back terms, such as *in front of* and *behind*, are learned before horizontal side-to-side terms, such as *beside* and *next to*. The order reflects the underlying concepts. Terms that denote order, such as *before*, *after*, *first*, and *last*, usually are learned before terms for simultaneity, such as *at the same time*, *during*, and *when*. Duration terms, such as *a long time*, generally are acquired last.

In general, it is better to begin with concrete definitions and progress to more abstract ones. For example, with *first*, *last*, *before*, and *after*, teaching can begin with objects in a line, such as a train. The adult can have the child touch individual train cars ("Which car is first?"), then progress to a short sequence of objects (*first*, *last*) and finally a reverse sequence. Sequenced objects should be used before sequenced events and the concept of time.

CHAPTER 11 SPECIFIC INTERVENTION TECHNIQUES

459

The greater the number of contexts, the more learning and generalization that will occur. Language can be used to help a child organize the environment by marking experiences of space and time. Table 11–9 includes common spatial and temporal terms.

The SLP can use direction-following games and activities to teach children about space and time. It might be best to begin with routines that the child knows, such as those that occur at home or in the classroom, and then move to less familiar activities, such as using an ATM machine, in which the child must rely more on linguistic input rather than physical memory. Activities involving making or cooking are excellent sequential tasks. (See Appendix G.)

Later, the SLP can use sequenced pictures or storytelling. Children can identify what happened first, next, and last.

Deixis and the use of deictic terms are very difficult concepts to teach. The adult who takes both the role of speaker and that of prompter for a child violates the roles in a conversation. The simple example of *here* and *there* is illustrative. The request "Put the ball here" is said from the speaker's perspective. To the listener, the speaker's *here* is most likely *there*. If the speaker then shifts to the listener's (the child's) perspective and says, "Yes, put it there," it may confuse the child further. How can it be both here and there for the speaker?

When teaching the child about deictic terms, it is best to sit next to the child so that you both can share a perspective. From this shared perspective, deictic terms for location would be similar. Another adult, puppet, or prerecorded tape may act as the other conversational partner. The teaching of deixis is discussed also under the topic of pronouns in the syntax section of this chapter.

Conjunctions. You can teach conjunctions by noting the relationships expressed in each. For example, *because* represents cause and effect and may not be fully acquired until approximately age 12 years. Table 11–10 presents the general order of conjunction acquisition. The conjunction *and* can first be taught to combine entities, as in "cats and dogs." In a cooking activity, the adult might say, "Which two types of cookies do you

Table 11–9. Common Spatial and Temporal Terms

Spatial			Temporal		
next to	under	in front of	next	today	days
before	over	behind	before	tomorrow	weeks
after	below	beside	after	calendar dates	hours
on, on top	corner	right	in, to	months	minutes
in, into	bottom	left	soon	seasons	through
in between	inside	through	later	numerals for years	away from
between	outside	high, tall	now	morning	toward
middle	side	upside down	above	afternoon	sometimes
above	end	together	yesterday	evening	

Table 11–10. A Rough Acquisition Order for English Conjunctions

And

And then

But, or, because

So, if, when

Until, before

After

Although

While, as

Unless, therefore

However

like best?" or "Tell me your two favorite types of cookies." Similarly, *but* can be used for like/dislike distinctions ("I like cookies, but not beets").

A *clause + conjunction + clause* format can be employed initially to help the child acquire the underlying relationship. For example, sentences might be presented as follows:

We like ice cream but I do not like pudding.

We want to have fun and I want to go to the park.

Once a child understands these relationships, other conjunctions can be introduced.

For conjunctions that order events, using the order of mention helps a child comprehend. For example, "Because it is cold, we wear a coat" or "If it's cold, I wear a coat" are easier that the reverse order, "I wear a coat because it's cold."

Next, the SLP can present clauses for the child to combine. The breakdown and buildup technique, described in Chapter 10, may be used to help the child identify clauses and conjunctions and then reconstruct the sentence. This can be accomplished conversationally.

Conjoining clauses with conjunctions is a natural occurrence within narratives and can be prompted through storybook retelling or with pictures. The SLP can reply to a child's utterance by supplying the desired conjunction and then asking for a restatement as in the following:

Child: And the whole bridge fell down.

Adult: Why? Because . . .

Child: 'Cause the water was going so fast.

CHAPTER 11 SPECIFIC INTERVENTION TECHNIQUES

Adult: That sounds very exciting, but I'm not sure I understand the whole thing. The bridge . . .

Child: The bridge fell down because the water was going fast.

Adult: The bridge fell down because the water was going fast. That's really scary. What happened next?

> **Food for Thought:** Have you pigeonholed semantics as just vocabulary words? That's common. But words are so much more as the surrounding sections indicate. For example, semantic classes are essential for sentence formation.

Word Retrieval and Categorization

Many of the lexical factors that affect word-finding or retrieval for children with TDL also affect those with word-finding difficulty. For example, the more frequently the word is used, the easier word-finding becomes to retrieve. Children tend to produce word substitutions that are shorter and have a higher frequency, neighborhood density, and phonotactic probability or likelihood than the target word.

Word-finding difficulties can result from two possible sources. The first is lack of elaboration or lack of a well-established, thorough representation of the word within the child's internal dictionary, or lexicon. Children who exhibit difficulties often have less extensive vocabularies and poor word knowledge.

The second source of problems is in retrieval. Although many elaboration difficulties occur alone, retrieval problems usually do not and may be an additional difficulty found in some children with elaborative problems.

Children with word retrieval problems appear to benefit from both elaboration and retrieval activities, but these can be fine-tuned through further exploration by an SLP. Word-finding activities can be incorporated easily into a number of everyday activities and conversations about these activities.

Prior to beginning intervention, it is important to determine the factors affecting the behavior. An SLP should derive naming data from a variety of activities to be certain of the cause of the problem. In general, children name real objects and colored pictures with a higher accuracy than black-and-white pictures (Barrow et al., 2000). Naming words in a meaningful context is also performance enhancing.

Children with storage problems have difficulty understanding and retrieving words that are not stable in their memory. Inadequate storage is the result of shallow meanings, reference-shifting (*here–there, me–you, come–go*) problems, and poor analytical and synthesizing skills. The goal of intervention for storage difficulties is to improve word knowledge and storage.

Those with retrieval-only problems have difficulty with search and recovery. Somewhere in the process of discriminating the desired word from among competing words and constructing the phonological specifications for production, the process breaks down. The goal of intervention for retrieval is improved access.

Memory storage seems to be affected by the depth or level of processing. In general, recall is best for words processed at the deepest levels. Acoustic processing, such as rhyming, is surface processing; categorical is mid-level; and semantic/syntactic is deep.

Words are remembered in relation to other words and form semantic networks. When one member of the family is accessed, it activates others. In other words, *ride* might elicit *drive* or *pedal* but not elicit *stride*, a phonological variation. Likewise, *cad* might elicit *villain* but not *cadet.*

Networks of semantic-related morphemes are also part of each individual's memory system. Thus, *stain*, *stained glass*, and *stainless steel* are perceived to be related.

Elaboration

Elaboration teaching focuses on organization of the child's lexicon and generalization of word meanings to everyday use. An SLP can use semantic focus strategies, such as nonidentical examples and word comparison tasks. Nonidentical examples of the word in several linguistic contexts enrich a child's definition and word associations. Examples for *house* might include *dollhouse, housefly*, and *greenhouse*. In comparative tasks, the SLP expects the child to identify similarities and differences between two words with related meanings, such as *house* and *hotel.*

A mnemonic or "key word" strategy also might be used to aid elaboration and recall of new vocabulary. New words are linked with acoustically or visually similar words with which the child is familiar. For example, *dogged* might be linked with *dog*. This initial superficial linkage is gradually modified through a semantic strategy with deeper processing.

Pictures and written descriptions may be used to link two words. A known word is used to aid learning and storage of an unknown one. In the previous example, a dog would be portrayed being stubborn or determined (*dogged*). Under the picture, it might read *The dog was dogged and would not give up*. Note also that the definition of *dogged* has been included. Other examples are given in Figure 11–3. The key word now becomes the retrieval cue.

Children using this approach reportedly are able to recall 50% more definitions than those taught vocabulary by a more traditional method. In addition, the combined picture and sentence format appears to be more effective than either used separately.

Children seem naturally to enjoy word games and word play, and these teaching strategies can be incorporated into many types of activities. As a communication partner, I like to get very "confused" and use words in silly ways. Children laugh and freely correct their somewhat slow-witted communication partner.

Taxonomic or Categorical Approaches

Data from children with TDL suggest that taxonomic or categorical relations, such as things to write with (*crayon, marker, pencil*), and thematic or event relations, such as the act of writing (*paper, pencil*), develop differently and can affect word recall (Hashimoto et al., 2007). In addition, taxonomic relationships are originally based by children on observable perceptual features (shape and size). For preschool and kindergarten children,

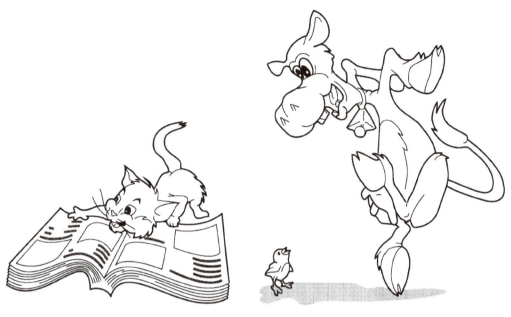

Figure 11–3. Examples of mnemonic strategies.

The **cat** is ordering from the **catalog**.   The **cow** is a frightened **coward**.

thematic cues might assist word recall. Taxonomic cues with school-age children should begin with obvious perceptual similarities.

Retrieval teaching may include categorization tasks, such as naming members of a category or identifying the category when given the members. Categories include animals, clothing, grocery items, and the like that can easily be introduced into functional methods. For example, "I heard you were going on a class trip. What will you put (clothing) in your suitcase?"

As a group, children with language disorder are less likely than children with TDL to discover semantic organization strategies on their own and usually require more examples to determine a basis for organization and for generalization of organizational skill. Word-substitution errors should demonstrate the predominant organizational framework of the child and alert the SLP to the patterns that need strengthening.

Categorization tasks, especially such familiar ones as favorite cartoon shows, in which the child names members of the category, facilitate recall by building associational and categorical linkages between words. Of course, the possibility still exists that a child will access the right category but retrieve the wrong member.

Categorization tasks can be elaborative in nature when members of more than one category are presented together. For example, the items chair, bed, and table can be classified as furniture; chair, swing, and bicycle are things on which you sit; and bicycle, car, and bus are vehicles. The adult could present these items together and ask the child to classify them in as many ways as possible.

Teaching might begin with actual objects and children making piles of objects that go together (Parente & Hermann, 1996). As a child, I sorted my comic books by main character and my baseball cards by team. Similar tasks are found in several everyday activities. After objects and pictures, then words can be used. Entities might be classified by description (e.g., cold) or by function (e.g., things that you ride on). The adult should encourage the child to use as many different sensory descriptions as possible.

After a sorting task, a child can be asked to recall the categories. Once the child has recalled categories, they can be asked to recall members and add new ones. Everyday tasks such as preparing grocery lists, organizing chores, or planning items to take on vacation or items that go in one's backpack or one's room have more relevance than arbitrary groupings.

Verbal teaching can begin with common words for everyday concrete objects. Familiar everyday objects and events should be used. I am reminded of a teacher who tried to teach zoo and farm animal categories but found the children very unresponsive. Both categories were outside their realm of everyday experience. When one child suggested the category of animals seen "squashed" on the highway, every child became a participant. Although the example is somewhat gruesome, the lesson for SLPs is very practical. Everyday natural environments, the ones functional intervention tries to use, provide specific cues that aid memory.

Retrieval

Word-retrieval difficulties can be helped by (a) naming/descriptive tasks ("It's a bicycle; you ride on it by peddling"), (b) associational activities ("Red, white, and _____"), and (c) sentential elaboration tasks based on syntactic characteristics of two words drawn at random ("The trailer was parked near the restaurant while the driver ate") and open-ended fill-ins and completions ("We eat with a _____") that involve deeper levels of processing. Word-sorting tasks can aid in the development of categorization and recall skills. Taxonomy charts, especially for newly introduced classroom content, also can help children develop categorization strategies.

Categorical identification seems to be the best cue for recall when a child is stuck or blocks on a word. By naming the category, the adult can help the child locate the desired word more easily. Other strategies include partial word cues; sentence completion; and nonverbal, gestural cues. Additional retrieval strategies are listed in Table 11–11. In intervention, retrieval units should move from single words to longer units.

With some children, a combination of phonological and perceptual strategies may also be effective, although semantic elaboration and retrieval activities produce better results than phonological strategies alone. In phonological teaching, the child participates in segmentation exercises such as rhyming, initial sound matching, and counting syllables and phonemes. The rationale for this method is that, in part, breakdown is the result of poor phonological representation of the word. Phonologically based treatment that focuses on words that begin with the same phoneme and words that sound alike can reduce semantic substitutions. Perceptual strategies involve imagery activities, such as simultaneous picture and auditory exposure, visualization with eyes closed, and silent name repetition.

The SLP can help a child note features and attributes that determine how members are categorized. One mediational strategy might be to teach the child to ask a set of ques-

CHAPTER 11 SPECIFIC INTERVENTION TECHNIQUES

Table 11–11. Word-Retrieval Strategies

Retrieval Strategy	Description
Attribute cue	Attribute of the word or meaning is presented.
	Types:
	Phonemic: Initial phoneme, vowel nucleus or syllable is presented, as in *It begins with /b/.*
	Semantic: Category name or function is presented, *boat* for *canoe* or *mixes* for *blender.*
	Visual: Picture or revisualization is presented.
	Gestural: Motor scheme is presented as in miming shoveling.
Associated cue	A word typically associated with the word is presented, such as *hiking* for *boot* or *orange* for *juice.*
Semantic alternative	Another word with a similar meaning is presented.
	Types:
	Synonym or category substitution: A synonym or other category members are presented, such as *afraid* to elicit *frightened* or *goats, cows,* and *horses* to elicit *pigs.*
	Multiword substitution or description is presented as in *It lives on a farm* or *You cut paper with them.*
Reflective pause	Child is reminded to pause and think in order to reduce competitive responses.

Source: Information from German (1992).

tions to establish an association between a new item and something familiar. Questions might include the following (Parente & Hermann, 1996, p. 50):

What does it look (sound, smell, taste) like?

What does it mean the same thing as?

What groups does it belong to?

Who is it commonly associated with?

It is important that children note a similar attribute on more than one object. Otherwise, children may begin to associate certain attributes with specific items. For example, several very different objects may be described as wet. This kind of task naturally leads to categorization. Attributes can appear also in many different linguistic forms, rather than just "It's . . . " in order to enhance storage and memory.

The relationship between responses to drill-like naming exercises and word-finding in conversation is unknown. At a minimum, therefore, it is essential that teaching include a strong conversational element to ensure generalization of word-finding skills.

Most word-learning methods include both study and retrieval. Continued retrieval after initial retrieval practice appears to be helpful even if further study is discontinued (Leonard et al., 2020). The most effective amount and type of retrieval have yet to be determined.

Comprehension

Language comprehension consists of a complex set of processes, including (Linderholm et al., 2000)

- encoding of facts;
- activation of knowledge; and
- generation of inferences.

Inferencing connects information in ways that make that information understandable and memorable. Comprehension difficulties occur when children have difficulty remembering what they have heard or read, applying their world knowledge to what they heard or read, or focusing on the important ideas and concepts presented (Kibby et al., 2004).

The goal of intervention is to teach the child to retrieve relevant word and world knowledge as a comprehension aid and to help the child decide how and what to remember from what they hear or read. Comprehension and memory are aided by familiar, meaningful contexts. The degree and type of experience the child has with events strongly shape their expectations and, thus, comprehension. Language within familiar play and role-play of everyday events can enhance comprehension.

The level of involvement also affects memory and comprehension. The more involved a child is, the more they comprehend and recall. Song lyrics, nursery rhymes, and finger play occur regularly in school classrooms and can be used to help a child make active associations between words and the nonlinguistic context. Repetitions aid comprehension.

Finally, comprehension intervention should be pleasurable. Fun activities keep children engaged, a necessity for comprehension and comprehension teaching.

Initial comprehension teaching may need to be very concrete and highly contextual. Preschool children benefit more from activities with more immediate recall versus narrative recall. The use of gestures and a slower rate of talking by the SLP also enhances comprehension by young children and children with DLD (Montgomery, 2005). As children approach school age, teaching can become more decontextualized, similar to many of the literate activities found in school.

Comprehension teaching might begin with recall from pictures or objects and progress to literal recall of one or more details from verbal sources. Gradually, an SLP can require a child to recall more details. Later, the child can detail these in sequence, possibly using sequential pictures, photographs of past events, or picture books as aids. Daily events can provide a script to aid comprehension. Next, the SLP can require the child to relate cause and effect from familiar or recently read narratives. Once able to

CHAPTER 11 SPECIFIC INTERVENTION TECHNIQUES

reconstruct these relationships, the child can begin to make inferences; draw conclusions; and predict outcomes from stories, riddles, and jokes. Finally, the child can learn to synthesize information and create subjective summaries of the meanings of narratives, TV shows, or movies.

To assist comprehension, you can shape question–response strategies by manipulating the semantic content, question complexity, context, and function. The therapy process moves from simple, context-embedded *yes/no* questions to the use of questions in more abstract contexts, while controlling the length of the questions and highlighting semantic content.

In the second stage, early developing *wh-* question forms might become the targets, with *yes/no* questions used to highlight the semantic content desired. Consider, for example, the question, "What is the girl wearing on her head?" A nonresponse, an inappropriate response, or an inaccurate response might be followed by "Is she wearing a shoe on her head?" If the child responds negatively, the prompt would be "That's right, what is she wearing on her head?" Print, pictures, or signs can be used to highlight the *wh-* words and, thus, emphasize the information desired. These prompts can be faded gradually.

In the third stage, new *wh-* forms are added systematically. Developmental data suggest a logical order for teaching *wh-* words and question types based on concept learning. Initial *wh-* words, concerned with things (objects), persons (agents), possession, and locations, include *what, who, whose,* and *where,* respectively. Soon, children learn distinctions between things, as expressed in the word *which.* Around age 4 years, they become aware of sequence, time, and causality, or the *wh-* words and questions *how, when,* and *why,* respectively. Content is shifted gradually from concrete, predictable, factually based academic topics to more abstract, less predictable conversational ones.

School-age children might manipulate objects or pictures and match them with the sentences heard. Similarly, the child might select a picture described by the adult from among a set of pictures. Written cues also could be used.

Figurative Language

Figurative language consists of idioms, metaphors, similes, and proverbs. Idioms are a form of figurative language that is particularly troublesome to comprehend for school-age children with language disorders and for children from CLD backgrounds. The most common error is literal interpretation. Children with language disorders may lack a strategy for determining meaning. Some common high- and low-familiarity idioms are listed in Table 11–12.

Intervention can begin with comprehension of transparent or easily decipherable idioms. Narratives may be the best teaching milieu because of the contextual support. The child can be instructed prior to the narrative that it will contain a certain idiom and that they will be able to figure out the meaning from the story. Questions can be used throughout the narrative to help the child attend to important information. After repeated exposure and the child's correct interpretation, they can be encouraged to invent their own narratives that illustrate use of the idiom. Finally, conversationally appropriate use can be discussed and role-played.

Table 11–12. Common American English Idioms

Animals

A bull in a china shop	Playing possum	Clinging like a leech
As stubborn as a mule	Go into one's shell	Grinning like a Cheshire cat
Going to the dogs	A fly in the ointment	Thrown to the wolves

Body Parts

On the tip of my tongue	Put their heads together*	Put your best foot forward
Raised eyebrows	Vote with one's feet	Turn heads
Turn the other cheek	Breathe down one's neck*	Put one's foot down*

Clothing

Dressed to kill	Talk through one's hat	Strait-laced
Hot under the collar	Fit like a glove	

Colors

Gray area	Tickled pink	Red letter day
Once in a blue moon	True blue	

Foods

Eat crow	That takes the cake	In a jam
Humble pie	A finger in every pie	Put all your eggs in one basket

Games and Sports

Ace up my sleeve	Paddle your own canoe	Get to first base
Cards are stacked against me	Rise to the bait	Keep the ball rolling
Got lost in the shuffle	Skate on thin ice*	On the rebound
Keep your head above water	Ballpark figure	Go around in circles*
Cross swords		

Plants

Heard it through the grapevine	Beat around the bush*	Shaking like a leaf
Resting on his laurels	No bed of roses	Withered on the vine

Vehicles

Fix your wagon	On the wagon	Missed the boat
Like ships passing in the night	Don't rock the boat	Take a back seat

Tools, Work, and School

Bury the hatchet	Throw a monkey wrench into it	Hit the roof
Has an axe to grind	Read between the lines*	Nursing his wounds
Hit the nail on the head	Doctor the books	Sober as a judge

Weather

Calm before the storm	Steal her thunder	Right as rain
Haven't the foggiest	Come rain or shine	Throw caution to the wind

Note: *Highly familiar.

CHAPTER 11 SPECIFIC INTERVENTION TECHNIQUES

469

Proverbs depend on context. The context in which the proverb is used facilitates understanding. In general, concrete proverbs are easier to interpret than abstract, and familiar proverbs are easier to understand than unfamiliar.

The ability to interpret and use proverbs develops during late elementary school, continues into adulthood, and is related to reading and metalinguistic abilities. With this in mind, an SLP is advised to teach proverb interpretation within the context of reading (Nippold, 2000).

Working in small groups, adolescents can discuss interpretations. The SLP can use contextual cues, questions, and analysis to help teens become independent learners. Through both asking and answering factual and inferential questions, adolescents learn to interpret the context. Analysis of the main characters' motivations, goals, actions, and feelings further aids interpretation. Finally, adolescents need help determining the relationship between the proverb and their own lives.

Verbal Working Memory

Although the depth and breadth of this topic is beyond the scope of this text and the topic fits only loosely—if at all—under semantics and comprehension, I would be remiss were I not to mention verbal working memory given the deficits mentioned in Chapter 2, especially for most children with DLD.

Before we begin, it's important to note our limitations here. Targeting processing skills, such as working memory (WM), in intervention is appealing because doing so offers the promise of improving language and learning deficits without having to directly target the specific language knowledge and skills (Kamhi, 2014). The reasoning is that if WM is a cause of language and learning problems, then improvements in WM should lead to changes in language function.

Unfortunately, a meta-analysis of 23 research studies found that memory teaching was not necessarily an effective intervention (Melby-Lervåg & Hulme, 2013). In addition, WM teaching may not lead to better performance outside of the training tasks.

The cautionary note is that all cognitive processing skills, including WM, are best taught within a language context if we want to improve language. In other words, teaching memory alone may have very little effect on language.

In addition, there is not a great deal of research on effective methods for teaching WM skills with children with language disorders. However, a critical component of successful intervention is placing significant storage and processing demands on WM and then systematically increasing or decreasing demands based on a child's performance (Boudreau & Costanza-Smith, 2011). Memory and awareness tasks for intervention are presented in Table 11–13.

Given the academic difficulties of children with WM deficits, it seems wise for the SLP in collaboration with classroom teachers to identify WM demands in the classroom that impact a child's academic performance and then modify the classroom environment to support each child. Let's discuss intervention in that order. See both Montgomery and colleagues (2010) and Boudreau and Costanza-Smith (2011) for more specifics than we have space to discuss here.

Intervention for children with DLD and WM deficits should focus on promoting stronger language abilities and be grounded in the principles of EBP. In the following

Table 11–13. Intervention for Working Memory and Awareness

Technique	Explanation
Rehearsal	Explicit training and rehearsal training can enhance the short-term memory storage and recall of children with SLI and other language impairments (Gill et al., 2003; Loomes et al., 2008). Older children and adolescents with SLI and/or WM deficits can be taught to rehearse information that is critical to a task. This, in turn, reduces WM demands. Memory strategies, such as systematically chunking words or information together, also make the information easier to remember (Minear & Shah, 2006).
Task analysis	Children can be taught to identify the current goal of a task and helped to systematically identify appropriate strategies.
Visualization	Using key words to organize verbal information into a visual representation can improve our ability to follow instructions and to remember complex information (Gill et al., 2003; Hood & Rankin, 2005). Visual representations constrain the amount and complexity of the information, reducing the amount of cognitive resources required (Alloway et al., 2009).
Study and organizational	Children with WM difficulties often struggle with organizing information. Organization and study skills might include visual or key word cues to represent steps in a process or instructions to follow.

sections, we briefly discuss intervention in three areas: phonological short-term memory (PSTM), WM capacity, and automaticity and rate.

Phonological Short-Term Memory

Interestingly, improving phonological memory seems to improve WM abilities overall as well as language. Repeating phonological forms that are unfamiliar may assist a child in perceiving the essentials of the phonological structure of language. Enhancing the efficiency of phonological encoding may improve the retention and the quality of phonological information in WM, as well as potentially improving reading ability (Maridaki-Kassotaki, 2002; Minear & Shah, 2006).

Phonological memory may also be improved through teaching of other phonological processes as well (O'Shaughnessy & Swanson, 2000). For example, intervention focused on rhyme and phoneme awareness improves phonological awareness skills as well as fostering significant improvement on new word recognition tasks.

Direct intervention through reading and writing can also improve phonological memory skills. For example, phonological spelling intervention, explained in Chapter 13, including specific teaching with syllable and phoneme segmentation of unfamiliar words as well as phoneme–grapheme relationships, can result in children's improved ability to spell, repeat, and read pseudo-words (Berninger, Winn, et al., 2008).

Working Memory Capacity

Working memory capacity teaching can increase reading comprehension accuracy, nonverbal reasoning, attention, and reading speed in young elementary school children (Klingberg et al., 2005; Loosli et al., 2008; Thorell et al., 2009). The purpose of WM capacity intervention for children with DLD is to allow them to better manage the dual demands of information processing and storage during language-related activities. It may be best to begin intervention with visuospatial WM teaching, given that children with DLD seem to struggle with verbal storage more than visuospatial storage (Archibald & Gathercole, 2006, 2007).

Visual stimuli might enable a child to learn to manage WM resources under more storage-friendly conditions (Montgomery et al., 2010). Once a child demonstrates good responses under these conditions, intervention could switch to auditory stimuli.

Several computerized teaching programs, such as Cogmed Working Memory Training (NeuroDevelopmental Center, 2013), Fast ForWord Language (Scientific Learning Corporation, 2021), and Soak Your Brain (Soak Your Head, n.d.), are available. In general, these programs require a child to complete a task while remembering rules, such as responding whenever a certain letter appears.

Although computerized programs are effective in producing gains in general language abilities and WM, traditional interventions seem equally effective, indicating that lower tech, lower priced interventions can yield comparable gains (Cohen et al., 2005; R. Gillam et al., 2008). Computerized programs alone, without direct SLP input, are less effective than a combination of both methods.

Automaticity and Rate

The SLP can help a child decrease WM demands by making some components of a learning situation more automatic. By analyzing learning situations in the classroom, the SLP and teacher can identify the knowledge and skills important for successful completion.

Through repeated practice, overlearning, and over-rehearsal, a task becomes automatic for the child. The SLP might focus on language abilities that are critical for assignments in reading and writing and also help support WM limitations. The SLP might also target vocabulary and syntax that are closely tied to a task, thus reducing the demands on available WM resources. For example, if a child has stored vocabulary terms on a certain topic and sentence frames for particular classroom activities, the task is easier and more automatic.

For young children with WM deficits, it is especially important to ensure that they can understand and follow directions. This may include learning sentence frames with causal or conditional clauses (e.g., *if/then, because*), temporal terms (e.g., *before, after, first, last*), or specific terms (e.g., *describe, explain, compare*).

Learning situations that require accessing prior knowledge place great demand on a child's WM abilities. By collaborating with the classroom teacher, the SLP can ensure that background knowledge is readily available to a child. This will result in greater resources dedicated to the task.

472 LANGUAGE DISORDERS: A FUNCTIONAL APPROACH TO ASSESSMENT AND INTERVENTION IN CHILDREN

Processing within actual use contexts is the goal of intervention. Each session can provide real conversational and academic activities within which the SLP can monitor each child's behavior and aid participation.

> ***Food for Thought:*** Have you truly noticed how quickly you process language in all its modes? For example, unless, you have memory challenges, words are withdrawn from storage so swiftly, you're unaware that it's even happening.

Syntax and Morphology

Although language use improves syntax, the reverse is not true. It is important, therefore, that syntactic teaching be as functional as possible. When language forms or constructions are taught devoid of a communication context, the forms may be mastered without the knowledge of how to express ideas within and across these forms. In addition, utterances produced in a context such as conversation strengthen cohesion and relationships across linguistic units. The linguistic techniques discussed in Chapter 10 are particularly applicable to syntactic and morphologic teaching.

During teaching, it is important that the SLP control for vocabulary and/or sentence length, especially when teaching new structures. If the adult changes too many variables at one time, it may confuse a child or make the task too complex for successful completion. The SLP also should be careful not to require metalinguistic skills beyond a child's abilities.

Although recognition and comprehension usually precede production, judgments of correct usage do not. Judging a sentence to be grammatically correct is a metalinguistic skill that develops in the middle elementary school years. Asking children to form sentences with selected words or to unscramble words to form a sentence (*coat john a yesterday new bought*) also requires metalinguistic skill and WM. In short, any task that requires the child to manipulate language abstractly takes some degree of metalinguistic skill. In addition, many of these tasks are never encountered in actual language use.

The development of syntactic and morphologic forms is well documented and provides a guide for intervention. In the following section, hierarchies for intervention with several different forms are discussed. The purpose is to offer general guidelines for the ordering of structures to be taught.

Morphology

Inflectional suffixes develop early and lend themselves well to teaching within a conversational milieu. Other morphemes may best be taught in a more explicit manner first, beginning with suffixes, followed by prefixes. Explicit rule learning is not recommended for preschool children. Common bound morphemes are listed in Appendix C. Because derivational relationships are complex and irregular, memorization is of little value as a learning tool. It is essential that the child understand the underlying changes in meaning and their effect on a listener.

CHAPTER 11 SPECIFIC INTERVENTION TECHNIQUES

Although data for school-age morphological development are scarce, some suggestions for teaching do exist. These are presented in Table 11–14. Teaching should begin with the most common, early developing morphemes and proceed toward those that are more complex and cause phonological and orthographic or spelling changes.

As you might imagine, deducing an underlying language rule is easier for children if they experience that rule in varied linguistic contexts. For example, it would be difficult to figure out the third person -s verb ending from only "She eats." If we varied the noun/pronoun and the specific verb, more and varied examples should lead to easier and quicker learning. This can be easily accomplished in a conversational milieu. When learning bound morphemes, children in high-variability contexts produce more unique utterances using the target morpheme (Plante et al., 2014).

Increasing syntactic difficulty decreases use of morphology for all children. In other words, processing demands influence morphological accuracy. Children with higher MLUs are less affected by sentence complexity.

Specially constructed "syntax stories" that provide numerous examples of forms, such as BE, can be used to increase language input of these forms. Stories tailored to the child and intervention target can serve as models for parents of how to provide intensive positive input for their child. A list of children's books for intervention is included in Appendix H. Westby (2005) provides several titles that can help clinicians and parents enhance the intensity of input for target forms.

Middle-school children can be taught complex derivational morphology in both the oral and written modes. Teaching for middle-school children also should include root words that frequently occur in science, math, and social studies.

Verbs and Verb Tensing

Children with language disorders don't usually have difficulty learning -ing, plural -s, or the locatives *in* and *on*. They do have difficulty learning grammatical morphemes that reflect verb tense and noun–verb agreement, such as past tense -ed, the auxiliary *do* forms (*do, does, did*), both copula and auxiliary BE forms (*is, are, am, was, were*), and third

---

Table 11–14. Suggested Order for Teaching Morphemes

1. Establish awareness of syllables and sounds. Practice counting both.

2. Identify roots and affixes. Practice pronouncing and defining roots and affixes in contrasting words that are similar in sound or appearance, such as *happy–sunny* and *include–conclude*.

3. Generate a formal definition in the form "A/An *X* is a (superordinate category) that (restrictive attributes)."

4. Discuss relationships with other words.

5. Use words in meaningful contexts and in analogies and cloze activities.

6. Use words in reading activities if appropriate.

7. Introduce spelling and spelling rules if appropriate.

person singular *-s*. Tense and agreement morphemes are significantly more difficult for children with DLD than for their peers with TDL (Gladfelter & Leonard, 2013).

Verb learning takes several years and is very difficult for children with language disorders, partly because of the many ways verbs are treated syntactically and morphologically. Studies with preschoolers with TDL suggest that verb learning is enhanced when specific movements, such as *jump* and *run*, are associated with verbs as opposed to general verbs, such as *do* (Brackenbury & Fey, 2003). In addition, children with DLD benefit from multiple and well-spaced presentation (Riches et al., 2005).

The teaching of verb tensing can be adapted easily to everyday activities in which children discuss what they are doing at present, did previously, or will do in the future. Art projects and building toys such as Legos are especially useful. Appendix G offers a number of activities for targeting verb tensing.

Teaching with very young children can begin with protoverbs, such as *up*, *in*, *off*, *down*, *no*, *there*, *bye-bye*, and *night-night*. These verb-like words usually are used in relation to some familiar action sequence.

More specific action verbs should be introduced in their uninflected or unmarked form. The language teacher can cue by asking what a child is doing or by directing the *child:*

> *Adult:* Let's color. Oh, SpongeBob SquarePants is sad. You better tell SpongeBob to color.
>
> *Child:* Color!

To facilitate learning, action word meanings might be taught with specific actions or objects, as in "throw ball." While playing, the adult can hide their eyes or turn away from the child and ask, "What are you doing?" Although the cue requires an *-ing* ending on the verb in the response ("Eating"), this form need not be required of the child at this very low level of teaching.

Familiar event sequences, such as play or routines, facilitate action verb usage because of the mental representations of the scripts that children possess. These event sequences enable the child to focus on the communication rather than on the extralinguistic elements of the event.

Once a child is able to form simple two- and three-word utterances with an action word, as in "Doggie eat," the present progressive verb form can be introduced without the auxiliary verb. The SLP can model this form through self-talk and parallel talk. The SLP can cue the child to use this form with "What's doggie doing?" or "What's he doing?" Pronouns should be used with caution at this level because many children with language disorders use very few.

Initially, a child only needs to deal with the immediate context. A sense of time beyond the present, however, is essential for further verb teaching.

Procedures for teaching verb tensing should make sense both semantically and pragmatically. Examples are asking the child to perform various tasks ("Will you please . . . ?"), problem-solving ("What will happen if . . . ?" "What might happen if . . . ?"), and role-playing ("What should we do if . . . ?"). Many children's books lend themselves to predicting tasks as well.

CHAPTER 11 SPECIFIC INTERVENTION TECHNIQUES

Past Tense. The SLP can use a few high-usage irregular past tense verbs, such as *ate*, *drank*, *ran*, *fell*, *sat*, *came*, and *went*, to introduce the past rather quickly and to forestall overgeneralization of the regular past *-ed* when introduced. With both past tense forms, storytelling, show-and-tell, and recounting past events are good vehicles for teaching and use.

Initially, the adult can ask the child a question such as "What did you eat (or other action verb)?" to teach the child the form. When the child responds with "Cookie" or another entity, the adult can reply, "What did you do with the cookie?"

Later, the sequence can begin with the question, "What did you do?" The child responds, "Ate cookie" or "I ate a cookie." It is important that question cues not violate pragmatic contingency, which requires that questions make sense. When possible, adults should not ask questions to which they already know the answers. This strategy is achieved easily by asking about unobserved actions or having a puppet ask questions.

Content plays a role in generalization and treatment efficacy. Although it may seem counterintuitive, at least one study suggests that SLPs select more difficult verbs for intervention for regular past tense *-ed* with late preschool and early school-age children (Owen Van Horne et al., 2018). Intervention using more difficult verbs resulted in children showing greater gains in follow-up testing and in conversational use.

Difficult verbs are considered those that do not have a definite end, are lower frequency, and phonologically complex. Verbs that are ongoing or incomplete include *rest*, *work*, *listen*, and *walk* as opposed to those with a definite end point, such as *cross*, *jump*, *close*, *answer*, and *sneeze*. Infrequent verbs include *exercise*, *rest*, *imagine*, *snore*, *paint*, and *squish*. More frequently used verbs include *close*, *scare*, *walk*, *close*, *remember*, and *turn*. Lists of both types of verbs are presented in Table 11–15.

Phonologically complex verbs end in obstruents, as in *close*, *slip*, and *imagine*, and in alveolars, as in *close*, *rest*, and *float*. In contrast, verbs ending in continuants, such as *play*, *whistle*, and *answer*, are more phonologically simple to mark with the past *-ed*.

Third Person Singular. Before teaching additional verb forms, the SLP should introduce singular and plural nouns and subjective pronouns because the child will need these for the third person singular present tense *-s* marker and for present tense forms of the verb BE.

The SLP can introduce the third person marker with singular nouns, contrasting "The dog eats" with "The dogs eat." Subjective pronouns can be introduced gradually with such cues as "What does he do every day (all of the time)?" or such fill-ins as "Every day, she (verbs)" or "All of the time, he (verbs)."

Table 11–15. Easy and Difficult Words to Use With Past Tense *-ed*

Easy: Actions With a Definite End	Difficult: Actions of Longer Duration
Close, cover, drop, dump, jump over, kick, knock, open, pop, scare	Brush, carry, chase, crawl, dance, hop, play, pull, push, rake

Source: Information from Leonard et al. (2007).

For preschool children, production of the third person singular *-s* is influenced by both utterance length and location within the utterance. In short, children with TDL make fewer errors in short utterances and when the third person marking is at the end of the sentence versus the utterance-medial position (Mealings & Demuth, 2014). In addition, 2-year-olds produce the third person singular *-s* markers more accurately in simple phonological vowel-ending words versus cluster-ending ones (*sees* versus *jumps*) (Sundara et al., 2011; Theodore et al., 2011).

Although children hear the third-person singular *-s* in sentence-medial position in conversation five times more frequently, they still selectively attend to the third person marker in sentence-final position. This suggests that the final position is more salient and should be where we place the third person marker when teaching. Perceptual factors also play an important role (Sundara et al., 2011). SLPs need to do everything possible to help a child note the third person marker.

Targeting of third person *-s* or the *is* form of BE in a focused stimulation story followed by a play period in which the SLP recasts the child's sentences containing the target result in significant gains in learning (Leonard et al., 2004, 2006). In a variation, the SLP can act out the story with toys as she tells it. Children generalize this learning to nontargeted forms.

Phonological Variations of Morphological Verb Endings.
Five-year-old children with TDL are still learning to generalize third person *-s* and regular past tense *-ed* to novel verbs. Low-frequency suffixes such as /əz/ (*kisses*) and /əd/ (*glided*) are challenging, especially for children with DLD (Tomas et al., 2017). These data suggest beginning teaching of third person and past tense markers with the /s, z/ and /t, d/ forms.

Initially, an SLP need not target the phonological variations. When the marker is first being emphasized in teaching, the SLP can use one form exclusively, such as the /d/ or the /s/. As the emphasis on the marker becomes more natural or lessens, its cognate /t, z/ can be introduced without any fanfare.

Be careful when talking with a child about morphological change. It's not the "D" or "S" sound being added but /d/ and /s/. Saying that "we add a 'D' . . . " may help spelling but is incorrect for speech.

The SLP should not expect a child to understand the phonological rules relative to ending sounds and added markers. Usually, de-emphasis of the marker's sound will allow the child to naturally produce either two voiced or two unvoiced sounds at the end of each word.

As noted previously, the /əd/ and /əz/ markers should be avoided until later. Children developing typically usually employ the cognates (/s-z, t-d/) by late preschool. It takes them a few more years to acquire the /əd/ and /əz/ forms.

Special Case of the Verb BE.
The verb BE is difficult to learn because of the many forms for various persons and tenses (*am, is, are, was, were*). These different forms should be introduced slowly.

The verb BE can be a main verb or an auxiliary verb, has multiple variations, and is used very frequently. For all these reasons, I suggest targeting BE in the form of

Noun + BE + *X*

The *X* can be just about anything—a noun, verb (*-ing*), adjective, adverb or prepositional phrase. BE as an auxiliary verb and copula can be taught together, thus facilitating carryover.

Use of pronouns and past tense by the child enables the SLP to teach different forms of the verb BE. This does not preclude earlier targeting of *is*, the most common form, with singular nouns. An SLP can contrast singular and plural nouns with *is/are*.

Children developing typically generally learn the *is* form first. As a rule, the uncontracted form is taught first to emphasize BE, as in "The dog is sleeping." Further emphasis can be added by a shortened repetition, placing BE in the final position as in

The dog is sleeping. He really **is**.

Teaching of the contracted form of *is*, as in "The dog's sleeping," can follow. Later, contrast *is* with one variation, such as *are*, then a second. An SLP should not attempt all variations at once.

Two thoughts:

- Auxiliary BE should not be attempted before a child has mastered the progressive *-ing* verb ending. Otherwise, learning the auxiliary BE doesn't serve the progressive verb form and learning it makes little sense.

- The distinction between singular and plural nouns is relatively simple and will be needed for *is* and *are*. The third person pronouns that can take the place of the nouns are more difficult and will need to be considered before you apply *is* and *are* to pronouns.

It's always wise not to introduce too many new targets at once. Intervention should be systematic and sequential.

The auxiliary BE (*He is eating*) is difficult for children with TDL, and mastery can take several years during preschool. One reason is that there are so many variations: *am, is, are, was, were*. A second factor may be inconsistent use by adults. In sentences involving a nonfinite subject–verb sequence in a subordinate clause, such as *The dad sees the boy eating*, and in elliptical responses, as in "Eating" in response to "What are you doing?" there is no auxiliary verb. As an SLP, you'll need to be mindful of your own use of the auxiliary BE.

In toy talk, mentioned previously, parents are encouraged to use a *Noun + is + X* format when talking about toys. With instruction, parents can increase their use of full *is* declaratives, thus providing good models for the verb BE. Diverse noun or noun phrase use by parents and children along with full *is* declaratives by parents are significant predictors of children's use of BE in sentences, suggesting a teaching format for BE (Hadley et al., 2017).

Auxiliary verb learning among children with DLD can be enhanced using an intervention model in which auxiliary BE appears next to the main verb. In one well-designed study, the authors successfully used a story retell model and sentence recasts to attain this proximity (Fey et al., 2017). Questions were of a yes/no variety in which the SLP made a statement followed by questions such as "Is that correct?" in which BE is the main verb. This is in contrast to "Is he eating a cookie?" in which the auxiliary verb is separated from the main verb.

Auxiliary Verbs. Omissions or errors with auxiliary verbs may, in part, be influenced by the way auxiliary verbs are treated in adult speech. For example, in the question, "Was mommy eating?" the auxiliary verb is separated from the main verb, resulting in a child hearing *mommy* and *eating* together. A similar effect may be operating when tense and person markers are moved from the main verb to the auxiliary verb (i.e., "She walks" and "Does she walk?") or omitted as in "Can she walk?"

Auxiliary verbs, such as *do*, can be introduced to facilitate the development of more mature negatives and interrogatives. For example, the negative form of *do* can be elicited with "Let's play school. Remember to tell me (some other person) not to (verb)."

Guidelines for teaching *can*, *do,* and *will/would* include the following:

- Allow some delay between mastery of one form and introduction of another in order to avoid confusion.
- Use self-reference in the form of either first person pronouns or the child's name initially because this is the first referent associated with these forms.
- Link these forms with actions because this is the first association of children developing normally.
- Initially, use short utterances with the word at the end in order to increase saliency ("Can you jump?" "Yes, I can"). Use the popular Bob the Builder refrain "Can we do it?" "Yes, we can."
- Provide meaningful situations in which the concepts and forms serve some purpose.

Children with DLD have particular difficulty with verbs, verb endings, tenses, and verb phrases. These children are more likely to use an auxiliary verb if it is included in the preceding sentence, but both the form and the location must be considered (Leonard et al., 2002).

Although the exact form of the verb does not need to be in the preceding sentence, some forms do facilitate others. For example, use of *are* facilitates *is*. The sentence-final position (*Yes, we can*) also facilitates learning, but the sentence-initial position as in questions (*Can we do it?*) does not (Fey & Frome Loeb, 2002).

After teaching other auxiliary verbs, the SLP can gradually introduce modal auxiliaries. These are helping verbs that express mood or feeling, such as *could*, *would*, *should*, *might*, and *may*. The shades of meaning across the various modal auxiliaries are often very subtle, and the adult should not expect mature usage for some time.

Future Tense. With the addition of the future tense, a child can discuss the past, present (progressive), and future. Language activities, such as baking cookies, can now include planning (*will mix*), execution (*am mixing*), and review (*mixed*).

Using the present progressive form *be* + *going*, the child can begin to form early future tense forms. Adults should be willing to accept this form because it marks the concept even though less mature than *will*.

Teaching should begin with *going to noun*, as in "going to the zoo," before *going to verb*, as in "going to eat." The former is more concrete and does not require use of an

CHAPTER 11 SPECIFIC INTERVENTION TECHNIQUES

infinitive phrase, such as *to eat*. The more mature *will* form of the future tense can be introduced later.

Verb Particles. Finally, the SLP may wish to target verb particles, which are multi-word units, such as *pick up* and *come over*, that function as verbs. Although verb particles emerge in early preschool years, they are not fully acquired and differentiated from prepositions until age 5 years.

The particle—*up*, *down*, *in*, *on*, *off*—may either precede or follow a noun phrase, as in *kick over the pumpkin* or *kick the pumpkin over*. The same words used as prepositions always precede noun phrases. The acquisition of verb particles is especially difficult for children with language disorder, possibly because they are unstressed units and may appear in either position vis-à-vis the noun phrase.

Particles should be introduced with a limited set of verbs used regularly by the child. It might be helpful to use position cues to teach the distinction between particles and prepositions. Particles could be taught following the noun phrase and prepositions preceding. Particles preceding the noun phrase could be introduced later.

Pronouns

Pronouns are extremely difficult to learn because the user must have syntactic, semantic, and pragmatic knowledge. In general, an SLP should teach the underlying concept first and should model appropriate use for the child. Use of pronouns requires an understanding of the semantic distinctions of number, person, and case. The noun in the sentence generally determines use, but the conversational context is also a determinant.

Children often avoid making an overt pronominal error by overusing nouns. This mistake can be avoided somewhat if the SLP limits the number of referents, thus reducing the difficulty of the task. For example, if the SLP uses too many characters in a story format, the child may overuse nouns in an attempt to remember who is being discussed. Using nouns may also help children who have memory challenges.

In general, the first person *I* should be taught before the second person *you*, followed by the third person *he/she/it*. This developmental order reflects increasing complexity with shifting reference and the number of possible referents.

Deictic terms, such as *I* and *you*, are difficult to teach. A second SLP, adult, or child can serve as a model to avoid confusing the child's frame of reference.

Development by typical children suggests that adults target subjective pronouns (*I, you, he, she, it, we, they*) before objective pronouns (*me, you, him, her, it, us, them*). Possessive pronouns would follow (*my, your, his, her, its, our, their*) and, finally, reflexive pronouns (*myself, yourself, himself, herself, itself, ourselves, yourselves, themselves*). Although there are exceptions to this hierarchy, it approximates typical development.

Subjective and objective case can be taught by location in the sentence. Similarly, possessive pronouns always precede nouns.

This hierarchy and the error patterns of young children suggest that reflexives might be taught initially as possessives (*myself*). The exceptions (*himself* and *themselves*) can be introduced later.

One exception to this suggested hierarchy might be third person singular pronouns. It appears easier for children to learn *her–hers–herself* than *him–his–himself* because of the consistency in the feminine gender. The three feminine pronouns might be taught as a unit before the masculine.

Conversational teaching with so many varied forms can be very confusing. Initially, the adult must target carefully the desired pronouns and practice cues to elicit these forms.

Pronouns can be taught in any context in which an object, toy, doll, action figure, character, or the child does something repeatedly, as in play or a narrative. After something or someone has been introduced, we use pronouns on repeat mention. For example, while telling a story from a book, a child might point and say, "He's running" or "They want to eat."

While directing play, a child may say,

> You be the boy and I be the girl. And this bes your fairy. He jump and he follow you everywhere. Now you both go sleep.

When pronouns are not used, they can be prompted or modeled for the child. For example,

> *Child:* And this bes your fairy. Fairy jump and fairy follow you everywhere.
>
> *SLP:* He does. He jumps and he follows me everywhere. What else?

Plural Nouns

To learn plurals, the child must have the concepts of *one* and *more than one*. Numbers or words such as *many* and *more* may serve as initial aids. Begin with comparisons of one item versus many. Cue with "Show me (touch block) more," then respond, "Yes, more blocks!"

Even something as seemingly simple as learning and producing the plural *-s* is affected by prosodic and articulatory factors that can complicate intervention. For example, among 2-year-olds, plural *–s* is easier to produce in the utterance-final than in utterance-medial position. Thus, the plural *-s* in *Give a cookie to the boys* (final) is easier than *Give the boys a cookie* (medial).

In addition, utterance-medial plurals are more articulatory complex if followed by a stop consonant, as in *cats bite*, than if followed by a vowel, as in *cats eat*. This seemingly easy articulatory context is not found when the following word has more than one syllable, as in *cats enjoy* (Theodore et al., 2015).

As with the past-tense *-ed* and third person *-s*, the adult should not expect mastery of the phonological rules until later. Again, teaching should begin with either the /s/ or the /z/, gradually introduce the other, and wait some time before introducing /əz/.

The SLP may wish to introduce a few common irregular plurals (*men*, *feet*) to avoid overgeneralization of plural *-s*. As mentioned in the semantics section of this chapter, words such as *water* and *sand* are not irregular plurals and present a special case, especially with the modifiers *many* and *much*.

CHAPTER 11 SPECIFIC INTERVENTION TECHNIQUES

481

Because so many toys have parts, play is almost a natural for teaching plurals. Use a key word such as *many* or *more* to signal the child to use the plural marker. Once a child is responding correctly with *many* or *more*, expand into more quantity words or counting. Use replica play of a birthday party or grocery shopping to elicit plurals. At birthday parties, there can be balloons, favors, treats, cookies, presents, cards, and games. Teaching of plurals lends itself nicely to a top-down approach.

Articles

Articles are extremely difficult for children to learn because of the two different operations they perform. Articles may mark definite (*the*) and indefinite (*a*) reference and also new (*a*) and old (*the*) information. When in doubt, preschool and early elementary school children tend to overuse *the*.

Articles and adjectives are acquired gradually along with development of the noun phrase (Kemp et al., 2005). Pragmatic reference (new/old) may be more difficult than the definite/indefinite distinction. Late preschool and early school-age children tend to use different articles with specific words, suggesting that individual words may influence use. For example, a child may use *the white kittie* but not *the white snow*. This suggests going slowly at first.

An SLP can use objects and pictures in play or books and instruct the child to describe what is seen ("A puppy"). Next, the SLP and the child can describe each object or picture, as in the following exchange:

Adult: What do you see?

Child: A duck. (New information)

Adult: A duck? Let's see. You're right. I can tell you that the duck (Old information) is yellow. What can you tell me?

Child: The duck is swimming.

Adult: Yeah, the duck is swimming. What else do you see?

The article *an* should not be introduced until a child is functioning at the early elementary school level.

Once pronouns have been introduced, the adult can switch back and forth between pronouns and articles, as in the following:

Adult: Here's a puppy. What can you tell me about him?

Child: He has a cold nose.

Adult: Who does?

Child: The puppy.

The possibilities are endless within a conversational paradigm. Remember that many Asian languages don't have articles, so this feature may be especially difficult for some ELL East Asian children.

Prepositions

Although nine prepositions (*at*, *by*, *for*, *from*, *in*, *of*, *on*, *to*, and *with*) account for 90% of preposition use, these nine have a combined total of approximately 250 meanings! No wonder some children with language disorders have difficulty with this class of words. ELLs will find prepositions especially difficult. Prepositions were discussed briefly in the semantics section. Here's more.

Development of prepositions suggests the following hierarchy of teaching:

in, on, inside, out of, under, next to

between, around, beside, in front of

in back of, behind

One promising strategy for teaching locational prepositions is to use contrasting states (Hicks et al., 2015). Many locational propositions are mutually exclusive. For example, an item can be *in* or *on* another object but not both at once. Some locational prepositions, such as *next to*, are less exclusive and may overlap with other prepositions, making them more difficult to learn.

More restricted prepositions can be taught within an "*X*–Not *X*" model, such as "In–Not in." An object cannot be *in* and *not in* at the same time. The contrast sharpens the meaning for the child. It's probably best to begin with a small group of items and locations and then to add more as a child grasps the concept.

In general, children will learn more easily when real objects are used in teaching. Spatial and directional aspects of prepositions should be taught with a number of objects and/or examples so that a child understands the concept separately from any specific referent. Variety may preclude the child's focusing on the objects and referents rather than on the relationship.

Large muscle activities also can be used as children go in and out of boxes or closets, on and off tables and chairs, and the like. Thus, the child's body becomes a referent and it's fun. Spatial terms may be taught in a naturalistic context of play with puppets, dolls, action figures, or the child's body. In one lesson, I played the tiger who pursued a preschool child into the cage ("The girl went **in**. And the tiger went **in**"), out of the cage, and so on.

> ***Food for Thought:*** Are some aspects of syntax daunting? You're not alone. As an SLP, you'll need to continue to learn and to manipulate different aspects of language on a daily basis.

Word Order and Sentence Types

Typical learners begin to produce two-clause or more sentences at age 2 years. By age 3 years, they are producing conjoined sentences and subordinate or dependent clauses.

CHAPTER 11 SPECIFIC INTERVENTION TECHNIQUES

This suggests that SLPs should target sentence elaboration early in a child's life. Word order and different sentence types are best taught within conversational give-and-take, although school-age children and adolescents also may benefit from both oral and written teaching.

Miniature linguistic systems have been used in initial teaching of word combinations. In these systems, a matrix is developed with one class of words on each axis. A child need not learn all possible combinations to acquire the rule. Good generalization to untrained combinations has been reported. Figure 11–4 presents some sample matrices and the teaching models that have been effective. A matrix can be used to tell a narrative or to direct play.

There are three basic ways to make sentences more complex:

- Noun phrase elaboration
- Verb phrase elaboration
- Conjoined and embedded clauses

Although we probably differ in the particulars, I can agree with Dr. Alan Kamhi's (2014) advice when teaching syntax to focus on meanings (semantics) and intentions (pragmatics) and then how to convey these by language form (morphosyntax) rather than just focusing on the structure or form itself. This is the essence of a functional approach.

Difficulties with syntax rarely occur alone. Most children struggling with grammar also have difficulties in other areas of language and literacy. Therefore, language can be taught in the service of daily tasks rather than in isolated drills. Sometimes called **contextualized language intervention**, this approach—often limited to literacy intervention—provides a therapeutic focus within a purposeful and meaningful activity and across activities (Ukrainetz, 2006).

Figure 11–4. Miniature linguistic systems.

	Cookie	Cake	Pudding	Pie	Bread
Eat	X	X	X	X	X
Bake	X				
Mix	X				
Want	X				
Give	X				

	Pet	Dog	Cat	Horse	Ferret
Feed	X	X			
Bathe		X	X		
Groom			X	X	
Walk				X	X
Brush	X				X

Verbs on one axis are combined with nouns on the other to form short phrases. Each combination taught is marked with an X. Rule learning will generalize to the untrained combination.

I set up verbal and nonverbal contexts in which a certain structure is needed and teach within that context. Kamhi focuses more on the linguistic function—for example, embedded clauses as the object in a sentence, as in *I hope **I get a bike for my birthday***. One purpose of this syntactic structure is to help the child discuss mental state verbs, such as *know*, *think*, *remember*, *wish*, and *forget*. In a second example, when teaching of conjoined clauses, as in *I ate lunch and then played on the playground,* the SLP could focus on the meaning of the coordinating conjunctions and how they can be used.

Noun Phrase Elaboration

Noun phrases initially can be expanded in isolation. A question–answer paradigm will enable an SLP to target specific aspects of the noun phrase (How many . . . ? Where . . . ? Can you tell me . . . ? Which one . . . ?).

Once placed within short sentences, the noun phrase can be expanded in the object position, followed by the subject position. Early expansion rarely goes beyond two elements, as in *a kittie* or *big horse*. The order of noun modifiers was discussed in Chapter 7 under analysis of the noun phrase (see Table 7–23).

It's worth recalling from the discussion of articles that children initially use both articles and adjectives with specific words, suggesting that individual words may influence use. To me, this means three things:

- Acquisition is gradual and intervention should be also.
- Contrastive teaching makes sense—for example, *the **white** kittie, the **brown** doggie*.
- Generalization won't just happen; it must be planned for.

Adjectives can be taught in contrastive situations in which the child must distinguish between two objects that differ along one parameter, as in *big ball* and *little ball*. Incorrect or inadequate adjective use in conversation would result in misunderstanding and the misinterpretation of the child's message, leading to some fun possibilities. Similarly, post-noun modifiers can be used with objects in different locations, as in *the ball in the box* and *the ball on the table*.

Verb Phrase Elaboration

Verb phrases and accompanying clause types should be chosen carefully. Specific verbs that clearly illustrate transitive and intransitive clauses might be chosen. Equitive verb phrases and the use of BE can be taught in elliptical answers to questions, as in *He is* and *We are* responses to questions such as "Who is going to the zoo?"

A similar method of teaching transitive and intransitive verbs can be used to teach auxiliary verbs, as in "Who should eat?" and "Who can jump?" The responses "We should" and "He can" place the auxiliary verb in the very salient final position in the sentence.

In acquiring new verbs, both 2-year-old children with TDL and those who are late talkers initially benefit more from hearing the word in consistent linguistic contexts than in varied ones (Horvath & Arunachalam, 2021). Children who are late talkers seem to benefit even more. It's possible that a consistent linguistic context provides both the verb meaning and information on its meaning and part of speech.

Infinitive phrases can be taught within play situations with dolls, puppets, or action figures or within storybook reading (Eisenberg, 2005). Of the two types of infinitives, noun–verb–to-verb (*Oscar wants to eat*) and noun–verb–noun–to-verb (*Oscar wants Ernie to eat*), the former is easier to learn and develops first. Early developing and frequently used verbs that take an infinitive complement in the N–V–to-V form include *want*, *like*, and *try*. A possible format for teaching is presented in Table 11–16.

Conjoined and Embedded Clauses

Using both oral and written techniques, an SLP can aid school-age children and adolescents to

- form longer sentences and more concise sentences; and
- use more low-frequency structures and intersentential cohesion.

Compound and complex sentences can be formed from a child's own simpler sentences.

Subordinate clauses, as in *The girl **who is driving the red car** from Iowa*, can be transformed later into more concise phrases, such as *The girl **driving the red car** is from Iowa*. Low-frequency structures, such as apposition (*Mary **my sister** is . . .* or *John **the psychologist** will . . .*), complex noun phrases (*the large red dog with the bushy tail* or *teachers such as Ms. Meeker or Ms. Lilius*), perfect aspect (*has been singing*), and passive voice (*The cat was chased by the dog*) can be targeted later. Finally, intersentential cohesion can be attempted by using adverbial conjuncts such as *therefore* and *however*. Acquisition is often very gradual. Less common types, such as *conversely* and *moreover*, should be introduced only to mature language users.

Several strategies discussed in Chapter 10 can be used very effectively to strengthen word order. For example, expansion can provide a more mature model than a child's utterance, and recasts can help the child analyze relationships.

Table 7–25 presents some guidelines on the acquisitional order of certain sentence types. By the time most children with TDL begin school, they are using adultlike declaratives, imperatives, and *wh-* and *yes/no* interrogatives in both the positive and negative forms.

Research has demonstrated that after hearing a particular syntactic structure, a child is more likely to produce the same sentence structure in their subsequent speech. This is referred to as syntactic or **structural priming**. Structural priming has been reported to aid in learning a variety of syntactic strictures (Bock et al., 2007; Messenger et al., 2012; Scheepers, 2003).

It's possible in structural priming that an abstract representation of the underlying syntactic form of an utterance remains active in memory for a short time after it's heard. This sentence pattern can then be quickly retrieved and used by the listener to create another sentence. In other words, a primed structure is more likely to be retrieved and

486 LANGUAGE DISORDERS: A FUNCTIONAL APPROACH TO ASSESSMENT AND INTERVENTION IN CHILDREN

Table 11–16. Top-Down Model of Intervention With Infinitives

Target Response	Adult Cues	Verbal Prompts in Order of Increasing Input*
N–V–to-V		
Want to	Nonverbal Playing house. Ernie stumbles around.	Verbal *Ernie says to Elmo, "I'm very tired. Can I sit?" You finish the story. Ernie wants . . . ?* *Ernie wants **to** . . .* *Does Ernie want **to eat**? No. What does Ernie want?* *Ernie doesn't want **to eat**. Ernie wants . . . ?* *Ernie doesn't want to eat. Ernie wants to . . . ?* *Ernie wants **to sit**. What does Ernie want?*
Like to	Nonverbal Playing with tools. Elmo wants the hammer.*	Verbal *Elmo says to Oscar, "I will hammer. That is my favorite thing to do. Elmo likes . . . ?* *Elmo likes **to** . . .* *Does Elmo like **to saw**? No. What does Elmo like?* *Elmo doesn't like **to saw**. Elmo likes . . . ?* *Elmo doesn't like **to saw**. Elmo likes to . . . ?* *Elmo likes **to hammer**. What does Elmo like?*
Try to	Nonverbal Playing eating. Cookie Monster wants to jump over the table.	Verbal *Cookie Monster says, "I will jump over the table." Cookie tries . . . ?* *Cookie tries **to** . . .* *Does Cookie try **to run**? No. What does Cookie try?* *Cookie doesn't try **to run**. Cookie tries . . . ?* *Cookie doesn't try **to run**. Cookie tries to . . . ?* *Cookie tries **to jump**. What does Cookie try?*
N–V–N–to-V		
Want N to	Nonverbal Play eating. Elmo won't eat.	Verbal *Ernie says to Elmo, "Eat your food." You finish the story. Ernie wants Elmo . . . ?* *Ernie wants Elmo **to** . . . ?* *Does Ernie want Elmo **to jump**? No. What does Ernie want?* *Ernie doesn't want Elmo **to jump**. Ernie wants Elmo . . . ?* *Ernie doesn't want Elmo **to jump**. Ernie wants Elmo to . . . ?* *Ernie wants Elmo **to eat**. What does Ernie want?*

CHAPTER 11 SPECIFIC INTERVENTION TECHNIQUES

Table 11–16. *continued*

Target Response	Adult Cues	Verbal Prompts in Order of Increasing Input*
Tell N to	Nonverbal Ernie is frightened by a big dog.	Verbal *Bert says to Ernie, "Let's run!" You finish the story.* *Bert tells Ernie . . . ?* *Bert tells Ernie to . . . ?* *Does Bert tell Ernie to sleep? No. What does Bert tell Ernie?* *Bert doesn't tell Ernie to sleep. Bert tells Ernie . . . ?* *Bert doesn't tell Ernie to sleep. Bert tells Ernie to . . . ?* *Bert tells Ernie to eat. What does Bert tell Ernie?* *Bert tells Ernie to run. What does Bert tell Ernie?*

Note: *The SLP provides more input only if needed by the child to be successful.
Source: Information from Eisenberg (2005).

then modified to create a new utterance because it was the most recently activated structure. Although priming can affect a variety of sentence structures, children with DLD perform more poorly, suggesting a deficit in implicit learning mechanisms (Evans et al., 2009; Hsu & Bishop, 2014; Tomblin et al., 2007).

A second strategy, called **focused recasting**, has also been used to improve learning of some syntactic structures. In focused recasting, a child's utterance is restructured to maintain its meaning while increasing its grammatical accuracy or modifying its structure. The recast utterance is modeled for the child. A systematic review suggested that recasting is an effective technique for increasing language ability in children (Cleave et al., 2015). Recasting in a conversational context is reportedly more effective than imitation by the child (Nelson et al., 1996).

Structural priming combined with a focused recasting procedure have been used successfully in intervention for subject- and object-focused relative clauses with both students with DLD and those with TDL (Wada et al., 2020). It appears that combining priming, an implicit procedure, with recasting, an explicit procedure, creates a more robust learning environment than the use of either technique separately.

Sentences can be primed and elicited using pictures. The child is shown a picture while the SLP verbally models the target syntactic structure. The child is then shown a second picture that depicts a related action and is asked to create a sentence that "sounds like" the previous sentence for the previous picture. If the child produces a sentence that contains the target structure, the SLP can repeat the child's sentence. If the child's utterance does not contain the target, the SLP can recast the child's sentence to include the target syntactic structure (Wada et al., 2020).

Children with DLD have difficulty learning and using complex sentences in both spoken and written language, with particular difficulty using relative clauses (Frizelle & Fletcher, 2014a, 2014b; Garraffa et al., 2012; Hesketh, 2006; Nippold et al., 2008; Novogrodsky & Friedmann, 2006; Scott, 2014; Zwitserlood et al., 2015). A relative clause is a subordinate clause found in the post-noun (noun-following) position.

Relative Clauses. In young children with TDL, the earliest relative clauses appear attached to isolated noun phrases, such as *The dog **who followed us***, and noun phrases introduced with phrases, such as *here is* or *there is* as in *Here's the toys **we can play with***. In general, these sentences express a single proposition and can be restated as a simple sentence. Thus, *The dog who followed us* can become *The dog followed us*.

Later developing relative clauses are most commonly attached to the direct object, such as *You saw the dog **I petted*** (Diessel & Tomasello, 2000, 2005). These sentences contain two propositions (*you saw* and *I petted*). Because noun phrases can occur in both the subject and object positions in a sentence, relative clauses can also.

We're safe in saying that the term *relative clause* represents a family of constructions that vary in difficulty. In general, children with DLD are significantly delayed in their ability to repeat all types of relative clause constructions (Frizelle & Fletcher, 2014a, 2014b, 2015). These children may lack the underlying syntactic representations or templates in their memory. The less syntactic knowledge a child has, the more they must rely on working memory (WM).

In general, children with DLD are more accurate with relative clauses attached to the subject (The dog *I like* is brown) than attached to the object (We bought the dog *I like*) (Adani et al., 2014). In addition, children have greater accuracy for sentences with dissimilar number features (i.e., one singular, one plural) on the noun and the embedded relative clause. For example, in "I liked *the cookie* that had *lots of chips*," cookie is singular and chips is plural.

Children with DLD perform best on subject relative clauses with intransitive verbs, as in *The girl **who walks to school** sits by me*. You may recall that intransitive verbs, such as *walk*, *stand*, *look*, *sleep*, and *stay*, do not take a direct object. More difficult are subject relative clauses with a transitive verb, such as *The girl **who picks up the papers** went home early*, and object and indirect object relative clauses, such as *My sister ate all the cookies **that mommy made*** and *I gave flowers to my teacher who teaches art*, respectively (Frizelle & Fletcher, 2014b). In general, the late-appearing relative clause types reflect the more difficult syntax and infrequent exposure of children to these forms.

These data suggest that an SLP initially confine intervention with children with DLD to subject relative clauses to reduce memory load. An SLP can reduce the length of the more difficult types of relative clause embedding. Given the relative ineffectiveness of targeting WM directly (Melby-Lervåg & Hulme, 2013), it is probably best to focus specifically on the syntactic structures involved.

Children With CLD Backgrounds

Contrary to popular belief, children with language disorders are perfectly capable, with appropriate support, of learning two languages (Paradis et al., 2003). Of course, the process will be less efficient than for ELLs with TDL. In addition, there is every reason to believe that children with language disorders are at greater risk for rapid regression or loss of their heritage language if it is not supported (Restrepo & Kruth, 2000; Salameh et al., 2004).

Although bilingual approaches have been found to be at least as effective as English-only approaches in regular education (Rolstad et al., 2005), there is a lingering fear among some professionals that intervention using a child's heritage language contributes to confusion or delays in development of English.

For children who are ELLs with language disorders, intervention in both home and school languages and support of both have been shown to have positive effects (Goodrich et al., 2013; Gorman, 2012; Lugo-Neris et al., 2010; Paradis et al., 2011; Pham et al., 2011; Restrepo et al., 2013; Riquelme & Rosas, 2014; Rosa-Lugo et al., 2012). Although optimal, intervention in both English and the heritage language is not always feasible, especially if the SLP does not speak the heritage language. However, a review of 18 studies on the effects of heritage language instruction on treatment outcomes for individuals with neurodevelopmental disorders concluded that there is a small effect favoring interventions delivered in both languages versus interventions delivered solely in the majority language (Lim et al., 2019).

Although bilingual language intervention would seem appropriate for many reasons, only a small percentage of SLPs in the United States are proficient in other languages (ASHA, 2013). In addition, very few SLPs speak many of the languages present in the United States, such as Hmong, Somali, and Karen. Thus, the vast majority of ELL U.S. children with language disorders receive services solely in English (ASHA, 2009, 2010).

Whenever possible, the SLP can refer to words or sentence forms in the heritage language. The SLP can learn relevant vocabulary and short phrases prior to an intervention session. Much of this information is available on translation websites.

With a little preparation, you as an SLP will be able to relate the learning objective in English to a word or structure in the child's first language. Teachers can do the same, especially if all ELLs in a class speak the same first language.

To support both languages at home, the SLP can add a home component to a child's intervention program. Family members can also be helped to craft conversations that incorporate both languages.

There is a growing body of research suggesting a bilingual approach to working with children with a variety of communication impairments (Gutierrez-Clellen et al., 2008; Hand, 2011; Kay-Raining Bird et al., 2005; Kay-Raining Bird & Trudeau, 2009; Paradis, 2007; Paradis et al., 2003). Although research findings from several studies suggest bilingualism does not have a negative effect on language development for children with ASD (Hambly & Fombonne, 2012; Ohashi et al., 2012; Yu, 2013), SLPs and other professionals predominantly advise parents against providing a bilingual environment (Drysdale et al., 2015). Discouraging families from using both languages at home can significantly impact interaction dynamics by decreasing the opportunities for communication and language learning (Soto & Yu, 2014).

Although SLPs may be focused on English with children who are ELLs, maintaining the heritage language is frequently as important for the family and community. Continued development of the heritage language depends on rich and frequent exposure and opportunities for practice, which usually occur in the home (Pham & Tipton, 2018).

Families differ in the amount of each language's use in the home. An SLP will need to design individualized intervention programs. Any bilingual approach will need to start with an accurate assessment of the child's communicative ability and the family's communication style and preferences. Close collaboration and cooperation are essential.

It is crucial that English-only SLPs collaborate with bilingual SLPs and colleagues, interpreters, and families to design and implement intervention programs that promote development of a child's heritage language alongside English. Collaboration might include

- team approaches;
- use of interpreters and family members;
- use of bilingual classroom teachers; and
- incorporation of technology or computer software.

The SLP can use a computer interface and prerecorded audio files in both the heritage language and English to teach vocabulary (Pham et al., 2011). Such a bilingual approach has the advantage of being just as effective as English-only approaches for English while having the additional benefit of promoting continued growth in a child's heritage language.

As little as 30 minutes of instruction in Spanish daily is enough to promote Spanish learning among prekindergarten ELLs (Restrepo et al., 2010). Effective programming might target 5 to 10 vocabulary words a week, dialogic book reading, phonemic awareness, and letter knowledge.

Although we have materials for bilingual Spanish–English children, similar tools most likely do not exist in most other languages. For example, *Improving the Vocabulary and Oral Language Skills of Bilingual Latino Preschoolers: An Intervention for Speech-Language Pathologists* (Gutierrez-Clellen et al., 2014) is an evidence-based intervention program in both Spanish and English for young children with language disorders. A monolingual SLP can use the program in collaboration with bilingual teachers or assistants. Lessons in the program manual use preschool books that are readily available commercially in both Spanish and English. Lessons are presented in both languages. Unfortunately, we have nothing similar for Urdu or Somali.

English vocabulary learning of 4- to 6-year-old Spanish–English speakers can be promoted by English vocabulary instruction enhanced with Spanish expansions (Lugo-Neris et al., 2010). Initial proficiency in both languages is important, and children with limited skills in both languages show significantly less vocabulary growth. Spanish expansions of novel vocabulary words during English storybook reading might include providing synonyms of words, using role-playing, and providing meanings or explanations. Over time, a bilingual child's vocabulary knowledge in both languages grows with multiple exposures and contexts. Children can associate additional semantic features with words and begin to recognize how words in English relate to the corresponding words in Spanish and vice versa.

Similarly, intervention with children speaking African American English (AAE) may be bidialectal (Stockman, 2010). African American children with language disorders are

CHAPTER 11 SPECIFIC INTERVENTION TECHNIQUES 491

likely to come to therapy with varying levels of competence in both AAE and the main-stream dialect. Therapy should focus on a child's level of dialect use.

Dialectal issues should influence the SLP's judgments of correctness and appropriate teaching contexts. For example, because the use of the plural *-s* is context sensitive in AAE, an SLP should be alert to the absence of a plural marker on nouns preceded by a quantifier, as in *two shoe*. It's best to first target noncontrastive or nondiffering AAE and majority dialect of American English patterns instead of contrastive or dissimilar patterns. Such a strategy recognizes that African American children with and without language disorders will use contrastive patterns typical of AAE. Language disorders should be most apparent on the noncontrastive patterns.

> ***Food for Thought:*** **Imagine, if only for a moment, the overwhelming task of being thrown into a classroom in which you only comprehend the minimum of what is being asked of you. That's the challenge for children who are ELLs, especially if they have a language disorder.**

Trust is especially important if faculty, staff, and parents from CLD backgrounds are going to act as language teachers. If, as an SLP, you know little of the local culture, you need to be proactive in seeking this information. It is not the child's or parent's responsibility to educate you.

Use of Microcomputers

Microcomputers can enhance language instruction when well integrated into an overall language program in a cohesive manner. The computer can complement—but should never replace—face-to-face learning situations.

Children enjoy using computers. Preschoolers prefer computer-based teaching to traditional therapy drills and desktop activities. Most interventive programs are user-friendly, lowering the threat to children with language disorders.

The goals of intervention and the methodology should be established prior to determining the role of the computer and integrating it into the overall plan. It is easy to fall into the trap of allowing the computer program to determine intervention goals. This *teach-for-the-program* approach is not individualized for each child, nor is it ethical or good practice.

Children with language disorders are best served by computers when both the child and the SLP actively participate, when computer use is individualized, and when software specific to the intervention goal is used. The most effective integration occurs when the SLP or other adult and the child interact around the program being used, commenting and discussing choices offered and the child's selections. In this way, computer programs can be tuned more to the needs of each child. Similarly, software designed to address specific language problems is better than generic, mass-market software. Computers seem especially useful for writing teaching and are discussed in Chapter 13. Possible intervention activities are presented in Table 11–17.

Table 11–17. Examples of Integrating Computer Activities Into Language Intervention

Language Objective	Computer Activity
Giving directions	Write directions for making or baking something.
Sequencing events	Explain how to accomplish a common task such as making a peanut butter and jelly sandwich.
Future tense	Write an announcement explaining what will happen at the Fourth of July celebration or the class party.
Past tense	Write a "news" story about the class trip. Write a narrative about some past event.
Questions	Plan an interview with questions for your favorite musical performer or actor.
Negatives	Compile a list of dos and don'ts for the cafeteria or the school bus.
Syntax	Write a letter inviting someone to your class and in it explain why you want that person to visit.
Summarizing/syntax	Write a synopsis of your favorite movie, TV show, or book.

Prior to using any program, the SLP should ask fundamental questions about its theoretical underpinnings, the design of studies reporting success, and the children who will seem to benefit most from program use. Of special concern for functional communication is the naturalness of the approach, its effect on overall communication, and generalization to real-life situations.

We have mentioned Fast ForWord–Language (FFW-L; Scientific Learning Corporation, 2021), a computer-based program, a few times in various contexts. FFW-L targets children's ability to process information from the speech stream by increasing the ability to rapidly process information. Unfortunately, although some children make substantial gains in language performance, recent studies have found either no treatment-related effects on language test performance or clinically significant gains not related to FFW-L (Cohen et al., 2005; R. Gillam et al., 2008; Pokorni et al., 2004; Rouse & Krueger, 2004).

In a study using FFW-L and narrative-based language intervention, FFW-L did not significantly improve language, nor did it enhance learning of subsequent language material (Fey et al., 2010). FFW-L does seem to improve attention, but the effects on subsequent language learning are not known (Stevens et al., 2008).

Conclusion

Although they cannot always use all elements of the functional model simultaneously, SLPs usually can employ several elements within any given teaching situation. Adults within the environment, everyday activities, and conversational give-and-take usually can be adapted to the individual child and language target(s). Some teaching may neces-

CHAPTER 11 SPECIFIC INTERVENTION TECHNIQUES

sitate the initial use of structured approaches. Generalization to conversational use, however, will require incorporating everyday settings and activities into the teaching.

Even though you may feel overwhelmed by all the recommendations in this and previous intervention chapters, we have discussed only a small percentage of the available intervention techniques. Limited space necessitates a rather cursory examination of these procedures. SLPs can seek further information in source materials, published clinical materials, professional journals, conferences, and online seminars.

In addition, they will conceive their own creative and innovative methods for intervening with children with language disorders. It is hoped that these methods will be adapted to fit the conversational model presented in Chapters 9 and 10.

Not all specific language problems are treated easily with a functional approach, but the entire model does not have to be discarded. For example, teaching can occur in meaningful contexts within everyday events. In Chapter 12, we explore one of those contexts—the classroom.

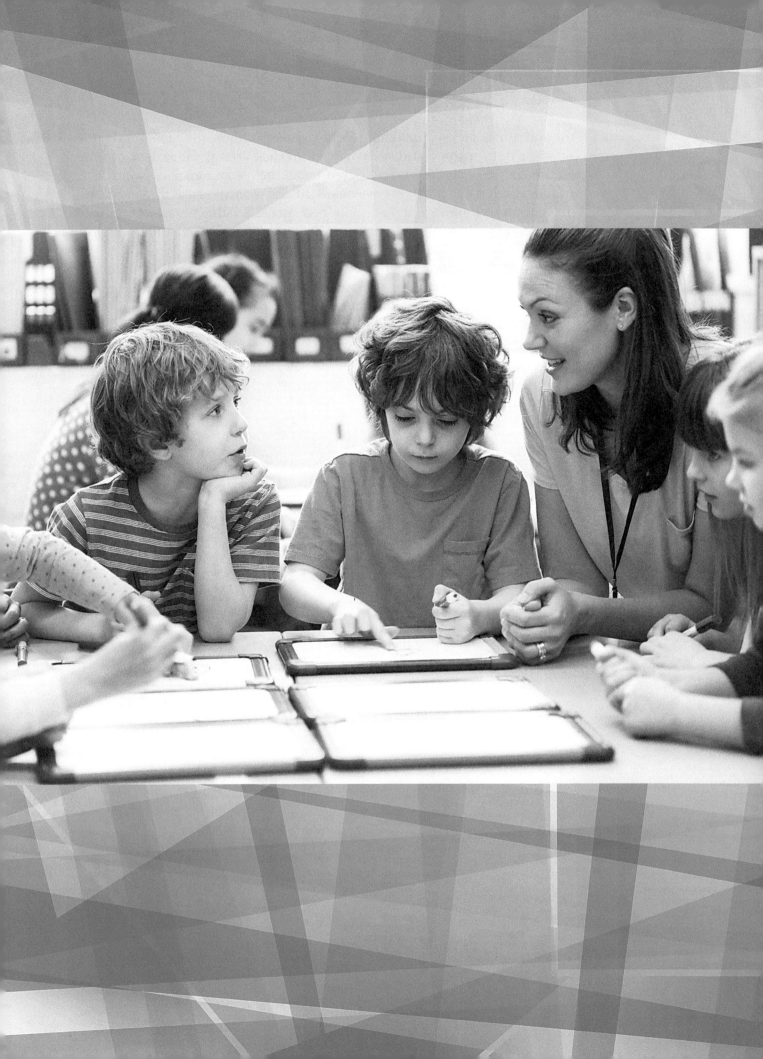

CHAPTER 12

CLASSROOM FUNCTIONAL INTERVENTION

*M*ikie *began to say words at about 13 months and seemed to develop language as a typical toddler and preschooler. His transition to kindergarten was difficult, and he had trouble adjusting to the more rigid instructional methods of school. He had difficulty following directions and carrying assignments through to completion.*

His parents reported even more resistance when he was required to read, write, and do mathematical problems. Even his drawings were minimal, lacking detail seen in his peers' renderings. After repeated complaining about his eyes, Mikie was taken by his parents to an optometrist who found no visual impairment.

As best the reading specialist could determine, Mikie read through a combination of memorization, guessing, and using pictures. By second grade, he was falling seriously behind. Reading comprehension was seriously compromised.

After being referred by both the teacher and the reading specialist to the school-based speech-language practitioner (SLP), Mikie was found to have deficits in several areas of language, including semantics and syntax. His language, whether in spoken or written form, was similar to that of a much younger child. The SLP reported that Mikie had a developmental language disorder characterized by deficits in verbal working memory.

Mikie's classroom teacher and the SLP collaborate on intervention for both oral and written language. In the classroom, the teacher is using visual aides to aid his language production and comprehension.

The SLP is targeting his working memory through functional language tasks within the classroom, such as following an instruction through changing circumstances and recalling increasingly more complex utterances in both print and reading, initially in both forms but now in each separately.

In school, children encounter the language of instruction, which is very different from the child's previous conversational interactions. In school, language is treated in the abstract. Children talk about it and manipulate it. Metalinguistic skills are very important. The child with inadequate language skills or inadequate strategies for making sense of different situations is apt to become lost.

On an oral-to-literate continuum, school tasks are at the extreme literate end, requiring the child to understand and express information displaced from their own experiential base. Language itself creates the context within which information is conveyed.

Although the language of most children with language disorders can be characterized by deficits in language form, many children also exhibit difficulty with vocabulary and discourse skills (Language and Reading Research Consortium, 2015). For example, early weaknesses in vocabulary, grammar, and comprehension and production have been linked to later reading comprehension difficulties (Nation et al., 2010). Discourse is the sequential organization of language beyond the sentence level.

School-age children with undiagnosed deficits in language and/or language processing may have behavioral issues in school (Moncrieff et al., 2018). A compilation of the data from 22 studies found that among children with emotional and behavioral issues, the prevalence of below-average language performance was 81% (Hollo et al., 2014).

Data indicate that throughout preschool and kindergarten, grammar, vocabulary, and use form a single construct. The separation of these three occurs in the first several grades of elementary school (Language and Reading Research Consortium, 2015). In other words, language ability is initially unidimensional but becomes increasingly multidimensional as children move through the primary grades and on to middle school. By third grade, vocabulary, grammar, and spoken and written discourse appear to be emerging as distinct skills.

One possible explanation for this emergent dimensionality is that a hierarchy of language exists, reflected in development from words to sentences to longer discourse (Tomblin & Zhang, 2006). As a dimension becomes consolidated and automatized in use, cognitive resources are freed up that can support more complex processing. The explanation may be as simple as vocabulary is needed for grammar and, similarly, grammar is needed to understand discourse or larger units. More likely, a child's language abilities are changing in response to the increasing demands of literacy and the classroom.

As an SLP, you can support a child's communication efforts in the following ways:

- Socially, by modifying their role and modeling appropriate roles and by creating contexts in which the child can take varying roles
- Emotionally, by preventing ostracism and by aiding the child to resolve conflict and to be tuned to the needs of others
- Functionally, by redesigning contexts when needed by the child and by helping all children achieve their communication goals
- Physically, by arranging the environment for maximum participation
- Communicatively, by providing scripts for participation

The goal is for each child to be successful in the classroom with diminishing adult support.

A functional approach to intervention shifts the focus from the child as the source and solution of the language problem to a holistic view that includes the child and the child's language uses and learning strategies, the contextual demands, the expectations and beliefs of other people within that context, the child's interaction, the context, and the child's communication partners. The classroom's cognitive activities are an excellent context for stimulating language growth. Within the classroom's constructive activities, children create, change, relate, and compare entities; set goals; encounter and try to

CHAPTER 12 CLASSROOM FUNCTIONAL INTERVENTION

overcome problems; make errors; reflect on success or failure; and note problem-solving procedures.

Context, especially in the school, has a significant effect on children's classroom skills, and several contexts should be included in language assessment and intervention with children with language disorders. For example, within a journal-writing activity, a small-group lesson, a peer play session, and sharing time, children with language disorders perform very differently in language productivity and complexity, use of self-monitoring strategies, and turn-taking patterns (Peets, 2009). For example, although there is a wide range, children generally produce the most words and utterances during peer play but speak most rapidly, take longer turns, and have higher type-token ratios during sharing time.

The functional model discussed throughout this text can be adapted to these differing classroom needs. In fact, some of the recent changes in education, such as the Common Core, response to intervention (RTI), inclusion, and collaborative teaching, espouse some of the same principles and goals we've been discussing. In this chapter, we examine these trends and propose some models of classroom intervention. Following that, we describe the new role of the public school SLP and elements of a classroom intervention model, including specific intervention targets for preschool and school-age children. Finally, we discuss implementation of classroom intervention.

Background and Rationale: Recent Educational Changes

Language training within the school classroom offers a special challenge for an SLP and a classroom teacher. School systems throughout the United States and Canada are adopting and modifying many models of intervention to provide more appropriate and effective intervention. These new models reflect recent educational trends.

Common Core State Standards

The Common Core State Standards (CCSS; Common Core, 2010) have been adopted by 43 U.S. states. The CCSS identify critical skills and outline development of these abilities from kindergarten through high school. CCSS further task all individuals working with students, including SLPs, to provide instruction in writing, speaking, listening, and language that helps students be successful. SLPs have important roles in literacy education and in supporting language and literacy for children with language disorders and for those at risk for school failure (American Speech-Language-Hearing Association [ASHA], n.d.).

The following six instructional practices for reading give the SLP a model for intervention (Gersten & Geva, 2003):

- Explicit teaching
- Promotion of English language learning
- Phonemic awareness and decoding
- Vocabulary development

- Interactive teaching that maximizes student engagement
- Instruction that produces accurate responses with feedback for struggling learners

These goals are inherent in CCSS (National Governors Association Center for Best Practices, 2010). In short, CCSS promote learning in all modes of language while supporting all children to succeed in the general curriculum (Justice, 2013; Roth et al., 2013). The role of the SLP in this process is critical.

> *Food for Thought:* Do you get a sense that as an SLP, you'll be expected to know much more than people might expect who view you as "the speech teacher"?

Response to Intervention

Response to intervention (RTI) is a multitiered, problem-solving approach to education that addresses the learning difficulties of all children, not just those with language disorders or other needs, incorporating both prevention and intervention. As such, RTI provides a structure within which educational teams can identify areas of concern and the need to provide appropriate levels of support for struggling children. Jackson et al. (2009) offer an excellent overview of RTI and its implications for early childhood professionals that is worth consulting.

Within the RTI model, SLPs have expanded opportunities to collaborate with teachers and other education professionals. From its beginning in early childhood education, RTI was envisioned as an interdisciplinary team approach within a comprehensive curriculum framework. RTI first appeared with the reauthorization of the Individuals with Disabilities Education Act (IDEA) in 2004. Decisions about when and how to implement RTI are left to individual states and local education agencies.

So far, this discussion seems rather vague, so let's examine RTI principles and how they affect the responsibilities of SLPs. Common principles of RTI include the following (Jackson et al., 2009):

- Many tiers of support for each child, incorporating different levels of instruction
- High-quality instruction from knowledgeable team members who use a variety of instructional approaches, ongoing assessment procedures, and experiences that match the needs of each child, and collaboration among professionals
- An evidence-based core curriculum that is evaluated for effectiveness
- A data collection system, including both formative and summative multiple informational sources, used to evaluate children's performance
- Evidence-based intervention, which uses validated practices across multiple environments to support individualized learning
- Family and professional procedures for identifying, selecting, and revising instructional practices based on child data and the learning context

- Measures to monitor and ensure effective and accurate implementation of instructional strategies and interventions

These characteristics of RTI offer SLPs new dynamics and standards for providing services and supports.

Most positive evidence for the effectiveness of RTI has come from smaller-scale controlled trials. The results from large-scale evaluation are less positive. The Evaluation of Response to Intervention Practices for Elementary School Reading (Balu et al., 2015), a study involving 146 elementary schools, implies that RTI is ineffective. This finding may reflect inappropriate implementation, such as students receiving instruction that is not appropriate for their skill level (Fuchs & Fuchs, 2017; Gersten et al., 2017).

Ensuring progress for all children has to be a collective effort involving families, educational professionals, related services providers, researchers, and legislators. SLPs play a crucial role in collaborating with other professionals and family members in the provision of language- and literacy-based services.

Deciding the most effective and efficient method of providing SLP services is important. According to research, the tiered approach to service delivery in RTI, presented in Figure 12–1, is a worthwhile model (Ebbels et al., 2018). Services become increasingly specialized and individualized as children demonstrate greater needs.

Most children will be in Tier 1 and not generally be in need of direct SLP services. Instead, these children receive any SLP services provided for the entire class, such as a lesson by an SLP on rhyming.

Tier 2 is made up of children with language weaknesses or vulnerabilities who may not be candidates for direct intervention services but can benefit from universal services and interventions by classroom teachers and aides who have been trained by the SLP.

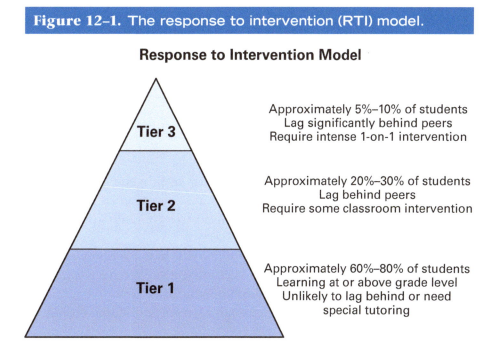

Figure 12–1. The response to intervention (RTI) model.

The third tier is for children with disorders. It is further divided into 3A and 3B. In 3A are children with milder or less pervasive language difficulties who can progress with intervention managed by an SLP but delivered indirectly by others. In contrast, 3B is meant for children with more complex or pervasive language impairments requiring direct individualized intervention by an SLP; Mikie, mentioned previously, would be classified as 3B.

Within the RTI model, an SLP might target direct narrative intervention, focusing on phonological awareness, phonics, vocabulary, and language development. Young children who are Spanish–English and Hmong–English English language learners (ELLs) with language disorders have gained emerging literacy skills through RTI, giving them the confidence to participate more in class and to engage more with literacy materials (Pieretti, 2011; Vaughn et al., 2006).

In part, RTI is a functional model because others in the child's environment are facilitating the child's language learning. In addition, learning is occurring for most children in the environment in which it is used.

If we assume that the school, district, and/or state curriculum sets goals, then those goals serve as a comprehensive guide for classroom instruction. By operating within this curriculum, SLPs can promote active engagement and learning, individualize and adapt practices, provide opportunities for learning within daily routines, and ensure collaboration and shared responsibilities (Grisham-Brown et al., 2005).

Operating within the framework of the curriculum enables various childhood professionals to work together and move away from traditional service delivery models. Implementing a curriculum framework provides a series of challenges—particularly challenges in reconceptualizing

- how to gather information on children's abilities;
- what to teach whom and in what order;
- how and when to teach; and
- where children are making progress.

This leads to four expanded and redefined professional roles for the SLP as collaborator, problem solver, interventionist, and coach.

Inclusion

The Individuals with Disabilities Education Improvement Act mandates that all students with disabilities have access to the general education curriculum. Inclusion is based on sound research documenting the benefits to both children with specific needs and their typically developing peers (Odom, 2000).

Inclusion is an educational philosophy that proposes one integrated educational system based on each classroom becoming a supportive environment much as we saw with RTI. Instead of separate systems of education, inclusive schooling proposes a unitary system of education adaptive enough to meet individual children's needs in a flexible manner. The result is

CHAPTER 12 CLASSROOM FUNCTIONAL INTERVENTION

- a shift in focus from the deficits to the abilities of children;
- collaborative learning;
- curriculum-based intervention; and
- placement of all children in regular-education classrooms, with special services as needed.

In an inclusive model, all aspects of speech and language services are built around the skills a specific child needs to function better in the classroom environment. That's functional language intervention!

The goal of inclusion is an educational continuum that extends from regular-education classrooms for most children through regular-education classrooms with special services to adaptive environments for a small majority of the children most severely involved. At the latter end of the continuum, children will require services from trained professionals and curriculum-based intervention services to enhance their classroom participation. For example, in reading readiness training, children with learning disability (LD) need explicit, systematic, and intense instruction in areas such as phonological awareness and letter–sound relationships (Silliman et al., 2000).

The notion of inclusion is predicated on the assumption that children can learn and thrive in general education settings. It is not inclusive education when children with special needs are simply placed in a general education classroom without making sure they have full access to the curriculum. Inclusive education only occurs when all children have the supports and assistance they need to be able to engage in meaningful learning opportunities throughout the day (Grisham-Brown et al., 2005). That's where RTI comes in.

Despite widespread support for inclusion, there is concern that children with disabilities are not provided specialized instruction by general education teachers (Markowitz et al., 2006). Teachers may lack the knowledge, specialized training, and confidence to provide inclusive care or early education that supports children's access to the general education curriculum (Chang et al., 2005). That's where you, the SLP, come in.

Collaborative Teaching

The possible negative effects of pulling children out of class to receive speech and language services are not found when these services occur in the classroom. Ongoing classroom activities can serve as the basis for intervention, with content coming from a child's assignments and projects and the interactions of the classroom. Thus, intervention is functional, relevant to the environment in which language is being used. In addition, a child can benefit from the social dynamics of the classroom.

Formats for classroom intervention include the following:

- An SLP team-teaches with a regular classroom teacher and other specialists.
- An SLP provides small group or one-on-one classroom-based intervention with selected students in the classroom by using course materials.

- An SLP acts as a consultant for a classroom teacher and other specialists, assisting primary caregivers with intervention strategies. Within a therapeutic partnership, the SLP helps the teacher set objectives, reinforce and modify behavior, and assess progress (Ehren, 2000).

The model for discussion in this chapter incorporates some elements of each of these, although primary emphasis is on the collaborative format.

Collaborative teaching is a combination of consultation, team teaching, direct individual intervention where needed, and side-by-side teaching in which a teacher and an SLP share the same goals for individual children. An SLP and classroom teacher combine their efforts. Parents are also members of the intervention team. The approach is a problem-solving one in which all participants share the responsibilities of decision making, planning, and implementation.

This model includes, but is not limited to, the following elements:

- An SLP provides in-service training for staff and parents.
- A classroom teacher helps identify potential children with language disorders through observation of classroom behavior. An SLP evaluates the speech and language skills of these children and others who fail speech and language screenings.
- An SLP, classroom teacher, and aide provide individual and small- and large-group intervention services within the classroom and the curriculum. In addition, the SLP continues to provide individual or small group therapy outside the classroom to children in need.
- A classroom teacher, aide, and parents interact daily with the children in ways that facilitate the development of language skills.

Classroom training has been shown to be effective in increasing both elicited and spontaneous language production. For example, with very young children, a classroom intervention model is superior to individual intervention methods in generalization of learned words. Providing language intervention in the classroom also has been shown to be effective in teaching some language concepts, such as key vocabulary, to elementary school children (Throneburg et al., 2000).

By working closely with classroom teachers, the SLP can become well-informed of the language demands of the curriculum. The SLP can gain this information by

- meeting with teachers to discuss classroom activities;
- listening to classroom instruction;
- observing classroom demonstrations;
- reviewing materials and upcoming assignments; and
- analyzing tasks to determine the skills needed to participate effectively.

Through this process, the SLP can gain insight into the lexical, syntactic, and discourse development required for students to succeed (Nippold, 2011). As teachers share their

CHAPTER 12 CLASSROOM FUNCTIONAL INTERVENTION

knowledge of the curriculum, the SLP can share their expertise in language development, language disorders, and language intervention techniques.

Inclusion of classroom content and vocabulary in intervention increases the relevance of language intervention. Ideally, the classroom provides an interactive model in which language features are modeled and embedded in familiar, ongoing activities. Real conversations and meaningful activities provide motivation and experiences that are usually not available in isolated individual intervention.

Despite the emphasis on classroom-based or "push-in" services, most SLPs use it sparingly. Challenges include lack of training in the inclusion model, the need for teacher "buy-in," too little time for planning, and limited administrative support (Green et al., 2019).

Summary

Educational trends have combined to change the teaching and remediation of language. In many schools, an SLP is working with children with language disorders within a naturalistic language curriculum in regular education classrooms. The principles we have been discussing in this book are a near perfect match to the demands of this intervention situation.

Role of the Speech-Language Pathologist

A classroom intervention model raises questions about your role as an SLP and about other team members' expectations. There are no quick answers. The model of intervention that evolves is a blend of the child's needs and the desires of the school, the individual teacher, and the SLP. Ideally, the SLP will assume the roles of co-teacher, consultant, and direct service provider and will be integrated fully into the classroom.

As an SLP, you'll be the school's language expert. As such, you'll advise administrators, teachers, and special needs committees about children and language impairment. The SLP is also responsible for speech and language assessment, for the planning and implementation of all speech and language programming, for record keeping, and for training personnel who will work with the children with language disorders.

Relating to Others

Functional intervention in the classroom necessitates coordination of intervention goals and schedules. This coordination requires that an SLP interact daily with a variety of individuals.

Classroom Teachers

As an SLP, you'll be uniquely qualified to assist classroom teachers in assessing each child's level of functioning, analyzing the language requirements of various activities and materials, and developing intervention strategies in conjunction with the classroom teachers. This is an ongoing process, accomplished through in-service training and individual consultation and training, as well as with co-teaching within the classroom.

Both teachers and SLPs rank team teaching and one teach/one drift as the most appropriate models for collaborative teaching. Team teaching is supplemental teaching in which one team member adapts the material for children with language disorders. In a one teach/one drift model, one member teaches and the other moves around the classroom assisting students as needed.

The SLP and the classroom teacher each have unique skills that they can use to help each other and a child with a language disorder. The SLP understands language development and the remediation of speech and language disorders. The classroom teacher knows each child and understands the use of large and small group interactions for teaching.

It is imperative that the SLP avoid the "tutor trap" in which they become a glorified classroom aide. Classroom requirements should not dictate clinical content. In addition, the SLP should work to enhance the classroom environment as well as to change the child's language.

It is important to retain a therapeutic focus. This requires the interrelated steps of planning and implementation (Ehren, 2000). Planning requires intervention services for children that target skills underlying the curriculum. In implementing intervention, the SLP should focus on the goals for children on the caseload and not on general educational activities. Examples of classroom dos and don'ts are presented in Table 12–1.

The SLP and the classroom teacher are part of the intervention team and should contribute in that fashion. Each has special expertise to impart. The role of the SLP is not to provide specific curriculum teaching or tutoring nor to relieve the teacher of the responsibility to teach all students in the class.

Table 12–1. Examples of Dos and Don'ts of Classroom Speech and Language Services

Do . . .	Don't . . .
Help child identify the important information on a math worksheet and decide on a way to perform the operation.	Help the child complete the math problems.
Teach relevant vocabulary by focusing on the words and figurative language of the science text that may be difficult for the child with LI, and encourage the teacher to establish a language learning center.	Preteach the science vocabulary of the next chapter.
Co-teach a social studies lesson by guiding the students with LI to practice the language strategies learned in therapy. Simple note cards containing reminders can be given to each child.	Co-teach a social studies lesson for all students without addressing the Individualized Education Plan goals of the children with LI.

Note: LI, language impairment.
Source: Information from Ehren (2000).

Classroom Aides

Not every school has classroom aides. If your school does, they can serve as language facilitators for students. Although evidence-based data are scarce, they tentatively suggest that highly trained language-teaching allies can provide effective services for children with language disorders under very specific conditions (Cirrin et al., 2010).

Parents and Caregivers

Not all parents and caregivers can or wish to participate in their children's speech-language intervention. Parents and caregivers tend to fall into three identifiable groups, the largest being those who desire participation. Next are those who do not desire to participate, and the smallest group is composed of parents and caregivers who only want more information. The first group can be involved in planning and implementation of intervention, and those who want information can be served through caregiver meetings and in-service training.

We must be fair here. Not every parent or caregiver is able to participate. Parents or caregivers may work, have health or transportation issues, or have other home-care responsibilities, to name a few. Those with low socioeconomic status (SES) backgrounds may work more than one job. Creative problem-solving may be needed to find ways to include parents or caregivers in intervention.

School Administrators

Administrators may not understand generalization and the need to provide language remediation within the classroom. Caseload dictates and contact hour requirements may have to be modified to accommodate the classroom model.

Both teachers and SLPs agree that finding enough consultative time is a major problem (Beck & Dennis, 1997). Discussion should center on how best to serve the children and how to use professional time commitments most efficiently.

Language Intervention and Language Arts

Classroom teachers and administrators are sometimes confused about the difference between language arts and language remediation. You may also be unclear on the distinction.

A lack of clarity can lead to misunderstanding of an SLP's role, especially as it relates to classroom intervention. Language arts accomplishes several things:

- Provides children with labels for the language units they have been using in their speech
- Requires children to stretch their language abilities into new areas, such as fictional and expository writing

- Enables children to have language growth experiences, such as performances
- Helps children reason and problem-solve by using linguistic units

All of these valuable accomplishments presuppose that each child has a well-formed language system.

Children with language disorders are at risk of failure. In language intervention, a child is taught language features that are not present or are in error. These problems can have a huge impact on a child's success within the curriculum.

Elements of a Classroom Model

As mentioned previously, the classroom model consists of identification and assessment, intervention, and facilitation. In each phase, the classroom teacher and the SLP, although a team, have individual inputs that affect the delivery of quality services for a child.

Identification of Children at Risk

Teachers play a vital role in identifying children with language disorders. Most teachers are not trained in language development or impairment, and the SLP must alert them to the behaviors that signal a possible impairment.

Teacher training can be accomplished through in-service sessions. Teachers also can be given help in identifying a potential language problem. Table 12–2 presents a list of some signs for recognizing children having difficulties in the classroom. Table 12–3 or its adaptation might be used by teachers for referral to the SLP.

Table 12–2. Recognizing Children With Language Impairment in the Classroom

The child may have some or all of the following:

Seems to fail to understand and follow instructions

Is unable to use language to meet daily living needs

Violates rules of social interaction, including politeness

Lacks ability to read signs or other symbols and to perform written tasks

Has problems using speech to communicate effectively

Demonstrates a lack of appropriate organization and sequence in verbal and written efforts

Does not remember significant information presented orally and/or in written form

May not recognize humor or indirect comments

Seems unable to interpret the emotions or predict the intentions of others

Responds inappropriately for the situation

Source: Information from N. Nelson (1992).

CHAPTER 12 CLASSROOM FUNCTIONAL INTERVENTION

Table 12–3. Teacher Referral of Children With Possible Language Impairment

____ Child mispronounces sounds and words.

____ Child omits word endings, such as plural -*s* and past tense -*ed*.

____ Child omits small unemphasized words, such as auxiliary verbs or prepositions.

____ Child uses an immature vocabulary, overuses empty words such as *one* and *thing*, or seems to have difficulty recalling or finding the right word.

____ Child has difficulty comprehending new words and concepts.

____ Child's sentence structure seems immature or overreliant on forms, such as subject–verb–object. It's unoriginal, dull.

____ Child's question and/or negative sentence style is immature.

____ Child has difficulty with one of the following:

____ Verb tensing	____ Articles	____ Auxiliary verbs
____ Pronouns	____ Irregular verbs	____ Prepositions
____ Word order	____ Irregular plurals	____ Conjunctions

____ Child has difficulty relating sequential events.

____ Child has difficulty following directions.

____ Child's questions often inaccurate or vague.

____ Child's questions often poorly formed.

____ Child has difficulty answering questions.

____ Child's comments often off-topic or inappropriate for the conversation.

____ There are long pauses between a remark and the child's reply or between successive remarks by the child. It's as if the child is searching for a response or is confused.

____ Child appears to be attending to communication but remembers little of what is said.

____ Child has difficulty using language socially for the following purposes:

____ Request needs	____ Pretend/image	____ Protest
____ Greet	____ Request information	____ Gain attention
____ Respond/reply	____ Share ideas, feelings	____ Clarify
____ Relate events	____ Entertain	____ Reason

____ Child has difficulty interpreting the following:

____ Figurative language	____ Humor	____ Gestures
____ Emotions	____ Body language	

____ Child does not alter production for different audiences and locations.

____ Child does not seem to consider the effect of language on the listener.

____ Child often has verbal misunderstandings with others.

____ Child has difficulty with reading and writing.

____ Child's language skills seem to be much lower than other areas, such as mechanical, artistic, or social skills.

Teachers can be trained to observe and describe classroom behaviors as precisely as possible. A trained teacher is a valuable source of raw data on classroom performance when they know what to observe and measure.

In addition, the SLP and the classroom teacher can identify the individual classroom's or grade level's curricular requirements as a gauge against which each child can be measured to assess achievement. Called curriculum-based assessment, this method uses a child's progress within the school curriculum as a measure of their educational success. When a child is assessed against the curriculum within which they are expected to perform, intervention can focus on changes in the child's behavior that are relevant to the educational setting.

> *Food for Thought:* Teaching within and through the curriculum is a very different proposition than teaching language as an abstract subject. This is a truly functional model.

From preschool through high school, the curriculum changes in the types of demands made on each student. Some of these changes are as follows:

Preschool: Learning focuses on sensorimotor, language, and socioemotional growth with materials that are manipulative, three-dimensional, and concrete.

Early grades (kindergarten–2): Learning focuses on perceptual–cognitive strategies with materials that are one-dimensional, abstract, and symbolic.

Middle grades (3–4): Learning places higher demands on linguistic and symbolic skills with less direct instruction. The child is expected to make inferences, analyze data, and synthesize information.

Upper grades (5–6): Learning focuses on content areas, with the child expected to recall past learning and display fluency with basic academic skills.

Middle and high school: Learning emphasizes lectures in content areas, with students expected to reorganize material as they listen and to gain the main or important points. From 75% to 90% of the school day may be spent receiving information.

Some school districts have identified specific skills that children need to succeed in each grade. Table 12–4 presents some of the skills needed in the first three grades.

The SLP can assess a child through a combination of interview and observation of the child's ability to meet the language demands of the curricula. The interview phase can provide information on the curricular expectations, and observation can focus on the specific linguistic demands made of a child and their response.

An analysis of the linguistic demands must consider all aspects of language and the many reception and production modes. Such an analysis also should note metalinguistic skills demanded in the classroom.

CHAPTER 12 CLASSROOM FUNCTIONAL INTERVENTION

Table 12–4. Some Possible Language Skills Needed in the First Three Grades

First Grade. The child will be able to:

Recognize correct word order auditorily.

Identify singular and plural common nouns and proper nouns.

Identify regular and irregular past and present verbs.

Identify descriptive and comparative adjectives.

Use nouns and pronouns, adjectives, and verbs correctly in sentences, including verb–noun agreement.

Give and write full sentences.

Categorize words by opposites, by sequence, by category, and as real/nonreal.

Retell a story.

Identify the main idea in a paragraph.

Classify narrative and descriptive writing.

Rhyme words and identify words that begin with the same sound.

Identify declarative and interrogative sentences and use correct ending punctuation for each.

Capitalize the first word in a sentence, days, months, people's names, and the pronoun I.

Alphabetize.

Give directions and explanations and follow two-step directions.

Read aloud.

Listen attentively and courteously to others.

Second Grade. In addition to the skills needed for first grade, the child will be able to:

Use correct word order.

Identify incomplete sentences.

Recognize singular and compound subjects of a sentence.

Identify possessive and plural nouns, contracted verbs, and superlative adjectives and use correctly.

Capitalize holidays, titles of people, books, stories, and places.

Identify correct comma use.

Use an apostrophe in contractions.

Identify the topic sentence and sentences that do not relate in a paragraph.

Write an explanation or set of directions.

Address an envelope.

Write rhyming words to complete a poem.

Identify figurative language and synonyms.

Recognize characters, plot, setting, and the major divisions in a story or play, and the difference between fiction and nonfiction.

Tell and write a clear, original story.

Use the title page and table of contents in a book.

Use the dictionary for spelling and meaning.

continues

Table 12–4. *continued*
Second Grade. *continued*
Read critically for sequence, main idea, and supporting details.
Use tables and graphs as sources of information.
Recognize types of poetry.
Listen discriminately for rhyming, sequences, and details.
Third Grade. In addition to the skills needed for first and second grade, the child will be able to:
Identify imperative and exclamatory sentences, simple and compound sentences, and run-on sentences.
Recognize compound predicates in a sentence.
Recognize articles and conjunctions in sentences.
Use an exclamation point.
Use an apostrophe in possessive nouns.
Define a paragraph and identify the main idea and supporting sentences.
Write a paragraph, a book report, and a letter with correct capitalization and punctuation.
Write a clear, original story with title, beginning, middle, and end.
Recognize the difference between biography and autobiography.
Use a dictionary for pronunciation.

An educational language assessment focuses on a child's oral and written abilities and capacity to learn. Data can be gathered by direct testing, dynamic assessment, and real-life observation within the classroom. The level of support necessary for learning is determined, including evaluation of the effectiveness of various instructional and intervention strategies. Most standardized tests are too global, and more specific measures can be used. The caregivers and the teacher, as well as the child and the SLP, should participate.

The SLP follows up these reports and collects further data within the classroom setting. These data can be corroborated by further testing and sampling.

Assessment With Preschool Children

With preschool children, an SLP is interested in pragmatic abilities; semantics, especially the child's lexicon or "personal dictionary"; language structure; and narrative forms needed for school. Additional areas of importance for literacy education include role-play and representational play, decontextualization, and adaptations for non-oral responding. Although there is overlap, these assessments are in addition to other assessments mentioned in Chapters 6 to 8.

Play is an important context within which to experiment with language. Of particular importance in play are the level of decontextualization, thematic content, organization,

CHAPTER 12 CLASSROOM FUNCTIONAL INTERVENTION

and self/other relations. Play can be very context-bound, using only real objects, or relatively decontextualized, using imaginary or symbolic objects. The familiar versus unfamiliar themes of play are also important for later intervention. The organization of play can demonstrate cohesion, logical connections with the theme, and planning. Finally, the roles a child takes and assigns may be important for later teaching and may tell an SLP something about the child's ability to take the perspective of others and to style switch.

Decontextualization in a child's language is particularly important for later reading and is demonstrated by reference to nonpresent entities and to past and future tense. Reading is very decontextualized because all meaning comes from print and little from the physical context.

Even though a child cannot read, pre-literacy skills are important for further development. An SLP is interested in a child's comprehension of text, knowledge and awareness of print, and sound–symbol associations and decoding abilities.

Finally, non-oral methods of communicating are also important. These include gestures, facial expression, and body posture, but also drawing and preschool "writing."

Assessment With School-Age Children and Adolescents

In addition to considering the language features mentioned in Chapters 6 through 8, the SLP is interested in the child's language as it relates to the specific requirements of the classroom. An assessment should include a dynamic *test–train–test* procedure, with both the SLP and the classroom teacher determining the best instructional strategies for an individual child.

An evaluation also consists of systematic observation of real teaching and learning in the classroom and might include rating scales and checklists, narrative records, and descriptive tools by the teacher, SLP, and student. Teacher logs, notes, journal entries, and student assignments and self-evaluations should be gathered to ascertain the child's oral and written language skills. Of interest is the amount of scaffolding or structure and assistance needed by a child for success.

Interviews with the student are also helpful. Students can be asked to describe their most difficult and easiest subjects and their strengths and weaknesses, to relate recent classroom events that made them feel bad, and to prioritize changes they would like to make in themselves and in the classroom and manner of instruction.

The SLP may gain additional information by informally sampling the child's performance. For example, the SLP might compare a secondary school child's notes with those of a higher performing student in the same class. Audio recordings of classroom instructions can be analyzed to determine the level of complexity that each child must be able to process. The SLP may want to collect samples of the child's oral reading or help the child complete assignments, noting the child's language-related work skills.

Within the classroom, children use language for self-monitoring, directing, reporting, reasoning, predicting, imagining, and projecting thoughts and feelings. Using a "speak-aloud" technique, a child can verbalize as they tackle classroom tasks. Also of interest is the breadth of functions demonstrated in conversation and narration.

School semantic features include abstract terms, refinement and decontextualization of word meanings, the ability to define words, multiple word meanings and figurative language, organization of a semantic network, and use of metalinguistic and metacognitive terms. Semantic networking, or relating ideas to a theme, is another important skill for children to acquire. Those with better formed, more extensive networks are better able to comprehend and follow a topic or theme. Networks can be evaluated by having the child name everything they can related to a given topic or category or place pictures and words into categories. Picture tasks can be made more challenging by the use of pictures with differing perspectives.

Success in the classroom requires that a child be able to explain decision making, to discuss mental processes, and to reflect on mental processes of others and themselves. Related metalinguistic and metacognitive terms are listed in Table 12–5. Some terms are acquired prior to school age, but many are not mastered until adolescence.

Syntax and morphology gradually change throughout the school years. Initially, structure is more complex in oral language than in written, but this reverses. Therefore, the SLP is interested in the structure of both. Analysis would include clause and T-unit length and elements of the noun phrase and verb phrase. Cohesive elements such as pronouns and conjunctions are especially important.

Narrative and expository writing and speaking also should be analyzed. Difficulty at these levels may signal underlying problems. Pictures can be used in an assessment to elicit both oral and written samples. Of interest are the clarity of cohesion and the types employed.

For children with word-finding difficulties, the SLP can analyze reading and writing errors to determine the strategies used by the child. Word substitutions may highlight the type of storage and retrieval being used by the child. Categorization strategies may also be revealed. A curriculum-based assessment should attempt to identify the discrepancy between the child's knowledge of classroom content and their ability to retrieve it.

Finally, auditory discrimination and articulation skills are important for spelling and should also be assessed. Similarly, phonemic awareness is important for writing and reading.

As language becomes more complex in school-age and adolescent years, the assessment and intervention tasks also become more challenging. Add to this the deficits found in reading and writing and the task becomes even more formidable. Reading and writing assessment and intervention are discussed in Chapter 13.

Table 12–5. Common Metacognitive and Metalinguistic Terms

afraid	assert	assume	believe	concede	conclude
confirm	disgusted	doubt	embarrass	feel	forget
guess	happy	hypothesize	imply	infer	interpret
know	mad	predict	propose	proud	remember
sad	surprised	talk	think	understand	

Curriculum-Based Intervention

School-based SLPs should contribute to the educational curriculum (ASHA, 2010). SLPs' language and literacy expertise make them well-suited for playing an important role in supporting curriculum-based language intervention (CBLI). I'll try to give you a brief overview of the many ways SLPs can contribute, but I urge you to read the very helpful tutorial by Bourque Meaux and Norris (2018) for a much fuller discussion and a plethora of helpful suggestions.

Children with language disorders may need assistance transitioning from preschool to kindergarten and elementary school (Prendeville & Ross-Allen, 2002), as did Mikie mentioned at the beginning of the chapter. Not only is the child-to-adult ratio increased but also children are expected to work increasingly in small groups and to negotiate using language. In addition, there is also increased expectation for a child to work independently while receiving less individualized support. The curriculum is different and language based, as is the manner of instruction. Children may need intervention to help them "bridge" to the curriculum.

Planning for each child's transition should be systematic, individualized, timely, and collaborative, involving the family, classroom teacher, and the SLP. Through collaborative intervention, the SLP can model interactive teaching styles and help the teacher combine listening, speaking, reading, and writing activities into each lesson but structured in such a way as to ensure success for children with language disorders.

CBLI Model

CBLI is the use of curriculum as a measure of a child's language intervention needs and abilities. This aspect of school-based language intervention has become increasingly important with the advent of the Common Core.

I feel safe in saying that every activity within the school day is a language activity, even lunchtime chatting. To that statement, I add that in both assessment and intervention, the school-based SLP must consider the needs of a child with a language disorder within the academic setting.

When we discuss the curriculum, it's important to realize that this term has several aspects. These consist of the following (Ehren, 2006, 2009):

- Official curriculum is what is to be learned in each grade as outlined in the CCSS.
- Cultural curriculum varies by culture and is what is considered necessary to become a literate, educated societal member.
- De facto curriculum is what is actually taught.
- School culture curriculum consists of the implicit and explicit rules governing student behavior.
- Hidden curriculum or hidden agenda behind the educational context.

These multiple curricula are the context for intervention and generalization. CBLI implementation places language and literacy intervention into this meaningful context

(Scheule & Ehren, 2016). Throughout this text, we have mentioned collaboration. CBLI can be the vehicle for doing that as SLPs, teachers, and others in the educational process generate creative solutions to problems of academic success.

Currently, the predominant model of intervention in schools is for SLPs to focus on foundational speech and language skills and hope for generalization to literacy. We've encountered this "bad case of the hopes" before. There is little or no evidence to support this approach (Bowyer-Crane et al., 2008). Unfortunately, only 33% of the SLPs focus on intervention for literacy (ASHA, 2016).

Let's change that statistic beginning now, beginning with you, me, and those SLPs who are already working within the curricular demands of children. An alternative is to teach language skills in the curricular context, which is a CBLI model.

The curriculum and curricular materials should be the context and the content for language and literacy assessment and intervention. CBLI assessment can be guided by the following (Nelson, 2010):

- The oral and written language skills required by the curriculum
- The oral and written language skills that a student currently possesses
- The future language skills and strategies a student will need to develop
- Ways in which the curriculum can be modified to make it more accessible

Ideally, language and literacy intervention in schools is a hybrid model that at the least includes traditional pullout therapy, individual or small group classroom-based interventions, and collaboration. Pullout is still the model of choice for many school-based SLPs (ASHA, 2016).

Within the classroom, called push in, an SLP can work with individuals or small groups of children and adolescents while the teacher works with the rest of the class. This is the essence of the RTI model.

Small group instruction is efficient and effective and increases generalization and interaction. Group projects can provide the context for intervention by using the techniques discussed in Chapters 10 and 11. Other children can serve as models.

Not all areas of language are equally served by push-in services. For example, although it's feasible for an SLP to provide narrative and vocabulary instruction in a classroom setting, children at high risk for academic failure seem to benefit more from narrative intervention and less from vocabulary instruction (S. Gillam et al., 2014).

Children's individual needs can be addressed if the SLP or teacher carefully interacts with each child in ways that foster the targeted aspects of language. With planning, adults can provide such training individually even in groups of children.

The goals of classroom intervention are for a child to learn new ways of communicating and to have ample opportunity to practice newly acquired skills. In a responsive environment, a child learns that language can have some effect. The language of effective classroom communicators is characterized by fluency of word-finding skill, coherence or content organization, and effectiveness and control.

A child's learning within the classroom is a function of individual learning style and the environment. Both must be considered when assessing or attempting to intervene

CHAPTER 12 CLASSROOM FUNCTIONAL INTERVENTION

with learning. The language of a child's classroom and materials can provide the context and content for intervention.

Barriers to CBLI

Change is often challenging. Barriers to implementing CBLI include time, place, participants, curriculum, school structure and culture, schedules, competing and overlapping programs, personnel, and many others (Bourque Meaux & Norris, 2018). Time is a major barrier in schools because CBLI requires frequent collaborations with several teachers. The heterogeneity of students may make it difficult to find time to address the individual needs of children, especially if treatment groups have students of different ages, disorders, and intervention goals.

One of the largest barriers is the school structure and culture. Approximately 80% of SLPs use a caseload approach to determine the number of students they serve (ASHA, 2016). SLP feedback suggested that administrators do not support other methods of determining which students are served. Teachers also differ in their attitude regarding interventions by the SLP within their classroom. Obviously, more needs to be done in this area to change school cultures.

Classroom Demands

With advancing grades, the emphasis shifts increasingly to independent work and to listening and note-taking abilities. Rules become implicit, and children are expected to work independently. Each of these tasks is extremely complex.

Intervention helps students learn strategies for analyzing various tasks and for determining the steps to take to accomplish them. The SLP might teach students with language disorders time management skills, study skills, critical thinking, and language use.

As an SLP, you could develop a book of listening activities for teacher use within the classroom. Other innovations that might help children with language disorders organize their day and make sense of the classroom include encouraging use of a daily planner, helping teachers add graphic input to lectures, defining concepts and vocabulary, cueing to guide reading comprehension, developing guided questions to help children make inferences, discussing how to answer questions, and helping children identify main ideas for note taking.

Study skills training might include text analysis, study strategies, note taking, test-taking strategies, and reference skills. Through text analysis, a child can be helped to understand the organization of texts and their more efficient use.

Study strategies might include active processes for reading, such as identifying the main ideas and reviewing periodically to organize the material. Children also can learn associative and other memory strategies.

Critical Thinking

Critical thinking is the collection, manipulation, and application of information to problem-solving. Language is an integral part of this process. Therefore, a child with a language disorder may experience difficulties with organizing information and with decision making. Likewise, sophisticated metalinguistic judgments also would be difficult. Critical thinking training might target three components: general thinking, problem-solving, and higher level thinking.

General thinking includes observation and description, development of concepts, comparisons and contrasts, hypotheses, generalization, prediction of outcomes, explanations, and alternatives. Problem-solving skills include analyzing the problem into smaller parts, developing options, predicting outcomes, and critiquing the decision. Higher level thinking includes deductive and inductive reasoning, solving analogies, and understanding relationships. These tasks become increasingly more abstract and require greater reliance on linguistic input.

Analogies (A is to B as C is to . . .) are particularly difficult for children with LD. Analogical reasoning can be taught through a two-phase model in which steps for solving analogies are taught in Phase I and bridging activities to specific academic areas are taught in Phase II. Phase I targets the following skills:

Encoding: Translating each term into an internal representation of its attributes

Inferring: Establishing the relationship of the first pair

Mapping: Using the first relationship to identify a similar one in the second pair

Applying: Picking the answer that has the same relationship as the first pair

Listening Skills

With increased emphasis on lectures in middle and high school, listening skills become more important. Good listening skills are highly correlated with good overall language performance.

Students can be taught to tune in to what they hear and to listen actively. Subsequent training can focus on recognition and understanding of lecture material.

The child's semantic, syntactic, and morphological repertoire can be expanded as a base for comparison with new information from lectures. Such training might include word meanings, relationships and categories, sentence transformations, active and passive voice, embedding and conjoining clauses, and segmentation. Through critical listening training, a child learns to supply missing information, complete stories, find important information, and recognize absurdities in spoken information. Children who have difficulty attending will need special help in listening to what they hear.

Oral Language in Support of Written and the Reverse

Through oral language production, a child can sharpen word-retrieval and figurative language skills. The SLP can teach children to verbalize important critical reasoning skills, such as questioning, comparing, and analyzing, and to discuss a task or topic and to give examples.

CHAPTER 12 CLASSROOM FUNCTIONAL INTERVENTION 517

Elementary school children and adolescents can also be taught metapragmatic awareness in order to judge inconsistencies, inadequacies, and communication failures. The SLP can help students with language disorders understand response requirements for relevancy and thoroughness.

An SLP can enhance written-language training by using computers and topics of interest to the child. Computer intervention can have a positive effect on language, especially vocabulary, and even can improve some social-interactive skills if the SLP mediates. Organizational skills gained in critical thinking training can be used in expressive writing training.

Finally, an SLP can enhance conversational skills by role-playing and practice. The child with a language disorder can be helped to identify different communication contexts and their requirements.

Written information can be used to train oral language skills. Within a conversational or small group framework, written scripts can be used for practice in communicating between speaker and listener. Written material can be controlled systematically to ensure that it is well organized and cohesive and that it offers a variety of topics, roles, and situations. The use of social interactions enables the child to learn language as an integrated social–cognitive–linguistic experience.

Adolescents

Adolescents can offer a special challenge. The structure of an adolescent's day highlights the need for some stability in the teen's language input. These students need more time than short classes allow. In addition, each teacher's contact with individual students is limited to class periods. No one teacher is responsible for the teen's overall language functioning and success.

Essential to any successful adolescent program is destigmatizating and the awarding of academic credit for intervention. The giving of credit aids motivation and gives the SLP clout and credibility. Group intervention classes should be mixed with other classes. Intervention classes can be given names similar to other classes, such as "oral communication skills" rather than "speech therapy."

Instructional Approaches

The overall intervention model might incorporate elements of two instructional approaches called strategy-based and systems models. The strategy-based intervention model assumes that learning problem-solving strategies is more powerful than learning factual content and will generalize more readily. Teaching includes strategies for verbal mediation and for the organization and retrieval of linguistic information. Verbal mediation is verbalizing the steps being used to accomplish a task. This model is highly appealing because of its potential for generalization outside the intervention setting.

In contrast, a systems model assumes that the source of the language disorder lies in the interactions of the child, the primary caregivers, and the content to be learned. Intervention strategies reflect the child's varying learning needs across several learning contexts.

Linguistic Awareness Intervention Within the Classroom

In addition to providing individual or group services within the curriculum and the classroom setting, as an SLP, you can increase linguistic awareness for all children. Within such activities, an SLP can be especially mindful of the needs of those children with language disorders. Each child should be encouraged to participate at their ability level.

Preschool

According to the National Center for Education Statistics (2021), approximately 61% of 3- to 5-year-old children in the United States attend center-based child care and education programs. Participation in high-quality preschool programs has the potential to equalize some early gaps in academic, social, cognitive, and language development for children who are at risk.

Although a language-intense preschool curriculum may provide some added benefit for children with language disorders in accelerating their expressive language growth, such programs alone are no substitute for intervention (Justice et al., 2008). Child language outcomes can be more readily improved through targeted intervention that is delivered within the preschool classroom setting's language-rich curriculum (van Kleeck et al., 2006; Wasik et al., 2006.)

Preschool teachers are a critical "first line" of intervention because they interact in an ongoing fashion with children. An SLP can provide professional development to teachers in the form of language-stimulating strategies for use within their classrooms (Girolametto et al., 2003).

Two contexts for intervention are classroom activities and instructional processes. Classroom activities occur across the school day through a combination of materials, props, and physical classroom organization. These may include art, dramatic play, storybook reading, large- and small-group activities, music, and free-choice centers such as a computer or discovery area.

Instructional processes complement the teachers' use of the specified activity contexts, especially the interactions that take place between adults and children, and might include use of strategies presented in Table 12–6. Some of these strategies have been discussed before in a more general context in Chapter 10.

Language-focused curricula are designed to improve at-risk preschool children's language outcomes through targeted improvements to both classroom activity contexts and instructional processes. Within these preschool classrooms, teachers find it easier to adhere to methods in activity contexts than to modify their behavior in instructional processes (Pence et al., 2008).

CHAPTER 12 CLASSROOM FUNCTIONAL INTERVENTION

519

Table 12–6. Strategies for Classroom Use

Strategy	Explanation	Example
Event casts	Adult provides a running description of an activity or event	*Now we're pouring the dough into the pan*
Expansions	Adult repeats the child's utterance in a more mature form, providing additional semantic information	Child: *I had birthday.* Adult: *Yes, you had a birthday party last week.*
Focused contrasts	Adult highlights contrasts between language targets	*Yes, I am eating cookies and you are eating a cupcake.*
Modeling	Adult emphasizes language targets not used independently by the child	*You rolled the ball and knocked over the dinosaurs.*
Open-ended questions	Adult asks questions with a variety of possible answers	*What should we do next?*
Recasts	Adult repeats the child's utterance with varied syntax	Child: *Sing song.* Adult: *That's right, yesterday we sang songs together.*
Redirects/prompted initiations	Adult prompts the child to initiate interaction with peer	*Juan is playing with the cars and you want to play. Ask Juan, "Can I play?"*
Scripted play	Adult provides appropriate verbalizations within familiar events	*Thank you. Here's your change. Drive to the next window.* (Playing fast-food drive-thru)

Source: Information from Pence et al. (2008).

> **Food for Thought:** Is it evident that preschool language intervention is critical to academic success in elementary school? Is your local school district or state supportive of a firm preschool foundation for all children?

To help teachers and other language facilitators acquire, refine, or enhance their intervention skills or strategies, the SLP can coach them through the use of modeling, demonstration, and feedback techniques mentioned elsewhere in this text. In general, coaching is a process of observing, demonstrating, and providing feedback that can result in the acquisition and use of the skills necessary to provide effective intervention. Coaching offers the opportunity for individualized instruction and assistance, and its positive outcomes are well documented in early childhood intervention (Hanft et al., 2004).

By training teachers and other adults, the SLP increases the chances that training will occur throughout the day in a variety of daily activities. In other words, *embedded learning opportunities* (ELOs) will occur in sufficient number and across sufficient numbers of activities to aid learning and generalization. The challenge is for the SLP and adult to create varied and multiple ELOs designed and implemented in a way that leads to improved outcomes for each child (Dinnebeil et al., 2009).

To be maximally effective, the teacher and SLP must create a classroom environment that is warm, inviting, and instructive, and one in which positive and productive social interactions between adults and children occur on a regular basis while actively engaged in multiple learning opportunities (Petersen, 2003; Pianta et al., 2005). In addition, adults with whom children spend the majority of their time must have the knowledge and skills and access to the resources necessary to support children's learning appropriately (Dinnebeil et al., 2009).

In order for SLPs and teachers to work effectively, they should have

- clear or consistent expectations of roles and responsibilities; and
- sufficient uninterrupted time to consult.

For their part, SLPs must be confident and comfortable in their role and able to do the following (Dinnebeil et al., 2009):

- Work well with other people
- Share and gather information appropriately
- Use active listening strategies and respond appropriately to their partners
- Accurately assess and respond to the needs of others

Effective SLPs assume that teachers come together with them in a collaborative spirit.

Preliterate Activities

Let's focus our discussion on preliterate activities as an illustration. Whole-class preliterate activities may include replica and role-play, narrative development, and the use of children's books. Each contributes to the general notion of narration and narrative form and is an important later development for literacy.

Replica and Role-Play. Play and narrative development are very similar. For children developing typically, the language of social make-believe play and the language of literacy have similar functions. For example, language must be modified for the audience or participants, meaning must be conveyed, language is elaborated, and there are cohesive ties and integrated themes.

The imaginative function of language is acquired during preschool through social interactional play. The language is very explicit in order to convey meaning crucial to directing such play ("You be the baby now"). Language is used to refer to objects within the situation ("This is my horse") and to negotiate and compromise ("Okay, you can talk like that if you're the baby"). Integrated themes are evident in the beginnings and ends of play episodes, in the temporal organization, and in the enactment of everyday events or previously heard or seen narratives.

CHAPTER 12 CLASSROOM FUNCTIONAL INTERVENTION

Imaginative language is heavily influenced by context. Both preschool boys and girls prefer replica toys, such as dolls, a simulated store, and dress-up. Replica toys reflect the real world and are used as props for their intended purposes.

Unfortunately, many children with disorders do not play like children developing typically. Sometimes, they do not have the experiential base for play. As a result, children with language disorders often are isolated in a typical preschool class, engaging in solitary play. Given the importance of play for later narrative development, it is essential that these children have normalizing play interactions.

Prior to beginning social play training, an SLP must plan the event carefully. First, the SLP must create a play script. Theme selection should be based on a child's familiarity with the theme or script and the child's level of play. It is best to begin with everyday events. Table 12–7 presents events based on familiarity. For a child unfamiliar with replica play, the SLP might select getting ready for school or going to the market. By providing a supportive context, familiar routines provide natural events within which language can occur.

Some events emphasize roles; others emphasize sequences. For example, grocery shopping is more role-dependent, whereas making a cake is sequential. Different types of events should be chosen over time to aid generalization.

A note of caution is in order. Event representations vary with cultures. A child in a preschool classroom from a different culture may not readily adapt to the event chosen.

The SLP determines each child's involvement and develops the script. Children can be involved in planning so that the play can be explained and some context provided. The script should begin with one sequence and progress to multisequence events. More detail can be added gradually, along with more story grammar components. Scenarios can be replayed and roles varied.

Table 12–7. Themes for Training Replica Play

Every Day	Once in a While	Very Seldom	Fantasy*
Getting ready for school	Baking a cake	Going to the zoo	Being the teacher (police, grocer, mommy, etc.)
Getting dressed	Having a birthday	Going to the circus	Being a dinosaur
Eating lunch	Going to a birthday party	Seeing a parade	Going to Mars
Riding on the school bus	Getting a haircut	Going on a boat ride	Piloting a plane
Going in the car	Going to the doctor	Going on an airplane	Being a caveman/cavewoman
Getting a bath	Going to the market	Visiting _____	Tracking a big animal
	Celebrating (holiday)	Going to an amusement park	Painting a huge canvas
	Going to church/temple	Going to a show/concert	
	Eating at a fast-food restaurant		

Note: *For preschool children.

Once children have progressed through several types of replica play, they can reenact selected texts from children's books. Appendix H includes a list of children's books for reading and enactment.

Decisions will need to be made about roles, props, repetitive elements in the narrative, and elaboration. In general, children with language disorders should be assigned initially to more familiar roles. Props should be real objects, such as empty product containers and clothing. Gradually, roles can be modified and reassigned, and prop use can become more decontextualized and symbolic.

Table 12–8 presents a possible format for the training of play. The script is presented first in such a way as to provide a context for play. General play and the specific theme of this particular play are discussed with children, with the children's help the adult models the appropriate roles, and children re-create the event. The event is replayed many times with varying roles and elaboration of the basic theme.

At each juncture, children are encouraged to describe and discuss the event enacted. The language of such group discussion and decision making is important for school success and helps more firmly stabilize learning.

Table 12–8. Sequence of Sociodramatic Script Training

Step 1: Present script.

Step 2: Model roles including spoken parts.

Step 3: Have children re-present event and script. If needed, teacher prompts children for turn changes and for what to say and do. Prompting decreases over time.

  Prompts for motor–gestural response

    Tell child what to do and give full physical prompt.

    Gradually decrease the prompt to a partial one and then to a physical assist.

    Tell child what to do and gesture or point.

    Tell child what to do.

    Point or gesture.

    Ask child, "What do you do next?"

  Prompts for verbal response

    Ask child to imitate and present child with model ("You say, 'I want a hamburger'").

    Ask child to imitate and present a partial model ("You say, 'I want . . . '").

    Tell child it's their turn and gesture or point.

    Point or gesture.

    Repeat prior child's behavior and ask, "What do you say?"

    Ask, "What do you say to X (other child's role)?"

Step 4: When children are familiar with roles, reassign. Offer fewer prompts.

Step 5: Modify roles and script.

CHAPTER 12 CLASSROOM FUNCTIONAL INTERVENTION

523

Narrative Development. Training for narrative development and production is similar in many ways to that for play, and it may occur at the same time or following more elaborate forms of replica play. Gradually, the events in play can become more decontextualized through the use of puppets or cutouts and imaginary or substituted objects. Children can take turns narrating the story as it continues.

After decontextualized enactment, the narrative might be repeated by the adult and retold by the children. With retelling, sequences can become even more elaborate so that a familiar event such as getting ready for school is modified with late arising, missing socks, burnt toast, no toothpaste, a flat tire, and so on.

Preschoolers may need help staying within the story frame. You typically aren't attacked by giants at the market nor rescued by Transformers on the school bus.

Gradually, the SLP can introduce stories with familiar event sequences that have not been enacted. These, too, can be retold and modified by the children. Finally, children's literature can be used and these narratives retold by the children.

Use of Children's Literature. Significant differences exist in the print interactions of many children with language disorders and those with typically developing language (TDL). These differences are reflected in the poorer letter knowledge, interactive reading skills, story-listening abilities, and discussion of reading skills of children with language disorders. The normalizing benefits of interactive reading with these children are very important.

Sharing children's literature with preschoolers is not just reading to them. Prereading, reading, and postreading activities can enhance the experience and make it more meaningful, while bonding the class together.

Children's literature must be presented to children within a framework that makes sense for each child. Books should be introduced by their title and related to world knowledge that children already possess. The following is an introduction to *Brown Bear, Brown Bear, What Do You See?*

> I'm going to read a book today called *Brown Bear, Brown Bear, What Do You See?* This is the cover. First, what is a bear? It's like a . . .
>
> That's right, Angel. Angel said a bear is like a big dog. Where does he live? Does he live in your house? No, he doesn't live in your house. Does he live in your neighborhood?
>
> Good, Antonio shook his head "No." He doesn't live in your neighborhood. I wonder if he lives in the woods.
>
> Yes, he lives in the woods. And in the zoo, good, Shawna.
>
> Now, this bear is brown; he has brown hair. Who has brown hair? John, point to someone with brown hair. That's your hair, John. Point to . . .
>
> Yes, Billie Sue has brown hair. Put up your hand if you have brown hair.

As is obvious, the children can bring a lot of world knowledge to the task. When the story is read subsequently, each child can use their knowledge to interpret the story.

Notice in my example that children responded as they could. The SLP can ensure that every child has an opportunity to participate and can facilitate their success by structuring participation.

Often, children with language disorders do not understand books, temporal and causal sequences, story grammars, or logical consequences. The SLP can guide them in constructing their narrative representation.

Within the classroom, books can be used for chanting, rhyming, or predicting activities or for specific language targets. Art activities, sequential memory, and consequential language (*if . . . then*) can follow reading. These activities and several resource books are listed in Appendix H. Books can be discussed with children at several levels of discourse and semantic complexity. These levels are presented in Table 12–9.

School-Age and Adolescent

Success in school requires extensive language skills. Reading and writing are an essential part of the educational system.

SLPs can encourage language use and aid development for those experiencing difficulties by actively engaging in classroom intervention. Skills targeted in intervention sessions can be enhanced in classroom application. Classroom linguistic awareness

Table 12–9. Levels of Discourse and Semantic Complexity

Discourse levels of book discussion	
Collection:	Relatively unorganized list
Descriptive list:	Utterances coordinated through a central topic
Ordered sequence:	Organized by temporal order
Reactive sequence:	Organized causally
Abbreviated structure:	Includes psychological intent and planning
Semantic complexity of book discussion	
Indication:	Nonlinguistic signals, such as pointing
Label:	Naming concrete, observable objects and agents
Description:	Characteristics and relationships
Interpretation:	Observable characteristics used to refer to internal states, motivations, and underlying qualities
Inference:	Own background used to go beyond observable characteristics in a situation
Evaluation:	Likes/dislikes, justifications, summarizations
Metalanguage:	Language applied to reflect on the way language is organized and used

CHAPTER 12 CLASSROOM FUNCTIONAL INTERVENTION

activities might include structuring classroom activities for success and metapragmatics. When asked to identify language targets that would facilitate successful communication interactions in high school, teachers highlight the following (Reed & Spicer, 2003):

- Relating narratives
- Presenting differing points of view or thoughts logically
- Employing conversation clarification and repair strategies
- Taking a conversational partner's perspective
- Taking turns appropriately

To be successful, adolescents must have the ability to use and understand spoken and written language at an advanced level. Throughout the school day and beyond, adolescents are expected to use and understand language in a sophisticated manner. So, it is not surprising that teens with language disorders frequently have poor academic performance and limited vocational options (Conti-Ramsden & Durkin, 2008; Nippold, 2007).

Structuring Classroom Activities

When children find school too frustrating and success too elusive, they give up. Different learning contexts within the classroom can reduce feelings of failure. For example, a noncompetitive environment can keep students task-involved rather than ego-involved.

Motivation is the key. Motivated students are more persistent.

An SLP can make all students aware of the metacognitive and metalinguistic aspects of learning and employ strategies that enhance their application. As an SLP, you can explicitly teach learning strategies and provide guided practice and feedback. Each student can be guided and encouraged to participate at their functioning level.

Students can be aided in recognizing the features that influence comprehension and recall and the processing and retrieval demands of a task. General comprehension strategies to be taught include self-monitoring, drawing inferences, and resolving ambiguities. Study strategies that might be targeted include paraphrasing, summarizing, and note taking.

Metapragmatics

Children with language disorders are often unpopular and may seem odd or out of place in the day-to-day communication so common in the classroom. Among teenagers, perspective taking, comprehension of tonal changes signaling emotion, and nonverbal communication are considered important communication skills. Everyday communication is important for classroom success and can be improved by intervention focusing on metapragmatics.

Metapragmatic awareness is a conscious awareness of the ways to use language effectively and appropriately. More precisely, it is the knowledge of common ways of communicating; the ability to detect and judge inconsistencies, inadequacies, and failures; and the flexibility to change communication behaviors in order to increase efficiency.

An SLP can improve metapragmatic awareness by presenting examples of good and poor communication, discussing the differences with students, and role-playing appropriate communication. Video-recorded examples of communication may also be employed. Gentle critiques and self-evaluation are essential.

With the entire class, an SLP helps students identify their communication goal and produce fluent, flexible, and efficient speech and language to reach that goal. The mature speaker is able to take and express another person's perspective and simultaneously formulate and test several communication hypotheses for effective language use. Within intervention, students can be taught to recognize patterns of social communication; develop options and evaluate their effectiveness; and organize communication behaviors to integrate communication goals, strategies, and perspectives.

Using scripted social drama as the vehicle for holistic training, an SLP can guide students through the following four steps of training (Wiig, 1995):

1. Awareness of pragmatic features and underlying plans, scripts, and schemes. For example, topic initiations can be signaled by phrases such as *That reminds me . . . , Speaking of . . . , You know . . . , Well . . . ,* and *By the way . . . .*

2. Extending pragmatic awareness to real-life situations.

3. Generalization training across different media, contexts, and partners.

4. Self-directed training to foster independence.

At each level and following each scripted drama, the SLP and students discuss feelings and reactions, identify alternative strategies, and apply the lessons learned to communication situations within their own lives. The SLP acts as coach while providing scaffolding and support.

With adolescents, communication skills that are important for employment success can be targeted, such as interviewing skills (Mathrick et al., 2017). Behaviors can be taught and consistently reinforced and then refined in mock interview role-plays.

Conversational narratives may be taught in a similar manner by first identifying the purpose of a narrative and then constructing the appropriate form to fulfill that function. Children can be helped to identify the cohesive ties, such as sequencing, word substitutions, use of nouns and pronouns, conjunctions, and topic–comment relationships.

Syntactic structures also can be taught within verbal interactions. Awareness activities might begin with modeling. The SLP can "think out loud" and discuss their options in a given conversation. Embedded within highly interesting conversations, other activities might include sentence combining and detection and correction of errors.

Summary

An SLP can provide classroom language instruction that addresses the needs of the entire class while enabling every child to participate. The SLP can provide the linguistic scaffolding, thus helping children become meaning makers and be successful. In addition, they can provide preteaching for the child with a language disorder, helping that child be successful.

Language Facilitation

The classroom is a special context with its own demands. Facilitative techniques can be used both in the classroom and in conversational interactions between children and their teachers, parents and caregivers, and peers. Language facilitation includes

- noting vocabulary of the classroom;
- identifying the needs of certain contexts and giving children the opportunity to experience these contexts successfully; and
- talking to children in ways that facilitate growth and highlight production.

Classroom Language Requirements

Often, the type of language used in the classroom is very different from what a child experiences at home. For example, the teacher's language consists of many indirect requests and statements. Questions or statements such as "Can you show us where the answer is written?" and "I can't hear Lori because others are being impolite" contain requests or demands.

In the classroom, the teacher asks questions that require responses. Certain question forms are difficult for children with language disorders.

The skill of knowing how to get things done in the classroom is not usually taught to children but, rather, is taken for granted by teachers. The lack of such knowledge can be problematic for children with language disorders, especially when asked to work with others to accomplish some task. Table 12–10 presents 10 rules for classroom participation.

Table 12–10. Rules for Classroom Participation
Teachers mostly talk and students mostly listen, except when teachers grant permission to talk.
Teachers give cues about when to listen closely.
Teachers convey content about things and procedures about how to do things.
Teachers' talk becomes more complex in the upper grades.
Teachers ask questions and expect specific responses.
Teachers give hints about what is correct and what is important to them.
Student talk is brief and to the point.
Students ask few questions and keep them short.
Students talk to teachers, not to other students.
Students make few unsolicited comments and only about the process or content of the lesson.

Source: Information from Sturm and Nelson (1997).

A child must be able to request and give information, action, and materials and to make judgments on the correct language and communication behaviors in and out of context. Each child is expected to be able to identify the information needed by all involved to complete a task and also to judge the appropriateness of information that is given.

Language Functions

Classroom language functions include the following:

- Relating socially to others while stating personal needs
- Directing others and self
- Requesting and giving information
- Reasoning, judging, and predicting
- Imagining and projecting into non-classroom situations

Relating socially to others while stating one's own needs includes referring to psychological or physical needs ("I want to leave now" or "I'm hungry"), protecting one's self and self-interest ("That's mine"), agreeing or disagreeing ("I think I'm right"), and expressing an opinion ("I love that dessert").

Directing self and others includes directing one's own actions, directing the actions of others, collaborating in the actions of others ("You be the mommy, and I'll be the daddy"), and requesting direction ("How do you do this?"). Self-directing can be elicited by requiring children to accomplish tasks of varying difficulty. There will also be a need to direct others and to follow others' directions.

Giving information includes labeling ("That's a piñata"), referring to events ("Yesterday, we got a kitty"), referring to detail ("That kitty is black and white"), sequencing ("We went to the party, and then we went to the movies"), making comparisons ("Yours is bigger"), and extracting the general point ("We're making Hanukkah presents"). This function occurs when a child shares an experience with someone who did not originally experience it, as in show-and-tell. If the classroom discussion involves activities in which the entire class has participated, children do not feel the need for relayed information to be as precise or detailed.

Requests for information vary with the type of information sought. For example, adults and children tend to use more direct requests when there are few, if any, obstacles to receiving the answer, as in checking short answers to problems. In this situation, the request is very direct: "What's the answer to number 4?"

As children mature, they learn to identify the type of information needed to help a requester. In general, children become more aware of the importance of information specificity.

Children are also more likely with maturity to provide information on the process of solving a certain problem rather than just the answer requested. In responding to the previous question about problem number 4, the child might try to presuppose the difficulties of the requester and respond "5/8ths; I converted to 8ths after solving the

CHAPTER 12 CLASSROOM FUNCTIONAL INTERVENTION

problem in 16ths." School-age children who provide specific information and process explanations are more likely to be high achievers.

The reasoning, judging, and predicting function includes explaining a process ("When you get lost, you should find a police officer"), recognizing causal relationships ("The bridge fell because it was weak"), recognizing problems and solutions ("This box is too small; get another one"), drawing conclusions ("We couldn't finish the project because there wasn't enough glue"), and anticipating results ("If we pull this cord, the bell should ring"). In general, problem-solving tasks, such as designing or building an object, will elicit this function. Problem-solving includes predicting, testing hypotheses, and drawing conclusions.

Finally, the imagining and projecting function includes projecting feeling onto others ("I think Carlos is afraid of the ghost") and imagining events in real life or fantasy ("I'm captain of the spaceship *Izits*. All aboard"). This function can be elicited by fantasy play.

Many activities can be projected into imaginings by asking children to imagine that they are some character in a story or what they would do in a particular situation. With older children, different situations can be role-played.

To be successful, children must be able to use all of these language functions with some facility. As noted previously, activities can be designed to aid this growth.

Talk and Language

As children transition to school, they must adjust to the expectations of the education system. One of the challenges children face is the transition to **academic talk** (AT), the language of the classroom. AT is fundamental to success with literacy (Nystrand, 2006; Uccelli et al., 2014). A child's ability to participate in classroom give and take is one factor in self-identity as a learner (Stables, 2003).

As an SLP, you'll need to consider this different way of talking and its relationship to a child's success in school. Ann van Kleck (2014) has written an excellent article on this topic, and those interested should read it for a much more thorough examination of this topic than we can do justice here.

AT is a broad style of talking with its own specific form, content, and use that differs from the pattern of language found in everyday casual communication. Whereas the largest factor in everyday language use appears to be heredity, the largest factor in development and use of AT is the environment (DeThorne et al., 2008).

We might also consider a second term, **Academic language** (AL), which refers to the highly useful language skills related to linguistic features prevalent across school content areas and increasingly used in texts as children progress through school (Schleppegrell, 2004; Uccelli et al., 2015). Aspects of AL include academic vocabulary, complex grammatical structures, and abstract concepts. Academic vocabulary refers to words common in academic textbooks for school-age children, such as *compare and contrast*, *represent*, *support*, *analyze*, and *research*.

> ***Food for Thought:*** Do your professors talk differently than your friends in casual conversation? That difference is academic language.

Academic words are often abstract. Experience or exposure to academic words in everyday communication is an important factor in vocabulary learning. Frequency of exposure varies with SES, culture, English proficiency, language ability, and access to print.

As an SLP working with preschool and kindergarten children, you'll need to consider the acquisition of AT in children with language disorders. AT is rarely explicitly taught in school and yet, it is vital to success. This circumstance creates challenges for children with language disorders, especially those from diverse backgrounds and/or lower SES families (van Kleeck, 2014). These children may have limited exposure to AT at home (Durham et al., 2007).

In general, preschoolers' proficiency with AT is strongly related to parental levels of higher education. When speaking with their preschool children, mothers with higher education and/or mid- to high-SES talk more and use greater sentence complexity and length, more elaborated language, more discussion of concepts, and more decontextualized language. As a result, these children come to school familiar with AT.

SLPs can foster foundations for later literacy and academic success by focusing explicitly on the features of AL. In addition, the adoption of Common Core by nearly all U.S. states focuses educators' attention on language and its centrality in academic success (Cummins, 2014). Because children with language disorders have deficits in their everyday communication, an SLP should expect that similar difficulties may arise with AL. Through consultation and collaboration with preschool, kindergarten, and elementary school classroom teachers, SLPs can also help teachers focus on explicitly fostering development of academic language (van Kleeck, 2014).

In general, ELLs and children with LD use academic words less frequently than their peers and have less variety in their academic word use (Wood et al., 2021). It is possible that acquiring academic vocabulary words is more challenging for ELLs and children with language disorders (Kan & Windsor, 2010; Ogle et al., 2016; Steele & Watkins, 2010; Townsend et al., 2012).

There's a significant relationship between a student's use of academic words and their academic achievement, especially reading comprehension (Townsend et al., 2012). Some of the gap in reading and writing skills is attributable to lack of academic vocabulary skills. Vocabulary skills also influence the writing process, writing productivity, and quality (Kim et al., 2011; Olinghouse & Wilson, 2013).

Although there are no definitive boundaries between more casual, everyday speech and AT or daily language and AL, I've tried to characterize them both in Table 12–11 (Scarcella, 2003; Schleppegrell, 2001, 2004; Snow & Uccelli, 2009). Differences are more one of degree or emphasis. Take a minute to note these differences.

Keep in mind that the characteristics of AT and AL will vary with culture. For example, mainstream American culture stresses the importance of the individual, and as a result, schools emphasize independence, self-reliance, personal achievement, and self-determination. In contrast, more collectivist cultures emphasize harmony, social reciprocity, obligation, and obedience (van Kleeck, 2013). A child who grew up in a home stressing cooperation and support may have difficulty with the more competitive and individualistic atmosphere in the classroom.

CHAPTER 12 CLASSROOM FUNCTIONAL INTERVENTION

Table 12–11. Characteristics of Academic Talk in Contrast to Everyday Communication

Social-interactive features	Rules for participation	Autonomy: Greater autonomy expected in AT.
		Verbal display: Language is used to display knowledge, thinking, and autonomy. Questions are as much as for a display of knowledge by the respondent as for fact-seeking.
		Topic participation: The topic is controlled by the adult with elicited participation, unlike everyday talk that has more equality.
	Degree of formality: AT has more literary content and vocabulary compared to everyday talk.	More unfamiliar words, especially those with Latin and Greek origin
		Longer words
		Fewer contractions and personal pronouns
		Fewer markers of interest and attitude
		Less variety in sentence types
		More declaratives
		More passive sentences
Cognitive features	More precise, decontextualized, metacognition and metalanguage	Less support from the immediate context with less indefinite reference (e.g., *it*) and fewer demonstrative (*this*, *that* used as pronouns) pronoun use but greater referential use of pronouns to refer to previous information
		Fewer active verbs and temporal and spatial adverbs, but more abstract concepts, nominalization, or converting verbs to nouns; more abstract subjects and abstract nouns; more categorization; and a higher level of vocabulary
		More precise and specific academic vocabulary and more morphologically complex words
		More globally coherent, topic-centered structure with a greater variety of conjunctions used in a more restrictive way
		More inferential language and more metacognitive references (*I think, I remember*)
		More metalanguage (metacognition and metalinguistics) along with more derivational morphological knowledge
		More expressions of certainty
Linguistic features	Greater complexity	More content words, higher lexical diversity
		More prepositional phrases and expanded noun phrases
		Longer sentences and more topic elaboration
		Carries a greater information load
		Contains fewer redundancies

Note: AT, academic talk.

Sources: Information taken from van Kleeck (2014), compiled from several sources (Scarcella, 2003; Schleppegrell, 2001, 2004; Snow & Uccelli, 2009).

The SLP's Role in Fostering Academic Talk. Academic talk can be learned by individuals, small groups, and entire classrooms. For children with language disorders, an SLP might want to include AT in a child's Individualized Education Plan (IEP). Other children might best be served through RTI and classroom instruction.

The tools for assessing AT (Blank et al., 2003; Uccelli et al., 2014) are helpful in determining general knowledge and use and the presence or absence of difficulties, but they do not highlight specific deficits in individual children. Task-oriented measures are better suited to determining specific weaknesses. SLPs can use actual classroom assignments and interactions. Observations and teacher collaboration can supplement this information.

For most children, if the SLP focuses on the social and cognitive features presented in Table 12–11, then the associated linguistic features seem to emerge easily to fit the need. This change may not be so automatic for children with language disorders. Children with language disorders may require additional reminders, practice, and gentle support.

In consultation with the teacher, the SLP can decide which structures are most important and should be the focus of intervention. All social–interactive features of AT (see Table 12–11) may not be as necessary as others. For example, preschool children may not be mature enough to understand the concept and linguistic feature accompanying formality. I recall working with a boy with high-functioning autism spectrum disorder (ASD) who had been schooled in the formality of AT. His formal bearing and elevated language were as odd as if he had been using echolalia.

Table 12–12 presents specific ideas for explicitly teaching of AT and AL. I encourage you to read van Kleeck and Schwarz (2011), from which the table is constructed, for a more in-depth discussion. Of importance is repeated practice and simplified instructions over time.

The most important preschool classroom factor in fostering preschoolers' language skills is teacher instructional interaction including many aspects of AT (Mashburn et al., 2008). Unfortunately, studies have found teacher instructional interactions to be typically poor quality, especially for teachers serving low-income children (Howes et al., 2008; LoCasale-Crouch et al., 2007; Pianta et al., 2005). SLPs can help teachers focus on the features of AT.

Expository Discourse. There are several types of discourse, including conversation, narration, persuasion, and exposition. Exposition is the discourse found in textbooks, classroom lectures, technical papers, and documentaries.

If you are interested in pursuing this topic in greater depth, I recommend the excellent tutorial by Lundine and McCauley (2016), from which I have taken much of the information that follows. In addition, Marilyn Nippold has conducted a number of fine studies of expository text, especially as it relates to adolescents with ASD.

In short, expository discourse is more linguistically complex than other forms of language use and more challenging to comprehend and produce (Nippold et al., 2005; Scott & Windsor, 2000). The vocabulary is more technical than that found in conversational discourse with the use of root words (e.g., *evolve*) and derivations (e.g., *evolution*, *evolutionary*). Table 12–13 presents the words and phrases used in different types of expository discourse.

CHAPTER 12 CLASSROOM FUNCTIONAL INTERVENTION

Table 12–12. Explicit Instruction in Academic Talk and Academic Language

Strategy	Examples
Verbal display	Teacher: *I'm going to ask you questions. If you know the answer, please raise your hand, and tell me so I can see if you do. If you don't know the answer, that's okay, because someone else might.* Show and tell teaches children how and how much to present. Teacher: *When you talk about your special X, you can quickly tell us why it is so special. I'll help you by asking some questions so we can all learn more about X.*
Thinking questions	Teacher: *Sometimes, we don't know the answer to questions. You can still listen to other students, think about the answer, and think about how to find the answer.* Demonstrations can pose questions and offer ways to find an answer. Think-alouds are the SLP's or teacher's response when a child is unable to effectively or correctly respond. These show children the thought process involved in making a logical guess. Think-alouds are potentially an "error-free" learning tool. If a child fails to or is unable to respond, the adult models a response, demonstrates a possible way to answer, and does so without being judgmental.
Level of certainty	A teacher's words can express certainty about information. Words include *wonder, don't know for sure, this is a guess,* and *maybe.*
Cognitive features	The level of language difficulty relates to the level of contextual support, level of thinking, and generality of topics. These variables can be manipulated by the teacher or SLP to make language use easier or more difficult. For example, book activities are decontextualized by their very nature, but the adult can control the difficulty by question formats. The adult can • Ask factual questions from a book • Ask about feelings of characters • Request that children predict what will happen next • Ask inferential questions • Elicit narration ("Can anyone tell us what happened so far in our story?") about read material and real events

Note: AL, academic language; AT, academic talk.
Source: Compiled from van Kleeck and Schwarz (2011).

Expository discourse often includes low-frequency, technical, and morphologically complex words and unfamiliar or abstract concepts (Nagy & Townsend, 2012; Nippold, 2014; Snyder & Caccamise, 2010). Prefixes and suffixes can alter a word's more familiar meaning and in turn affect syntactic complexity (Nippold & Sun, 2008). Word meanings may be difficult to deduce from context and may depend on prior knowledge. In addition, highly technical words are often discipline-specific (e.g., *isosceles triangle, heat index, cardiac*). In addition, these words are used repeatedly and with great

Table 12–13. Words and Phrases Used With Types of Expository Discourse	
Expository Type	**Words and Phrases**
Descriptive	*An example of, such as, to illustrate*
Procedural	*First, second, last, then, next, during, while, before, after*
Enumerative	*The following, another, similarly, likewise, also, another*
Cause and effect	*Because, as a result, consequently, thus, therefore, so, due to, for this reason, if . . . then*
Compare and contrast	*As opposed to, in contrast, both, either. . . or, but, in comparison, alike, dissimilar, similar, instead of*
Problem/solution	*The reason for, as a result, so that, the solution is, a possibility, one issue*

variation compared to narratives discourse (Fang, 2008; Schleppegrell, 2001; Westby et al., 2010).

The expression of complex ideas and relationships requires more complex syntax (Berman & Nir-Sagiv, 2007; Nippold et al., 2005; Scott & Windsor, 2000). Varying word classes—verbs become nouns and vice versa (e.g., *survive, survival*)—require accompanying changes in language form. Referral to past information means increased use of pronouns. Other changes are expanded noun phrases and increased use of embedded clauses in complex multiclausal sentences that require skill to comprehend and produce (Fang et al., 2006; Scott & Balthazar, 2010).

Although narratives use a sequential structure focused on the actions of one individual, each expository type has its own internal organization or macrostructure. Knowledge of these differing macrostructures is central to comprehending and producing expository discourse (Westby, 2005; Wolfe, 2005). As we might expect, children and adolescents perform differently depending on the type of exposition (Culatta et al., 2010).

Use of expository discourse depends on prior knowledge from long-term memory and on executive function. Prior knowledge is often content-specific; thus, a discussion on climate change requires different background knowledge than a discussion of free trade. New information gained through expository discourse is integrated into memory (Nippold, 2010). As might be expected, children with greater background information produce more complex expository discourse and comprehend expository text better (Helder et al., 2013; Nippold, 2009). Prior knowledge of macrostructure helps listeners identify central points, key ideas, and supportive information.

Processing complex syntax and concepts requires attention and working memory (WM) skills. While information is held in WM, information is updated and related to knowledge stored in long-term memory.

Children with WM and executive function deficits have significantly poorer comprehension skills with syntactically complex sentences (Leonard et al., 2013). In part, this deficit is believed to reflect the reduced cognitive capacity of these children. Mikie, mentioned at the beginning of this chapter, may have deficits in these areas.

CHAPTER 12 CLASSROOM FUNCTIONAL INTERVENTION

Although preschoolers and kindergarteners are able to create simple expository passages, generalize simple learning strategies, and understand the difference between narrative and expository discourse, their skills are minimal, still evolving, and dependent on the growth of cognition and language (Culatta et al., 2010; Donovan & Smolkin, 2002; Ehren et al., 2014; Scott, 2005). Development depends on the complex interaction of changes in all these areas.

Vocabulary develops over time as a result of multiple exposures. Usually, by age 10 to 12 years, children have a general proficiency in the use of academic words, collectively called the academic lexicon (Nagy & Townsend, 2012).

Children with low-SES backgrounds often are limited in the experiences needed to build background knowledge for vocabulary growth because experiences provided to these children are more limited overall than for those with greater economic resources. Early differences in children's vocabulary knowledge grow into larger ones in school-age and may be difficult to modify without intervention (Biemiller, 2001; National Institute of Child Health and Human Development Early Child Care Research Network, 2005).

Children from socially, culturally, and linguistically diverse backgrounds often struggle because of exposure to different vocabulary and to different emphasis on which words are central to their life experiences and ways of understanding. As children learn language, they learn the meanings of their culture. Children's early word learning reflects the values, expectations, and rules of their microculture. These children may be at risk of academic failure because their word meanings differ from those of the school environment.

Children with language disorders generally have smaller vocabularies and poorer definitions that their peers with TDL. The heavy reliance of expository discourse on technical vocabulary poses a special challenge for children with language disorders. Struggles with words and word meanings can act as a hindrance to a child's inferencing and higher level cognitive skills, such as identifying the main idea in written text (Adlof & Perfetti, 2014).

Both cognitive and linguistic skills seem to continue to develop in tandem. These changes enable a child to handle the more complex requirements of expository discourse (Montgomery, 2002; Westby & Clauser, 2005). The complexity of expository discourse can be difficult for children with language disorders regardless of the primary cause (Catts & Hogan, 2003; Ehren et al., 2014; Moran & Gillon, 2010; Nippold, 2014; Nippold et al., 2008).

As noted previously, children with language disorders tend to produce less syntactically complex oral and written language than their peers with TDL (Dockrell et al., 2007; Mackie & Dockrell, 2004; Nippold et al., 2008, 2009). This disparity continues into the high school years accompanied by a decreased ability to comprehend complex sentences, such as those found in expository discourse (Montgomery & Evans, 2009). In general, the writing of children with language disorders exhibits reduced grammatical complexity and increased grammatical errors compared with that of students with TDL.

The SLP's Role in Fostering Expository Discourse. As children develop and share more complex thoughts, they require more complex syntax (Nippold, 2010). By age 11 or 12 years, adolescents have the ability to write sentences found in complex expository texts, including multiclausal sentences (Verhoeven et al., 2002). For children having difficulty, grammar instruction alone is not enough. Children require practice in creating multiclausal sentences (Graham & Perin, 2007). Composing those sentences within an actual writing task is of the most value in training for children with language disorders.

Given the complex demands of each subject area, the modality (e.g., speaking, reading), and the expository discourse type, an SLP needs to recognize the increased language demands of expository discourse on children with language disorders. In addition to unique, technical vocabulary and specific syntactic features, different academic subjects have specific macrostructural features. For example, history or social studies depends heavily on sequencing of events and causes/consequences, whereas science relies more on compare/contrast and description. Textbooks may use multiple expository types. Finally, an understanding of a child's language, the requirements of an expository task, and the workings of memory and executive function is important for any SLP considering curriculum-based intervention.

Learning to produce and comprehend various types of expository discourse is a slow, maturational process. Working with children with language disorders, the SLP will want to remind a student of the overall purpose of the expository discourse type as each sentence is written or read. For example, when children are taught explicit text-structure organization such as summarization, they produce statistically improved summaries in expository discourse (Westby et al., 2010). Students with language disorder may also need help in determining the main idea and linking newly learned information with previously learned facts. Not all facts have equal importance, so an SLP can also help a child eliminate all but the most relevant facts.

As children's language and cognition mature, basic low-level skills become automatic, enabling a child to devote more cognitive resources to higher level skill, such as inferencing. Weakness in orthographic and phonological processing makes it more difficult for a child with a language disorder to automatize these parts of expository discourse. This suggests that an SLP may also need to continue to pay attention to a child's lower level skills.

Inferential information and relationships between concepts may not be obvious to children with language disorders. Some success has been reported in explicitly teaching children how to identify relationships among facts and concepts and their relationship to the overall theme and purpose of an expository passage. For example, graphic organizers have been used successfully to help children with language disorders identify relational connections (DiCecco & Gleason, 2002).

Poor readers have more difficulty identifying central ideas, summarizing, and relating newly learned information to background knowledge (Miller & Keenan, 2009). Children and adolescents with language disorder may exhibit rapid deterioration in their performance with increased task demands. These demands require children to process information more quickly, use multiple mental steps, activate prior knowledge, and integrate new information (Cain, 2013; R. Gillam et al., 2002). By walking children with language disorders through these mental processes and through the use of learning and memory aids, SLPs can help these children maximize the available resources.

CHAPTER 12 CLASSROOM FUNCTIONAL INTERVENTION

Talking With Children

Adult interactions with children should facilitate language growth and learning. In a nonthreatening way, whenever possible, the SLP can observe and comment on the use of language by teachers and parents. Teachers are often unaware of the effect their language has on the processing of children with language disorders. For example, teachers' oral directions can contain a large proportion of figurative expressions and indirect requests that are difficult for these children.

Teachers tend to respond to children with language disorders below the optimal level. In general, teachers reply infrequently and, often, in a manner that terminates the interaction. The teacher's frequent use of directives also may limit child–teacher interactions.

The SLP can efficiently introduce teachers, aides, and parents/caregivers to facilitative conversational techniques at in-service training sessions or parent meetings. The SLP can help teachers, aides, and parents/caregivers understand the importance of adult modeling and responding to communicative behaviors.

Examples of good interactive styles, such as those in Table 12–14, may provide a helpful handout for teachers, aides, and parents/caregivers. The SLP should stress the importance of different facilitator behaviors and the need to tailor techniques to the

Table 12–14. Guide for Parents' and Teachers' Interactive Style

Talk about things that the child is interested in.

Follow the child's lead. Reply to the child's initiations and comments. Share the child's excitement.

Don't ask too many questions. If you must, use questions such as *how did/do . . ., why did/do . . .,* and *what happened . . .* that result in longer explanatory answers.

Encourage the child to ask questions. Respond openly and honestly. If you don't want to answer a question, say so and explain why. (*I don't think I want to answer that question: It's very personal.*)

Use a pleasant tone of voice. You need not be a comedian, but you can be light and humorous. Children love it when adults are a little silly.

Don't be judgmental or make fun of a child's language. If you are overly critical of the child's language or try to "shotgun" all errors, the child will stop talking to you.

Allow enough time for the child to respond.

Treat the child with courtesy by not interrupting when the child is talking.

Include the child in family and classroom discussions. Encourage participation and listen to the child's ideas.

Be accepting of the child and of the child's language. Hugs and acceptance can go a long way.

Provide opportunities for the child to use language and to have that language work for the child to accomplish goals.

Peers as Language Models

Classmates with TDL can serve well as models and can be taught functional strategies that promote interaction. Sociodramatic or replica play can provide a basis for interaction for preschoolers. With school-age children, many alternative activities can foster interaction and carryover.

One small set of facilitative principles to use with preschool peers can be stated as *stay, play, talk* (Goldstein et al., 1997):

> *Stay* close to your buddy.

> *Play* together, use the other child's name, and attend to the same objects.

> *Talk* while you stay and play.

This phrase plus adult modeling, guided practice, and independent practice with feedback and discussion of what it means to be a buddy and of the unconventional communication of some children can provide a model for effective peer training.

School-age typically developing classmates can be taught to increase communication interactions using a few simple steps. Questions seem to facilitate naturally occurring communication more than directive prompts, although males with intellectual developmental disorder respond more to comments by peers. Although specific techniques for cueing and prompting can be taught to peers, these are relatively ineffective and time-consuming to teach. The fewer strategies taught, the better.

One effective method, presented in Table 12–15, is to teach interactive strategies rather than teaching specific techniques to the peer with TDL and then to prompt and reinforce these strategies. This approach can increase interactions and on-topic responses by children with language disorders. Several precautions seem relevant. Strategies should do all of the following:

- Include only behaviors observed in high-quality interactions
- Have a high likelihood of inducing the subsequent behavior
- Not place the child with a language disorder in a subservient role
- Not target language features that take a great deal of effort or time to teach
- Have the potential to produce balanced and sustainable interactions
- Optimize typical social interaction, not simplify it

Peer strategies reportedly continue when teacher prompts decline. Peers can also serve as effective tutors in narrative learning (McGregor, 2000).

School-age peers can be encouraged to interact through cooperative learning, homework monitoring, and language contracts. Cooperative learning fosters interdependence and individual accountability while encouraging face-to-face interactions and

CHAPTER 12 CLASSROOM FUNCTIONAL INTERVENTION

Table 12–15. Training Peers as Facilitators in Preschool Classrooms

Step 1: Teach peer to interact.

Introduction

Explain purpose: To help friend "talk" better.

Model with another adult.

Direct instruction

Children rehearse and adults critique.

Adults take role of child with disabilities.

Posters provide reminders.

Step 2: Prompt and reinforce use of strategies taught.

Gradual change with less adult input and fewer peer facilitators and more children with disabilities.

Teacher prompts ("Remember to have your friend look at you first," "Remember to point").

Adults should try not to interrupt too much—inhibits children.

Whisper or point to posters.

Source: Information from Goldstein and Strain (1988).

interpersonal skills. Students with different language abilities are paired for classroom language projects and rewarded for group achievement.

In homework monitoring, a child who has the skills needed to accomplish the assignment helps a child with language disorder. As the SLP, you'd work with both to help them complete their homework, use role-play to teach the tutor and tutored roles to the tutoring peers, and critique role-played interactions between the tutors. In addition, the SLP monitors the peers when actual tutoring begins.

Finally, language contracts can be used to decrease inappropriate language behavior. Both the child with a language disorder and the classroom peers must be able to identify the behavior and understand the need to decrease its occurrence. The contract with the entire class defines the behavior and specifies the ways to reduce it and to elicit a more desirable one. It's helpful in eliciting peer cooperation that the class be solicited for suggestions for decreasing the behavior. The contract is reviewed periodically, and peers are reinforced for success.

Classroom Support for Children With Working Memory Deficits

A first step for the SLP in supporting a child with WM deficits in the classroom is observing and analyzing the WM demands of both classroom discourse and assignments (Boudreau & Costanza-Smith, 2011). Most important is identifying learning contexts in which WM limitations are most likely to influence performance. A child is most likely to experience difficulties with classroom instruction that is lengthy and does not reflect a routine classroom activity, activities that require both storage and processing of information, and writing activities that involve generating sentences or writing to dictation (Gathercole et al., 2006).

The SLP will want to pay particular attention to the language of classroom instruction, noting how much information is delivered, assignments communicated, and participation facilitated (Boudreau & Costanza-Smith, 2011). It's important to remember that WM demands are not limited to reading and writing activities.

Singer and Bashir (2018) have done a fine job of summarizing intervention for children with WM deficits. I encourage you to read their tutorial in full, but I will do my best to summarize their main points and add in the work of others. Given the complex nature of cognition, it's not surprising that that attention, executive function, and other processes affect a child's WM.

Rather than treating verbal WM as a separate cognitive process, it seems prudent to use a comprehensive, multidimensional intervention model that incorporates both a child's knowledge and abilities and the language-learning demands in the classroom. Thus, Singer and Bashir (2018) offer five intervention principles that are summarized in Table 12–16.

As an SLP, you'll also want to consider the WM demands within classroom texts and other materials. For example, complex narratives result in poorer performance in both narrative production and comprehension (Boudreau, 2007). Narratives used in the curriculum can be analyzed for the difficulty of language, the number of episodes, and the intricacies of plot and interaction of characters. Texts can be especially problematic if they contain complex sentences that place greater demand on WM (Montgomery & Evans, 2009; Thordardottir, 2008).

Mental resources for comprehension of words or structure leaves fewer resources for integrating content with previous information. As oral and written processes become automatized, the resources required for word recognition decrease, allowing more cognitive resources for comprehension monitoring.

Similarly, knowledge of various domains of language increases spoken language comprehension and reading comprehension abilities. Thus, intervention should target vocabulary (Bryant et al., 2003), morphology (Wolter & Green, 2013), syntax (Saddler & Graham, 2005; Scott & Balthazar, 2008; Singer & Tamborella, 2018; Tamborella & Singer, 2015), narrative comprehension and formulation (S. Gillam et al., 2015; Peterson et al., 2010; Swanson et al., 2005), spoken and written discourse (Bashir & Singer, 2006), and literacy (Derewianka & Jones, 2016; Fang & Schleppegrel, 2008), as noted previously.

To target verbal WM in isolation flies in the face of a functional approach to intervention. Analysis of classroom demands can also include identifying supports and strategies currently in place that reduce WM demands (Boudreau & Costanza-Smith, 2011). These include visual supports and teaching practices that can reduce memory load. In turn, the SLP can inform teachers of ways in which these supports facilitate learning for children with WM deficits. Wisely, Mikie's SLP from the opening of this chapter has opted to target WM within everyday classroom language requirements.

External language factors within the classroom influence verbal WM. These may include the rate of speech, the use of stress to highlight key words, utterance length,

CHAPTER 12 CLASSROOM FUNCTIONAL INTERVENTION

Table 12–16. Singer and Bashir's (2018) Five Intervention Principles for Verbal Working Memory

Principle	Support
Underlying neurodevelopmental status and WM cannot be modified directly.	Little evidence that computer-based WM training improves WM capacity (Melby-Lervåg & Hulme, 2013; Shipstead et al., 2016). Computer-based training demonstrates no direct transfer to other, more academically relevant tasks.
Increasing efficiency and automaticity with language improves WM capacity for functionally.	Increasing a child's awareness of and automaticity with fundamental patterns of language frees up resources for active processing. Children with DLD and stored linguistic knowledge recognize linguistic patterns more readily, alleviating verbal WM demands for language processing. Intervention for children with verbal WM challenges should focus on enhancing metalinguistic awareness and establishing language knowledge (Singer & Bashir, 2018).
Visual anchors can support verbal WM storage and effective processing.	Visualization in support of verbal WM is shown to be effective. Functional intervention can use visual strategies that maximize a child's ability to use language within authentic learning experiences that require verbal WM (Gill et al., 2003). Strategies that represent concepts graphically alleviate demands on verbal WM and support language use.
Heightening linguistic structure and salience can support verbal WM.	External language factors influence verbal WM. Adults monitor a child's comprehension for understanding and can adjust speaking style accordingly.
Professional collaboration aids in identification and accommodation of a child's verbal WM challenges across different contexts.	Through collaboration with teachers, school-based SLPs can enhance a child's language performance. Other professionals may have little understanding of how language and verbal WM can constrain attention, cognition, executive functions, and self-regulation systems and the effect on language and academic outcomes.

Note: DLD, developmental language disorder; WM, working memory.

semantic and syntactic complexity, the use of short pauses to highlight grammatical elements, and the use of gestures that enhance meaning (Singer & Bashir, 2018).

Four ways that SLPs can support the learning of children with WM deficits are by addressing teacher discourse strategies, visual support, preteaching, and breaking learning tasks smaller steps (Boudreau & Costanza-Smith, 2011). Teachers can present material in a manner that directs a child's attention and reduces overload on WM. Possible strategies are presented in Table 12–17.

Children with WM deficits are likely to do better if tasks can be broken into smaller steps. By reducing the amount of information a child must process or store, complex

Table 12–17. Strategies to Aid Working Memory in the Classroom

- Repeat key points to assist child in knowing what is most important from a story, lecture, or discussion, and provide child an opportunity to store key information in memory.
- Chunk information, such as periodic summarization of key content, to help reduce WM demands.
- Set clear expectations of what is expected in a task or assignment or what a child will be asked to do with information being presented or discussed. The child with WM deficits may also benefit from an example of the expected outcome of an assignment.
- Check a child's perceived understanding of an assignment.
- Request that a child restate the directions in their own words or demonstrate what the child believes are the directions.
- Provide checklists or written lists of key steps to be accomplished in a classroom assignment or task.
- Reduce the rate of instruction, especially when new concepts are introduced. Slower rate results in better word learning in children with language impairment.
- Modify discussion characteristics to allow the child with WM deficits to be an early contributor or to recap key points before asking the child to contribute. Asking a student to contribute after several contributors requires a child to hold prior information while formulating a response.

Note: WM, working memory.

Sources: Information from Boudreau and Costanza-Smith (2011), Gathercole et al. (2006), Horohov and Oetting (2004), and Rankin and Hood (2005).

tasks can be accomplished one step at a time, with each part being a small piece of the larger whole (Gathercole & Alloway, 2008).

Visual Supports

The use of visual supports can reduce WM demands in some learning contexts. Children with poor WM skills may be more successful if a teacher uses gesture, written instructions, keyword lists, check-off forms, and object manipulation (Quail et al., 2009). Interestingly, physical manipulation of objects that correspond with written text can enhance reading comprehension in elementary-age children (Glenberg et al., 2005, 2007).

Graphic Organizers. Graphic organizers (GOs) can be used to depict the key concepts and ideas visually prior to learning. Use of GOs has positive effects on learning and retention.

GOs visually portray not only key concepts, such as vocabulary, but also the relationships between those concepts. Although much research is needed to explore the variables that affect learning and retention, GOs do provide a method for visually representing linguistic information in a manner that "holds" language external to a child's verbal

CHAPTER 12 CLASSROOM FUNCTIONAL INTERVENTION

543

WM (Singer & Bashire, 2018). Research suggests that GOs serve as an external WM space enhancing permanent information storage (Lenz et al., 2007).

If children construct graphic schemes or "frames" by hand, they take ownership of the content, its organization, and the relationships within (Singer & Bashir, 2000). As information is processed, the graphic frame develops further. Ideally, the associations and relationship represented graphically aid processing, comprehension, and memory. In this way, GOs can functionally support children's WM in tasks with high language and memory demands.

SLP and the Curriculum

As an SLP, you can offer valuable insight about the language of the curriculum and the ability of students to meet the linguistic and processing demands of academic tasks (Ehren, 2012). You can collaborate with educators in a team effort on modifying curriculum materials to decrease the linguistic complexity and, thus, lighten the load on verbal WM.

Teacher styles conducive to easing verbal WM load include the following (Singer & Bashir, 2018):

- Moderate speaking rate
- Redundance and repetition
- Periodic summaries woven into lessons to consolidate new concepts
- Controlled pace at which new terms are introduced
- Visual enhancements

Teachers' instructional styles can also be a factor.

Last, some children with developmental language disorders have situationally induced social anxiety (Beitchman et al., 2001). Anxiety restricts performance on WM tasks (Moran, 2016). In these cases, SLPs will want to coordinate services with school psychologists and classroom teachers. Learning tasks can be analyzed and monitored for the level of language and WM needed and then modified accordingly.

> ***Food for Thought:*** **Did you think that you as an SLP might have a hand in decisions about the curriculum? Is it now evident why you are an important team member?**

Instituting a Classroom Model

The transition from pull-out service to classroom-based or push-in service takes careful planning. Central to success is the resolution of the following issues:

- Training of the SLP
- Training of other professionals

- Establishment of a clear source of authority and responsibility for intervention
- Administrative support in the form of adequate space, scheduled time slots, and financial commitment
- Identification criteria for students to receive services based not on standardized test scores but on classroom language processing and use
- Responsibility for IEPs

It may take 3 to 5 years to fully implement a collaborative classroom intervention model. The process is one of evolution. It is essential to begin slowly and to prepare parents and other professionals for the change.

The final model will vary with student needs and teacher/SLP flexibility. The teacher and SLP will need to consult for general language activities and for specific language support of individual children.

First, an SLP must train themself. This training includes education in the use of a functional approach and in the school curriculum. This text provides one step in that education. Workshops, convention presentations, observation, and further professional reading are also essential. In addition, the SLP should role-play the use of various techniques because they differ considerably from the more traditional behavioral patterns.

Classroom teachers can help the SLP become familiar with small and large group instruction. Possibly, the SLP could spend an hour per week in some group activity within a classroom.

Second, the SLP will need to recruit teachers and enlist administrative support. Informational meetings, breakfasts, and parent/caregiver meetings can be used with demonstrations and video-recorded presentations. Administrators can be approached individually. The SLP can present a rationale for collaborative teaching, share scheduling, send brief memos of very successful interventions, invite administrators to attend sessions, and request time for discussion at parent events.

Once convinced of the need for such a model of intervention, teachers can begin to learn specific intervention techniques. These techniques may be introduced through in-service training, with individual instruction to follow. Videotaped lessons including children with language disorders are excellent training vehicles to demonstrate the use of various techniques. Professionals conducting the training should be credible, knowledgeable, and practical. Appropriate materials and hands-on experience are essential to teacher training.

Third, the SLP must train other people. The initial purpose of this training is to educate teachers and administrators about the need for classroom intervention. This is best accomplished with in-service training stressing

- the importance of the environment for nonimpaired language learning;
- questions of generalization;
- the verbal nature of the classroom;
- the practicality and efficiency of classroom intervention strategies; and
- the need for and desirability of team approaches.

CHAPTER 12 CLASSROOM FUNCTIONAL INTERVENTION **545**

A possible in-service training model is presented in Table 12–18.

It is also important to remember that some children still will require pull-out services for specific language skills teaching. Collaborative teaching is better suited to training of general communication skills.

Table 12–18. In-Service Training Model for Collaborating Teachers and SLPs	
Sessions	**Description**
1	Normal communication development and communication disorders in the classroom Help teachers understand development and the ways in which a communication disorder affects every aspect of classroom participation.
2	Language of the classroom Explain the collaborative model and the roles of the teacher and SLP. Help teachers understand how a communication problem makes participation difficult.
3	Scripts and identifying and managing classroom language demands Differentiate language arts from language intervention. Emphasize school "curriculums" and role of scripts in aiding participation. Stress (a) the process of language versus the product and (b) the need for a process approach to language problems.
4	Collaborative approach to identifying communication problems in the classroom Explain a curriculum-based approach. Describe the roles the teacher and SLP play in identifying students with potential communication problems.
5	Strategies for managing language Help teachers recognize the complexity of classroom language. Learn to adapt the curriculum to individual student needs. Learn strategies for collaborating to enhance a child's performance.
6	Literacy problems Explain the oral language–written language link. Learn to recognize literacy problems. Learn strategies for using literacy in the classroom with children with literacy problems.
7	Issues in collaboration Discuss roles, barriers, and issues of collaboration.

Source: Information from Prelock et al. (1995).

Administrators may be reluctant to change current one-on-one pull-out services. A more functional classroom model can be presented emphasizing both inclusion and RTI.

Goals and objectives, probably modest at first, can be established prior to implementation. At each step in implementation, administrators need to be kept informed of progress.

Several alternative models for collaboration are available. Peer coaching and co-teaching seem especially promising. In peer coaching, the SLP and the classroom teacher work as a team, coaching each other through observation and feedback, commenting on effective teaching strategies.

In co-teaching, each professional focuses on their component of instruction on the basis of the curriculum goals of the class. The teacher and the SLP jointly determine student needs, develop goals and objectives and activities to meet them, implement these plans, and evaluate progress.

Fourth, clear lines of authority for language intervention must be established. It is vital to the success of this model that roles and responsibilities, as well as authority, be clearly established. This step requires administrative support and a definite statement of policy. New roles and responsibilities should be written into the curriculum, budget, and job descriptions. Responsibility is shared, and roles shift within the classroom.

Fifth, administrative support in the form of space, scheduled time, and necessary financial outlays must be established. It is easy for administrators to declare a change in procedures without giving adequate support to ensure success.

The largest single impediment to implementation is the lack of time. The SLP and the classroom teacher must allow time each week to discuss each child's success and to review targets and techniques.

Frequently, administrators have difficulty seeing the need to lessen dependence on standardized measures of language that offer a quantifiable measure of behavior. Similar measurement can be made against the curriculum and from conversational samples. The implementation of this step requires the joint educational effort of the SLP and the classroom teacher.

Finally, IEPs will need to be written or modified to reflect the change in service delivery. Other members of the intervention team, including parents and caregivers, will need to be educated on the rationale for such changes. Parents and caregivers usually accept the classroom model when shown the increased service that their child will receive if the classroom teacher is also a language trainer. Many parents are also happy with the decreased amount of pull-out time.

The implementation phase can progress slowly and carefully because it is new to both the SLP and the classroom teacher. It's best to choose the initial child and classroom carefully to ensure some measure of success and to minimize friction with the classroom teacher. Once the SLP and the teacher begin to experience success, other teachers will be more willing to adopt the model.

The selection of the first classroom is critical. The SLP might begin with a best friend on the faculty, someone willing to learn, grow, and make mistakes. Teacher training should include SLP critiques of teacher use of training techniques. A checklist can ensure objectivity.

CHAPTER 12 CLASSROOM FUNCTIONAL INTERVENTION

At first, one child in one classroom can be targeted. This can gradually be expanded to include several children in this classroom or one child in each of several classrooms. It might be best for teachers to begin by attempting to integrate a child's newly acquired skills into the daily routine rather than trying to teach new language skills.

The first class taught by the SLP should, likewise, begin cautiously. One goal per lesson is recommended. Later, individual IEP goals can be introduced through focused lessons with the whole class.

There will always be administrators, classroom teachers, and/or parents who refuse to accept or cooperate with the implementation of the classroom model. Rather than become discouraged, you, as the SLP, can work with those individuals who accept the model and continue to try to educate those who do not. Usually, success with a few children is all that is needed to convince the foot-draggers. The key to success is your rapport with the educators involved.

Conclusion

Functional environmental approaches, as represented by the classroom model, are among the most progressive trends evidenced today. In many school districts throughout Canada and the United States, this model is a reality. Some districts are mandating the change from above, whereas others are experiencing a quiet revolution from below. Relax; no change as radical as this one can be accomplished without some difficulties.

The role of the SLP is changing too. In many cases, SLPs are being asked to implement intervention models for which they have minimal training. Although such requests are expected in a professional field that is changing and growing as rapidly as speech-language pathology, it does highlight the need for continuing professional education.

Still, the SLP is the language expert responsible for identifying children with language disorders and for implementing intervention. In this new role of consultant, the SLP enhances this intervention process through others.

By itself, going into the classroom is only the most minimal of changes. In fact, data indicate that many SLPs engaged in a collaborative model are now modifying their intervention style to a more functional one.

Although location, such as a classroom, was one of the variables of generalization addressed in Chapter 1, it was not the only one. Functional intervention is conversational intervention. A truly functional approach uses language scaffolding techniques within real conversational contexts to accomplish communication goals.

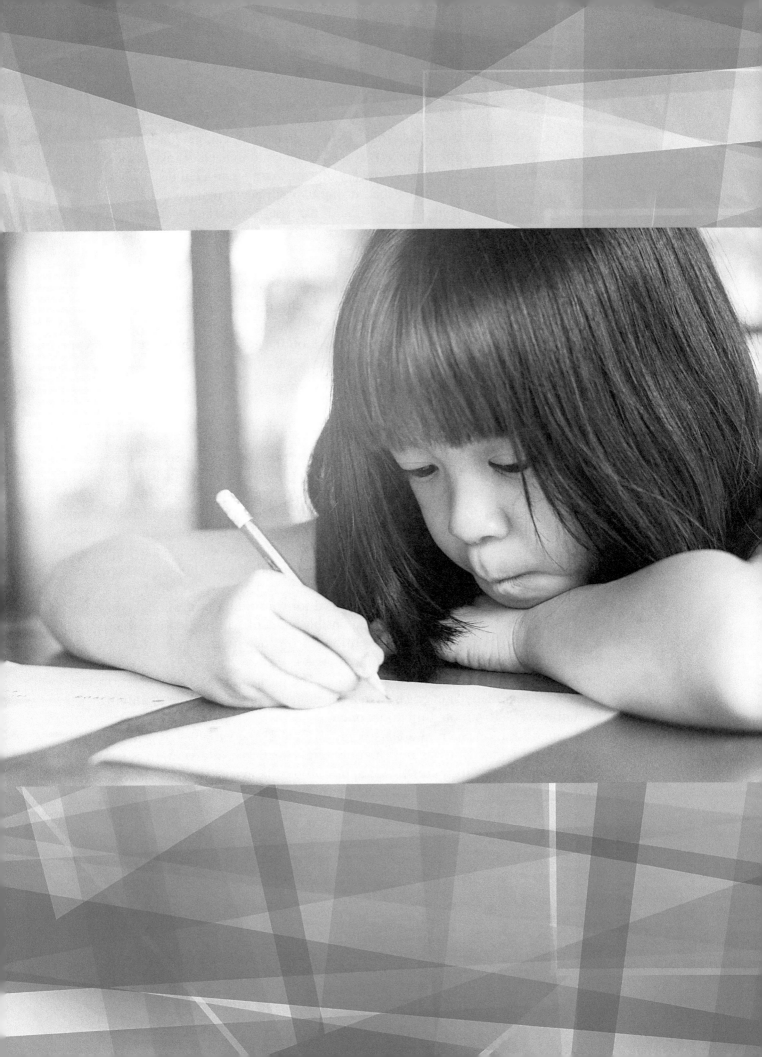

CHAPTER 13

LITERACY IMPAIRMENTS: LANGUAGE IN A VISUAL MODE

Michael is in third grade and having a miserable time. His teacher expects him to read quickly and to learn new words as he reads. Reading was difficult but still fairly easy until now. He had compensated for his lack of ability to sound out words by a combination of memorizing word shapes, guessing, and using the pictures to help. It feels as if the teacher has unreasonable expectations.

Memorizing words isn't working so well. There seem to be too many words. And many of the pictures have been replaced by even more words. His spelling is also poor, and he spells phonetically, so "photo" is spelled F-O-T-O and "apple" is A-P-U-L. The other day, he said in frustration, "I hate words!"

His reading comprehension is suffering too. It takes so long to figure out what the words are that he loses his train of thought and can't recall what he's just read.

The school reading specialist assessed Michael as having dyslexia and asked the speech-language pathologist (SLP) to help. Now Michael has to go twice weekly to "speech therapy," adding to his embarrassment. And his teacher has spoken to his parents about his repeating third grade.

As a preschooler, Michael had difficulty with speech sounds. Close-sounding phonemes were often confused, and he had difficulty recognizing a sound in connected speech. For this reason, phonics was also difficult. Although his overall language was low-normal, no one seemed overly concerned.

In class, he's become disruptive. He teases other kids and is somewhat of a bully to the girls. His behavior is making Michael an outcast, and he's getting a reputation as a troublemaker.

Reading and writing are essential for full participation in society. Unfortunately, children who begin school with poor reading abilities usually either continue to be behind their peers or fall even further behind. As a consequence, these children often have less exposure to written text, which further hinders development, and their ability to learn from what they read is reduced (Mol & Bus, 2011).

The importance of oral language for reading cannot be overemphasized. Oral language delays that persist through preschool are associated with higher risk of poor literacy by age 8 years (Jin et al., 2020).

This oral–literate relationship is true for both monolingual English-speaking and bilingual Spanish–English speaking children. For example, in the early stages of reading development, oral language in both the heritage language and English makes a significant and independent contribution to word reading (Language and Reading Research Consortium et al., 2019). The strongest predictors of English word reading in first grade are English letter knowledge and oral language proficiency.

Unfortunately, in the United States, only approximately 35% of all fourth graders can read on grade level (National Assessment of Educational Progress [NAEP], 2021). Among children of color and those with low socioeconomic status (SES) backgrounds, this rate is only 18% to 21%. These grim statistics are even more alarming when we realize that 67% of students with disorders read below even a basic level (NAEP, 2021).

National statistics for writing are similarly sad. In the United States, a majority of students in Grades 4, 8, and 12 do not demonstrate grade-level writing skills (National Center for Education Statistics, 2021). In the most recent assessment, only 28% of 4th graders and 27% of 8th and 12th graders meet grade-level writing expectations on the NAEP writing assessment. Among children with disabilities, only 7% of 4th graders and 5% 8th and 12th grade students perform at or above grade-level expectations.

Children with language disorders are at far greater risk for reading disability compared to children with typically developing language (TDL) (Catts et al., 2002; Lewis et al., 2000, 2002). From 40% to 65% of children with language disorders are diagnosed in the early grades with a reading disorder (Catts et al., 2002). Rather than decrease with maturity, early literacy deficits continue to persist throughout the school years.

Because they lack preliteracy skills, children with language disorders are unprepared for reading and writing. Key indicators of this lack of skills can be found in their oral language and narrative ability, phonological awareness, alphabet knowledge, phoneme–grapheme (sound–letter) knowledge, spelling and orthographic knowledge, and word awareness (Justice et al., 2002).

In preschool and kindergarten, children with language disorders are less able to recognize and copy letters and less likely to pretend to read or write, to engage in daily preliteracy activities, or to engage adults in question–answer activities during reading and writing compared to their peers with TDL. Unfortunately, many school-based SLPs are not providing any written language services to students with written language weaknesses (Fallon & Katz, 2011).

Usually, reading and writing intervention is the responsibility of special education teachers and reading specialists. However, an SLP's specific knowledge of language disorders is vital in assessment, decision making, and intervention in support of these children's reading and writing needs (American Speech-Language-Hearing Association [ASHA], 2001, 2010).

Within a preschool or kindergarten setting, an SLP should

- alert parents to the oral language–literacy relationship;
- identify children at risk and notify parents;

CHAPTER 13 LITERACY IMPAIRMENTS: LANGUAGE IN A VISUAL MODE

- refer parents to good literacy programs, and

- recommend assessment and treatment in preliteracy skills, such as phonological awareness, letter knowledge, and literacy activities, when needed (Snow et al., 1999).

Within the school-age population, the SLP

- continues to help children or adolescents develop a strong language base;

- addresses difficulties in phonological awareness, memory, and retrieval; and

- addresses difficulties individual children are encountering with both narrative and expository texts.

Al Otaiba et al. (2018) have done an excellent job assembling much of evidence-based intervention information. I encourage you to read their article, from which I've taken some of the intervention methods in this chapter.

As we progress through the chapter, I shall address all the topics mentioned so far. For clarity, I have divided the chapter into two major sections, reading and writing. Within each, I've organized the information into sections on literacy challenges for children with language disorders, assessment, and intervention. I have tried to be judicious and not include regular reading and writing instruction, subjects more appropriately taught by classroom teachers and reading specialists.

Throughout this text, I have tried to take a functional approach. A similar strategy can be used in intervention with reading and writing. Obviously, some minimal phonics skills as well as phoneme–grapheme (sound–letter) knowledge are needed.

Within guided reading practice, students can confront unknown words or grammatical structures and attempt to decipher the meaning from the surrounding text. They can be helped to read actively and to ask themselves questions about what they know, to summarize, predict, and interpret as they go.

Reading

The relationship of early speech and language skills to later literacy attainment is complicated. Studies with twins indicate that both genetic and environmental factors are important in the relationship between early language and reading (Hayiou-Thomas et al., 2010). Taken together, these facts highlight the importance of early language experiences for children.

Development of reading is a complex process based on the integration of its diverse components into a smooth and automatic foundation on which fluent reading and comprehension are based (Wolf, 2007). In order to read fluently and comprehend, multiple processes must be managed simultaneously (Bashir & Hook, 2009).

Phonological and orthographic processing are essential to word identification, and linguistic and cognitive requirements are essential for fluent reading and comprehension. At another level of processing, language and world knowledge are combined to derive an understanding of the text. This comprehension process and the message being decoded are monitored automatically to ensure that the synthesized information makes sense.

Fluency occurs as the rapid and accurate reading of a connected text is enabled by rapid retrieval of orthographic, phonological, and semantic processes, leading to an effective speed of reading to allow comprehension to occur (Wolf & Katzir-Cohen, 2001). The reallocation of attention from subword units, such as phonemes, to higher language and cognitive processes is essential for comprehension (Wolf & Katzir-Cohen, 2001). It would be simplistic to think of word identification abilities morphing automatically into text comprehension (Katzir et al., 2006; Torgesen et al., 2001; Wolf, 2007). The development of reading fluency depends on the interaction of multiple factors.

As you may recall, a part of metalinguistics is the ability to consider language out of context. Reading is also closely related to metalinguistics in that the entire context of reading is constructed by the text itself.

Given the metalinguistic abilities underlying both reading and figurative language, it should not be surprising that the two skill areas are related. In general, good reading comprehension and idiom interpretation go hand-in-hand (Potocki & Laval, 2019).

When something goes wrong, the reading process becomes less automatic and less fluent. Reading becomes labored and slow. The entire process may not make sense to some children, who may become frustrated and feel helpless.

Reading Comprehension and Inferencing

Reading comprehension is multidimensional and not a single ability that can be assessed by one or more general reading measures (Catts & Kamhi, 2017). Nor can it be taught using a small set of strategies or approaches. Performance will vary by individual child, specific texts, and reading tasks.

Readers vary considerably in cognitive–linguistic abilities, motivations, interests, and background knowledge brought to the task of reading. These factors interact within a sociocultural context, such as where the reading occurs; how much support there is; and the cultural value placed on reading by a child's family, peers, and racial–ethnic group. Because reading comprehension depends on the interaction of these factors, it is a fluid or dynamic process.

The multidimensionality of reading comprehension can be seen in the low correlation found across standardized reading tests used to assess reading comprehension. Variability in student performance on reading tests is a function of the interaction of these factors and should be interpreted in relation to the specific reading demands of the assessment (Keenan & Meenan, 2014).

Development of Inferencing

Comprehension consists of a complex interplay of factors, making inferencing difficult for individuals with language disorders (Catts et al., 2006; Humphries et al., 2004; Moran & Gillon, 2005; Nation et al., 2004). Unlike their peers with TDL, preschool children with language disorders often fail to infer speakers' emotions from their speech and facial expressions during conversation, leading to less socially competent behavior (Ford

CHAPTER 13 LITERACY IMPAIRMENTS: LANGUAGE IN A VISUAL MODE **553**

& Milosky, 2008). Similarly, comprehension during reading is affected by these same inferencing skills.

Inferential language in which the answer is not explicitly stated in the story contributes to reading comprehension (Cain et al., 2004a, 2004b). With preschool children, inferential questions may include

- story predictions and reasoning;
- questions about character emotions and reasoning about why a character may feel a certain way; and
- questions about why a character acted a certain way.

Think-alouds by adults can provide a model for the children's responses.

Inferencing skills develop throughout the preschool years and into early school age (Filiatrault-Veilleux et al., 2016). Although there is considerable individual difference, inferential comprehension emerges between ages 3 and 4 years.

> ***Food for Thought:*** **Is inferencing a new concept? Can you recall times when you've used inferencing while reading?**

Beginning at age 4 years, children can infer the problem in the story and the internal response of a character, and they can make predictions about narratives. By age 5 to 6 years, children are able to infer a narrative character's goal, the attempt to solve the problem, and the resolution. In addition, the quality of children's responses improves with age.

For mature readers, inferencing may occur in two phases:

- Constructing inferences
- Integrating the inferences into a coherent text base

Reading Problems

Good readers guide and control their behavior. It's purposeful and flexible. In contrast, poor readers lack such strategies.

Many children who read poorly become passive, lacking persistence and accepting low self-esteem, and they display apathy and resignation. Others will become aggressive or display acting-out behaviors. These affective problems interfere with subsequent learning and development.

Risk Factors for Reading Impairment

Reading difficulties result from the interaction of a combination of risk factors that vary across individuals, including the following:

- *Genetic*. Reading difficulties are inheritable, so SLPs should consider family history and monitor reading among children with close relatives with reading difficulties. Among children with a parent or sibling with reading difficulties, 40% to 66% will also develop reading difficulties, compared with 6% to 14% of other children (Catts, 2017; Snowling et al., 2003).

- *Oral language skills*. As noted previously, poor oral language is associated with reading difficulties (Catts et al., 2002; Snowling, 2014; Snowling et al., 2016; Thompson et al., 2015). Specifically, poor talkers often have deficits in phonological skills, vocabulary knowledge, and morphological awareness (MA). We'll briefly discuss each of these in the following section.

- *Hearing difficulties and speech sound disorders*. Deafness and hearing loss can affect both the nature and the quality of spoken language input, which in turn affects oral language skills important for reading. Children with acute otitis media are also more likely to experience reading difficulties (Carroll & Breadmore, 2018).

- *Environmental*. Children not exposed to print and to a literacy-rich environment early in life tend to have poorer reading skills later.

- *Cognitive*. In addition to the cognitive skills underlying language, other factors include rapid automatic naming, short-term memory, working memory (WM), and executive functions (Alloway & Alloway, 2010; Gathercole et al., 2006; St. Clair-Thompson & Gathercole, 2006). Interestingly, interventions that specifically target these broader cognitive skills are not effective in improving reading (Banales et al., 2015; Jacob & Parkinson, 2015; Kirby et al., 2010; Melby-Lervåg & Hulme, 2013; Melby-Lervåg et al., 2012).

Let's focus briefly on some of the risk factors, including deficits in phonological skills and letter knowledge, vocabulary knowledge, and MA (Colenbrander et al., 2018; Murphy et al., 2016). These same factors, in addition to signed or spoken language skills, also predict literacy attainment for children with deafness (Kyle et al., 2016; Mayberry et al., 2011).

Phonological Skills. **Phonemic awareness** (PA) is the ability to manipulate sounds in speech and to analyze the sound structure of language. A set of skills of varying complexity and depth, PA draws on an underlying knowledge base (Anthony & Lonigan, 2004; Justice & Schucle, 2004). These skills include

- the ability to attend to and make judgments about the sound structure of language, such as dividing words into syllables, identifying and generating rhymes, and matching words with the same beginning sound; and

- the ability to isolate and manipulate individual sounds or phonemes, called phonemic awareness, which is important in early word decoding.

PA is often confused with phonics, which is the relationship between print symbols or letters and the sounds of oral language they represent.

CHAPTER 13 LITERACY IMPAIRMENTS: LANGUAGE IN A VISUAL MODE **555**

To be proficient in phonics, a child needs PA. Alphabetic script makes little sense if a child does not appreciate that words are composed of sounds.

PA is the strongest single predictor of word reading ability. Deficits in phonological processing are strongly associated with difficulties in decoding, word reading, and spelling (Carroll et al., 2014; Melby-Lervåg et al., 2012; Pennington et al., 2012; Snowling et al., 2003). However, phonological difficulties are usually not the sole cause of dyslexia (Carroll et al., 2016; Pennington et al., 2012; Snowling, 2008, 2014).

Letter Knowledge. Letter knowledge or **orthographic awareness** is an individual's conscious attention to print. A metalinguistic skill, orthographic awareness is active consideration of this aspect of language.

Orthographic knowledge informs how we represent spoken language in written form. I suggest reading the excellent tutorial by Apel (2011). The term **mental graphemic representations** (MGRs) refers to the stored mental images of specific written words or word parts (Apel, 2010; Wolter & Apel, 2010). This is similar to the stored phonological representations that underlie spoken words. MGRs contain specific allowable sequences of graphemes or letters representing written words.

Orthographic knowledge is an individual's knowledge of orthographic patterns, including

- how a letter or letters may represent speech sounds;
- how we represent sounds that go beyond one-to-one correspondence, such as spelling of long vowels and use of consonant doubling;
- how letters can and cannot be combined; and
- positional and contextual constraints or orthotactic rules.

Positional constraints in English govern the use of letters, such as not beginning a word with *tch*, the imported Yiddish *tchotchke* excluded. If we don't follow the orthographic patterns, we make spelling errors.

You read and spell either by accessing stored knowledge of specific words or by using knowledge of orthographic patterns. Figure 13–1 presents a graphic representation of the manner in which the components of orthographic knowledge relate to one another.

Letter knowledge is a strong predictor of word reading and spelling abilities (Caravolas et al., 2001; Pennington & Lefly, 2001; Thompson et al., 2015). Evidence suggests that letter knowledge may be a causal factor in reading difficulties (Hulme & Snowling, 2014).

Vocabulary Knowledge. Poor oral vocabulary knowledge is strongly related to poor reading comprehension (Elwer et al., 2013; Nation et al., 2007). In short, a child must be able to understand the words in order to fully comprehend.

Vocabulary knowledge aids children's decoding attempts (Dyson et al., 2017; Tunmer & Chapman, 2012). In addition, vocabulary skills may influence word reading by affecting phonological processing.

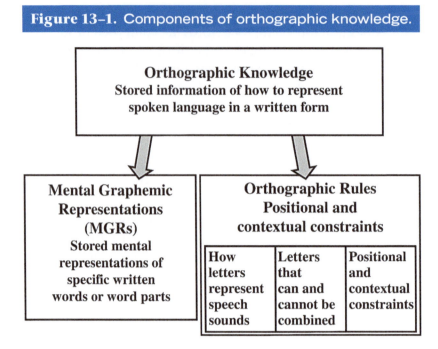

Figure 13–1. Components of orthographic knowledge.

Again, as with other factors, preschool or kindergarten oral vocabulary knowledge alone is not a reliable predictor of later word reading ability and varies by grade level (Duff et al., 2015; Muter et al., 2004; Nation & Snowling, 2004; Ricketts et al., 2007, 2016). Nevertheless, children are better at reading irregularly spelled words when they know or can predict their meaning (Wang et al., 2013).

Morphological Awareness. Morphological awareness—understanding the effects bound morphemes have on root words, such as adding *un-* to *happy*—is associated with word reading, spelling, and reading comprehension (Deacon et al., 2013, 2017). Although PA is essential for learning to read and write, by age 10 years, if not earlier, awareness of and knowledge about the morphological structure of words is a better predictor of decoding ability (Mann & Singson, 2003). Children with speech sound disorders, and thus poorer PA, also have poor MA, suggesting a general insufficiency in linguistic awareness (Apel & Lawrence, 2011).

Children as young as first graders are capable of generating morphologically related words to fit a linguistic context, demonstrating some level of explicit awareness of both derivational and inflectional morphology (Wolter et al., 2009). Morphology plays a key role in reading and spelling from the beginning (Breadmore & Deacon, 2018; Pacton & Deacon, 2008; Treiman, 2017).

Food for Thought: Before you became a communication sciences and disorders major, had you even heard the word "morpheme"? And yet did you probably notice similarities in word endings and wonder about them?

CHAPTER 13 LITERACY IMPAIRMENTS: LANGUAGE IN A VISUAL MODE

As children progress through the elementary grades and into middle school, morphologically complex words make up an increasing proportion of the words they encounter. If teachers and SLPs introduce children to awareness of morphemic structure from an early age, then they can provide children with additional strategies for use in spelling and reading morphologically complex words.

Children With Culturally Linguistically Diverse Backgrounds

For many children from culturally linguistically diverse (CLD) backgrounds, especially those from low-SES environments, school and family cultural notions of the value of literacy may differ greatly. This mismatch potentially places a child at risk of poor literacy development, especially if they are experiencing oral language difficulties with English.

Many children in publicly funded preschool and prekindergarten programs exhibit elevated risks for later reading problems. The results of a survey of children in Head Start programs reveal that maternal education and the frequency of home literacy activities are strong factors in children's vocabulary and reading abilities (Scheffner Hammer et al., 2010). Frequent book reading in the home has a positive effect for the overall narrative quality of children from Spanish-speaking homes who are learning English (Bitetti & Scheffner Hammer, 2016).

Children who speak non-mainstream dialects of American English (NMAE), such as African American English (AAE), will be expected to learn to shift from their dialect to MAE across the early elementary grades, when they are first exposed to formal instruction in reading. Maturity of metalinguistic skills and executive function are important factors in this linguistic adaptation (Craig et al., 2014). This is not surprising given the close relationship between metalinguistics and literacy.

AAE-speaking students who learn to use MAE for literacy tasks, such as writing, outperform their dialect non-adapting peers in reading tasks (Craig et al., 2009). Among AAE-speaking children, higher dialect density or use of more AAE features is related to slower growth in reading (Washington et al., 2018). In fact, the rate of AAE use is inversely related to reading achievement scores.

In contrast, the MA skills of African American children do not seem to be associated with the amount of AAE used by the children in their speech (Apel & Thomas-Tate, 2009). Students' performance on MA tasks is related to their performance on the word-level reading, spelling, and receptive vocabulary measures.

Meta-analysis demonstrates that among children using non-mainstream dialects, there is a negative relationship between dialect use and literacy performance (Gatlin & Wanzek, 2015). Dialectal variation alone cannot account for these literacy differences. SES is also a large contributing factor, with low SES negatively impacting literacy skills (Patton Terry et al., 2010).

As an SLP, you'll want to be aware of ethnic and SES factors affecting both parenting and shared book reading behaviors. Remember that difference is difference, not a cause of disorders.

Mexican American mothers use a variety of communication behaviors during shared book reading, including interactive reading strategies such as *wh-* and *yes/no* questions, directives/requests, labels, descriptions, positive feedback, and vocally directing their children's attention. Compared to White non-Latino mothers, the Mexican American mothers rarely engage in interactive reading that supports comprehension, nor do they use literacy strategies, such as elaborating on their children's ideas as they share books. In general, middle-SES Mexican American mothers use more positive feedback and *yes/no* questioning than do low-SES mothers (Rodríguez et al., 2009).

Kindergarten English vocabulary, phonological awareness, letter–word identification, and Spanish word reading skills are significant predictors of English reading skills by first grade (Páez & Rinaldi, 2006). Although ELL children from low-income backgrounds who have TDL initially perform poorly in all three areas, they can acquire these abilities quickly in kindergarten (Hammer & Miccio, 2006).

Whereas oral language skills in English are a predictor of reading in English, oral language skills in the heritage language are not (August et al., 2006). Rather, reading skills in the heritage language are closely related to future reading ability in English. Specifically, children with high Spanish letter–name and sound knowledge tend to also show high levels of both in English (Cárdenas-Hagan et al., 2007). PA skills seem to transfer directly from Spanish to English.

Letter–name and sound knowledge in heritage languages with different alphabets (Cyrillic, Arabic) or sound systems may not transfer skills as readily. The good news is that all these skills—letter–name, sound knowledge, and phonological awareness—can be taught to these children easily.

Reading and Language Disorders

Although children with developmental language disorder (DLD) and others with reading disorders share common reading difficulties, the underlying processes seem to be different (Spanoudis et al., 2019). In addition to several of the important factors mentioned previously, children with DLD also evidence deficits primarily in semantics, nonverbal short-term memory, and spelling.

Typically, children with DLD and those with learning disability (LD) are slower in learning oral language during the preschool years. In contrast, children with autism spectrum disorder (ASD) may exhibit uneven development predictive of reading behaviors (Sénéchal et al., 2001). For example, a child with ASD may be able to decode words very effectively but not comprehend what is read.

Risk of difficulty with reading is greatest among children with a history of problems in both articulation and receptive and expressive language (Segebart DeThorne et al., 2006; Werfel & Krimm, 2017). Poor reading comprehension is related to deficits in oral language comprehension but normal phonological abilities (Hulme & Snowling, 2014). In contrast, the development of decoding or word reading skills depends heavily on phonological language skills, phoneme awareness, letter–sound knowledge, and rapid automatized naming. Children who are poor decoders have poor phonological abilities but little or no oral language comprehension difficulties (Catts et al., 2006). Remember Michael? He had no recorded language difficulties prior to school.

The relationship of early language difficulties and literacy problems may be more nuanced. There seems to be an interaction between children's early reading abilities, their conversational language abilities, and their history of language difficulties (Segebart DeThorne et al., 2010). Conversational language skills contribute a small but significant amount to children's early reading.

Children with language disorders who have average or above-average intelligence may read initially by memorizing word shapes. By second grade, having failed to develop word attack or decoding skills, these children begin to fall behind. Serious reading comprehension problems may go unnoticed among beginning readers who may compensate by using other information to guess words (Nation et al., 2004).

Children with language disorders tend to use compensatory strategies. For example, they may initially have overall reading growth that is faster than that of children with TDL as they try to compensate for their lower starting point. Unfortunately, by fifth grade, these children exhibit reading skills that are substantially lower than those of children with TDL.

Children with both speech and language difficulties, especially those who lack phoneme awareness at age 6 years, are at greater risk for literacy difficulties (Nathan et al., 2004). Those whose spoken language abilities improve have better reading outcomes than those whose language disorder persists (Catts et al., 2002). As adolescents, poor readers also exhibit vocabulary, grammar, and verbal memory deficits in comparison with their peers with TDL (Rescorla, 2005).

Phonological problems are often more severe in children with a reading-based learning disorder than in children with other forms of language disorder (Catts, Hogan, et al., 2005). Children with LD or DLD generally have impaired reading comprehension even in the absence of phonologically based associated word reading problems (Catts et al., 2006; Silliman & Scott, 2009). Children with DLD exhibit graphophonemic (letter–sound), syntactic, semantic, and pragmatic miscues or misreadings.

We shouldn't move on without mentioning children with speech sound disorders or persistent difficulties with speech production not due to sensory, motor, or other physical conditions (American Psychiatric Association, 2013). As you might guess, these children are also at an increased risk of developing reading difficulties, especially if their speech sound disorders persist until school entry and they are at risk for the other factors mentioned (Hayiou-Thomas et al., 2017).

Contribution of Linguistic Awareness

As mentioned previously, a number of types of linguistic awareness contribute to the acquisition of literacy. Some have a heightened role in literacy disorders:

- Phonological awareness: The ability to think about, reflect on, and manipulate the sound structures of a language

- Orthographic awareness: The ability to translate spoken language into its written form based on the allowable spelling sequences of a language

- Syntactic awareness: The ability to arrange words and morphemes in patterns that help a reader or listener understand novel word meanings and larger concepts not encountered before

- Semantic awareness: The understanding that words have meanings
- Morphological awareness: The recognition that words can be divided into their component morphemes, enabling listeners to identify families of words and their shared meanings

Children with expressive phonological delays have poorer phonemic perception and poorer phonological awareness skills compared to their TD peers (Rvachew et al., 2003). Difficulties seem to be related to failure to analyze words into syllables and these, in turn, into smaller phonological units.

Before we move on, one last thought on phonological processing. Decoding skills for both children with TDL and those with language disorder are strongly correlate with two factors—phonological processing and environmental or classroom quality in first grade (Tambyraja et al., 2015). It's important therefore that as an SLP, you assess for PA in struggling readers, but it is equally critical that you advocate for a language-rich, quality curriculum.

Children with language disorders are less robust at developing initial MGRs than are their peers with TDL (Wolter & Apel, 2010). Children, such as many of those with LD, who have little interest in print, may fail to extract recognizable patterns.

Children with dyslexia often have weak or atypical morphological skills (Breadmore & Carroll, 2016a, 2016b; Carroll & Breadmore, 2018). As might be expected, given their oral language deficits, children with DLD also evidence weak MA.

Deficits in Comprehension

Deficits in comprehension may not be evident in the early stages of reading acquisition when phonics is extremely important. Although phonics-based problems often decrease by third grade, comprehension problems persist for many children (Foster & Miller, 2007). Poor reading comprehension is associated not with phonics but with poor oral language (Nation & Frazier Norbury, 2005).

The situation compounds itself as children mature (Stanovich, 2000). Students with poor reading comprehension are likely to read simpler texts, often below grade level, and to read less frequently. This lack of exposure to print containing more mature structure and content results in poor readers becoming poorer as they fall farther behind.

Comprehension and ASD

Children with ASD are likely to have persisting reading comprehension, spelling, and composition difficulties unless they receive instruction in morphological and syntactic awareness and comprehension strategies (Berninger, 2008). In contrast, children with a reading-based LD usually have difficulty with phonological and orthographic coding in WM, phonological decoding, and spelling, not with reading comprehension or syntax (Berninger, 2007a, 2007b, 2008).

Young children with ASD demonstrate wide variability in their emergent literacy ability (Davidson & Ellis Weismer, 2014; Westerveld, Paynter, et al., 2020). These

CHAPTER 13 LITERACY IMPAIRMENTS: LANGUAGE IN A VISUAL MODE

children often have high print-related skills, such as alphabet knowledge, but lower meaning-related ability (Westerveld & Roberts, 2017). It's possible that this difference in print-related and meaning-related skills results from the fascination of a child with ASD with letter shapes relative to a lack of shared book reading skills and understanding mental states and viewpoints of others. Of most importance is that we not assume a nonverbal child is incapable of learning emergent literacy skills (Afacan et al., 2018; Allor et al., 2010; Mirenda, 2003).

Reading comprehension is poor among many school-age children with ASD and may be affected by one or more components in an individual child (Davidson, 2021). Many children and adults with ASD, even mildly affected or high-functioning individuals, have difficulty inferencing and comprehending metaphoric expressions and ambiguity (Dennis et al., 2001; Diehl et al., 2005; Griswold et al., 2002; Smith-Myles et al., 2002). Unfortunately, most children with ASD do not become skilled readers because of difficulties interpreting text.

Children with high-functioning autism are able to understand words that convey an internal state, such as *know*, *remember*, *forget*, *think*, and *believe*, but they fail to infer what these same words mean in context (Dennis et al., 2001; Wahlberg & Magliano, 2004). Although able to answer factual comprehension questions, they may be unable to inference, which is important for true reading comprehension.

Deficits in Inferencing

Inference construction within spoken and written narratives and texts is an important social and educational tool. Constructing inferences can facilitate the coherent representation necessary for comprehension (Cain et al., 2001; Virtue et al., 2006; Virtue & van den Broek, 2004). Children with language disorders tend to find inferencing challenging, although not every child with a language disorder will have the same issues.

Children with DLD find reading comprehension especially challenging. These children are significantly poorer at elaborative inferencing compared to both their peers with low language proficiency and those with TDL. Furthermore, a positive association exists between inferencing ability and vocabulary knowledge, single word reading accuracy, grammatical skill, and verbal WM (Gough Kenyon et al., 2018).

> *Food for Thought:* Do you ever read something and then find that you cannot recall anything you read? It happens when we're stressed or distracted. Imagine if that was the norm for you.

Interestingly, although only 12.5% of children with TDL find answering inferential questions challenging relative to answering literal questions, more than 50% of children with language disorders demonstrate inferencing deficits (Lucas & Frazier Norbury, 2015). For children with high-functioning ASD, language ability may be an even bigger factor than the presence of ASD.

Dyslexia

Although we mentioned dyslexia in Chapter 2 and have referred to it throughout this text, we have not described dyslexia in detail. We'll remedy that now.

There is no consensus among professionals on precise diagnostic criteria for dyslexia (Adlof & Hogan, 2018), although most definitions include difficulties in reading, decoding, and spelling. These difficulties are somewhat independent of general intellectual abilities (American Psychiatric Association [APA], 2013; Lyon et al., 2003; National Institute of Neurological Disorders and Stroke, 2017; Tunmer & Greaney, 2010). There is less clarity about other aspects of language that are affected in individuals with dyslexia.

Because of the lack of clarity in the definition, considerable variation in estimated prevalence exists. It's estimated that 3% to 20% of the population exhibits dyslexia (Adlof & Hogan, 2018; Rutter et al., 2004; Spencer et al., 2014). Not much to go on, so let's try to be more specific.

According to the fifth edition of the *Diagnostic and Statistical Manual of Mental Disorders* (*DSM-5*; APA, 2013), dyslexia (called "specific learning disability with impairment in reading" in DSM-5) is defined as a neurodevelopmental disorder typified by impairments in

- decoding;
- word reading accuracy and fluency; and
- spelling.

Interestingly, spelling is closely associated with word reading. Difficulties often result from deficits in similar underlying skills. This sounds like a description of Michael mentioned at the beginning of the chapter. As you might expect, children with dyslexia read less, which is unfortunate because reading is one way to increase language skills.

According to the APA (2013), dyslexia must have persisted for at least 6 months despite adequate intervention for this diagnosis to be made. In addition, the disorder is unaccompanied by a range of related factors, such as intellectual disabilities, psychosocial adversity, or inadequate instruction, which may also cause reading impairment.

Children with a family history of dyslexia experience delayed language development as infants and toddlers. In the preschool years, they have significant difficulties in phonological processes and with broader language skills and in acquiring the foundations of decoding skill, such as letter knowledge, phonological awareness, and rapid automatized naming (RAN).

RAN is the ability to quickly name aloud a series of familiar items, such as letters, numbers, colors, or objects. Children with dyslexia often have poorer RAN compared to children with DLD (DeGroot et al., 2015).

Summarizing data from studies of young children, prior to beginning to read, we can say the following (Adlof & Hogan, 2018; Snowling & Melby-Lervåg, 2016):

- Children with dyslexia have a family history of dyslexia and persistent deficits in phonology (Snowling & Melby-Lervåg, 2016).

CHAPTER 13 LITERACY IMPAIRMENTS: LANGUAGE IN A VISUAL MODE 563

- Children with a family history who then develop dyslexia have not only more severely impaired phonology but also more severely impaired semantics (vocabulary) and syntax (Carroll et al., 2014; Plakas et al., 2013; Snowling et al., 2007; Torppa et al., 2010).

- Few studies have examined language abilities other than phonology and receptive vocabulary.

Thus, children diagnosed as having dyslexia display more severe impairments in preschool language compared to those who are classified as typical readers, even those with a family history (Snowling & Melby-Lervåg, 2016).

For gifted children with dyslexia, although phonology is still a risk factor, it's moderated by skills in other areas, such as WM, grammar, and vocabulary. These children use these other skills to compensate for the deficit and to mask literacy difficulties (van Viersen et al., 2016).

Dyslexia and DLD

Dyslexia may or may not occur comorbid with DLD. Adlof and Hogan (2018) thoroughly explore this relationship in their excellent tutorial, which I encourage you to read. A sizeable proportion of children with DLD are identified in later school grades because of problems with reading comprehension (Catts et al., 2006; Conti-Ramsden et al., 2006; Nation et al., 2004; Tomblin et al., 1997).

Although dyslexia and DLD are two separate disorders that frequently co-occur, some children with dyslexia who do not have DLD may still have relatively weak language skills compared with peers with TDL. These might include poorer word learning skills, vocabulary, sentence repetition, and syntactic comprehension even when they display above-average standardized language test scores (Adlof et al., 2017; Alt et al., 2017; Bishop et al., 2009; De Groot et al., 2015; Kim & Lombardino, 2013; Ramus et al., 2013).

Obviously, there are overlaps in the definitions of dyslexia and DLD (Adlof & Hogan, 2018). First, their deficit is "unexpected" given the absence of intellectual deficits or other medical explanations. Second, in both, there is adequate environmental stimulation.

They differ in that the deficits in dyslexia are in perception and word reading. In DLD, the deficit is in overall language development. Phonological deficits are generally more closely associated with dyslexia than with DLD.

Word-learning characteristics vary across children with differing diagnoses. For example, children with both dyslexia and DLD demonstrate word-learning deficits relative to both phonology and semantic processing, whereas children with dyslexia only primarily struggle with the phonological aspects of word learning (Alt et al., 2019).

In one study, 55% of children with dyslexia could also have been classified as having DLD, and 51% of children with DLD could have been classified as having dyslexia. In addition, 90% of children with dyslexia scored below average on standardized language assessments, and 80% of children with DLD scored below average on reading measures (McArthur et al., 2000).

564 LANGUAGE DISORDERS: A FUNCTIONAL APPROACH TO ASSESSMENT AND INTERVENTION IN CHILDREN

A large study of 500 children supported a notion of dyslexia and DLD as fully distinct disorders, with different underlying deficits (Catts, Adlof, et al., 2005); this has been supported by several follow-up studies (e.g., Adlof et al., 2017; Bishop et al., 2009; Fraser et al., 2010; Ramus et al., 2013). In addition, 17% to 36% of children with kindergarten DLD are later identified as having dyslexia in the second through eighth grades (Catts, Hogan, et al., 2005).

Assessment of Reading

Language deficits associated with reading are often present during the preschool years. Prereading and reading assessment should be a portion of any thorough language evaluation.

It is critical that SLPs accurately identify reading difficulties as early as possible. Research evidence indicates that effective early schooling has long-term benefits (Catts et al., 2015; Dion et al., 2010; Scanlon et al., 2005; Tymms et al., 2018).

Data Collection

Just as all children do not require an oral language assessment, neither do they all require a reading assessment. As mentioned in Chapter 3, language assessments begin with an initial data-gathering step that may include use of questionnaires, interviews, referrals, and screening testing. Table 13–1 presents a checklist designed to identify kindergarten and first-grade schoolchildren at risk for language-based reading difficulties. No one item alone will indicate a possible problem.

Teacher and Parent/Caregiver Reports

Teacher reports are a moderately accurate predictor of children's literacy behaviors during assessment. In other words, teachers are moderately good predictors of children who will experience reading difficulties in elementary school (Cabell, Justice, Zucker, et al., 2009).

On an early literacy parent/caregiver questionnaire, parental reports of early literacy skills of their preschool children with language disorders compare favorably with professional assessments (Boudreau, 2005). Questions on reports typically concern the frequency of book-reading behaviors, responses to print, language awareness, interest in letters, and early writing.

Screening

Early literacy can be screened using SLP-designed tasks such as those presented in Table 13–2 (Justice et al., 2002). Children who are good and poor readers can be accurately identified at the end of first grade using a screening battery containing measures of letter-naming fluency, phonological awareness, rapid naming, or nonword repetition (Catts et al., 2015). For a wider view, data from these tasks can be combined with parental information on home literacy materials and activities.

CHAPTER 13 LITERACY IMPAIRMENTS: LANGUAGE IN A VISUAL MODE

Table 13–1. Early Identification of Children With Language-Based Reading Impairment

The following checklist can be used by teachers to refer children to the SLP who exhibit possible language-based reading disorders

The child has difficulty . . .

____ Counting and identifying syllables in words

____ Rhyming

____ Recognizing words that begin with the same sound

____ With sound–letter identification

____ Retrieving words and/or names

____ With specific words, preferring words such as *one* and *thing*

____ Recalling word sequences (alphabet, months of the year)

____ Recalling directions or instructions

____ Giving directions or instructions

____ Saying words

____ Confusing words that sound similar

____ Understanding questions and comments

____ Understanding simple stories

____ Telling stories, especially sequential events, clearly

____ With the give-and-take of conversations

____ Understanding the motivations and feelings of others

____ Initiating conversation

The child does not show an interest in . . .

____ Books   ____ Play with others   ____ Talking with others

The child's speech is characterized by frequent . . .

____ Word substitutions   ____ Sound errors

____ Pauses and fillers, such *as you know* and *like*

____ Requests for repetition, such as *What?* and *Huh?*

____ Repetitions of words and phrases

____ Short sentences   ____ Grammatical errors

Child has . . .

____ History of speech and language problems

____ Family history of speech and language problems

____ Limited home literacy

Sources: Information from Catts (1997) among others.

Table 13–2. Clinician-Designed Tasks of Early Literacy Screening

Area	Tasks
Print awareness	During shared book experience, differentiates written-language units, such as letter, word, and sentence, and identifies direction of print flow, location of cover, functions of books, etc. (Clay, 1979; Justice & Ezell, 2000; Lomax & McGee, 1987) Reads common environmental words (R. Gillam & Johnston, 1985)
Phonological awareness	Finds one in three words that differs on the basis of an onset or rime or tells how two words differ on the same basis (Maclean et al., 1987) Produces words that begin with a certain sound or rhyme (Chaney, 1992) Produces a "new" word after one sound has been deleted, as in "Say cat without the /k/ sound" (Lonigan et al., 1998) Takes a word apart, then puts it together again Identifies the number of phonemes in a word
Letter name knowledge	Says the names of upper- and lowercase letters or points to letters named in two modes at own pace or as fast as possible (RAN) (Blachman, 1984; Justice & Ezell, 2000)
Grapheme–phoneme correspondence	Produces sound that goes with letter or names the letter that goes with a sound (Juel, 1988); could also be accomplished with pointing to letter when sound is heard
Literacy motivation	Engages in a variety of literacy events and level of involvement is rated along a continuum from no engagement to high engagement (Kaderavek & Sulzby, 1998)
Home literacy	Parents complete checklist or questionnaire on home literacy activities and materials to determine child's access and participation (Allen & Mason, 1989; Dickinson & DeTemple, 1998)

Source: Information from Justice et al. (2002). Readers are advised to read this article for a fuller explanation of the tasks mentioned.

Interviews

Children who read poorly may exhibit learned helplessness or have negative attitudes toward the reading process. This information can be gathered from interviews with teachers, parents, and the child and by observation within the classroom.

Interview questions should include the child's perceptions of the importance of reading and different types of reading and difficulties, along with self-perceptions. Scaled responses, such as a 0–5 disagree–agree scale, can be used with statements such as "Reading is difficult for me" or "My teacher helps me learn to read better."

Observation

Observation can confirm the child, teacher, and parent responses. Behavioral changes related to learned helplessness, such as nervousness, withdrawal, and aggression, may

CHAPTER 13 LITERACY IMPAIRMENTS: LANGUAGE IN A VISUAL MODE

be noted. Lack of task persistence can be recorded as the amount of time or the number of attempts made in decoding a word or longer unit. A very high or very low number of requests for assistance also can be a good indicator. In addition, self-verbalizations blaming themself ("I'm so dumb") or others ("This story is stupid" or "Why didn't you tell me I was next?") rather than stating alternative strategies for success ("Oh, this word is spelled like _____, so it's pronounced '_____' ") also may signal helplessness.

Testing

During more formal testing, either the SLP or the reading specialist can use standardized testing to determine if the child is functioning within normal limits. For example, the Test of Early Reading Ability, Fourth Edition (Reid et al., 2017) is designed for children ages 3 to 8 years and assesses alphabet knowledge, phonological awareness, and ability to derive meaning from parts. In contrast, the Gray Oral Reading Test, Fifth Edition (Wiederholt & Bryant, 2012), is a timed instrument useful with slow readers. Finally, the Woodcock Reading Mastery Tests, Third Edition (Woodcock, 2011) assesses sight vocabulary, nonsense-word decoding, and comprehension.

Word-level WM tasks may be appropriate for assessing reading of word-level written language skills. In contrast, sentence-level WM tasks may be appropriate for assessing sentence- and text-level reading and writing skills, such as reading comprehension (Berninger et al., 2010).

Assessment of sentence repetition has been proposed as a measure of AAE use and prediction of reading (Maher et al., 2021). This task may also prove useful with other NMAE dialects.

Morphological dialect differences may be an important factor in later literacy, although more data are needed. It's important to keep in mind that dialectal speakers are not the origin of the problem, which rests in our ability as teachers to make MAE more accessible for these children.

Functional Tasks

In a more functional task, a child might also be asked to read aloud curricular materials in an attempt to assess their ability to function within the classroom (N. Nelson & Van Meter, 2002). The material should be new to the child to ensure that it has not been previously taught.

Reading aloud gives the SLP information on decoding and can be digitally recorded for later analysis. If curricular materials seem to be too difficult, the SLP or reading specialist could use graded passages, such as those found in the Qualitative Reading Inventory, Seventh Edition (Leslie & Caldwell, 2021). Regardless of the method of collection, some portion should be read aloud and recorded.

Comprehension can be assessed by using questions based on the text. Alternative forms include retelling or paraphrasing. Most standardized tests include a comprehension subtest.

Think-Alouds. The ability to paraphrase reading passages is closely related to measures of expository text comprehension (Laing Gillam et al., 2009). For this reason, data obtained during think-aloud sessions may be a useful supplement to traditional measures of comprehension.

Think-aloud methods can reveal metacognitive processes that occur during thinking or reasoning. In think-alouds, children verbalize their thoughts or thought processes while reading, listening, or problem-solving (Braten & Stromso, 2003).

During a think-aloud task, the SLP periodically asks a child to report thoughts while problem-solving during tasks and to talk about why or how they arrived at particular solutions. A child's response might be classified as follows (Laing Gillam et al., 2009):

- *Exact repetition:* Utterance matches exactly or differs by only one word from the focal sentence.
- *Paraphrase:* A transformation of the focal sentence that preserves its meaning.
- *Explanation:* Utterance provides an answer to why questions.
- *Prediction:* Utterance provides answers to causal consequence questions. Predictive inferences may be produced in chains in which one prediction is necessary for and/or enables another one to occur.
- *Association:* Utterance in which content occurs concurrently with the event, state, or activity depicted in the focal sentence in the form of generalizations, specifications of procedures, and expressions of manner, features, and properties of characters or objects, as well as specification of temporal or spatial information.

Although this list is not a strict hierarchy of comprehension, it does provide a systematic way to characterize a child's level of comprehension processing.

Data Analysis

Passages can be photocopied and used by the SLP to record discrepancies noted on the recorded reading samples. All attempts at word decoding, repetitions, corrections, omitted words and morphemes, extended pauses, and dialectal usages should be noted by the SLP and analyzed for possible strategies used by the child. There is little danger that children with DLD or LD will inflate their performance by guessing words correctly, because a part of their reading difficulty is an inability to integrate syntactic, semantic, and textual information (N. Nelson & Van Meter, 2002).

The percentage of words correct on the first attempt can be calculated. Usually, children who experience less than 90% correct on their first attempt demonstrate frustration (Leslie & Caldwell, 2000).

Miscues or words read incorrectly can be analyzed by type at the word level. These include

- reversals, in which word order is changed;
- semantic substitutions, in which an acceptable but different word is substituted;
- syntactic substitutions, in which a syntactically appropriate but semantically nonsensical word is substituted;

CHAPTER 13 LITERACY IMPAIRMENTS: LANGUAGE IN A VISUAL MODE

- insertions, in which a word is added; and
- deletions.

The percentage of incorrect but linguistically acceptable words can also be calculated. These words indicate the use of linguistic cues to predict words.

The SLP can note the way in which the child sounds out unknown words (N. Nelson & Van Meter, 2002). Good readers use several strategies. Common strategies include the following:

- Sound by sound
- By consonant clusters including digraphs ("sh," "th," "on," "ch," "ay")
- Common rimes ("-ack," "-ent," "-ite," "-at")
- Morphemes ("un-," "dis-," "-ly")

Assessment of Phonological Awareness

Given its prominence, I've given PA its own section. Assessment for PA can be accomplished within an overall assessment of reading that includes measurement of reading, spelling, PA, verbal WM, and RAN. One caution: African American children from low-income families may score below expected norms on some phonological awareness measures even though their reading performance is within normal limits (Thomas-Tate et al., 2004).

A thorough assessment of PA includes rhyming, sound isolation, segmentation, blending, deletion, and substitution. The rhyming portion is only predictive of reading with preschool and kindergarten children.

Formal testing can be accomplished using the Comprehensive Test of Phonological Processing (CTOPP; Wagner et al., 1999), Test of Phonological Awareness, Second Edition (TOPA-2+; Torgensen & Bryant, 2013), or the Phonological Awareness Test (PAT; Robertson & Salter, 2017). Designed for ages 5 through 21 years, the CTOPP includes subtests on deletion of sounds, sound and word blending, segmentation, and phoneme reversal, a difficult memory task. In addition, tasks on the CTOPP also assess verbal WM and RAN.

The TOPA-2+ is a group- or individual-administered, norm-referenced measure of phonological awareness for children ages 5 through 8 years. The PAT, designed for children ages 5 through 9 years, includes testing of rhyming, segmentation, phoneme isolation, deletion, substitution, blending, sound–symbol association, and word decoding.

Assessment of Morphological Awareness

Children with DLD often omit morphological endings in their speech. This is also true in their aloud reading. This consistency points up the relationship of oral language and literacy. For example, a score of less than 90% accuracy on reading regular past tense verbs yields moderate sensitivity and specificity for identifying second and third grade students with DLD (Werfel et al., 2017).

Textbooks for adolescents and young adults contain a variety of morphologically complex words, such as *regeneration*, *reptilian*, and *strenuous*. Given the importance of derived words for academic success, MA should be assessed, especially in older children (Nippold & Sun, 2008).

At the very least, you as an SLPs should examine adolescent students' understanding of *-able* (*acceptable*), *-ar* (*molecular*), *-ic* (*genetic*), *-ful* (*powerful*), *-less* (*speechless*), *-ment* (*concealment*), *-ship* (*citizenship*), *-tion* (*prediction*), *-ness* (*weariness*), and *-ity* (*diversity*). Additional suffixes might include *-ous*, *-like*, and *-ish* for adjectives and *-ian*, *-ster*, and *-ology* for nouns. Actual word choice should be based on frequency of word use in curricular materials and in textbook glossaries.

Assessment of Comprehension

Assessment for comprehension is difficult because of the multifaceted character of the process. Kindergarten and first-grade screening tests focus on phonological awareness and phonics, thus identifying only children who will have difficulty with early reading. Comprehension deficits manifest themselves later and are not based on an inability to sound out words.

A single silent reading comprehension test is insufficient to identify those who are slow readers from those who have language-based comprehension problems (Snyder et al., 2005). At the very least, a thorough evaluation must include the following:

- Oral language skills, especially vocabulary and listening comprehension
- Narrative skills from conversational samples
- Standardized assessment of all aspects of comprehension beyond simple recall of text content, including paraphrasing, summarizing, predicting, and inferencing
- Sampling of grade-appropriate reading comprehension

Early Assessment of Dyslexia

Let's focus on the identification of word reading difficulties of children from preschool through second grade, the very beginning of reading instruction. For a fuller discussion, see the wonderful tutorial by Colenbrander et al. (2018), from which I have borrowed some of the ideas.

Given the complexity of reading and the young age of beginning readers, it's difficult to identify those who will become poor readers (Bishop, 2015; Snowling, 2013). In addition, during preschool and kindergarten, reliable assessment of reading potential can be extremely difficult (Colenbrander et al., 2018). It's important, therefore, to consider a broad range of reading-related skills and risk factors (Pennington et al., 2012). Remember that no individual risk factor accurately predicts reading ability.

The most widely researched framework for early identification is response to intervention (RTI). Recall that RTI uses a three-tiered model of instruction and assessment to determine which children need additional academic support.

CHAPTER 13 LITERACY IMPAIRMENTS: LANGUAGE IN A VISUAL MODE 571

Ideally, RTI doesn't involve "waiting to fail" (Fletcher et al., 2004; Fuchs & Fuchs, 2006). Because children's progress is monitored right from the start of reading instruction, problems can be identified and addressed early on. Success relies on the methods of instruction within each tier; the choice of sensitive, specific, and reliable assessment of reading achievement; and the extent of RTI adoption by a specific school district (Catts et al., 2015; Fletcher & Vaughn, 2009; Fuchs & Fuchs, 2006).

Successful early identification rests on the following (Arden et al., 2017; Fuchs & Fuchs, 2017; Gersten, Jayanthi, et al., 2017):

- Sensitive and specific assessments with clear links to instructional recommendations
- Appropriate cutoff points for identification
- Regular progress monitoring
- Ongoing training and support for teachers and SLPs

As an SLP, you'll play a vital role in this process. Ideally, you'll be part of a schoolwide, multidisciplinary approach to RTI (Justice, 2006).

In kindergarten, assessments of PA, letter naming, and/or letter–sound correspondence knowledge and vocabulary are appropriate. In first and second grades, the ability to read simple nonwords and frequent regular and irregular words, in addition to passage reading fluency, can also be assessed (Gersten et al., 2009). Multiple assessments tend to be more sensitive than information from only one (Gersten et al., 2009). Performance differences across assessments may help highlight areas of strength or weakness.

A stepped or gated assessment procedure will likely be most efficient (Compton et al., 2010; Fuchs et al., 2012). In this procedure, a single assessment or a set of brief assessments can be used to determine which children definitely are not at risk of reading impairment. Of those who are left, children below the cutoff score in the first screening assessment can be further assessed within the RTI model.

Most SLPs have access to PA measures, many of which contain tests of nonword reading. In addition, researcher-designed assessments of reading are available online for free, such as the MOTif (http://www.motif.org.au).

An SLP may need to construct their own assessments in some areas of concern. In these cases, it's important to keep records of children's performance so these can be compared to developmental reading skills. This will also require consistency of testing combined with flexibility in exploring areas of concern and teachability. Dynamic assessment is encouraged.

Some children with reading difficulties will already be on your caseload because of language disorders. As an SLP, you can adapt these children's intervention program to include written language.

PA can be expanded to include letter–sound correspondence. This additional knowledge is more effective for improving a child's reading than PA alone (Ehri et al., 2001). Similarly, vocabulary intervention can include exposure to written forms of words, which leads to better learning of both written forms and meaning (Parsons & Branagan, 2014;

Ricketts et al., 2009, 2015). Language intervention activities can include discussion of books or other written texts such as websites, magazine articles, and newspapers. Finally, an SLP, as part of the RTI team, can offer instruction to all students or can work with selected students within the classroom on curricular written materials.

As a last note, I offer a caution. A child's progress should be monitored throughout their school years. Early gains may fade over time (Tymms et al., 2017), and short-term intervention is likely not to be enough for those with the poorest word reading ability or the highest levels of risk. As the demands of the curriculum change, these children will probably need ongoing support (McMaster et al., 2005).

> ***Food for Thought:*** **Do there seem to be many pieces to assessment of reading? Why is that? Are there many related factors?**

Reading Assessment for Children With ASD

It is easy for some professionals to dismiss literacy concerns in children with ASD or to assume that all deficits are similar for these children. Differences exist that reflect severity of ASD and comorbid conditions (Westerveld et al., 2018).

As many as 65% of children with ASD have difficulty with literacy (Arciuli et al., 2013; Jones et al., 2009; Nation et al., 2006; Westerveld et al., 2018). Assessment of emergent literacy skills is therefore essential. Clendon et al. (2021) offer a very thorough tutorial on emergent literacy assessment for these children. The assessment should include all members of the educational team and be comprehensive and individualized.

In line with a functional approach, an assessment should extend beyond a child's skills and include the child's literacy environment at home and/or (pre)school (Clendon et al., 2021; Westerveld et al., 2017, 2018; Westerveld, Paynter, & Wicks, 2020). Emergent literacy skills are generally nurtured in these environments through interactions between a child and a parent/caregiver or educator.

Thorough literacy assessment of children with ASD is transdisciplinary and, in addition to the SLP, includes educators, school psychologists, reading specialists, and parents. Information can be collected using a variety of sources, such as a comprehensive assessment battery, informal questionnaires on home literacy, standardized parent questionnaires, teacher evaluations, and prior speech-language assessment. Additional information can include the child's communication skills at home and school, their interests and strengths, and the strategies and supports that help them learn best.

A comprehensive assessment battery should include both the (emergent) literacy skills of children with ASD (e.g., Nation et al., 2006; Westerveld et al., 2016) and the key emergent literacy skills important for supporting children's literacy learning as discussed in this chapter. These include the following:

- Letter name and letter sound knowledge
- Print concepts

- Early name writing
- Early developing phonological awareness
- Vocabulary knowledge
- Syntactic knowledge
- Text-level language skills

Clendon et al. (2021) offer a sample of such an assessment and considerations and guidelines for its use.

Given the nature of ASD, an assessment must take into consideration the individual child and be adapted accordingly. For example, a child who is nonverbal may use an augmentative and alternative communication device that should be included in the assessment process. Other considerations include who should participate in the evaluation, environmental supports, where the evaluation is to occur, modes of response, and the manner and time of the assessment.

Language-Based Reading Intervention

Language-based reading intervention focuses on areas of language that underpin and are essential for reading development. These may include oral language development, listening, and reading comprehension. Oral language development can focus on semantics or vocabulary, morphology, syntax or grammar, and pragmatics or language use. A more traditional area for SLPs, this type of intervention targets language disorder as it relates to reading and writing difficulties.

As we've seen throughout this text, it's never too early to begin. We'll start our discussion with early intervention and proceed through preschool to school age.

Early Literacy Intervention

A rich home literacy and oral language environment provides an important foundation for the more structured literacy environment of school (Terrell & Watson, 2018). A variety of direct and indirect practices in the home, child care, and preschool can support and enhance all aspects of oral and written literacy.

Emergent literacy (EL) consists of "literacy-like" behaviors that are acquired prior to formal reading and writing instruction (Saracho, 2017). Some of those behaviors develop prior to age 3 years, whereas others emerge in the preschool years.

The first experiences with print and early reading usually occur in the home within parent/caregiver–child interactions. Although young children are exposed to print in electronic media, the cornerstone of EL is shared picture book reading in which a young child learns about picture and symbol representation. Shared reading exposes a child to print and print concepts. Educators can use similar literacy experiences with young children who may not have this exposure at home.

Early literacy exposure can have a significant impact on a child's later literacy and academic development. In addition to other communication concerns, an SLP can help families and day care centers recognize the importance of early literacy experiences (Terrell & Watson, 2018). ASHA (2008a, 2008b) recognizes the importance of EL and recommends that literacy be addressed as both a prevention and an intervention measure.

Coaching is a recognized early intervention parent-teaching model (Rush & Shelden, 2011). Literacy coaching might involve modeling a technique to the caregivers. A few strategies are presented in Table 13–3. For a fuller list, see the tutorial by Terrell and Watson (2018).

As mentioned in Chapter 3, working with parents and caregivers includes minimal instruction accompanied by modeling, coaching, soliciting of caregiver comfort and feelings, and providing evaluative feedback, along with a healthy dose of encouragement. The SLP will most likely need to remind caregivers that the goal is vocabulary building, narrative skills growth, and "grammar" expansion, not reading per se.

Preschool Emerging Literacy

Preschool intervention may occur in a variety of settings. Some children will have a history of print exposure and well-developed EL skills, whereas others may have had only limited exposure to print and may lag behind their peers.

Table 13–3. Strategies for Early Shared Reading

Strategy	Example
Use engaging books	Shorter more limited text
Supply background knowledge	*This book is about a brown bear. You have a bear. Do you know about any other bears? Where do bears live? Yes, some live in the zoo.*
Engage children in conversation, making predictions, asking questions, pointing, commenting, "co-reading" familiar books	With young child: *I see a cow. Do you see a cow? Show me the cow. Yeah, that's a cow. What's a cow say?* With older child: *You know this one; what's he say? Let's read it together. You point to the words and I'll read.* With older child: *What do you think happens next?*
Follow the child's lead	Younger child: *That one? He doesn't look happy. He's . . . . Yes, sad. He's sad. He's sad because he lost his hat.*
Play interactively with the book	*This book is called "Where's Spot." The mommy dog can't find Spot. She's looking. Is he in the closet? Look; open the closet. No! He isn't in the closet. Who is? Who's in the closet?*
Use paralinguistics and nonlinguistics to increase interest	Vary intonation and loudness. Role-play different characters in the book. Use facial expression and gestures.
Use your finger to highlight words	*If I move my hand like this, it touches all the words I read. Listen. Now you move your finger and I'll read your words.*
Show younger children book conventions	*We hold a book this way. And we turn pages like this so we can read the story. We're finished reading this page. Can you gently turn the page?*

Source: Information taken from Terrell and Watson (2018), where you will find a wealth of ideas.

CHAPTER 13 LITERACY IMPAIRMENTS: LANGUAGE IN A VISUAL MODE

The Common Core State Standards (National Governors Association Center for Best Practices, 2010) state that by kindergarten, a child should recognize and name alphabet letters, associate sounds with letters, and be proficient in such phonological awareness tasks as identifying phonemes in simple words and substituting phonemes in single words to create new words.

Unfortunately, not all preschool classrooms are providing learning opportunities necessary to foster EL skill development (Mihai et al., 2017). An SLP can collaborate with teachers to develop and adapt teaching strategies for children's oral and written language skills, including a classroom literacy environment. Intervention may be direct; through collaboration, modeling, and coaching with teachers; and/or within an RTI model.

I'd be remiss if I didn't at least acknowledge the role of digital media. Thirty-eight percent of children younger than age 2 years have used a smartphone or tablet, and 80% of 2- to 4-year-olds have done so (Common Sense Media, 2013). Although digital media seem omnipresent, it's important to keep in mind that television, the Internet, and videos are no substitute for real-life interactions with people (Anderson & Pempek, 2005; Kirkorian et al., 2016; Kremar et al., 2007). Digital literacy is an important skill in today's world, but it's not the same as print literacy. Currently, there is no strong evidence for the use of apps or electronic media in intervention or the home for teaching EL skills.

Evidence-based practice (EBP) suggests that four possible preschool target areas are strongly related to later reading development (Justice & Kaderavek, 2004):

- Alphabet knowledge
- Print and word knowledge
- Phonological awareness
- Literate language

Alphabet knowledge consists of knowing the features and names of letters in both upper- and lowercase. In contrast, print and word knowledge is knowledge of how letters form words and the ways that pages (left to right) and books (front to back) are organized. PA, as mentioned previously, involves awareness of the sound and syllable structure of oral language. Finally, literate language differs from oral language in its use of vocabulary and syntax, such as elaborated noun phrases, to create text.

These written conventions differ from those used in speech. Although primary responsibility for EL instruction falls upon the classroom teacher, the SLP has expertise in some areas in which teachers are unprepared.

SLPs can collaborate with early childhood teachers to use print-focused read-alouds with children with language disorders to improve early literacy skills, such as children's alphabet knowledge, print concepts, and name-writing skills. Print knowledge gained in this way has both short-term and long-term benefits; results do not fade over time (Justice et al., 2017).

Print and Word Knowledge

By age 3 years, most children in the majority culture are familiar with books; can recognize their favorite books; and have the rudiments of print awareness, such as knowing the direction in which reading proceeds across a page and through a book, being interested in print, and recognizing some letters (Snow et al., 1999). **Print awareness** includes these skills plus later-developing ones, such as knowing that words are discrete units; being able to identify letters; and using literacy terminology, such as *letter*, *word*, and *sentence*.

Print knowledge can be conceived as encompassing both print concept knowledge and alphabet knowledge (Justice et al., 2006). Print knowledge is a generalized concept of what print does and how it is organized. In contrast, alphabet knowledge is the ability to identify and name letters or orthography. Print knowledge can be taught through verbal and nonverbal means that help a child attend to the shapes of words and letters and the function of written symbols.

These strategies can easily be adapted into shared book reading. For example, a child could move their hand across a page and the adult can read words as the child points. Techniques such as this have been found to improve the print knowledge of children with language disorders and those from low-SES backgrounds (Justice et al., 2017; Lovelace & Stewart, 2007).

Print knowledge activities can occur throughout the day in a variety of contexts. Teachers and parents can be taught to effectively use these techniques while engaging in shared book reading (Justice & Ezell, 2000, 2004).

Print knowledge can be increased among preschool children with print-focused reading activities that emphasize word concepts and alphabetic knowledge (Justice & Ezell, 2002). Print-focus prompts are presented in Table 13–4.

Print-focused prompts are easy to teach, and parents and caregivers have been successful with only minimal training. For example, the adult can easily point to words as they read to a child. As a result, the child learns about print through the behavior of the parent or caregiver. Print referencing has been shown to facilitate development of word concepts and alphabet knowledge as well as print concepts (Ezell et al., 2000; Justice & Ezell, 2002).

Curriculum supplements such as Read It Again! (RIA; Justice & McGinty, 2016) offer downloadable materials (https://www.pdfdrive.com/read-it-again-prek-e21697951.html) for use with 15 commercially available children's books and are an alternative to high-cost language and literacy curricula, which often require ongoing intensive professional development. RIA and similar material offer a viable means of enhancing the language and literacy instruction within preschool classrooms and increasing children's grammar and vocabulary and literacy skills, such as rhyming, alliteration, and print awareness (Justice et al., 2010).

For emergent readers who fail to achieve adequate reading, intervention is different from that addressed with prereaders and includes phonemic awareness, phonics, fluency, vocabulary, and reading comprehension. As in prereading difficulties, some of these areas are best addressed by an SLP. To date, Early Interventions in Reading (Vaughn et al., 2006) is the only literacy intervention with demonstrated effectiveness for children who are English language learners (ELLs).

For preschool and kindergarten children with language disorders, the transition from emergent readers to readers can be facilitated by an integrated multitiered intervention approach using both embedded and explicit approaches. Children demonstrate widespread EL gains with both explicit and implicit methods that can occur within embedded approaches, which we'll now explore (Justice et al., 2003).

CHAPTER 13 LITERACY IMPAIRMENTS: LANGUAGE IN A VISUAL MODE

Table 13–4. Print-Focus Prompts

Print-Focus Strategy	Examples	
Nonverbal	Point to print in text or to print in illustrations.	
	Follow print with finger while reading.	
Verbal		
Print conventions	Ask questions	Do you read this way or this way?
		And this one says?
		Where would you read if you were telling this story?
	Comment	We start here and turn the pages this way.
		That one tells you what the boy says.
	Requests	Show me how to hold a book to read.
		Call you show me where it says "Help"?
Word concepts	Ask questions	Where is the last word on the page?
		Is "cat" a word?
	Comment	This word says "cow."
		This says "hungry" and this says "caterpillar." We put them together to make "hungry caterpillar."
	Request	Show me the first word.
		You point to the words and I'll read.
Alphabet knowledge	Ask questions	Do you know this letter? What does it say?
		What's the first letter in "bear"?
	Comment	That's a B. It makes the /b/ sound.
		Where's Spot. Bet we can find her. Spot begins with S, just like your name, Susan.
	Request	Show me where the P is.

Source: Adapted from Justice and Ezell (2002, 2004).

Embedded Approaches

In embedded approaches, children's growth is fostered through high-quality daily literacy experiences and interactions with print that are placed within meaningful literacy activities. The goal is to maximize children's use of print through a literacy-rich environment (Towey et al., 2004). Other elements may include the following:

- Morning message board with words to count and segment and sounds to blend into words, or for finding words that begin with a selected sound or rhyme

- In-school breakfast and lunch menus with printed words and picture

- Matching games throughout the day using sounds and rhyming
- Recipes with words and pictures
- Music, finger play, and rhyming
- Identifying beginning sounds within themed activities, such as the names of different kinds of trucks (e.g., *F-iretruck*, *M-ixer*, *D-umptruck*)
- Sorting tasks by rhyming

Embedding might include labels on items in the classroom, increased availability of children's books, and shared story reading with adults. These approaches may be more effective than more explicit models in increasing young children's positive orientation to reading.

Interestingly, language difficulties of young children with DLD are not sufficient to account for their poor print knowledge. Instead, the quality of home literacy experiences seems to play an important role in fostering their print knowledge (McGinty & Justice, 2009). These findings suggest a strong home literacy component to any intervention with young children with DLD.

Book Sharing. One frequently suggested early literacy intervention is *interactive reading*, in which an adult reads a text to a child (or children) while making use of specific linguistic strategies, including asking questions, commenting on pictures, and expanding on the child's utterances. Also called shared reading, interactive reading as an intervention tool incorporates three key features (Kaderavek et al., 2013; Mol et al., 2008):

- It can be provided in the home and school environment by parents and education professionals.
- It uses familiar and engaging books.
- It is often a part of family and school routines.

Preliminary results suggest that digital texts can be used similarly (Boyle et al., 2017).

Individual book sharing accompanied by targeted questions can improve both literal and inferential language skills among Head Start preschoolers with language disorders (van Kleeck et al., 2006). Examples of questions and prompts for correct answers are presented in Table 13–5. Book sharing accompanied by dialogue is an excellent activity for promoting oral language, including syntax, semantics, and language comprehension (van Kleeck, 2003). And it can be fun!

Sustained and intensive preschool, kindergarten, and first- and second-grade intervention can reduce reading difficulties among at-risk children (Justice, 2006). As little as a 15- to 20-minute daily block of dedicated literacy time in preschool may be sufficient to forestall reading difficulties for many children (Kame'enui et al., 2000). This increases to 30 to 45 minutes in kindergarten and 90 minutes by first grade.

Books are a stable source of linguistic forms and content. Adults can use a variety of strategies, such as open-ended questions, repetition, modeling, expansion, and cloze techniques, to facilitate the child's participation and learning. Used appropriately, shared

CHAPTER 13 LITERACY IMPAIRMENTS: LANGUAGE IN A VISUAL MODE

Table 13–5. Literal and Inferential Questions and Prompts for Use in Guided Reading

Question	Feedback/Prompt
Level I (literal) What's that?	*Correct:* Repeat correct answer and "Yes, it's a X." *Incorrect:* Build a bridge to the correct answer. "Yes, it's a kind of Y called a . . . " *No response:* Prompt with the beginning sound or syllable, and if still no answer, tell the child and provide more information.
Level II (literal) What's the bunny doing?	*Correct:* Repeat correct answer and "Yes, he's X-ing (*running, jumping*, etc.)." *Incorrect:* Build a bridge to the correct answer. "Yes, that's the bunny and he's . . . " *No response:* Prompt with the beginning sound or syllable, and if still no answer, tell the child and provide more information.
Level III (inferential) How do you think the bunny feels when he finds all his friends are hiding?	*Correct:* Repeat correct answer and "Yes, I think he feels X because Y. Do you ever feel X? *Incorrect:* "I think he feels X because . . . " After child gives reason, add "Yes, the bunny feels X because (repeat child's reason)." *No response:* "Bunny feels . . . " If no response, "Bunny feels X because Y. Do you ever feel X?"
Level IV (inferential) What do you think the bunny will do next to find his friends?	*Correct:* "I think so too. The bunny wants to X so he can Z. Shall we keep reading and see?" *Incorrect:* "I think he's going to do X so he can . . . " After correct response, "Yes, I think so too. He's going to X so he can Y." *No response:* "Bunny wants to Y, so he's going to X."

Source: Information from van Kleeck et al. (2006).

book reading has been shown to increase vocabulary and overall language and literacy development (Justice & Kaderavek, 2004; Justice et al., 2005).

Intervention techniques for the home should not only be effective but also must be accomplished with minimal disruption to family routines. Although we may expect families to participate in their child's intervention and become agents of change, it is too much to expect that most parents will be able to carry through with very structured teaching programs that place an undue burden on the family.

Parents from CLD backgrounds who are participating in family literacy programs based on European American practices may encounter programs that do not approximate their patterns of interaction with their children. This could jeopardize success with their children. This is where collaboration and flexibility come into play.

An SLP would need to exercise caution when attempting to get parents to change their interactive style. Disregarding differences between a program's inherent interaction practices and those of families can result in poor intervention outcomes and limited parent participation (Janes & Kermani, 2001; Kummerer et al., 2007). Culturally relevant intervention programs are essential.

Book sharing is one of a series of prereading suggestions for children with ASD. Frequent and repeated shared book reading can increase oral language and attention (Bellon et al., 2000; Koppenhaver & Erickson, 2003). Books for children with ASD should contain simple pictures; predictable stories with clear cause-and-effect relationships or goal-directed behavior; events that can be related to everyday experiences; and elements that can easily be contextualized with manipulative props, such as puppets or action figures (Bellon et al., 2000).

Phonological Awareness

Phonological awareness skills progress along a continuum that can be used to create instruction within the preschool curriculum. It's recommended given the age of the children and the potential difficulty of the concept that lessons be short but frequent (Callaghan & Madelaine, 2012), possibly by integrating PA into classroom activities. That's called functional intervention.

Multimodality instruction, including visual input and physical movement, can be combined with auditory input. Phoneme identification and letter identification should be separate initially and later combined for maximum effectiveness, especially in word decoding (National Early Literacy Panel, 2008). Many ideas for PA intervention can be found in the tutorial by Terrell and Watson (2018).

Preschool children with early literacy delays can benefit from a supplemental PA curriculum such as PAth to Literacy (Goldstein, 2016), which consists of 36 daily scripted 10-minute lessons with interactive games (Goldstein et al., 2017).

Response to Intervention

Literate language skills of preschool children without identified language disorders but with low oral language skills can be addressed within an RTI model. For example, intervention might occur in frequent 20-minute blocks across the curriculum and target sentence-level syntactic and semantic features, such as prepositions, conjunctions, adverbs, and negations (Phillips et al., 2016). Children receiving this supplemental instruction are reported to show significantly educationally meaningful gains. To read about such an approach in more detail, see Phillips and colleagues (2016).

Embedding vocabulary instruction into shared book reading within early childhood educational settings is an effective way to teach challenging vocabulary to small groups of high-risk preschoolers (Goldstein et al., 2016). The wide range of language skills among preschoolers requires that a multitiered approach similar to RTI be used (Gettinger & Stoiber, 2008; VanDerHeyden et al., 2007, 2008). It's important that intervention

- uses existing classroom resources;
- is explicit;
- teaches important instructional targets;
- supports learning through scaffolding; and
- provides opportunities for children to participate (Foorman & Torgesen, 2001).

CHAPTER 13 LITERACY IMPAIRMENTS: LANGUAGE IN A VISUAL MODE   581

Adherence to these principles is important for change.

Story Friends is a supplemental preschool intervention program in which prerecorded vocabulary and comprehension instruction are embedded in specially designed storybooks (Greenwood et al., 2016; Kelley et al., 2015; Spencer et al., 2012). Although we discuss the curriculum briefly, I suggest you read the expanded discussion in Kelley and Goldstein (2014).

Designed to accompany a variety of curricula, Story Friends has been used effectively with RTI Tier 2 vocabulary instruction, although the program seems less effective with story comprehension (Goldstein et al., 2016). In vocabulary intervention, sophisticated vocabulary words were targeted using explicit instruction.

Vocabulary words may come from individualized lists that conform to curricular needs. Selection criteria might include vocabulary words that

- are unlikely to be familiar to preschool children with limited vocabulary;
- are likely to occur frequently in sophisticated spoken and written language;
- can be defined with a simple, child-friendly explanation; and
- can be supported in the story context with explicit instruction (Spencer et al., 2012).

Explicit instruction can include reference to a story and to children's everyday routines and experiences and provide opportunities for children to use the word.

Summary

Preschool EL intervention is important for children with language disorders and for those without. Some children with language disorders will not be identified until school age. In addition, despite programs such as Head Start, a need for intense exposure to literacy in preschool continues to exist, especially for children from CLD backgrounds (Hammer et al., 2003).

School-Age Intervention

Language-focused intervention can positively impact students' performance on curricular measures of vocabulary, comprehension monitoring, and understanding narrative and expository text, and also on reading comprehension measures (Language and Reading Research Consortium et al., 2019). An example of language-focused intervention is the Let's Know curriculum (Language and Reading Research Consortium et al., 2017), which includes instruction targeting vocabulary, narrative ability, and listening comprehension and integration of text skills.

Given the increasing popularity of ebooks and multimedia input, we might wonder if these forms are as effective as typical (static) books for word learning. Although both static and video books are effective in increasing knowledge of unknown words, static books are most effective (Smeets et al., 2014). The presence of background music or sounds decreases word learning for children with language disorders, possibly due to attention-allocation problems with speech perception in noisy conditions.

RTI has mostly been implemented for reading and math. Within an RTI framework, an SLP can help teachers focus on critical reading concepts, such as print knowledge, alphabet skills, and PA. As an SLP, you can then provide Tier 2 instruction supplementing classroom learning opportunities. Tier 2 interventions can target more rapid EL skill development. Two critical components are strategies and techniques to foster children's acquisition of phoneme awareness and print concept knowledge.

The most effective language and literacy intervention centers on knowledge deficits rather than processing limitations. Although intervention targeting basic perceptual or cognitive processes, such as attention and memory, often has more rapid gains than knowledge-based interventions, such as language skills, these gains show less retention and generalization (Kamhi, 2011).

Explicit Approaches

Explicit approaches include direct instruction. Some areas, such as PA, may be best suited to an explicit approach. Ideally, explicit instruction would be provided in the classroom, in small groups, and individually.

The classroom teacher is primarily responsible for embedded learning and for explicit whole-class instruction. Through collaboration, intervention team membership, and classroom activities, the SLP can support the classroom teacher while fostering children's growth in literacy.

Children with dyslexia need specialized instruction to develop their phonological, orthographic, and morphological awareness and their ability to coordinate this knowledge in word decoding and spelling (Berninger, Raskind, et al., 2008; Berninger & Wolf, 2009a, 2009b). Those with DLD, LD, or other print deficits may need specialized instruction in word retrieval to overcome their difficulty in applying executive functions to long-term memory search, and in syntactic awareness and text inferencing (Cain & Oakhill, 2007; Silliman & Scott, 2009).

Let's begin our discussion with a two-stage conceptualization of reading intervention and then look at specific language targets, such as vocabulary and phonological awareness. Of particular interest are reading comprehension and identifying main ideas.

Two-Stage Intervention. In a two-stage intervention model (van Kleeck, 1995), stage 1 establishes a meaning foundation where an adult reader scaffolds the reading for a child by placing the text in context and asking questions to guide comprehension. The child learns that print contains the meaning and gains PA and letter knowledge.

In stage 2, form foundation, PA and alphabetic knowledge are emphasized. Phonological teaching includes syllables and subsyllabic units, such as initial phonemes, or onsets, and rimes, or the remaining part of the word. Rhyming and alliteration activities also would be used. Training in alphabetic knowledge would include learning uppercase letters, followed by lowercase, copying shapes and letters, sound–letter correspondence, and knowledge of meaning found in books read to the child by others.

Four levels of abstraction of meaning are presented in Table 13–6. The first two require concrete skills, such as naming and describing, whereas the latter two require children to make inferences and to reason.

CHAPTER 13 LITERACY IMPAIRMENTS: LANGUAGE IN A VISUAL MODE 583

Table 13–6. Levels of Abstraction

Level	Intervention Strategies
I: Matching perception	Name and label characters, objects, and actions Find characters or objects named Direct adult's attention to a character, object, or action
II: Selection analysis/integration of perception	Describe characteristics, parts, or personal qualities of characters or objects Describe scenes and actions Recall previous information from the text
III: Reorder/infer	Summarize two or more events or actions in the text Describe similarities or differences in characters, actions, or events in text
IV: Reasoning	Predict what will happen next in text Consider causes for actions or events in text Explain actions or events in task Describe emotions of characters in text and possible influence on behavior

Sources: Information from van Kleeck (1995) and others.

Later reading intervention might target both linguistic and metalinguistic skills, including recognition of key words, use of all parts of the text such as the glossary and the index, and application of general learning strategies such as graphic organizers.

Each child brings a sense of self to the therapeutic situation. In part, this self-concept has grown out of their interactions with family and immediate community members. If as an SLP you fail to recognize and include these dimensions of an individual's social identity, it can negatively impact intervention (Demmert et al., 2006).

Intervention for Vocabulary. A strong correlation exists between vocabulary and reading comprehension (Biemiller, 2005). Understanding word meanings would seem to be essential for comprehension. In fact, children with lower-than-average reading comprehension make greater gains in text comprehension following robust vocabulary instruction than do typical readers (Duff, 2019).

An SLP can prioritize vocabulary words as we discussed in Chapters 11 and 12. A multi-pronged approach would consist of direct instruction with repeated exposures, modeling of word meanings and relationships, direct teaching of synonyms and antonyms, and discussion to promote word usage. Although the research is limited, use of a word's written form when teaching a word leads to improved learning of its spelling and spoken form (Colenbrander et al., 2019).

Intervention for Pragmatics. The ability to comprehend and produce narratives appears to be particularly important for academic success (Catts et al., 2006; Clarke et al., 2010; Colozzo et al., 2011; Larney, 2002; Nation et al., 2004). Both production and understanding of the complex language found in narratives can be improved with intervention, as noted in Chapter 11 (Clarke et al., 2010; S. Gillam et al., 2012; Petersen, 2011; Petersen et al., 2010, 2014; Spencer et al., 2014; Spencer & Slocum, 2010).

Intervention for Phonological Awareness.

In emergent reading, a child is focused on sounding out words by matching sounds to letters and then blending these sounds into words. This ability depends on both phonemic awareness and phonics.

Simply stated, phonemic awareness is the ability to manipulate sounds in speech. Phonics is an understanding of how letters represent sounds.

As a child progresses, the reading process becomes more automatized and fluent. As an SLP, you can support students who are experiencing difficulty with speech sounds and reading.

> ***Food for Thought:*** Would Michael benefit from phonological awareness teaching? Or does he need something more based on comprehension strategies?

SLPs have distinct and extensive knowledge related to PA and can play a critical role on educational teams (Cunningham et al., 2004; Moats & Foorman, 2003; Spencer et al., 2007). For example, SLPs can contribute to their school teams' efforts to enhance children's PA acquisition in several ways (Schuele & Boudreau, 2008):

- Boost other team members' knowledge by contributing their expertise
- Provide a unique perspective in assessment decisions
- Collaborate with classroom teachers and reading specialists to enhance PA instruction within the general education curriculum
- Provide small-group PA intervention to struggling students

Although classroom instruction focuses on children's achievement of specific curricular outcomes, an SLP's intervention focuses on the individual learning needs of children who are not achieving these desired classroom goals. I suggest that you read the excellent article by Schuele and Boudreau (2008) for a more in-depth discussion of PA and EBP than we can have in a text.

Direct, explicit instruction has been found to be effective, especially for students in the primary grades (Gersten et al., 2009; Torgesen, 2004; Wanzek et al., 2010; Wanzek & Vaughn, 2007). SLPs typically begin with manipulating phonemes in spoken language and relating these manipulations to print. Visual input can be used along with the SLP's "If we take /d/ away from . . ." as the child manipulates the corresponding letters.

Phoneme Awareness. Intervention for phoneme awareness can be effective with preschool children, even those with speech sound disorders (Gillon, 2005). Developmental intervention for phoneme awareness can include the following:

- Phoneme awareness and identification
- Letter identification
- Encoding and decoding print

Phoneme awareness teaching activities can be placed within play activities and can include the following (Gillon, 2005):

- Phoneme detection (*Find the word that starts with . . . or Does . . . begin with . . . ?*)
- Phoneme categorization (*Find all the toys that begin with . . .*)
- Initial phoneme matching (*Ball begins with /b/. Find the one that begins the same sound as ball. Book or Doll?*)
- Phoneme isolation (*What sound does pony start with?*)

Letter–name and letter–sound intervention can begin with recognition of letters that vary widely in their appearance and accompanying sound. Within words, it's best to begin with the letter in the initial position. Picture cards should contain the word written under the picture so children can begin to match sound and letter.

Phonological Awareness. As a child masters letter–sound correspondence, the SLP can shift emphasis to blending and segmenting words and then to decoding and encoding. Next, a student uses spellings of parts of words to read multisyllabic words and to begin to automatically recognize words with irregular patterns.

Fluency is the ability to read connected text smoothly, rapidly, and with minimal errors. As you might assume, if a child is spending more cognitive energy on sounding out words, fluency and comprehension suffer. After a child develops some automaticity in word recognition, they practice to achieve fluency. Once a child can read fluently and with prosody, it's easier to self-monitor comprehension.

Teaching PA is akin to teaching problem-solving and can be accomplished through the SLP's repeated modeling with multiple examples and guided practice by the child. The SLP provides a framework for accomplishing the task. This might take the following form (Schuele & Boudreau, 2008):

- SLP introduces a word and comments on a sound or syllable, as in "The first sound in the time is /t/."
- SLP repeats the process and has the child repeat the sound or syllable.
- SLP asks the child a question, as in "What's the first sound in time?"

Although this is a bare-bones example, it can be spruced up with some fun and silliness, such as "Is the first sound in time a (cough)?"

Through this or a similar step-by-step process, the child learns the task as well as the correct answer. Using words in the child's environment or favorite books makes the entire process more functional.

Ideally, each step supports subsequent steps. For example, data suggest that segmenting a word into phonemes may be easier if the child has used the word in rhyming and matching initial sounds. Previous exposure to the word may provide the child with practice analyzing the characteristics of the word even though the child has never been asked to segment the word's component sounds.

Whenever possible, PA should be taught within meaningful text experiences. In this way, the emergent nature of both literacy and phonological awareness can be used. Environmental signs, such as *stop*, *women*, and *Main Street*, can be used to enhance training.

Multisensory approaches are also helpful and can make the training interesting. For example, during auditory training, children can respond to target sounds by dropping objects into cans, stacking toys, playing hopscotch, or taking turns in any number of child games. Although typically developing children seem to benefit more than most children with DLD from computer-supported phonological awareness intervention, the method still holds promise as one aspect of a comprehensive intervention plan (Segers & Verhoeven, 2004).

Within *rhyming*, the SLP can use a variety of tasks that vary in the amount of support provided to the child (Adams et al., 1998; Anthony et al., 2003). The child can be asked if two words rhyme, choose one of three words that does not rhyme, match rhyming words, or generate their own rhymes (Schuele & Boudreau, 2008).

Rhymes may be more easily recognized by children when articulation of the final sounds are visible, such as labial sounds. Rhyming words that end in consonants (*stop*) seem to be easier than rhyming words that end in vowel sounds (*stay*).

Segmenting and blending are based on broader PA skills. It seems to make sense to target low-level skills, such as rhyming, to the extent that they facilitate development of more complex PA skills, such as segmenting into syllables and sounds and blending into words.

SLPs and teachers should work to ensure that each child has a sufficient foundation in PA to enable them to benefit from general education decoding instruction (Schuele & Dayton, 2000). At the very least, this involves the following (Schuele & Boudreau, 2008):

- The ability to consistently and independently segment and blend consonant–vowel (CV), VC, and CVC words
- An emerging ability to segment and blend words with consonant clusters or blends (CCVC, CVCC)

Once blending and segmenting are established, the SLP can provide a link between PA skills and classroom decoding and spelling instruction by providing practice that facilitates the application of phonemic awareness knowledge to spelling and decoding words (Blachman et al., 2000).

Teaching segmentation is easiest for children if the SLP begins with larger units, such as words, and proceeds to smaller units, such as syllables and then phonemes. Within words, however, shorter words with fewer syllables and single consonants are easier than multisyllabic words with blended consonants. When progressing to multisyllabic words, obvious units, such as syllables in compound words, as in *football* or *cupcake*,

CHAPTER 13 LITERACY IMPAIRMENTS: LANGUAGE IN A VISUAL MODE **587**

are easier than compound words, such as *telephone*, in which the units are not readily identifiable (Schuele & Dayton, 2000). When segmenting words or separating them into their constituent sounds, note the following (Blachman et al., 2000):

- Consonants are easier to segment than vowels.
- Initial sounds are easier to segment than final sounds.
- Syllable final /r/ is particularly difficult.
- Continuing phonemes, such as /s/ and /ʃ/, seem to be easier to analyze than stop phonemes, such as /p/ and /t/. It's possible to elongate continuing sounds to make them more salient for children.
- Shorter words, such as CV, are easier to segment than longer words, such as CVC.
- Initial sounds are easier to segment than final sounds.
- Single consonants, as in CV words, are easier to segment than blended consonants, as in CCV.
- Blended consonants may be easier to segment if the phonemes are produced in different locations, as in the /st/ in *stop*, than if they are produced in the same location, as in /mp/ in *stamp*.
- Segmenting words with blends, such as *bring*, may be easier when the child has had practice segmenting a subunit of that word, such as *ring* (Blachman et al., 2000).

Letter representations can be physically manipulated to add another element to training.

Regarding *letter–sound knowledge*, printed letters can be used to support phoneme learning, especially if letters are used in the classroom. Again, a functional approach tries to incorporate use contexts, such as the classroom, as much as possible. Letters give additional input, are a potential memory aid, and are functional for generalization to reading. For children with deficits in verbal WM, letters can offer a compensatory visual aid.

It is important to remember that intervention is for phonological awareness, not reading per se. It is very tempting to try to teach reading, but that is not the job of an SLP.

Letter–sound knowledge can be viewed as consisting of recognition, or pointing to a letter or letters when a sound or consonant blend is presented; recall, or saying a sound or sounds when a letter or consonant blend is presented; and reproduction, or writing a letter or consonant blend when the sound or sounds are heard. In general, recognition is easier than recall, which in turn is easier than reproduction (Dodd & Carr, 2003).

Vowels offer a particular problem because of the number and inconsistent spelling in English. An SLP can begin with short vowels because they are the nucleus of the longest syllables, called closed syllables. Closed syllables have rimes that end in at least one consonant and may have a maximum of six phonemes in the word, as in *scrimp*. Children can be taught common rimes such as *-ent*, *-old*, and *-ick*.

Long vowels can be introduced later, first in the VCe form, in which the "e" is silent, as in *ate*; followed by the open syllable with no consonant in the coda, as in *tray* or *she.* Appearing in short syllables or syllables with unusual spellings, long vowels can be taught as intervention assumes more of a reading focus. The inconsistent spelling of long vowels can be seen in *day*, *weigh*, and *raise*.

Training of the phoneme–grapheme relationship should be approached cautiously following the previous outline. Some sound–letter relationships, presented in Table 13–7, are particularly difficult.

Intervention for Morphological Awareness. Reading and spelling accuracy can be improved through instruction in MA together with other forms of linguistic awareness, including knowledge of phonology, orthography, syntax, and semantics (Kirk & Gillon, 2009). For example, MA intervention has resulted in improved reading and spelling performance for late elementary school students (Berninger et al., 2003).

Intervention focuses on increasing awareness of the morphological structure of words, with particular attention to the orthographic rules that apply when suffixes are added to the base word. For example, the "y" in *happy* and *crazy* changes to an "i" before the *-ly* marker in *happily* and *crazily*. Intervention tasks might include the following (Kirk & Gillon, 2009):

- Segmenting words into syllables and morphemes.
- Combining affixes and base words. For example, comparing the agentive *-er* suffix and the comparative *-er* suffix, as in *healer* versus *bigger*, helps children understand that suffixes are more than just graphemes, and that they alter the meaning of a word in predictable ways.

Table 13–7. Difficult Phoneme–Grapheme Relationships

Phoneme	Examples	Explanation
/r/-controlled vowels	Thr*ough*, tr*ue*, cr*ew*	Inconsistent spelling
diphthongs	Fl*y*, h*eigh*t, r*igh*t	Inconsistent spelling
/ɛ/	Sof*a*, t*e*lephone	Stress and spelling interact
/ʌ/	F*u*n, w*o*n, *o*ne	Multiple spellings
Grapheme	**Examples**	**Explanation**
-nk	Tha*nk*s, ri*nk*	Two phonemes /ŋk/
x	Ta*x*i, ma*x*imum	Two sounds /ks/
u	t*u*ne, f*u*n	Two pronunciations /ʊ/ and /ʌ/
Plural *-s*	Dog*s*, cat*s*, kisse*s*	Multiple pronunciations
Past *-ed*	Walk*ed*, jogg*ed*, collid*ed*	Multiple pronunciations
-pt	Ke*pt*, sle*pt*	Final blend has short stop

Source: Information from Hambly and Riddle (2002).

- Generating new words for each morpheme in a given word.
- Identifying base words and common affixes, such as *un-, non-, dis-, -er, -est, -ing, -y, -ed, -iest, -ier, -ly, -ish, -en*, and *–ened*.
- Identifying orthographic changes to the base word when a suffix is added, as in consonant doubling in *shopping*, e-dropping in *riding*, and y → i in *funniest*.
- Recognizing semantic relationships between morphologically complex words.

The transparent or opaque nature of morphological derivations affects both reading speed and accuracy. In transparency relationships, a base word does not change when a morphological affix is added, as in *active–actively*. In opaque relationships, the base word changes, as in *piano–pianist*. The more opaque the relationship, the more difficult the word is to read.

As an SLP, you can help older students by "morphing" words into parts and helping children hear the sound changes while appreciating the spelling consistencies, as in *sign–signature*. A fun activity is "Comes From," which employs underlying semantic relationships (Green, 2004). In this activity, the SLP poses questions such as "Does *mother* come from *moth*?"

Teaching morphology along with variations in the related English phonology and orthography results in improvement in the reading and/or spelling abilities for mid-elementary-age children (Murphy & Diehm, 2020). For example, a root word such as *please* changes little in pronunciation or spelling when modified to *pleased, unpleased, displease, displeased*, and *pleasing*. Pronunciation of the root does change, however, with morphological endings such as *-ant* and *-ure*, as in *pleasure, displeasure, unpleasant*, and *pleasant*. Phonological training is enhanced with the use of orthography.

Intervention for Comprehension. Comprehension relies on many different aspects of processing. When we read, our knowledge and experience blend with the information on the page to form a mental representation of the meaning. An active reader makes inferences from the text and past knowledge and experience that bridge these gaps.

One strategy for developing oral language comprehension is shared book reading. For example, the SLP can preteach essential vocabulary and then, while reading, ask questions to engage a child, encourage use of vocabulary, and help with recalling information and drawing inferences.

Text Comprehension

An SLP can provide instruction to develop background knowledge; focus on strategy instruction, such as predicting, clarifying, monitoring, and summarizing; and incorporate story grammar for narrative text comprehension and structure for expository comprehension. This instruction can occur before, after, and throughout the reading process.

An SLP or teacher can facilitate this process through instruction, questions, visual and verbal cues, explanations, and comments (Crowe, 2003). Shanahan and colleagues (2010) report strong evidence for the use of evidence-based reading comprehension strategies, which include activating background knowledge, questioning, visualization, monitoring, inferencing, and retelling.

> *Food for Thought:* Are you an active reader, checking what you know and comparing it to what you knew before? Do you draw in other sources of information and summarize what you know?

The variability in reading comprehension strongly suggests that effective instruction should be tailored to a child's abilities across specific texts and tasks. In other words, intervention is not a one-size-fits-all model.

As an SLP, in addition to thoroughly assessing a child's reading ability, you'll need to identify educationally relevant reading comprehension activities and directly address the component skills and knowledge bases involved in these activities (Catts & Kamhi, 2017). For example, reading comprehension within academic reading tasks might be addressed by teaching a general reading comprehension strategy. This would include learning to identify the main idea, evaluate the evidence, and consider the bias of both the author and the reader.

Comprehending Word Meanings. When we analyze children's eye movements while reading, we begin to understand that their eyes are bounding ahead and back, trying to check the accuracy of words within the surrounding meaning. Children are sense-makers, and when they read, they are trying to make sense of the words on the page.

In similar fashion, they can be taught to use this information to determine word meaning (Owens & Kim, 2007). They can also be helped to use dictionaries and glossaries, to analyze words into roots, and to use sentence structure to acquire word meaning.

The effect of different adult strategies is dependent on when they are used. For example, whereas semantic strategies prior to reading reduce reading miscues or errors, graphophonemic strategies are more effective during reading (Kouri et al., 2006).

Semantic strategies consist of giving a definition or synonym for key words. In contrast, graphophonemic strategies include encouraging a child to "sound out" a word, calling a child's attention to phonetic regularities, or asking a child to identify initial or final sounds or consonant blends.

Activation of prior knowledge improves comprehension, especially for children with LD. As a student reads, they gather information that is kept current and used to interpret following passages. Once students can successfully access this knowledge, they can be helped to use it to predict subsequent information from the text. In addition, children can be helped in applying past learning and experience to the comprehension task.

Comprehending Content. By providing contextually supported intervention, such as establishing the content and setting the scene prior to reading, establishing relationships, and discussing unfamiliar vocabulary and concepts, an SLP or teacher assists students in constructing meaning from print.

CHAPTER 13 LITERACY IMPAIRMENTS: LANGUAGE IN A VISUAL MODE

Using a conversational style, the adult provides cues and feedback as oral group reading occurs. It's important that questions used by adults reflect the level of comprehension targeted and not simply ask all students to recount facts from the page. The strategy can be accompanied by more direct vocabulary instruction, especially for words related to specific curricular topics, such as *ecology* or *geometry* (Ehren, 2006).

Intervention for comprehension of written narratives with younger children could include learning narrative structure and the use of mnemonics to aid retrieval. Older students could be taught about characterization and plot development. These general skills will be tailored for the specific book and task.

As young adolescents enter middle school, they are expected to read informational texts, summarize the details, answer questions related to the texts, and make inferences. An SLP can target strategies for accomplishing these tasks. In addition, the SLP can provide more information about the topic, which is critical to understanding informational texts. For example, the SLP can supplement the text with other sources of print and digital information, such as YouTube videos; enactments; or demonstrations. Effective readers use knowledge and multiple strategies to comprehend text.

Poor reading comprehension in adolescence is often related to deficits in word reading ability, lexical development, and syntactic development (Nippold, 2017). All the strategies mentioned previously may have limited results if a child has difficulty reading at the word level. Improving the accuracy and/or fluency of word reading improves reading comprehension (National Institute of Child Health and Human Development, 2000). These data suggest that intervention should target the underlying areas of deficiency as well.

Comprehension can be enhanced by inferential thinking that goes beyond the text and helps children integrate their world knowledge with the information on the page. This may consist of dialogue between the teacher and students to help students construct meaning as they read, not just at the conclusion of the story. The teacher can provide background information or encourage students to use their own knowledge sources.

Periodically during reading, you can help students summarize the story and/or select the main idea or ideas. Finally, they can contemplate alternatives, explain motives, personalize the story, and predict what will happen next in the story based on the information to this point.

Active Goal-Specific Strategies. Ideally, students will internalize comprehension strategies and use them as they read actively. Three types of strategies are goal-specific strategies, monitoring and repair, and packaging (Ehren, 2005, 2006). Goal-specific strategies include the following:

- Using context to analyze word meaning
- Activating prior knowledge
- Rereading difficult passages
- Self-questioning to help frame key ideas
- Analyzing text structures to determine type of reading
- Visualizing content

- Paraphrasing in one's own words
- Summarizing

These strategies are used in tandem with monitoring and repair strategies, in which a reader decides if a reading passage makes sense and, if not, what repairs need to be made so that it does. On the basis of these answers, a reader decides which of the goal-specific strategies to continue, discontinue, or modify. Finally, packaging strategies organize the entire process, planning what to do and how to do it through the other two types of strategies. It's this active aspect of reading that truly constitutes self-regulated reading. Let's take a look at some goal-specific strategies in more detail.

Good readers recognize when they have not comprehended a written passage and therefore reread it. Poor readers may not realize that they have missed key points. Several of the strategies presented here will help students with language disorders recognize what they don't know. When this is highlighted for them, a teacher or SLP can guide them to reread portions of the text.

Self-questioning is a strategy that encourages a reader to be active and to make inferences that the author hopefully intended the reader to make. Students should be encouraged to ask questions about the structure, such as when and where a narrative occurred, and about specific content, such as why a character acted a certain way.

Text structure provides information that assists readers in determining overall organization and important points. Students can be instructed in the use of text structure to assist comprehension, modeling, and guided and independent practice, including "think-alouds" to evaluate one's progress. Explorations to be made by a reader include

- the type of text, expository or narrative;
- visual cues that aid in figuring out the organization, such as headings, introductory paragraphs, and topic sentences;
- overall organization;
- the most important ideas; and
- devices that signal how ideas are connected.

By helping children with language disorders visualize the content, written material, especially narration, comes alive. Imagery can be taught as a strategy for increasing comprehension.

Paraphrasing and summarizing can occur at various points in reading, such as the end of a paragraph or a passage. Good readers do this automatically as they read. Paraphrasing demonstrates a child's comprehension by forcing a child to focus on the meaning and to replace content words and/or syntactic structure with equivalent forms. In order to paraphrase and summarize, students with language disorder may need to be helped in identifying the main idea in what they read.

Identifying the Main Idea

Children with language disorders often cannot find the main idea or organizing frame even in simple texts. This task is fundamental to comprehension and academic success.

Structure of narrative and expository texts differs greatly and affects comprehension and memory. Readers or listeners go through a process of deleting, generalizing, and integrating a text until they reach a macrostructure that summarizes the propositions presented. This process is dependent on underlying cognitive classification skills and world knowledge.

Understanding develops as the readers progressively revise their expectations until they approximate the meaning of the author. Organizational clues supplied by the author enable the reader to interpret the passage and determine the main ideas. Several textual features signal important information, including graphic features, such as italics, boldface, and type size; syntactic features, such as word order; semantic features, such as summaries and introductions; and schematic features, such as text structure.

Good readers are sensitive to the text organization. Many children with language disorders fail to realize the internal organization of the text. These children may fail to integrate new information with prior knowledge or fail to use the author's clues. Poor readers use a fragmented organization or impose an unrelated structure.

Intervention might include active comprehension strategies, such as predicting, questioning, clarifying, and summarizing; semantic networking; generative tasks in which the child generates a summary sentence; and familiarization with different text structures. Summarizing strategies used by older children include deletion of unimportant and redundant information, categorical organization of information, and selection or creation of a topic sentence. Helping children organize and reorganize structure into semantic networks during and after reading improves reading comprehension, writing cohesion, retention, and recall.

Adult-aided scaffolding or the construction of character and plot maps can aid comprehension. Scaffolded character event maps paired with a review of the previous chapter's map aids comprehension for adolescents with ASD (Williamson et al., 2015). The review of the previous map aids prediction about the upcoming chapter.

Ideas can be displayed in semantic networks as clusters resembling spiders. Major ideas are circles or other shapes. Lines form related ideas or connect major ideas. Semantic clusters can be taught with a guided study approach that helps the child develop generalizable strategies. Slowly, students adapt and internalize the methods for reading comprehension and for writing.

Organizational patterns are of two types: cluster and episodic. Cluster patterns are for superordination and subordination. In Figure 13–2, the topic, or superordinate aspect, is in the center. Related ideas radiate outward. Episodic organizers representing change move from event to event as in narration. These also can be used for problem–solution and cause–effect diagrams.

Children can begin to use semantic organizers in kindergarten or first grade, drawing pictures for the sequence of events in a narrative. Older children can write events in each cluster, either to aid recall or to structure narratives for telling or retelling.

Variations, such as the story map, can help children develop story grammars. Similar diagrams, such as the mind map, can be adapted to various purposes, such as a book report, newspaper article, or argument. Likewise, classroom brainstorming can help children realize their prior knowledge by examining all they know about a given topic.

Summarizing expository and narrative passages is an important academic skill for adolescents. The type of expository text may impact student performance. In addition,

Figure 13–2. Examples of semantic networks.

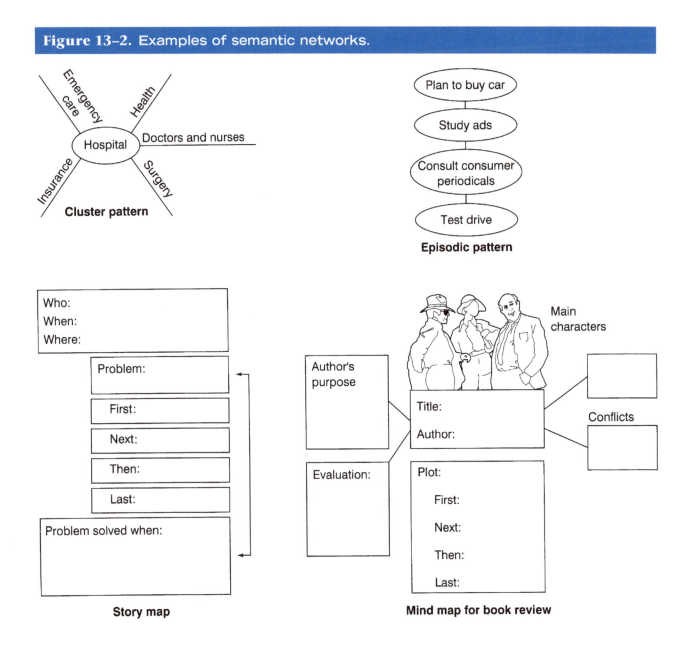

cognitive ability heavily impacts summary quality (Lundine et al., 2018). For example, cause–effect summaries seem to have better syntax and be of a higher quality than compare–contrast summaries.

As SLPs, we are interested in language and in helping children make sense of the language they receive and produce. This includes both what they hear and read. Now let's discuss children with CLD backgrounds and then proceed to writing.

Children With CLD Backgrounds

Providing culturally responsive intervention is extremely important for children with CLD backgrounds. For example, an SLP can integrate culturally based stories into shared storybook intervention (Inglebret et al., 2008).

CHAPTER 13 LITERACY IMPAIRMENTS: LANGUAGE IN A VISUAL MODE

Responding to children from CLD backgrounds means much more than simply having pictures of children of color in the materials being used. Even books translated from another language may have been unintentionally altered to reflect a Eurocentric perspective. Being culturally responsive may involve the SLP collaborating with people in the community.

Although materials for use with children from CLD backgrounds may already exist, not all stories accurately reflect a culture's norms or values. Again, it is best to consult with members of the ethnic community before using such materials.

For bilingual Spanish–English ELLs, structured intervention including emphasis on grammatical elements in the broader context of both speech and reading intervention can lead to significant gains in the production of morphosyntax in conversation and narration (Bedore et al., 2020). This change can be seen across both languages.

Writing

As with all language modes, writing is a social act. Just like a speaker, the writer must consider the audience. Because the audience is not present when the writing occurs, writing demands more cognitive resources for planning and execution than does speaking.

Writing is a complex process that includes the generation of ideas, organization and planning, action based on the plan, revision, monitoring, and self-feedback. More abstract and decontextualized than conversation, writing also requires internal knowledge of the writing form. Forms can be divided into narrative and expository writing.

Expository texts have several forms. The easiest type, especially with familiar content, is sequential or procedurally organized. A typical sequential text explains how something is accomplished. Problem-solving, cause-and-effect, and compare-and-contrast genres are more difficult.

Writing consists of several processes: text construction, handwriting or typing, executive function, spelling, and memory (Berninger, 2000). Text construction is the process of going from ideas to written texts. The author selects words and sentences that support their ideas.

Executive function is the self-regulatory aspect of writing. It's the ability to select and sustain attention, organize perception, and flexibly shift perceptual and cognitive setup, as well as control social and affective behavior. Furthermore, executive function includes

- realistic self-appraisal of strengths and weaknesses and the difficulty of tasks;
- the ability to set reasonable goals;
- planning and organizing to achieve each goal;
- initiating, monitoring, and evaluating one's performance in relation to each goal; and
- revising plans and strategies based on feedback.

Language use and executive function are interdependent.

Young writers must first develop a foundation in text generation and transcription (spelling, handwriting, and punctuation) before they can divert cognitive resources to higher level processes, such as planning and revising. Among upper-level elementary school children, the process of encoding thoughts and ideas into meaningful words, phrases, clauses, and sentences generally limits the planning and revising components of writing seen among older adolescents and adults (Berninger, 2000).

Spelling is a complex process with multiple components and skills, including the following (Bear et al., 2016; Williams et al., 2017):

- Mastery of letter-to-sound relationships
- Understanding letter and syllable spelling patterns
- Understanding the meaning layer, including word roots and affixes

The more effective a speller becomes, the more automatic the writing process. Automaticity frees a student's WM to enable greater focus on other writing processes.

Research has consistently shown that spelling and writing, which are both difficult retrieval tasks, benefit reading (Graham & Hebert, 2010; Shahar-Yames & Share, 2008), but the reverse is not true. For example, spelling has been shown to be a powerful self-teaching tool for the formation of word-specific orthographic information necessary for fluent reading (Shahar-Yames & Share, 2008).

The writing of Spanish-speaking early adolescent ELLs demonstrates similar lexical, syntactic, and discourse sophistication across both languages, indicating that these teens are emerging writers in both Spanish and English (Danzak, 2011). This implies the potential transfer of writing skills across languages.

Memory serves the writer in many ways. WM stores ideas as they are worked and reworked by the writer. Short-term memory is used for word recognition while writing. Long-term memory provides content and word knowledge as well as overall format. Automaticity of retrieving letters and words from memory and producing them contributes to the quality of text generation.

Writing Problems

Children with oral language disorders will most likely have writing disorders too. For many children with language disorders, writing difficulties do not decrease with age, and the gap widens between their writing abilities and those of children with TDL. The content and organization of their writing suffer because more of their cognitive capacity is used for the lower level mechanics of writing, such as spelling.

> ***Food for Thought:*** **Why haven't we discussed writing by hand? Is that outside the scope of SLP practice and better left to an occupational therapist? Will computer typing solve all the problems of letter formation that a child may have?**

Children with LD have difficulties with all aspects of the writing process. In general, children with LD fail to plan, make few substantive revisions, and write very little on a given task. Cognitive capacity is expended on low-order mechanics. Spelling often follows a maladaptive pattern in which words that can be spelled are substituted for those that cannot. In the process, meaning suffers.

In narrative writing as in oral storytelling, children with language disorders lack mature internalized story schemes. As noted in Chapter 7, the oral narratives of children with language disorders are often shorter with fewer episodes, contain fewer details, and often fail to consider the needs of the listener. Listeners are only rarely given cause and effect or character motivation.

In general, children with language disorders exhibit reduced written productivity as measured by total number of words, total number of utterances, or total number of ideas (Puranik et al., 2007; Scott & Windsor, 2000). Similarly, these same children exhibit deficits in writing complexity as measured by average length of T-units, number of different words, and percentage of complex sentences (Fey et al., 2004; Mackie & Dockrell, 2004; Nelson & Van Meter, 2003; Puranik et al., 2007). Finally, children with language disorders exhibit reduced accuracy as measured by number of spelling or mechanical errors and number of syntax errors (Altmann et al., 2008; Mackie & Dockrell, 2004; Nelson & Van Meter, 2003; Puranik et al., 2007).

Deficits in Executive Function

When executive function is impaired, as is often the case with traumatic brain injury (TBI), communication abilities are diminished, especially in socially demanding or complex linguistic tasks, such as writing. Executive function is especially important for the pragmatic aspects of communication, memory and retrieval, strategic thinking, perspective taking, and generalization. Several language disorders discussed in Chapter 3 evidence difficulty with executive function.

Executive function impairment is most evident in children with TBI. The high frequency of frontal lobe injury makes executive function particularly vulnerable in these children. Children with attention-deficit/hyperactivity disorder (ADHD) have been described as inattentive and impulsive, disorganized, unable to inhibit behavior, and ineffective learners—characteristics of those with impaired executive function.

When children with LD write, they follow a "retrieve-write" strategy in which they write whatever comes to mind, each sentence stimulating the next, with little thought to planning. The result is that they produce and elaborate very little. Revisions are ineffective and can be characterized by seeming indifference to the audience, inept detection of errors, and difficulty executing intended changes (Graham & Harris, 1999).

Deficits in Spelling

Writing and spelling are separate but correlated processes. Children with written-language deficits due to LD, DLD, or other causes may have problems in either or both.

Children with spelling difficulties may view spelling as arbitrary and random. To them, spelling is difficult and ultimately unlearnable. Poor spellers may also have parallel deficits in reading, especially in word attack or decoding skills. This sounds like Michael.

Spelling deficits represent poor phonological processing and poor knowledge and use of phoneme–grapheme information. The misspellings of the poorest older spellers suggest the following patterns (Moats, 1995):

- Omission of liquids and nasals in rime or noninitial positions, as in *SEF* for *self* and *RET* for *rent*
- Omission in consonant clusters, especially in the syllable and word-final positions, as in *FAT* for *fast*
- Omission of unstressed vowel, as in *TELFON* for *telephone*
- Vowel substitutions, as in *TRI* for *try*
- Consonant substitutions that share some articulatory features, as in "t" for "d" or "m" for "n"
- Omission of plural inflections
- Omission or substitution of past tense inflections
- Misspelling of difficult common words, such as *their/there* and *to/too/two*

Many poor spellers demonstrate primitive phonologically based errors even when they have high levels of orthographic knowledge.

Although most typical spellers shift to greater use of analogy (e.g., *pillage* is spelled like *village*) between second and fifth grade, poor spellers continue to rely on visual matching skills and phoneme position rules because of limited knowledge of sound–letter correspondences (Kamhi & Hinton, 2000). In other words, they continue to use the visual approach to learning that characterizes much younger spellers.

SLPs have expertise in the key areas, such as phonology, morphology, and semantics, that are important links between language and spelling. Although we discuss many of these links, you may want to read the tutorial by Carol Moxam (2019).

Assessment of Writing

One method of assessing writing in the classroom is through the use of portfolios of children's writing. Portfolios are a collection of meaningful writing selected by a child, SLP, and teacher that contains samples of the child's writing over time, enabling the child to demonstrate progress.

A wide variety helps increase the validity of the sample. Allowing children to contribute fosters self-growth and monitoring. In addition, selection of teacher and SLP choices fosters collaboration. Items to be included in a portfolio may include SLP observation notes; work samples; first drafts of writing samples, such as journal or learning log entries, and projects/papers and final drafts of the same; and peer and teacher evaluations.

Data Collection

A variety of formal and informal assessment methods exist. Although standardized tests can provide valuable information about a student's written language skills compared to

CHAPTER 13 LITERACY IMPAIRMENTS: LANGUAGE IN A VISUAL MODE

peers and are often necessary to demonstrate a written language disorder and to determine eligibility for intervention services, these tests do not typically provide the information needed to describe a child's specific difficulties and establish intervention goals.

Written language sampling can be used as an informal measure (ASHA, 2002; Nelson et al., 2004). A written language sample can be a rich source of information and a more holistic approach. In addition, written samples can be adapted to satisfy assessment needs and to reflect the curriculum in the classroom.

There's little consensus in the professional literature on the best way to collect a written language sample (Hudson et al., 2005). Writing samples have been gathered using a variety of methods.

Although adolescents acquire greater skill with expository writing, it seems appropriate with younger children to use narrative writing, such as spontaneous stories or story retelling from a book or video. In addition to reflecting the demands of the curriculum, including comprehending read-aloud material, holding key concepts in memory, and reformulating the information, a narrative retelling format gives the SLP some control of the stimulus input and a more reliable gauge of the accuracy of information recalled and the propositions and inferences made (Puranik et al., 2008).

Executive function is best assessed within an overall writing assessment or through dynamic assessment techniques. There is a risk in separating the various functions and considering them separately from functional communication tasks.

Whenever possible, the SLP can observe the writing process for evidence of planning and organizing, drafting, writing, revising, and editing. Samples should be written in pen to allow the SLP to note revisions. The teacher or SLP should inform children that edits are fine and encourage them to do their best. It's helpful to allow children to plan and to write drafts. Notes and plans can be encouraged and collected along with the finished product. These can be added to the portfolio.

Added information can be obtained if children read their paper aloud while being recorded. This procedure aids the SLP in interpreting garbled or poorly spelled words.

Narratives

Narrative tasks may be in response to the following (Price & Jackson, 2015):

- Storybook pictures, including wordless picture books
- The content of a video
- An oral prompt about a specific topic, such as a funny memory or special holiday
- An oral prompt about a nonspecific topic or topic of choice

A student can be asked to write a narrative for someone who isn't present at an event or did not view the book or video. Specific procedures will vary with the task.

Written narratives can be sorted into two broad categories: personal and fictional. An SLP will want to sample both due to their prominence in the curriculum.

Personal written narratives can be elicited using a format found on many states' fourth-grade writing examination (Puranik et al., 2008). This generally takes the following form:

Think about your favorite thing to do . . . . Maybe you like to . . . . Write a story about a fun time that you had doing your favorite thing. Give enough details to show the reader what happened and why it was fun. (Massachusetts Department of Education, 2006)

Of course, this information may need to be simplified for children with language disorders.

Expository Writing

Expository texts can be elicited by a number of procedures. For example, sequential/procedural texts can be elicited by asking the child, "Tell me how you make *X*." With the cause-and-effect genre, the SLP might say, "Tell me what might happen if *X*." Problem-solving genres can be encouraged with "How would you *X*?" It is important to pose familiar and unfamiliar themes. Key words, such as *describe*, *compare*, *contrast*, *cause*, and *solve*, can cue the child for the type desired.

Expository writing, called informational/explanatory writing in the Common Core, is a broad category that includes compare–contrast, problem–solution, procedural directions, descriptions, and cause–effect (Singer, 2007; Ward-Lonergan, 2010). Students are expected to be able to write a variety of types of informational/explanatory texts.

Tasks that might be used for eliciting informational/explanatory writing samples include (Price & Jackson, 2015)

- describing isolated pictures;
- describing and explaining without pictures, such as using a newspaper or magazine article;
- comparing–contrasting tasks similarities and differences; and
- retelling of expository text, such as a prerecorded passage or podcast.

Obviously, students will need some instruction, discussion, and verbal prompting.

Data Analysis

As with spoken language, several aspects of written language can be analyzed, including word level, sentence level, discourse, and genre-specific measures. Some of this analysis will be familiar based on our discussion of oral samples. Table 13–8 provides a summary of possible analyses at each level (Price & Jackson, 2015).

Word-level analysis includes vocabulary and spelling. Vocabulary could be analyzed in general or based on the specific course or content relative to the topic. One cautionary note is that students may avoid writing words they can't spell, so additional measures may be needed.

Sentence-level measures should focus on syntax, including length, complexity, and correctness. One measure of syntactic length is the T-unit or C-unit. As you may recall, a T-unit is a main or independent clause plus the subordinate or dependent clauses

CHAPTER 13 LITERACY IMPAIRMENTS: LANGUAGE IN A VISUAL MODE

Table 13–8. Levels of Writing Analysis

Word-level measures	Vocabulary use
	
	    Number of different words (NDW); type–token ratio (TTR)
	
	    Specific: Common Core Standards
	
	Spelling
	
	    Orthographic patterns
	
	    Words and word parts (syllable patterns)
	
	    Grade-level words (Common Core Standards)
	
	    Percent correct
	
	        Characterize spelling errors based on phonology, orthography, and morphology

Sentence-level measures	Syntactic length (MLU_W of T-units or C-units) Syntactic complexity (subordination index/clausal density; clauses/T-units) Syntactic correctness (percent grammatical T-units; percent correct complex sentences)
Discourse-level measures	Punctuation and writing conventions (Common Core Standards) Capitalization at the beginning and use of period at the end (percent correct sentences) Overall productivity Length (total number of written words or total number of T-units or C-units)

Source: Information taken from Price and Jackson (2015).

attached to it or embedded within it (Hunt, 1970). Examples of T-units can be found in Chapter 7. For written samples, C-units, which include elliptical utterances, may be very similar to T-units given that these are highly unlikely to occur in writing, unless the child is using dialogue.

Syntactic complexity can also be measured by calculating the subordination index (SI), also called clausal density and clausal complexity by some authors. SI is the total number of independent and dependent clauses in the writing sample divided by the total number of T-units in the sample. In essence, we're calculating the average number of clauses per T-unit.

Discourse-level measures may include punctuation and writing conventions, overall productivity or the amount written, and features specific to each writing genre or type. Writing convention would include use of capitalization.

Genre-specific measures include both organization and structure. Each genre has a unique overall organization and structure. To become effective writers, students need to learn to convey information within these constraints. For example, narratives consist of event sequences not typically found in other types of writing. An SLP could calculate the number of story grammar elements present in several narratives.

Expository writing can have a variety of organizational structures related to the purpose of the writing task. For example, compare–contrast writing has different requirements than cause–effect explanations. Structure of expository writing might include the following (Hall-Mills & Apel, 2013):

● Easily identifiable structure appropriate for the task
● Well-developed structure
● Logical, clear sequence of ideas
● Clear, identifiable introduction with thesis, body containing supporting ideas and evidence, and a conclusion

Although few specific measures exist for persuasive writing, an SLP can note effectiveness and clarity.

In general, persuasive writing tasks use complex language to analyze and discuss topics clearly and to make one's case convincingly. This skill has application to work and life in general (Nippold et al., 2005).

Persuasive arguments are written by kindergarten through grade 12 students in a variety of classes. Students can be presented with a thought-provoking question requiring a persuasive answer. Topics could range from climate change to the best fast-food restaurant.

By adolescence, the expository writing of typically developing children has made several strides. Changes found in persuasive writing include increases in essay length, mean length of utterance measured in words, relative clause production, and use of literate words (Nippold et al., 2005). Literate words include adverbial conjuncts, discussed earlier (*however, finally, in conclusion, personally*), abstract nouns (*kindness, loyalty, benefits, pleasure*), and metalinguistic and metacognitive verbs (*think, remember, reflect, agree, persuade, confess*).

The greater flexibility of older writers is seen in presentation of greater numbers of reasons and acknowledgment of diverse perspectives and differing opinions. Average values are presented in Table 13–9.

Individual variation is great, and there is much overlap. It's important to recognize that the values in Table 13–9 will vary by task and represent a 20-minute writing sample based on a presentation of three diverse points of view and the instructions to state one's own perspective supported by several good reasons for the opinion.

Finally, overall effectiveness of a child's writing might be measured by a holistic scale of the entire sample. For example, the 6+1 Trait Writing Rubric (Education Northwest, 2018), used with both narrative and expository samples, rates a student's writing for ideas, organization, voice, word choice, sentence fluency, conventions, and presentation.

As discussed with oral samples, written samples can be analyzed by hand or using a computer. Computer-aided analyses can be accomplished using Systematic Analysis of Language Transcripts (Miller & Iglesias, 2015), the Computerized Language Analysis program of the Child Language Data Exchange System (MacWhinney, 2022), and Microsoft Word. Although not designed for written samples, Sampling Utterances and Grammatical Analysis Revised (SUGAR) (Owens & Pavelko, 2021) may also be used for quick measurement of some of the less complex features. All of these have been discussed previously.

CHAPTER 13 LITERACY IMPAIRMENTS: LANGUAGE IN A VISUAL MODE

Table 13–9. Parameters of Persuasive Writing by Age

	Age 11 Years	Age 17 Years	Age 24 Years
MLU-W (mean length of utterance in words)	11.3	13.9	15.9
Range	5.5–19.3	8.9–23.8	11.1–27
Below 1 SD	5.5–8.3	8.9–11.9	11.1–14.6
Total words	146.9	188.5	262.9
Range	33–297	86–321	146–481
Below 1 SD	33–88	86–139	146–215
Word types as percentage of total words			
Adverbial conjuncts	0.30%	0.77%	0.83%
Range	0–3.9%	0–2.8%	0–2.5%
Abstract nouns	2.70%	5.70%	7.80%
Range	0–6.3%	1.8–17.3%	3.7–16.4%
Metaverbs	1.30%	1.90%	2%
Range	0–3.7%	0–5.9%	0–4.6%
Total utterances	13.6	14.7	17.3
Range	4–30	5–33	7–37
Below 1 SD	4–9.8	5–10.6	7–12.7
Relative clauses as percentage of total utterances	11.70%	16.70%	20.80%
Total reasons	6.8	7.9	12.7

Source: Information taken from Nippold et al. (2007).

> ***Food for Thought:*** Would a written sample contain many language features found in speaking? Would there be additions? Deletions?

Spelling Assessment

Although it may seem straightforward, spelling deficits are very complex and can be difficult to describe. Collection should be of sufficient quantity to allow for a broad-based analysis of error types.

Data Collection

Spelling deficits can be assessed through both dictation and connected writing (Masterson & Apel, 2000). In dictation, either within standardized testing or from word inventories, the SLP or teacher reads words while the child writes them. Standardized tests include the Test of Written Language, Fourth Edition (Hammill & Larson, 2009); the Test of Written Spelling (Larson et al., 2013); and the Wide Range Achievement Test, Fifth Edition (Wilkinson & Robertson, 2017).

Word inventories, either preselected—such as those found in Bear et al. (2016)—or SLP-designed, should be developmental in nature and include several phoneme–grapheme variations, including, but not limited to, single consonants in various positions in words, consonant blends, morphological inflections, diphthongs, digraphs or two letters for one phoneme such as "ch" and "sh," and complex morphologic derivations as in *omit–omission*. The choice of words will vary with the age and functioning level of the child. The number of words should be sufficient to identify patterns of functioning. Using 50 to 100 words is probably adequate, although more is desirable (Masterson & Apel, 2000).

Single-word spelling may be of little real value because decontextualized spelling does not measure a child's ability in a real communicative context. More functional connected writing can be generated in response to pictures or narratives or provided portfolios. In a variation, the child can write an original sentence or narrative using representative words taken from word lists.

Testing tasks that require a child to select correctly spelled words may seem like a good assessment tool but may be of little actual value (Ehri, 2000). These tasks occur infrequently in the real world of the child and thus are not functional for either assessment or intervention.

Data Analysis

Descriptive analysis should focus on orthographic patterns evident in the child's spelling (Bear et al., 2008). Although individual errors are significant, error patterns are important for intervention. Of interest are the most frequent and the lowest level patterns.

As an SLP, try to determine the type of error reflected in the child's spelling of each incorrect word. It's helpful to analyze base words (*teach*), inflected words (*teaches*), and derived words (*teacher*) separately to see if errors are related to any specific word or morphological form. Spelling is the result of segmenting a word into phonemic elements and selecting the appropriate graphemes.

In analyzing the spelling sample, the SLP can note consonant blends by location within the syllable and word and by the presence of other phonemes. The SLP can seek phonemic (*EKWAT* for *equate*), morphologic (omits morphologic markers), or semantic (confuses similar sounding words, as in *there, their*, and *they're*) explanations for error patterns (Bourassa & Treiman, 2001).

Phonological processing and spelling are related for elementary school children, less so for older students who use multiple spelling strategies. If the child uses an incorrect letter, the error most likely represents a problem in phonological awareness. Inserted or deleted letters may represent a speech perception problem.

In addition, the SLP can look at each error to determine the child's orthographic system knowledge. This includes letter selection and position constraints. For example, "ts" is an acceptable blend but is constrained by position and is not acceptable at the

CHAPTER 13 LITERACY IMPAIRMENTS: LANGUAGE IN A VISUAL MODE

beginning of a word, with the exception of the Russian "tsar" and the Japanese "tsunami." Such knowledge addresses the question, *Could this be a word?* Has the child's error violated acceptable English spelling or would the resultant word be an acceptable one?

Language-Based Writing Intervention

SLPs can help students acquire writing skills relevant to the requirements of the Common Core State Standards (National Governors Association Center for Best Practices and Council of Chief State School Officers, 2010) and have a vital role in supporting students' literacy (ASHA, 2001, 2010). Although space precludes the in-depth discussion needed, I urge you to read the thorough and informative tutorial by Price and Jackson (2015).

Extended Writing

Ideally, writing instruction would

- be explicit and systematic;
- promote student practice; and
- provide ongoing scaffolding and feedback prior to students practicing writing skills on their own (Graham, 2006; McMaster et al., 2017).

Intervention for writing may involve both general training and more specific techniques for narrative and expository forms. Generalization is enhanced if intervention is functional, curriculum-based, and within authentic writing projects.

Children developing typically are able to print their first names by approximately age 4½ years, suggesting that emergent literacy/writing tasks be considered in late preschool language assessment and intervention. Children with DLD consistently display delays in PA, alphabet knowledge (AK), print awareness, and emergent writing. PA, AK, and letter writing are all important factors in name writing, suggesting that in intervention, all three areas of literacy can be taught simultaneously (Pavelko et al., 2018).

These skills are not singular entities to be treated in isolation but, rather, can all be taught in an integrated approach within developmentally appropriate activities. In other words, as SLPs teach one, they need to incorporate the others. Merely having children copy their names will not be as effective. All letters in a child's name can be used simultaneously to develop PA, AK, and letter-writing skills. *Emergent Literacy: Lessons for Success* (Cabell, Justice, Kaderavek, et al., 2009) provides evidenced-based emergent literacy intervention activities.

Executive function can be targeted within the writing process of older children using a *goal–plan–do–review* format. Although there is little SLPs can do to alleviate the root causes of TBI, ADHD, or other impairments relative to executive function, they can provide external support to enable children with these impairments to experience some level of success (Ylvisaker & DeBonis, 2000).

This should not be interpreted to mean that the SLP acts as the child's executive function. In that situation, little changes for the child. SLPs give children the tools to facilitate their lives by changing behaviors and processes.

Intervention can begin by allowing children to select their own topics. This increases motivation and shifts the focus to ideas. Mechanics will come later. Topic selection works well with small groups of children, and the sharing process often generates more ideas.

In the planning phase, the SLP and children can brainstorm ideas for inclusion in the writing. Drawings and ideational maps or spider diagrams can help. For narratives, children might draw a few simple pictures and organize them in the appropriate order. It is also useful for the child to focus on the potential audience. The SLP can ask questions such as the following:

Who will read your paper?

What do your readers know?

What do your readers need to know?

Why are you writing your paper? (What's your purpose?)

Computer programs can also be helpful but are no substitute for adult guidance.

Computer software, such as Inspiration-10 (TechEd Marketing, 2022), can aid text generation, and the result is easily modifiable by the child or teacher. Although the technology itself is unlikely to improve writing, it does remove the handwriting difficulties for some children.

Typing can also detract from text development, and computer use can result in new burdens for WM. However, note that children with LD who receive training in executive function along with word processing make greater gains in the quality of their writing compared to children instructed only in executive function. Word processing experience alone, however, does not improve overall quality.

A word about spellcheckers and grammar checkers seems in order. Neither are foolproof, as I'm sure you know. Spellcheckers are discussed in the section on spelling. Grammar checkers miss many errors, especially if there are multiple spelling errors, and can easily confuse the writer, who is left to figure out just what is the error.

Word-prediction programs, such as Co:Writer (Johnston, 2022), Write Away (Thoughtful Learning, 2017), and Clicker 8 or Clicker Writer (Crick Software, 2022a, 2022b), may be helpful, but mostly for spelling. Most have speech synthesis too. Inputs vary from spelling only to spelling plus grammar.

It is important that the word-prediction program's vocabulary match the writing task of the child. Some programs allow for assignment- or teacher-specific words.

Finally, speech recognition software allows children to compose by dictation, resulting in longer and higher quality papers by children with LD. Children must be instructed to speak clearly in order to improve speech recognition and to dictate punctuation and formatting. Speech-recognition software cannot overcome oral language difficulties, although these can be moderated with the additional use of grammar checkers.

Narrative Writing

A correlation exists between oral language and written language ability. We cannot stress enough the implications of this relationship for writing intervention. Oral narrative instruction has a positive effect on children's writing (Spencer & Petersen, 2018).

Narrative writing may require explicit instruction in story structure, as outlined in Chapter 11. Story maps using pictures or story frames may be necessary initially but should be faded gradually as the child assumes more responsibility for the narrative. Story frames are written starters for each main-story grammar element. The child completes the sentence and continues with that portion of the narrative. Cards or checklists can also be used to remind the child of story grammar elements. Some software also has story elements to guide composition.

During the writing process, the SLP can use story guides, prompts, and acronyms to aid the child. Story guides are questions that help a student construct the narrative, whereas prompts are story beginning and ending phrases. Acronyms, such as SPACE for *setting*, *problem*, *action*, and *consequent events*, can also act as prompts for guiding writing. Children can be encouraged to write more with verbal prompts such as "Tell me more" or "What happened next?"

Feelings and motivations found in mature narratives are often missing from the stories of children with language disorders. These elements can be targeted with pictures and questions such as "How do you think she felt?" (Roth, 2000).

Expository Writing

Procedures for intervention with expository writing include collaborative planning; individual, independent writing; conferencing with the teacher/SLP and peers; individual, independent revising; and final editing (Wong, 2000). Whatever the expository genre involved, collaborative planning is important, including planning, writing, and revising. In the first step, the child should think aloud and solicit opinions. This is an opportunity for the child to hear alternative views and to reconcile these with their own.

For opinion papers, the child first needs to choose a topic. These might come from a prepared list, from the child, or from topics discussed in class. Once the topic is selected and discussed in small groups, with a peer, and/or with the SLP, the SLP can give the child a planning sheet to help organize their thoughts. It might include two columns: *What I believe* and *What someone else believes* (Wong, 2000). After the child has completed the sheet, either with help or working alone, the SLP can help the child form dyads of opposing views. This is a great time for verbal repartee, challenging, and helping the child clarify their views and prepare for independent writing.

Writing, although independent, can be fostered through the use of a prompt card containing key words for each major section of the paper. Table 13–10 presents a sample prompt card. After the child has completed the paper, the child conference with peers for feedback while the SLP mediates. The child revises the paper based on feedback.

At each stage in the process, the child should record progress on a checklist. In addition to providing a model for the writing process, the checklist can motivate the child as they finish each step.

Table 13–10. Sample Prompt Card for Opinion Writing	
Section of Paper	**Examples**
Introduction	In my opinion . . .
	I believe . . .
	From my point of view . . .
	I agree with . . .
	I disagree with . . .
	Supporting words: first, second, finally, for example, most important is . . ., consider, think about, remember
Counter Opinion	Although . . .
	However, . . .
	On the other hand, . . .
	To the contrary, . . .
	Even though . . .
Conclusion	In conclusion . . .
	After considering both sides, . . .
	To summarize, . . .

Source: Information from Wong et al. (1996).

For compare-and-contrast writing, the planning process can be similar. Again, the topic—which entities are to be compared—can come from prepared lists, the child, or the curriculum. Through brainstorming, the child and the SLP try to answer the question, "How can we compare them?" Be prepared for some comparisons that are very "original," especially from children who have perceptual deficits and may view the world quite differently from adults. Again, the child can be helped with writing prompts, such as the following:

In this essay, I'm going to compare and contrast . . .

I have chosen two (any number) features: . . .

In conclusion, . . .

As mentioned previously, peer, teacher, and SLP review and feedback can help the child revise.

In a study investigating the efficacy of teaching expository reporting skills through an intervention called Sketch and Speak, the authors reported that fourth to sixth graders with language disorders made significantly better improvement with this intervention (Ukrainetz, 2019). The intervention employs two types of note-taking and oral practice. The students in the intervention group received six 30-minute individual or paired sessions from an SLP. During treatment, students

CHAPTER 13 LITERACY IMPAIRMENTS: LANGUAGE IN A VISUAL MODE **609**

- reduce statements from grade-level science articles into concise ideas;
- record the ideas as pictographic and conventional notes; and
- expand from the notes into full oral sentences that are then combined into oral reports.

Student progress may be attributable to the treatment's simplicity, use of visuals, oral practice exercises, repeated learning opportunities, and visible progress.

Spelling

The SLP is not the "spelling teacher." It is as inappropriate for the SLP to teach this week's spelling list as it is to teach this week's vocabulary. Rather, the SLP's role is to help children learn to spell. *Reread this paragraph.*

Spelling interventions differ depending on the type of words a student is expected to learn. For example, strategies for memorization may be appropriate for irregular words that don't follow regular patterns.

> ***Food for Thought:*** **Do you rely on your laptop's spellchecker? Why does it work for you but less so for a child with a spelling deficit?**

Use of Computers

Computers are helpful and encourage editing, although spellcheckers are not foolproof and the child may learn little. In general, spellcheckers miss words in which the misspelling has inadvertently produced another word. Suggested spellings may also confound the child with poor word attack skills. In addition, suggested spellings may be far afield if the original word has multiple misspellings.

Spellcheckers help only approximately 37% of the time for children with LD, a lower percentage than found among children with TDL (MacArthur et al. 1996). On the other hand, word-prediction programs reduce spelling errors of children with language disorders by more than half, although the user must get the initial letters correct for the program to work effectively.

If children with language disorders are taught to spell phonetically when unsure of the correct spelling, spellcheckers generate more correct suggestions. Proofing and editing on a hard copy also seem to increase the number of correctly spelled words. Internet searches can foster spelling learning because correct spelling is needed to complete searches successfully.

Effective Spelling Intervention

Effective spelling interventions include the following (Berninger et al., 2000; McLaughlin et al., 2013; McMaster et al., 2017; Schlesinger & Gray, 2017; Wanzek et al., 2017; Williams et al., 2017):

- Direct and systematic instruction in letter–sound correspondences, such as the spelling of syllable patterns, morphemes, and irregular words.

- Monitoring and self-correcting spelling errors that provide immediate corrective feedback. A common method is one in which a student looks at a spelling word, covers it, copies it from memory, and then compares the written word to the correctly written version.

- Including strategies for spelling words and for self-monitoring their learning. Strategies might include word sorting, word hunts, flashcards, and peer practice with spelling words.

- Applying newly learned spelling skills in sentence writing and in written compositions. Typically, these activities begin with spelling to dictation in increasingly longer forms.

- Using multisensory activities, such as tracing three-dimensional letters with their fingers while saying the letters aloud to spell a given word.

These effective spelling interventions have been reported to improved spelling and also writing quality, writing fluency, and word reading skills (Berninger et al., 2000; McLaughlin et al., 2013; McMaster et al., 2017; Williams et al., 2017).

Much of our previous discussion of PA intervention is also applicable here. The benefits of early PA learning for spelling are well documented. In addition to spelling better by mid-elementary school than children who did not receive preschool PA teaching, children who did receive such teaching are more likely to employ MA—knowledge of root words and affixes—when spelling (Kirk & Gillon, 2007).

Words selected for intervention should be individualized for each child and reflect both the curriculum and the child's desires. Spelling intervention should be integrated into real writing and reading within the classroom. It is best if intervention can occur when the child is actually writing. During writing tasks, the child can be reminded of alphabetic and orthographic principles (Scott, 2000). Words misspelled in class can be analyzed by the SLP. Spelling strategies can be discussed with the child using these words.

Spelling can be taught within teaching of general executive function in which the child is taught to proofread, correct, and edit. Peer editing can also be effective.

Prompted spelling is helping a child identify the sounds in the word, such as the length of the vowel, and the orthographic pattern. With bound morphemes, the SLP might ask the child to recall what happens when the morpheme is added to certain words with long and short vowels, as in *roping* and *ripping*. Notice that many types of word knowledge are being activated. More on that later.

If needed, spelling intervention should begin with alphabetic principles, connecting sounds and letters. Targeted words can be taught as explained in the next few paragraphs but expanded into onset-rime training to facilitate overall spelling ability.

Children with LD benefit from multisensory input such as pictures, objects, or actions (Graham, 1999). Several multisensory study techniques have been proposed. For example, the child (1) says the word; (2) writes it while saying it again; (3) checks spelling; (4) if correct, traces it while saying it again; and finally, (5) writes the word and checks the spelling. In a variation, the child pronounces the word carefully. Letters are

CHAPTER 13 LITERACY IMPAIRMENTS: LANGUAGE IN A VISUAL MODE 611

pronounced in sequence, then recalled. The child then writes the word, checks, and if incorrect, respells and checks again.

In the 8-Step Method (Berninger et al., 1998), first, the SLP sweeps their finger over the word and pronounces it out loud. Next, to call attention to the phoneme–grapheme correspondence, the SLP says the word again, emphasizing sounds that correspond to colored letter groupings. For example, saying /b/-/i/-/d/ for "b"-"ea"-"d." On the third pass, the child names the letters as the SLP points to each in sequence. The child then closes their eyes and visualizes the word. In step 5, while their eyes are closed, the child spells the word out loud. Following this step, the child writes the word and then compares it to the sample. In the final step, the SLP reinforces the child's correct spelling. If the child's spelling is incorrect, the SLP points out the difference between the sample and the child's attempt and repeats the previous steps.

Word analysis and sorting tasks can be used to strengthen the alphabetic principle (Scott, 2000). Patterns to be taught should be identified from the child's misspellings. Minimum pairs that differ on the bases of these processes can be used to demonstrate the lexical consequences of misspelling (Masterson & Crede, 1999). The SLP should use known and unknown words to facilitate generalization.

Sorting tasks will differ based on the spelling level of the child (Scott, 2000). Sorting may be of various patterns:

- Morphological (*magic, magical, magically, magician*)
- Phonological (e.g., words that were phonologically identical except for the length of the vowel, as in *-ke* and *-ck* in *bake* and *back*, respectively)
- Orthographic (e.g., length of the vowel or consistent orthographic shape despite phonological variation as in the three variants of *-ed* in *walked, jogged,* and *glided*)
- Syntactic (e.g., by word class as noun, verb, or adjective and learning how these categories interact with various suffixes)
- Semantic (e.g., *to, too, two*)

At the letter–name level of development, words can be sorted or grouped by sounds and location, as in initial consonants or initial digraphs (two letters = one sound, "sh" = /ʃ/). Minimal pairs might contrast short vowels, long and short vowels, single consonants and blends, and one digraph with another.

With more mature spellers, the SLP can sort by orthographic patterns, such as vowel patterns, rimes, and homophones. In later stages, words can be grouped by syllable juncture principles and meaning, including inflectional suffixes and simple prefixes and derivational suffixes, consonant doubling with open and closed syllables, compound words, changing final "y" to "i," and word roots. Minimal pairs may contrast variants of inflectional suffixes, such as "-s" and "-es," and base words with derivational suffixes, as in *teach/teacher*.

Orthographic knowledge or knowledge on acceptable letter patterns, such as *sh, st, br,* and *er,* are a component of spelling. When you look at a word you've just typed, part of your evaluation is the way the word looks. Are the letter combinations allowable? In part, this knowledge comes from reading and seeing words in print.

Although children with DLD acquire the general knowledge of a written language's orthography, they have less well-represented word-specific orthographic knowledge compared to their peers with TDL (Williams et al., 2021). Because children with DLD are able to extract the orthographic features of a clue word (*bead*), such as vowel order, and use these to produce more accurate spellings (*dead*, *tear*, *deaf*), an orthographic approach to spelling instruction seems warranted with these children.

Spelling intervention is more meaningful if it occurs within authentic writing exercises, such as curriculum-based writing. Within these activities, children can be taught to ask themselves if they can identify word part or initial or final sounds. They can try to identify similarly sounding words or identify locations where the word has appeared. These can be checked for the correct spelling.

When all else fails, the student should try to find the word in the dictionary. This may be facilitated by use of a personal or class dictionary or dictionaries produced for different classroom topics. Computer spellcheckers may also be helpful.

Sentence Construction and Composition

Many children with language disorders struggle with both the cognitive demands of sentence construction and the skills needed to carry out the writing process (Datchuk & Kubina, 2013; Lienemann & Reid, 2008; MacArthur & Graham, 2016; Saddler, 2013). Composing a sentence is complex and cognitively demanding, requiring a writer to consider lexical, syntactical, grammatical, mechanical (e.g., punctuation), and rhetorical aspects of a sentence (Fayol, 2016). Lacking the linguistic skills for this task, children with language disorders often produce compositions that are less coherent and less complex (Saddler et al., 2008).

Effective intervention practices for sentence construction include the following:

- Direct instruction through modeling, guided practice, and independent practice in how to develop and write simple and complex sentences. Picture–word prompts, in which the child uses an illustration along with several related words, enable a student to describe the illustration without having to recall writing content on their own.

- Sentence-combining activities during sentence construction interventions. An SLP can aid a child by underlining parts of each kernel that should be retained in the combined sentence and highlighting connector words, such as conjunctions.

- Teaching of grammar skills within the functional context of actual writing assignments.

- Mnemonics for remembering steps in creating complete and interesting sentences.

Of most importance is providing opportunities for a child to apply sentence construction skills in their own writing and to get feedback from the SLP and/or peers.

Unlike skilled writers, children with language disorders may not consider what they know about a topic, how to present this knowledge to an intended reader, important elements, and the best text structure to convey these ideas (Graham, 2006; MacArthur & Graham, 2016). Thus, they require targeted interventions to address each of these areas of weakness. The following are common effective practices:

- A writing process approach, including planning, drafting, editing, revising, and publish; writing with a specific audience in mind; collaborative writing with peers; and mini-lessons as needed (Graham & Sandmel, 2011)
- Direct instruction during the writing process and the use of mnemonics for remembering steps in writing (Harris et al., 2008).
- Explicit instruction in writing strategies, instruction in self-regulation strategies needed, and provided background knowledge and writing knowledge, such as vocabulary used in a specific writing genre, elements of specific genres, and examples of the types of texts a student is learning (Harris et al., 2008)
- Frequent writing feedback during composition

Reported results of these types of intervention are increased writing quality including increases in the number of genre elements present and in the length of written texts (Gersten & Baker, 2001; Gillespie & Graham, 2014; McMaster et al., 2017).

Common instructional characteristics of evidence-based writing interventions are explicit, direct, and systematic (Berninger et al., 2000; Datchuk & Kubina, 2013; McMaster et al., 2017). SLPs and teachers can offer multiple opportunities for guided practice within an authentic or functional context, leading to increasing independence by a child (Berninger et al., 2000; Datchuk & Kubina, 2013; Graham, 2006; Troia, 2013).

Conclusion

Learning to use print is much more than just using another mode for transmitting language. Reading and writing demand new skills and tax a child's language in different ways. You the SLP are as vital in literacy intervention as you are in oral intervention. You are the language and language disorders expert.

Even in the area of literacy, functional communication is important. Using real reading and writing samples, training occurs within the kinds of reading and writing that the child is encountering in the classroom.

Keeping literacy intervention as functional as possible is especially important. For example, words are easier to spell in context. Remember, decontextualized training routinely fails at the level of memory and generalization.

Afterword

And so, we reach the end of this text. I hope that I have challenged your thinking along the way and that you'll use this book as a reference.

Functional language assessment and intervention require thinking. They're not easy. But the results are real.

Intervention in the classroom is about as close as a speech-language pathologist in the schools can get to the actual use environment of a child. Other aspects of the functional model that we have discussed may also be present. For example, parents or caregivers may be involved in their children's learning. Cues and consequences can still be as natural as possible. And the use environment is right there in the classroom and the content.

I hope our paths will cross someday, at a conference or a professional workshop. I wish you all the success possible as a future speech-language pathologist. You can have a rich, rewarding career if you choose to make it so.

APPENDIX A

Formal Language Measures

Assessment Measure	Date	Age	Statistics
Ages and Stages Questionnaire (ASQ)	2009	1–66 months	
Assessment of Literacy and Language (ALL)	2005	Pre-kindergarten–Grade 1	R = .88; Sn = .96; Sp = .89
Assessment, Evaluation, and Programming System for Infants and Children, 2nd edition (AEPS-2)	2002	Birth–6 years	
Bilingual English–Spanish Assessment (BESA)	2018	4–6;11 years	Sn = >.8; Sp = >.8
Carolina Curriculum for Infants and Toddlers with Special Needs, 3rd edition	2004	Birth–36 months	
Children's Communication Checklist, 2nd edition (CCC-2)	2006	4–16;11 years	
Clinical Evaluation of Language Fundamentals, 4th edition, Spanish (CELF-4 Spanish)	2014	5–21 years	
Clinical Evaluation of Language Fundamentals, 5th edition (CELF-5)	2013	5–20;11 years	R = .9; Sn = 1.0; Sp = .86
Clinical Evaluation of Language Fundamentals, 4th edition Screening Test (CELF-4 Screening Test)	2004	5–20;11 years	
Clinical Evaluation of Language Fundamentals–Preschool, 2nd edition (CELF-Preschool 2)	2004	3–5;11 years	
Communication and Symbolic Behavior Scales Developmental Profile Sample	2002	6–24 months	
Comprehensive Assessment of Spoken Language (CASL)	1999	3–21;11 years	R = >.9
Comprehensive Receptive and Expressive Vocabulary Test, 3rd edition (CREVT-3)	2013	5–89 years	
Computerized Profiling 9.7.0 (CP9.7.0)	2012	—	
Diagnostic Evaluation of Language Variance (DELV)–Norm Referenced	2005	4–9 years	

continues

Appendix A. *continued*

Assessment Measure	Date	Age	Statistics
Diagnostic Evaluation of Language Variance (DELV)–Screening Test	2003	4–9 years	
Early Language Milestone Scale, 2nd edition (ELM Scale-2)	2001	5–12;11 years	
Early Social Communication Scales	2003	8–30 months	
Expressive Language Test, 2nd edition (ELT 2)	2010	5–11;11 years	R = .91; V = .75
Expressive One-Word Picture Vocabulary Test: Spanish-Bilingual Edition (EOWPVT-SBE)	2013	2–70+ years	
Expressive One-Word Picture Vocabulary Test, 4th edition (EOWPVT-4)	2010	2–80+ years	
Expressive Vocabulary Test, 2nd edition (EVT-2)	2007	2;6–90+ years	R = .92; V = .77
Fluharty Preschool Speech and Language Screening Test, 2nd edition (FPSLST-2)	2000	3–6;11 years	
Fullerton Language Test for Adolescents, 2nd edition (FLTA-2)	1986	11–18 years	
Get Ready to Read–Revised	2001	4–4;11 years	
Language Processing Test 3: Elementary (LPT 3: Elementary)	2005	5–11;11 years	
Language Use Inventory (LUI)	2009	18–47 months	
McArthur–Bates Communication Development Inventories (MB-CDIs)	2006	8–30 months	
Montgomery Assessment of Vocabulary Acquisition (MAVA)	2008	3–12;11 years	
Peabody Picture Vocabulary Test, 4th edition (PPVT-4)	2007	2;6–90+ years	R = .9; V = .82
Phonological Awareness Test, 2nd edition (PAT-2)	2007	5–9 years	
Pragmatic Language Skills Inventory (PLSI)	2006	5–12;11 years	
Preschool Language Assessment Instrument, 2nd edition (PLAI-2)	2003	3–5;11 years	
Preschool Language Scale, 5th edition (PLS-5)	2011	Birth–7;11 years	R = .89; Sn = .83; Sp = .8
Preschool Language Scale, 5th edition (PLS-5) Spanish Edition	2013	Birth–7;11 years	
Rapid Automatized Naming and Rapid Alternating Stimulus Tests (RAN/RAS)	2005	5–18;11 years	

APPENDIX A FORMAL LANGUAGE MEASURES

Assessment Measure	Date	Age	Statistics
Receptive One-Word Picture Vocabulary Test: Spanish-Bilingual Edition (ROWPVT-SBE)	2013	2–70+ years	
Receptive One-Word Picture Vocabulary Test, 4th edition (ROWPVT-4)	2010	2–80+ years	
Receptive–Expressive Emergent Language Test, 4th edition (REEL-4)	2020	Birth–3 years	
Rossetti Infant–Toddler Language Scale	2006	Birth–36 months	
Social Communication Questionnaire (SCQ)	2003	4+ years	R = .71; V = .88; Sn = .85; Sp = .75
Social Language Development Test Elementary	2008	6–11;11 years	R = .85; V = .88
Spanish Language Assessment Procedures, 3rd edition (SLAP)	1995	3–9 years	
Spanish Test for Assessing Morphologic Production (STAMP)	1991	5–11 years	
Structured Photographic Expressive Language Test, 3rd edition (SPELT-3)	2003	4–9;11 years	
Structured Photographic Expressive Language Test–Preschool, 2nd edition (SPELT-P 2)	2005	3–5;11 years	
Test for Auditory Comprehension of Language, 3rd edition (TACL-3)	1999	3–9;11 years	R = .94; V = .7; Sn = .77; Sp = .84
Test of Adolescent and Adult Language, 4th edition (TOAL-4)	2007	12–24;11 years	
Test of Early Communication and Emerging Language (TECEL)	2011	Birth–24 months	
Test of Early Language Development, 3rd edition (TELD-3)	1999	2–7;11 years	
Test of Early Language Development, 3rd edition: Spanish	2007	2–7;11 years	
Test of Language Development–Intermediate, 4th edition (TOLD-I:4)	2008	8–17;11 years	
Test of Language Development–Primary, 4th edition (TOLD-P:4)	2008	4–8;11 years	
Test of Narrative Language (TNL)	2004	5–11;11 years	R = .92; V = .87
Test of Pragmatic Language-2 (TOPL-2)	2007	6–18;11 years	
Test of Problem Solving, Adolescent, 2nd edition (TOPS–2)	2007	12–17;11 years	R = .9; V = .94

continues

Appendix A. *continued*

Assessment Measure	Date	Age	Statistics
Test of Semantic Skills–Intermediate (TOSS-I)	2003	9–13;11 years	
Test of Semantic Skills–Intermediate (TOSS-I)	2003	9–13;11 years	
Test of Word Finding–2nd edition (TWF-2)	2000	4–12;11 years	R = .89; Sn = .83; Sp = .8
Test of Word Knowledge (TOWK)	1992	5–17;11 years	
Token Test for Children, 2nd edition (TTFC-2)	2007	3–12;11 years	
Transdisciplinary Play-Based Assessment, 2nd edition (TPBA-2)	2008	Birth–6 years	
Wiig Assessment of Basic Concepts (WABC)	2004	2;6–7;11 years	R = .93; V = .92
Wiig Assessment of Basic Concepts–Spanish (WABC-S)	2006	3–7;11 years	
WORD Test, 2nd: Adolescent	2002	4 years +	R = .89; V = .91
WORD Test, 2nd: Elementary	2014	6–11;11 years	R = .93; V = .87

Note: R, reliability; Sn, sensitivity; Sp, specificity; V, validity.

APPENDIX B

SUGAR (Sampling Utterances and Grammatical Analysis Revised) Procedures

Collection: SUGAR Robust Sampling

Collect only 10 minutes of conversation. This amount of time should be more than enough.

The most important aspect of talking with the child is to **avoid as many yes/no or product (one-word answer) questions as possible and to ask process question (How did/do . . .) or use "Tell me . . ." or "I wonder . . ." statements. Practice before collecting.**

- Turnabouts = Comment + Cue for child to talk
- Process Questions
  - *How did . . .*
  - *What happened . . .*
  - *Tell me . . .*
  - *I wonder what you . . .*
  - *Why did . . .*
    - More than one-word "why" questions
    - Not appropriate for kids below 4.5 yrs
- Use narrative elicitations instead of yes/no questions
  - Build on what the child says or on what you know
  - Begin with . . .
    - *Your mom says you. . . . That sounds like fun. Tell me what happened.*
    - *I know that you. . . . Tell me what happened.*
    - *Did you ever. . . . Tell me what you did.*

622   LANGUAGE DISORDERS: A FUNCTIONAL APPROACH TO ASSESSMENT AND INTERVENTION IN CHILDREN

If you have ten or more one-word child utterances preceded by a wh- product question or a yes/no question, your sample should **NOT** be considered to be robust.

SUGAR Rapid Transcription

Transcribe the sample directly onto your computer. Only type the child's utterances, NOT yours. Do NOT include identifying data. Set "Numbering," found on the tool bar in the "Paragraph" section, to ensure that you only type 50 utterances. Remember that an utterance is a sentence or less, separated by a pause, drop in voice, inhalation or combination of these. Do not belabor the process of utterance determination. Stop when you have 50 utterances.

Procedures For Transcribing (Think *Speed!*)

- Type in plain English as spoken.
- Omit immediate child imitations of the other speaker.
- Highlight all utterances that are imperative or elliptical so when you analyze each you will know that some information has been omitted by the child.
- Omit punctuation to save time.
- Do NOT embellish the child's utterance. In other words, don't add morphemes that are missing.
- Type words in full even when pronunciation omits portions as follows:
  - *Talkin'* should be transcribed as "Talking"
  - *Gonna*, *wanna*, *gotta*, *hafta* should be transcribed as "going to, want to, got to, have to"
- Type contractions as is. In other words, *don't* should be typed as "don't" and *I'm* as "I'm."
- Do NOT include fillers (uhhhh, ummm, like, you know).
- Do NOT include disfluences. **Only include the fullest form of what the child actually said**. Example: "He said . . . he says . . . he tell me secrets" becomes "He tell me secrets."
- Do NOT include repeated words unless it is for emphasis, as in "He went down down down in the cave."
- Don't spend an inordinate amount of time deciphering unintelligible utterances. If the entire utterance is unintelligible, omit it. If a word is unintelligible, type nonsense, such as "XX" in place of the word. If an utterance contains two or more unintelligible words, omit the entire utterance.
- If an utterance contains more than two clauses joined with *and*, consider it a run-on sentence and divide as follows:

  We went to the circus and I saw clowns and there were elephants and I got this sweet sticky stuff. but I didn't like it so I gave it to my sister.

APPENDIX B SUGAR (SAMPLING UTTERANCES AND GRAMMATICAL ANALYSIS REVISED) PROCEDURES **623**

Becomes . . .

We went to the circus and I saw clowns.

There were elephants and I got this sweet sticky stuff but I didn't like it so I gave it to my sister.

An utterance has only one "and" joining clauses. Do NOT do this with other conjunctions. Note in the previous example that the initial "and" was omitted in the second utterance.

Stop at 50 utterances. Save the document. Come out of your document. Hit Control-S for PC or Command-S for Apple/Mac to save.

SUGAR Analysis

Word Count

Before doing any actual analysis, make sure the "Numbering" function is off. Nothing else should be on the page except the child's 50 utterances. Turn "off" the "Numbering" function by highlighting the entire document (Control-A for PC, Command-A for Apple/Mac), going to the "Paragraph" section of the Toolbar and clicking on "Numbering."

Word count is on the tool bar at the bottom of your screen. Record the number of words before moving on.

MLU

Words are already separated by a space. Now set off bound morphemes in the same way. For example, "unhappily" would be "un happi ly," "bunnies" would be "bunnie s," and "can't" will be "ca n t." **Don't worry about the spelling of the pieces or about leftover apostrophes . . . time is of the essence here.** For example, "I' m un happi ly marrie d" counts as 7 words, although we know it's 7 morphemes were counting. **Follow the rules below for counting morphemes.**

Rules for Morpheme Counting (in order to speed the process)

- Count as one morpheme (Do not separate with a space)
    Ritualized reduplications (*choo-choo*)
    Irregular past tense verbs (*went*)
    Diminutives (*doggie*)
    Auxiliary verbs
    Irregular plurals (*men*)

- Count as two morphemes (Separate with a space)

  Possessive nouns (noun + *'s* or *s'*)

  Plural nouns (noun + *s*)

  Third person singular present tense verbs (verb + *s*)

  Regular past tense verbs (verb + *ed*)

  Present progressive verbs (verb + *ing*)

- Count as one morpheme each word in Proper names

- Additional bound morphemes to offset with a space

Morpheme	Example	Morpheme	Example
-ing Adjective Gerund	*Smiling girl* *I love hiking*	-ed Adjective	*Powdered sugar*
-ly	*Mostly*	-ment	*Entertainment*
dis-	*Dislike*	re-	*Refill*
-er Comparative	*Bigger*	-y Adjective	*Bumpy*
-est Superlative	*Biggest*	-sion -tion	*Discussion* *Invitation*
-ful	*Thoughtful*	Un-	*Unhappy*
-ish	*Foolish*		

- Count contractions (*do n't, I' d, he' s, we' ll, they' ve*) as two morphemes

- Count the traditional *uh-huh* (yes) and *uhn-uh* (no) as 1 word and 1 morpheme each. These forms are not fillers and do carry meaning.

Separate contracted words even when the stem violates traditional spelling. We're not grading for spelling, so just leave the pieces as is in order to save time. For example, *won't* will end up as the two morphemes "wo" and "n't." Although this seems odd, go with it.

The number of morphemes will appear in the word count on the tool bar at the bottom of the screen. Record the number of morphemes. Divide the number of morphemes by 50. Or . . . Multiply by 2 and use 2 decimal places. For example, 208 morphemes × 2 = 416. Two decimal places = 4.16.

Pull out of the document by clicking the X in the upper right corner. A pop-up will ask if you want to save. DO NOT SAVE THE DOCUMENT. The sample now reverts to its original form.

APPENDIX B SUGAR (SAMPLING UTTERANCES AND GRAMMATICAL ANALYSIS REVISED) PROCEDURES **625**

Words/Sentence

Reopen the sample. Before doing any actual analysis, make sure the "Numbering" function (In the paragraph section on the toolbar at the top) is off. Nothing else should be on the page except the child's 50 utterances.

Delete all utterances that are NOT sentences. Follow the rules for determining a sentence.

Both a sentence and a clause contain a subject and a verb, as in *Mommy walked*. A sentence can have more than one clause, as in *Mommy walked* but *I ran* (2 clauses, 1 sentence). The critical element in a sentence is a verb.

Procedures for Determining a Sentence

- Count imperatives as sentences. In an imperative, the subject is understood to be *you*.

  Come here. ([*You*] *come* here.) (1 clause, 1 sentence)

- Count as a clause and a sentence when either *the subject or a portion of the verb is omitted* because of ellipsis.

  Examples:

    Who can go with me?

      I can = 1 clause (S + aux. verb, so 1 clause, I sentence)

    What did you do?

      Ran home. (Main verb, so 1 clause, 1 sentence)

- NEVER count as a clause or a sentence if the entire verb is missing, as in "Me" in response to "Who ate the cookies?" Other examples include "What?", "Why?", "Okay", "Yes", "Sure", and the like.

Once you have only sentences represented, note the total words from the word count section on the toolbar at the bottom of the screen. Record this number.

Switch on the "Numbering" function again, found in the paragraph section of the tool bar at the top of the screen. With this on, you can tell how many sentences you have.

Divide the number of words by the number of sentences to get the mean words/sentence. Record this value somewhere.

Leave the "Numbering" function on.

Clauses/Sentence

You know the number of sentences, so now all you need is the number of clauses. **Locate the clauses. At the beginning of each clause within a sentence, hit the "Enter" key.**

Remember that the definition for a clause and a sentence are similar so again use the RULES FOR DETERMINING A SENTENCE.

Procedures for Determining a Clause

- Clauses may be either conjoined (Compound sentence) or embedded (Complex sentence).

  Conjoined: I like ice cream but I don't like the kind with nuts.

  Because I was sick, I stayed home.

  Embedded:

  Noun phrase complement (Finishes the verb): I know you ate my cookie = I know + you ate my cookie [Often found with cognitive verbs such as *know, remember, forget, think*, and verbs such as *say* and the slang *like* (Mom was like you better come here.)]

  Relative clause (Modifies a noun): I want the one you have = I want the one + you have.

- Count *compound subjects or verbs* as a single clause/sentence.

  Mommy walked and ran all the way home = 1 clause, 1 sentence (1 subject but 2 verbs).

  Bobby and Jim ran fast = 1 clauses, 1 sentence (2 subjects but 1 verb).

  I ate cookies and milk. Combined objects don't count as separate clauses either.

No one is looking over your shoulder to see if each clause is exactly correct or that the remainder may be a partial clause. Time is of the essence. For example, "The boy who's in my class is yukky" consists of two clauses, "The boy is yukky" and "Who is in my class." Separate these as follows:

The boy   *who's in my class is yukky*

Are these correct grammatically? Of course not. Does it count correctly as two clauses? Yes, and that's our purpose here. We can go back later and decide on the grammar just as we would go back and interpret test results.

When you have separated the clauses, **note the number and divide it by the same number of sentences as in the previous step.**

SUGAR Guidelines for Determining Language Impairment

Before you make a decision about a child having a language impairment, ask yourself the following questions:

- Is the sample truly robust?

APPENDIX B SUGAR (SAMPLING UTTERANCES AND GRAMMATICAL ANALYSIS REVISED) PROCEDURES **627**

- Did the examiner ask fewer than 10 questions that could be answered with yes/no or a one-word response?
- Was the sampling activity one that offered the child an opportunity to provide extended utterances?

If you can answer "Yes" to all of these and standardized test results and other methods also suggest a language impairment, do a sub-analysis to determine areas for possible intervention.

Interpreting the SUGAR Metrics

After calculating the four SUGAR metrics, use the Pavelko and Owens (2019) article to guide decisions in determining evidence-based cutscores. The highest diagnostic accuracy was a combination of –1 SD for MLU_S and a –1.25 SD for CPS.

SUGAR Sub-Analysis

To do a sub-analysis, select the appropriate sub-analysis form based on the chronological age of the child. Each form is different, depending on the structures seen in 70% of the samples of children that age or younger.

Open the language sample file for the child.

If the utterances are numbered, highlight the entire document (Control-A or Command-A),), go to the "Paragraph" section of the Toolbar and clicking on "Numbering" to delete all numbers.

With the sample still highlighted, select Control-C or Command-C.

Go to the Sub-analysis form, highlight all utterance spaces, then select Control-V or Command-V. The sample should appear in the utterance spaces.

You are now free to begin locating structures in the sample. A guide is below.

Here's a freebie:

Calculating Type/Token Ratio: Go to http://www.usingenglish.com/resources/text-statistics.php. Copy and paste the entire sample without numbering. Typically functioning 3–8 year old children should have a TTR of .45–.55. Scores below .45 indicate that the child is using the same words over and over. Be cautious because TTR is situationally variable. If you are playing a game, the word "Turn" may occur many times.

Source: Owens and Pavelko (2021). https://www.sugarlanguage.org

APPENDIX C

Comparison of Computer-Based Language Sample Analysis Methods

In this appendix, you'll find a brief description of three computer-based language sample analysis (LSA) methods that range from SALT, which is automated, requiring encoding of data, to SUGAR that uses the conveniences of a computer to facilitate the analysis process. As one of the authors of SUGAR, I'm somewhat biased but will try to be fair and honest. I have no financial motives because SUGAR is free . . . but we'll get to that in due time. I'll explore the three methods in alphabetic order.

CLAN (Computerized Language Analysis) (MacWhinney, 2000)

Designed initially as a research tool, CLAN is a cost-free, customizable program that can be used across 49 different languages. Samples are collected in a play situation. CLAN is designed for children younger than age 6 years and compares their language samples to those of children in the Child Language Data Exchange System (CHILDES) database. In addition, the CLAN manual includes values for mean length of utterance (MLU), number of different words (NDW), and other measures for English-speaking children only (Bernstein Ratner & Brundage, 2018).

CLAN uses KIDEVAL, a subset of the CHILDES database, for comparison. This collection consists of approximately 450 typically developing children from more than 30 different studies. Some studies used are longitudinal, resulting is some children being included multiple times.

Unlike SALT but similar to SUGAR, CLAN does not require manual coding of morphological markers. Instead, a command that is 94% accurate compared to hand scoring is available (Bernstein Ratner & MacWhinney, 2016).

As with hand scoring, unintelligible segments, fillers, repetitions, and mazes are excluded from analysis. This is accomplished by using an asterisk to indicate an error.

Transcription is made easier by linking the transcription and audio files. Using keyboard commands, the transcriber can stop and start the audio portion while typing.

The CLAN can be accessed at https://talkbank.org/manuals/CLAN.pdf

SALT (Systematic Analysis of Language Transcripts)
(Miller & Iglesias, 2015)

SALT rates several quantifiable language measures in both English and Spanish. Results can be automatically compared to a built-in database for children aged 2 to 18 years in the several contexts, such as play, conversation, narrative, expository, or persuasive. The SALT comparison database samples also feature additional coding to capture the overall structure of the sample separated by sample type.

Currently, SALT cost $209 for program software. The software is updated approximately every 2 years. Users must encode morphemes in each transcript to perform analysis such as MLU. Similarly, fillers, repetitions, unintelligible utterances, and mazes/abandoned utterances must be encoded to be excluded from analysis. Errors may also be marked for error type.

For some age groups, such as preschool, the number of samples in the database are small. At the same time, SALT contains both narrative and expository databases for adolescents. The normative database is strong through the school-age years.

The most widely used computerized LSA program, SALT has a sensitivity of .78 and a specificity of .85. I say this with some caution because the data are not presented in those terms.

SALT is available at http://saltsoftware.com/products/software

SUGAR (Sampling Utterances and Grammatical Analysis Revised)
(Owens & Pavelko, 2021)

The impetus for SUGAR, the newest LSA entry, is somewhat different than that for the others. The developers found that speech-language pathologists (SLPs) sampled little primarily because LSA takes too long and because they doubted its validity. Deciding to meet SLPs where they were, Pavelko and Owens (2017) devised an LSA method that was easy, quick, and used only 50 utterances.

Reasoning that comparing a 50-utterance sample to a 50-utterance database was more accurate than comparing a 50-utterance sample to a longitudinal database, Owens and Pavelko (2021) set out to redesign LSA. Samples are collected using robust collection methods, and values such as MLU_{SUGAR} are based on morphological markers seen in older children. The robust collecting protocol encourages SLPs to use process questions and narrative elicitations, intended to increase a child's language complexity during conversation.

Samples are typed in plain English with fillers, repetitions, and reformulations omitted. Unintelligible words are left in and utterances omitted only when more than two words are unintelligible.

Compared to both CLAN and SALT, SUGAR encoding is minimal, consisting of spaces between morphemes and line breaks between clauses. Collection, transcription, and quantitative analysis can be accomplished in less than 30 minutes. Sub-analysis highlights features likely to be seen in a 50-utterance sample and can guide decisions on intervention targets (Owens et al., 2018).

APPENDIX C COMPARISON OF COMPUTER-BASED LANGUAGE SAMPLE ANALYSIS METHODS

Cost-free, SUGAR has both high sensitivity and high specificity of .98 and .83, respectively (Pavelko & Owens, 2020). Normative values for four measures—MLU_{SUGAR}, total number of words, words per sentence, and clauses per sentence—are available for children aged 3;0 to 10;11 years.

SUGAR is available at https://www.sugarlanguage.org

APPENDIX D
Selected English Morphological Prefixes and Suffixes

Table D–1. Prefixes and Suffixes		
	Derivational	**Inflectional**
Prefixes	**Suffixes**	
a- (in, on, into, in a manner)	-able (ability, tendency, likelihood)	-ed (past)
bi- (twice, two)	-al (pertaining to, like, action, process)	-ing (at present)
de- (negative, descent, reversal)	-ance (action, state)	-s (plural)
ex- (out of, from, thoroughly)	-ation (denoting action in a noun)	-s (third person marker)
inter- (reciprocal between, together)	-en (used to form verbs from adjectives	-s' (possession)
mis- (ill, negative, wrong)	-ence (action, state)	
out- (extra, beyond, not)	-er (used as an agentive ending)	
over- (over)	-est (superlative)	
post- (behind, after)	-ful (full, tending)	
pre- (to, before)	-ible (ability, tendency, likelihood)	
pro- (in favor of)	-ish (belonging to)	
re- (again, backward motion)	-ism (doctrine, state, practice)	
semi- (half)	-ist (one who does something)	
super- (superior)	-ity (used for abstract nouns)	
trans- (across, beyond)	-ive (tendency or connection)	
tri- (three)	-ize (action, policy)	
un- (not, reversal)	-less (without)	
under- (under)	-ly (used to form adverbs)	

continues

633

LANGUAGE DISORDERS: A FUNCTIONAL APPROACH TO ASSESSMENT AND INTERVENTION IN CHILDREN

Table D–1. *continued*

Prefixes	Derivational Suffixes	Inflectional
	-ment (action, product, means, state)	
	-ness (quality, state)	
	-or (used as an agentive ending)	
	-ous (full of, having, like)	
	-y (inclined to)	

APPENDIX E

Non-Majority American English Dialects and English Influenced by Other Languages

For many reasons, rather that discuss English, it may be more appropriate to talk about "the Englishes." Obvious differences exist between British and American English. But in our day-to-day use of American English, we each speak a dialect. In the United States, we each speak an American English dialect that is influenced by several variables, such as socioeconomic status (SES) and region.

I, for one, grew up speaking low-SES Middle Atlantic American English. Although I may have sounded different to someone from California, we were still intelligible to each other because the differences were minimal. Middle American English, found roughly in the mid-Atlantic states of eastern Maryland, Delaware, eastern Pennsylvania, and southwestern New Jersey, is a regional dialect of American English, and although it has its own peculiarities, it's close enough to the mainstream dialect to be classified as such.

Some dialects of American English differ more and have been classified by linguists as non-mainstream or NMAE. African American English (AAE), spoken by some but not all African Americans and some non-African Americans, is one of these, as is Appalachian American English.

In addition, many Americans originally spoke another language, either in another country or right here in the United States. Often, the original or heritage language influences the manner in which the person uses American English. We can, therefore, speak of Spanish-influenced English or Mandarin-influenced English.

As a speech-language pathologist, it's important that you not conflate these natural language differences with language disorders. Remember that natural language differences are not disorders. It's also good to keep in mind that race or ethnicity does not equate with use of NMAE. That's why we assess children's language.

In this appendix, I lay out the major characteristics of AAE and Spanish-influenced American English. I also make a few comments on the myriad Asian languages spoken in the United States and their influences. Please keep in mind that the influence of a

636 LANGUAGE DISORDERS: A FUNCTIONAL APPROACH TO ASSESSMENT AND INTERVENTION IN CHILDREN

language varies with the language and there are simply too many—Hindi, Mandarin, Korean, Japanese, Vietnamese, Tagalog, Karen—to mention each individually.

It's important to keep in mind that every speaker is an individual. The characteristics mentioned in this appendix do not necessarily represent any one individual. Children may have some but not all of the characteristics. With these cautions in mind, let's begin.

African American English

Although this is not a course in phonology, it's worth noting that some phonological variations, such as the weakening or no or zero (Ø) marking of final consonants, will have an effect on morphological markers. Some of the features of spoken AAE represent natural phonological processes, such as cluster reduction.

It's also important to note the national nature of AAE, meaning that regional dialects also influence. Thus, the rules evident in an AAE speaker will affect both AAE and the region of the country where a person lives, similar to what we find in MAE speakers (Baranowski, 2013; Eberhardt, 2008).

Young AAE speakers do not have all the language features mentioned in the following Table E–1. The most consistent syntactic features found in the speech of many African American preschoolers are zero marking or a lack of the copula and the third person -*s* marker (Washington & Craig, 1994).

Many syntactic rules of AAE reflect the redundant nature of MAE constructions. For example, the plural *'s* is unnecessary when a numerical term (*six*) or quantifier (*some*) occurs before the noun, as in *six shirt*. In another example, context (*yesterday*) often signals the verb tense. Examples of features of AAE are presented in Table E–1.

Spanish-Influenced English

Within the United States, the largest ethnic population is Latino/Latina. Many, but not all, individuals with a Spanish surname speak English. Some are natural-born U.S. citizens, such as those from or currently residing in Puerto Rico, who may have spoken Spanish at home or school. Others emigrated from Spanish-speaking countries, such as Mexico and others in Central and South America or the Caribbean.

Just as we should not assume that all African Americans speak AAE, we must not assume that all those with a Spanish surname speak Spanish. It's important to remember that many families with a Spanish family name have been in the United States for hundreds of years and may consider American English to be their native language.

Spanish dialectal differences also influence comprehension and production of American English. The dialect of American English spoken in the surrounding community will also have an effect. The general characteristics of Spanish-influenced English (SIE) are presented in Table E–2.

Structural contrasts between SIE and the mainstream dialect (MAE) also reflect many of the redundant MAE markers. Other AE markers, such as possessive -*'s*, do not exist in

APPENDIX E NON-MAJORITY AMERICAN ENGLISH DIALECTS & ENGLISH INFLUENCED BY OTHER LANGUAGES **637**

Table E–1. Grammatical Features of AAE	
Grammatical Structure	**AAE Grammatical Structure**
Copula and Auxiliary BE	Ø* use in MAE contractible BE form, as in *He happy*. Marked in MAE uncontractible BE form, as in *He is*. The governing factor seems to be meaning or intention, getting one's message across. Therefore, the absence does not occur when BE is emphasized.
Past tense *-ed*	Ø when reference understood from context, as in *Last night, she cook dinner*.
Possessive *–s*	Ø when meaning is conveyed by word order, as in *This is Brenda bracelet*.
Irregular past tense	A past tense verb (*went*) may be used in place of a past participle (*gone*) and vice versa, as in *James seen her*.
Plural *-s*	Ø when numerical term or quantifier precedes noun, as in *He got two bike* but *Where are my books?*
Negation	Use of *ain't* is permissible. Multiple negation is acceptable within the same sentence, *I don't have none*.
Habitual use of BE	BE used unmarked to describe a habitual/continuing action or state, as in *She be working all the time*.
Use of Been	*Been* may be used to mark the distant past, as in *She been sick*.
Auxiliary modal verbs	Use of double modals, as in *She might could go*.
Third person singular *-s*	Ø marking, as in *She eat her lunch at work*.

Note: *Feature not marked. Ø signifies no marking or use.

Sources: Information from DeBose (2015), Mufwene et al. (1998), Washington and Craig (1994, 2002), and Wolfram and Schilling (2016).

Spanish. In the case of possession, Spanish uses post-noun possessive (house *of Maria*). In addition, adjectives follow the noun. Also, the SIE speaker of LE may use Spanish words depending on the size of their English vocabulary and on the context.

The Influence of Asian Languages on English

Space does not permit an in-depth exploration of all the many Asian languages currently spoken in the United States, but let's discuss the effects of a few on American English. Asian languages have many variations. For example, Mandarin and Thai are tonal, meaning that different tonal patterns determine a word's or a sentence's meaning. Other languages, such a Tagalog, spoken in areas of the Philippines, have a complex morphological system.

638 LANGUAGE DISORDERS: A FUNCTIONAL APPROACH TO ASSESSMENT AND INTERVENTION IN CHILDREN

Table E–2. Grammatical Features of Spanish-Influenced English

Grammatical Structure	SIE Structure
Possessive -'s	Use post-noun modifier, as in *This is the dress of my sister.*
	Article used to identify body parts, as in *I cut the finger.*
Plural -s	Non-obligatory use, as in *The girl are playing.*
Past tense -ed	Non-obligatory when understood by context, as in *I talk with her yesterday.*
Third person singular -s	Non-obligatory, as in *She eat too much.*
Articles	Ø marking, as in *I going to store.*
Subjective pronouns	Ø marking when subject identified in previous sentence, as in *My father is happy. Bought a new car.*
Future tense	Use of *go to*, as in *I go to dance.*
Negation	Use *no* before the verb, as in *She no eat candy.*
Questions	Ø noun–verb inversion, use intonation, as in *Maria is going?*
Copula BE	Occasional use of *have*, as in *I have ten years* [old].
Negative imperatives	*No* used for *don't*, as in *No throw stones.*
DO insertion	Non-obligatory in questions, as in *You like ice cream?*
Comparatives	Frequent use of *more* form, as in *He is more tall.*

Note: Ø signifies no marking or use.

The most widely used languages in Asia are Mandarin Chinese, Cantonese Chinese, Filipino, Hindi, Japanese, Khmer, Korean, Laotian, Thai, and Vietnamese. Of these, Mandarin has had the most pervasive influence on the evolution of the others. Indian and colonial European cultures, as well as others, have influenced these languages. Each language has various dialects and features that distinguish it from the others. Nonetheless, the English of Asian language speakers has certain characteristics in common. Grammatical features are presented in Table E–3.

APPENDIX E NON-MAJORITY AMERICAN ENGLISH DIALECTS & ENGLISH INFLUENCED BY OTHER LANGUAGES 639

Table E–3. Grammatical Characteristics of Some Asian Language Speakers

Grammatical Structure	Structures Used by Some Asian Language Speakers
Plural -s	Ø use with numerical term, as in *I see three cat.* Used with irregular plural, as in *I want to buy sheeps.*
Auxiliary BE and DO	Ø marking, as in *I going home.* Uninflected, as in *I is going to school.*
Verb HAVE	Ø marking, as in *She been there.* Uninflected, as in *He have one.*
Past tense -ed	Ø marking, as in *We talk yesterday.* Used on irregular past tense verbs, as in *I eated yesterday.* Double marking, as in *I didn't walked yesterday.*
Interrogative	Ø noun–verb inversion, as in *You are late?* Omitted auxiliary, as in *You like ice cream?*
Perfective marker	Ø marking, as in *I have write letter.*
Verb–noun agreement	Ø agreement, as in *He go to school* or *You goes to school.*
Article	Ø, as in *Please send gift.* Overgeneralization, as in *She go the school.*
Preposition	Ø use, as in *He go bus.* Misuse, as in *I am in home.*
Pronoun	Subjective–objective confusion, as in *Him go quickly.*
Demonstrative	Confusion, as in *I have them there.*
Conjunction	Ø marking, as in *You I go together.*
Negation	Double marking, as in *I don't see nobody.* Simplified form, as in *He no go.*
Word order	Adjective following noun (Vietnamese), as in *She wearing clothes new.* Possessive following noun (Vietnamese), as in *She lost book her.* Ø object with transitive verb, as in *I want.*

Note: Ø signifies no marking or use.

Sources: Information from Bolton et al. (2020) and Honna (2005).

APPENDIX F

Indirect Elicitation Techniques

There is an infinite variety of indirect elicitation techniques, although we tend to rely on two old favorites:

Tell me what you see.

Tell me in a whole sentence.

Here are a few conversational techniques that came to mind one day. The list is not exhaustive, merely illustrative.

Table F–1. Indirect Elicitation Techniques

Technique	Target	Example
The emperor's new clothes	Negative statements	*Clinician:* Oh, Shirley, what beautiful yellow boots. *Child:* I'm not wearing boots!
Pass it on	Requests for information	*Clinician:* John, do you know where Linda's projects is? *Child:* No. *Clinician:* Oh, see if she knows? *Child:* Linda, where's your project?
Violating routines ("Silly rabbit")	Imperatives, directives	*Clinician:* Here's your sandwich. *Child:* Nothing in it. *Clinician:* Oh, you must like different sandwiches than I do. What do you want? *Child:* Peanut butter. *Clinician:* How do I do it? (There's your opener)
Nonblabbermouth	Requests for information	*Clinician:* (Place interesting object in front of child) "Boy is this neat. *Child:* What is it? *Clinician:* A flibbideejibbit. (Now STOP. Don't give any more info) *Child:* What's it do?

continues

641

Table F–1. *continued*

Technique	Target	Example
What I have	Request for action	*Clinician:* Oh, I can't wait to show you what I have in this bag. It's really neat. (Wait child out)
Guess what I did	Request for information, past tense verbs	*Clinician:* Guess what I did yesterday in the park. *Child:* Jogged? Picked flowers? Had a picnic?
Mumble	Contingent query	At height of an interesting story or punchline of a joke, clinician should mumble so that the child doesn't receive the message. If needed, increase the pressure by asking questions about what was said.
Ask someone else	Request for information	*Clinician:* What do you need? *Child:* Sugar. *Clinician:* I don't know where it is. Why don't you ask Sally where the sugar is?
Rule giving	Requests for objects	*Clinician:* I have the athletic equipment for recess. If you need some, just ask me. *Child:* I want jump rope.
Request for assistance	Initiating conversation	*Clinician:* John, can you ask Keith to help me?
Modeling with Meaningful intent	I want _____	*Clinician:* We have lots of colored paper for our project. Now let's see who needs some. I want a green one. (Take one and wait) *Child:* I want blue.
"Screw up" #1	Locatives, prepositions	*Clinician:* Can you help me dress this doll? (Place shoe on doll's head) How's that? *Child:* No. The shoe goes *on* the doll's foot. *Clinician:* But now the foot's all gone. *Child:* No. It's *in* the shoe.
"Screw up" #2	Negative statements	*Clinician:* Here's your snack. (Give child a pencil) *Child:* That's not a snack.
Requests for topic	Statements	*Clinician:* Now let's talk about your birthday party. (Not shared information)
Expansion of child utterance into desired form	Infinitives	*Child:* I want paste crayon. *Clinician:* You want crayon to *sing with*? *Child:* No, to color *Clinician:* What? *Child:* I want crayon to color.

APPENDIX G

Intervention Activities and Language Targets

Begins on following page.

Activities and Targets

Activities	Nouns	Plurals	Verb tensing	Adjectives/descriptive words	Adverbs	Pronouns	Articles and demonstratives	Prepositions/spatial terms	Requests for objects	Requests for assistance	Requests for information	Negatives	Interrogatives	Following directions	Giving directions	Sequencing	Turn taking	Topic intro and maintenance	Categorization	Register	Presupposition	Conversational repair	Variety of pragmatic features	Auditory processing/memory	Word association	Vocabulary
Barrier tasks														X	X	X					X			X		
Body tracing	X		X					X		X				X	X	X										X
Cellphone play		X		X		X	X				X	X	X				X	X		X	X	X	X			
Cooking*	X	X	X	X					X		X		X	X	X				X							X
Describe hidden pictures	X	X		X			X														X					
Dolls, clothing, furniture	X	X		X				X												X						X
Dressing	X	X							X																	
Dress-up			X	X		X	X	X						X	X											
Explaining how-to				X	X			X							X	X										
Farm or zoo play	X	X		X	X																					
Guiding others												X		X	X	X		X	X	X	X	X	X			
Interviewing				X				X			X	X	X				X	X		X	X	X				X
"I see something that's . . ."											X		X				X	X							X	

APPENDIX G INTERVENTION ACTIVITIES AND LANGUAGE TARGETS

Targets

Activities	Nouns	Plurals	Verb tensing	Adjectives/descriptive words	Adverbs	Pronouns	Articles and demonstratives	Prepositions/spatial terms	Requests for objects	Requests for assistance	Requests for information	Negatives	Interrogatives	Following directions	Giving directions	Sequencing	Turn taking	Topic intro and maintenance	Categorization	Register	Presupposition	Conversational repair	Variety of pragmatic features	Auditory processing/memory	Word association	Vocabulary
Jeopardy											X	X	X												X	
Kitchen play	X	X		X					X	X							X	X					X			X
Making things**	X		X	X	X	X	X	X	X	X	X	X		X	X	X	X									X
Map following								X		X	X	X	X	X	X											
Mime														X		X		X			X					
My "ME book"				X	X	X												X								
Music and action songs														X	X	X										
Nature/science				X	X	X	X	X	X	X	X		X	X	X	X	X		X					X	X	X
Obstacle course			X	X	X	X		X		X			X	X	X	X										
Planning an activity			X	X				X										X			X					X
Planting seeds			X	X		X	X	X						X	X											X
Playhouse			X																	X			X			
Playing teacher												X			X			X		X	X	X	X			
Pretend errands	X									X	X	X	X				X	X	X	X	X	X	X			X

continues

Appendix G. *continued*

Activities	Nouns	Plurals	Verb tensing	Adjectives/descriptive words	Adverbs	Pronouns	Articles and demonstratives	Prepositions/spatial terms	Requests for objects	Requests for assistance	Requests for information	Negatives	Interrogatives	Following directions	Giving directions	Sequencing	Turn taking	Topic intro and maintenance	Categorization	Register	Presupposition	Conversational repair	Variety of pragmatic features	Auditory processing/memory	Word association	Vocabulary
Puppet show																X				X			X			
Putting object in order				X				X											X						X	
Simon says	X	X	X											X	X	X									X	
Simulated restaurant	X	X							X		X		X				X		X	X	X		X			X
Sorting clothing			X			X	X		X					X					X							
Storytelling																X		X				X		X		
Treasure hunt								X						X	X						X					
TV commercials				X														X		X	X	X	X			
"Twenty questions"				X							X	X	X													
Washing dishes	X	X		X	X	X			X	X				X	X											
"What am I?"				X	X	X	X	X			X	X	X				X	X				X				
"What do you do . . . ?"			X		X	X	X	X			X		X				X	X				X				

APPENDIX G INTERVENTION ACTIVITIES AND LANGUAGE TARGETS 647

Note: *Possible cooking activities
Be sure to check for food allergies (dairy, nuts, flour)

- Cookies, cupcakes, muffins
- Cornbread and butter
- Edible honeybees: ½ cup peanut butter; 1/3 cup + 1 T honey; 2 T sesame seeds, and 2 T wheat germ. Roll into balls. Make stripes by dipping a toothpick into cocoa powder and pressing onto surface of ball. Use slivered almonds for wings.
- English muffin pizza
- Fruit salad. Try to add a few vegetables to stir discussion.
- Ice cream sundaes
- Milkshakes: lots of varieties and dairy substitutes
- Fruit smoothies
- Peanut butter and jelly sandwiches
- Peanut butter balls: ½ cup honey; ½ cup peanut butter; 1 cup dry milk powder; and 1 cup oatmeal. Roll into balls and refrigerate.
- Yoghurt faces in the cup with raisins or chocolate chips for mouth, eyes, nose and coconut flakes for hair.
- Picnic lunch
- Popcorn and popcorn balls

**Possible things to make

- Cereal box instruments: Use a strong cereal box with a circular hole cut on the broad side similar to a guitar. Stretch different thickness rubber bands around the box and across thin strips of wood near the hole like bridges on a guitar. Now play your heart out.
- Costumes from grocery bags: Cut head and arm holes, decorate, and wear.
- Decorate a box as a room with wallpaper scraps.
- Food sculptures held together with toothpicks or peanut butter
- Holiday cards
- Kites
- Paper bag puppets: always a favorite
- Paper butterflies
- Paper flowers or better yet, edible flowers made from fruit pieces
- Potato and sponge prints
- Sachets for mom or gran'ma: Add cloves, crumbled bay leaves, and/or cinnamon stick pieces together in the center of a square cloth. Bring the ends of the cloth together and tie with a fancy bow.

- Nos People from Styrofoam balls, pipe cleaners, cloves for the face, and toothpicks. Jazz them up with colorful cloth scarves and gumdrops for mittens.
- Stained-glass windows: Cut out the holes from a solid piece of cardboard, tape aluminum foil to one side, and place this side down. Fill the open portions with Elmer's glue, swirl in food coloring. Allow to dry thoroughly, peel the foil, and voila—a stained-glass window. Cool!

APPENDIX H

Use of Children's Literature in Preschool Classrooms

Books and Their Uses in Intervention

Targets

Auditory Skills

Auditory Awareness

Rhyming

Aardema, *Bring the rain to Kapiti Plain* (M)

Ahlberg, *Each peach pear plum*

Alborough, *Where's my teddy?*

Anholt & Anholt, *Here come the babies*

Bang, *Ten, nine, eight* (M)

Deming, *Who is tapping at my window?*

deRegniers, *Going for a walk*

Jonas, *This old man*

Kandoian, *Molly's seasons*

Lear, *The owl and the pussycat*

Lotz, *Snowsong shistling*

Lyon, *Together*

Martin, *Brown bear, brown bear, what do you see?*

Martin, *The happy hippopotami*

Martin, *Polar bear, polar bear, what do you hear?*

Patron, *Dark cloud, strong breeze*

Philpot, *Amazing Anthony Ant*

Polushkin, *Mother, mother, I want another*

Seuss, *Hop on pop*

Stickland & Stickland, *Dinosaur roar!*

Wood, *The napping house*

Auditory Memory

Bennett & Cooke, *One cow moo moo*

Hayes, *The grumpalump*

Hutchins, *Don't forget the bacon*

Hutchins, *The surprise party*

Numeroff, *If you give a mouse a cookie*
Auditory and visual memory

Numeroff, *If you give a moose a muffin*
Auditory and visual memory

Neitzel, *The jacket I wear in the snow*

Offen, *The sheep made a leap*
Following directions

Smalls-Hector, *Jonathan and his mommy* (M)
Following directions

Auditory Attending and Other Skills

Brown, *The noise book*
  Discrimination

Calmenson, *It begins with an A*
  Attending and synthesis

Carle, *The very hungry caterpillar*
  Sequencing, auditory memory

deRegniers, *It does not say meow*
  Auditory attending and processing

Word Play

Barrett, *Animals should definitely not act like people*

Calmenson, *It begins with an A*

Carle, *The secret birthday message*

Hutchins, *Don't forget the bacon*

Syntax and Morphology

Verb Tensing

Present Progressive

Allen, *A lion in the night*

Barton, *Harry is a scaredy-cat*

Brown, *The runaway bunny*

Burningham, *Jangle, twang*

DePaola, *Pancakes for breakfast*

Ets, *In the forest*

Gelman, *I went to the zoo*

Hutchins, *The very worst monster*

Keats, *Over in the meadow*

Keats, *Peter's chair*

Krauss, *Bears*

Krauss, *The carrot seed*

Lear, *The owl and the pussycat*

Martin, *Brown bear, brown bear, what do you see?*

Martin, *Polar bear, polar bear, what do you hear?*

Martin & Archambault, *Here are my hands*

Mayer, *There's an alligator under my bed*

Noll, *Jiggle, wiggle, prance*

Peppe, *Odd one out*

Rockwell, *First comes spring*

Rockwell & Rockwell, *At the beach*

Sendak, *Alligators all around*

Van Laan, *Possum come a-knockin'*

Wood, *The napping house*

Future Tense

Allen, *A lion in the night*

Zolotow, *Do you know what I'll do?*

Past Tense

Aardema, *Bring the rain to Kapiti Plain* (M)

Arnold, *Green Wilma*

Arnold, *The simple people*

Baker, *The third-story cat*

Charlip, *Fortunately*

Chorao, *Kate's box*

Cole, *Monster manners*

DePaola, *Charlie needs a cloak*

DePaola, *The knight and the dragon*

Ehlert, *Red leaf, yellow leaf*

Ets, *Play with me*

Everitt, *Frida the wondercat*

APPENDIX H USE OF CHILDREN'S LITERATURE IN PRESCHOOL CLASSROOMS

651

Ginsburg, *Good morning, chick*

Hayes, *The grumpalump*

Hutchins, *Goodnight owl*

Hutchins, *Rosie's walk*

Keats, *Over in the meadow*

Keats, *Peter's chair*

Kent, *There's no such thing as a dragon*

Knowlton, *Why cowboys sleep with their boots on*

Krauss, *The carrot seed*

Lear, *The owl and the pussycat*

London, *Froggy gets dressed*

London, *Let's go, froggy!*

Mayer, *Just me and my little sister*

Mayer, *There's an alligator under my bed*

Peppe, *Odd one out*

Ruschak, *One hot day*

Scieszka, *The true story of the 3 little pigs*

Tojhurst, *Somebody and the three Blairs*

Wells, *Noisy Nora*

Noun–Verb Agreement

Barton, *Airplanes*

Barton, *Airport*

Barton, *Boats*

Brown, *Goodnight moon*

Lewin, *Jafta's mother* (M)

Sendak, *Alligators all around*

Prepositions

Ahlberg, *Each peach pear plum*

Appelt, *Elephants aloft*

Baker, *The third-story cat*

Banchek, *Snake in, snake out*

Brown, *The runaway bunny*

Brown, *A dark dark tale*

Carle, *The secret birthday message*

Chorao, *Kate's box*

Hill, *Spot's birthday party*

Hutchins, *Rosie's walk*

Krauss, *Bears*

Lillie, *Everything has a place*

London, *Let's go, froggy!*

Mayer, *There's an alligator under my bed*

Noll, *Jiggle, wiggle, prance*

Westcott, *The lady with the alligator purse*

Wheeler, *Marmalade's yellow leaf*

Pronouns

Brown, *Arthur's nose*

Brown, *The runaway bunny*

Chorao, *Kate's box*

Mayer, *Just my friend and me*

Mayer, *Just me and my little sister*

Roffey, *Look, there's my hat*

Adjectives/Descriptor Words

Asch, *The last puppy* (first/last)

Asch, *Little fish, big fish* (big/little)

Baker, *Hide and snake*

Baker, *White rabbit's coloring book*

Brown, *A dark dark tale*

Collington, *The midnight circus*

Davol, *Black, white, just right* (M)

Day, *Good dog, Carl*

Day, *Carl goes to daycare*

Day, *Carl goes shopping*

Day, *Carl's afternoon in the park*

deRegniers, *It does not say meow*

Geisert, *Oink, oink*

Gill, *The spring hat*

Glassman, *The wizard next door*

Graham, *Full moon soup or the fall of the Hotel Splendide*

Guarino, *Is your mama a llama?*

Guarino, *Tu mama es una llama?* (M)

Hoban, *Is it rough, is it smooth, is it shiny?*

Hoban, *Exactly the opposite*

Hoban, *Is it larger? Is it smaller?*

Hudson & Ford, *Bright eyes, brown skin* (M)

Hutchins, *The very worst monster*

Jonas, *Reflections*

Jonas, *The 13th clue*

Jonas, *The trek*

Jonas, *Where can it be*

Kandoian, *Molly's seasons*

Keats, *Peter's chair*

Lester, *It wasn't my fault*

Martin, *Brown bear, brown bear, what do you see?*

Martin, *When dinosaurs go visiting*

Marzollo & Pinkney, *Pretend you're a cat*

Reiss, *Colors*

Rockwell, *Big wheels*

Viorst, *My mama says*

Wood, *The napping house*

Possessive -'s

Brown, *Arthur's nose*

Chorao, *Kate's box*

Gibbons, *The season of the Arnold's apple tree*

Keats, *Peter's chair*

Kraus, *Whose mouse are you?*

Yabuuchi, *Whose footprints?*

Plurals (Regular -s & Irregular)

Brown, *Goodnight moon*

Ehlert, *Red leaf, yellow leaf*

Ets, *In the forest*

Gibbons, *The season of the Arnold's apple tree*

Hoban, *Is it larger? Is it smaller?*

Kandoian, *Molly's seasons*

Keats, *Over in the meadow*

Lionni, *A color of his own*

Lukesova, *Julian in the autumn woods*

Third person singular -s

Gibbons, *The season of the Arnold's apple tree*

LeSaux, *Daddy shaves*

Lester, *Clive eats alligators*

Loomis, *In the diner*

Tafuri, *This is the farmer*

Verbs

LeSaux, *Daddy shaves*

Lester, *Clive eats alligators*

Loomis, *In the diner*

APPENDIX H   USE OF CHILDREN'S LITERATURE IN PRESCHOOL CLASSROOMS   653

Lyon, *Together*

Martin, *When dinosaurs go visiting*

Marzollo & Pinkney, *Pretend you're a cat*

Mayer, *Just my friend and me*

Numeroff, *Dogs don't wear sneakers*

Offen, *The sheep made a leap*

Shaw, *Sheep in a shop*

Shaw, *Sheep on a ship*

Shaw, *Sheep out to eat*

Smalls-Hector, *Jonathan and his mommy* (M)

Westcott, *The lady with the alligator purse*

Zolotow, *Do you know what I'll do?*

Negative and/or Interrogative Sentences

Burningham, *Mr. Gumpy's outing*

Kraus, *Whose mouse are you?*

Numeroff, *Dogs don't wear sneakers*

To Elicit SVO Sentences

Burningham, *Skip, trip*

Burningham, *Sniff, shout*

Comparative

Hoban, *Is it larger? Is it smaller?*

Superlative

Ruschak, *One hot day*

But Clauses

Scott & Coalson, *Hi*

And then Clauses

Wolf, *And then what?*

When Clauses

Schecter, *When will the snow trees grow?*

Because Clauses

Porter-Gaylord, *I love my daddy because*

Zukman & Edelman, *It's a good thing*

Relative Clauses

Wood, *Silly Sally*

Pragmatics

Cole, *Monster manners*

Corey, *Everyone takes turns*

Meddaugh, *Martha speaks*

Describing

Graham, *Full moon soup or the fall of the Hotel Splendide*

Lester, *It wasn't my fault*

Marzollo & Wick, *I spy*

Mayer, *Ah-choo* (No words)

Mayer, *A boy, a dog, a frog and a friend* (No words)

Mayer, *Frog goes to dinner* (No words)

Mayer, *Frog on his own* (No words)

Mayer, *Hiccup* (No words)

Mayer, *The great cat chase* (No words)

McCully, *Picnic* (No words)

McNaughton, *Guess who just moved in next door*

McPhail, *Emma's pet*

Novak, *Elmer Blunt's open house*

O'Malley, *Bruno, you're late for school* (No words)

Raskin, *Nothing ever happens on my block*

Raschka, *Yo! Yes?*

Rathman, *Good night, gorilla*

Roe, *All I am*

Russo, *The great treasure hunt*

Schories, *Mouse around* (No words)

Spier, *Dreams* (No words)

Turkle, *Deep in the forest* (No words)

Discussion

Porter-Gaylord, *I love my daddy because*

Roe, *All I am*

Small, *Imogene's antlers* (What if . . .)

Zukman & Edelman, *It's a good thing*

Imagining

Barrett, *Cloudy with a chance of meatballs* (If . . . then)

Small, *Imogene's antlers*

Spier, *Dreams* (No words)

Noticing the "Ridiculous"

Slepian & Seidler, *The hungry thing returns*

Question/Answer

Charles, *What am I?*

Graham, *Full moon soup or the fall of the Hotel Splendide*

Marzollo & Pinkney, *Pretend you're a cat*

Raschka, *Yo! Yes?*

Semantics

Vocabulary

Barton, *Airplanes*

Barton, *Airport*

Barton, *Boats*

Burningham, *Skip, trip*

Burningham, *Sniff, shout*

Carle, *The secret birthday message*

DePaola, *Charlie needs a cloak*

DePaola, *Pancakes for breakfast*

King, *Gus is gone*

King, *Lucy is lost*

Krauss, *Bears*

Marzollo & Wick, *I spy*

Marzollo & Wick, *I spy mystery*

Noll, *Jiggle, wiggle, prance*

Peppe, *Odd one out*

Reiss, *Colors*

Rockwell, *Big wheels*

Rockwell, *My kitchen*

Rockwell, *Things that go*

Rockwell, *Things to play with*

Rockwell & Rockwell, *At the beach*

Viorst, *Alexander and the terrible, horrible, no good, very bad day*

Yabuuchi, *Whose footprints?*

Antonyms

Butterworth & Inkpen, *Nice or nasty: A book of opposites*

Hoban, *Is it rough, is it smooth, is it shiny?*

Hoban, *Exactly the opposite*

Wildsmith, *What the moon saw*

Categories

Barton, *Airplanes*

Barton, *Airport*

Barton, *Boats*

Martin, *Brown bear, brown bear, what do you see?*

APPENDIX H   USE OF CHILDREN'S LITERATURE IN PRESCHOOL CLASSROOMS

Martin, *Polar bear, polar bear, what do you hear?*

Rockwell, *Big wheels*

Rockwell, *My kitchen*

Viorst, *Alexander and the terrible, horrible, no good, very bad day*

Yabuuchi, *Whose footprints?*

Zolotow, *Some things go together*

Word Associations

Zolotow, *Some things go together*

Verbal Absurdities

Allard, *The Stupids die*

Allard, *The Stupids have a ball*

Allard, *The Stupids step out*

Barrett, *Animals should definitely not act like people*

Gwynne, *A chocolate moose for dinner*

Gwynne, *A king who rained*

Johnson, *Never babysit the hippopotamuses*

Synonyms

Wood, *The napping house*

Figurative Language

Barrett, *Cloudy with a chance of meatballs*

Gwynne, *A chocolate moose for dinner*

Gwynne, *A king who rained*

Lewin, *Jafta*

Macaulay, *Why the chicken crossed the road*

Numeroff, *If you give a mouse a cookie*

Numeroff, *If you give a moose a muffin*

Publications to Assist in Classroom Use of Books

Charner, K. (2000). *The giant encyclopedia of theme activities for children 2 to 5*. Gryphon House.

Devlin, N. (2015). *Read to me, talk with me (Revised): Your child first three years with books*. Author House.

Gebers, J. (2003). *Books are for talking, too!* Communication Skill Builders. https://recommendationpopularmedia.blogspot.com/book91.php?asin=0890799024

Jett-Simpson, M. (Ed.). (1989). *Adventures with books: A booklist for pre-K–grade 6*. National Council of Teachers of English.

Raines, S. C., & Canady, R. J. (1989). *Story s-t-r-e-t-c-h-e-r-s: Activities to expand children's favorite books*. Gryphon House.

Raines, S. C., & Smith, B. S. (2011). *Story s-t-r-e-t-c-h-e-r-s for the primary grades: Activities to expand children's books*. Gryphon House.

Trelease, J., & Giorgis, C. (2019). *Jim Trelease's read-aloud handbook* (8th ed.). Penguin.

Glossary

Academic lexicon: A child's story of words used in texts and in the classroom.

Alexithymia: Limited ability to predict and interpret the intentions of others and to self-regulate their own language use found in some maltreated children.

Alphabet knowledge: Knowing the features and names of letters in both upper- and lowercase.

Applied behavior analysis: Used with children with autism spectrum disorder in which specific intervention targets are addressed through grouped multiple trials of *antecedent–behavior–consequence* chains. Many programs teach individual skills one at a time through drill-based repetition.

Assessment: The ongoing process, using multiple tools and methods, of identifying a child's unique needs; the family's priorities, concerns, and resources; and the nature and extent of the early intervention services needed by both. Usually less formal than evaluations and rely on the use of multiple tools and methods with the close cooperation of families and professionals.

At-risk: A broad category of children served by early intervention programs in which there is the potential for both biological and environmental factors to interfere with a child's ability to interact in a typical way with the environment and to develop typically.

Attention-deficit/hyperactivity disorder (ADHD): Characterized by overactivity and an inability to attend for more than short periods of time. Although related to learning disability, the disorder does not manifest itself in severe perceptual and learning difficulties.

Augmentative and alternative communication (AAC): A form of assistive technology and an intervention approach that uses other-than-speech means to complement or supplement an individual's communication abilities and may include combining existing speech or vocalizations with gestures, manual signs, communication boards, and speech-output communication devices.

Breakdowns and buildups: Dividing the child's utterances into shorter units and then combining them and expanding on the child's original utterance in order to help the child understand intrasentential relationships.

Cerebrovascular accident (CVA): A portion of the brain is denied oxygen, usually because of a blockage or rupture in a blood vessel serving the brain, resulting most frequently in damage that is specific and localized.

Childhood schizophrenia: A serious psychiatric illness that causes strange thinking, odd feelings, and unusual behavior. It is uncommon, occurring in approximately 1 in every 40,000 children younger than age 13 years.

Code switching: A complicated, rule-governed shifting from one language to another within and/or across different utterances.

Collaborative teaching: An educational method that combines consultation, team teaching, direct individual intervention, and side-by-side teaching in which the teacher and speech-language pathologist share the same goals for individual children.

Communication event: An entire conversation or narration and/or the topic or topics included therein.

Comprehension monitoring: Device used by communication participants to help them detect that a problem has occurred and to attempt to correct it and thus improve the accuracy of their representation of the meaning.

Contextualized language intervention (CLI): Language taught in the service of daily tasks rather than in isolated drills, providing a therapeutic focus within a purposeful and meaningful activity and across activities.

Contrast teaching: Teaching method that teaches a child to discriminate between structures and situations that obligate use of the feature being trained and those features that do not.

Critical thinking: Collecting and manipulating information, and applying it, often via language, to problem-solving.

Cultural congruency: Synchrony of intervention strategies and techniques with the cultural values, beliefs, and behaviors of the cultural/linguistic community.

Cultural humility: Recognizing one's own lack of cultural knowledge and maintaining an interpersonal stance that is open to others in relation to aspects of their cultural identity that are most important to them.

Culture: A shared framework of meanings within which a population shapes its way of life.

C-unit: A main clause plus any attached or embedded subordinate clause and also nonclausal structures, such as elliptical responses.

Deafness: A profound hearing loss of 90 dB or greater.

Deductive teaching procedures: Presentation of a rule guiding the use of a morphological inflection or marker along with models of use.

Developmental disabilities (DD): A severe, chronic disability of an individual aged 5 years or older that is attributable to mental or physical impairment or a combination of impairments; manifested before age 22 years; likely to continue indefinitely; results in substantial functional limitations in three or more areas of life activity; and reflects the individual's need for a combination and sequence of special, interdisciplinary, or generic services, individualized supports, or other forms of assistance that are of lifelong or of extended duration.

Dialectal scoring: An alternative method for scoring a test or analyzing a language sample, considering the dialectal structures and uses of a child.

Direct reference: Speaker considers the audience and clearly identifies the entity being mentioned.

Dual language learner (DLL): Term often used to refer to multilingual preschool children rather than the more inclusive English language learner (ELL).

Dynamic assessment: Adult-mediated assessment tasks that emphasize ability to communicate and learn language.

Dyslexia: A literacy disorder, characterized by difficulties with accurate or fluent word recognition, poor spelling, and deficits in coding abilities; referred to as "specific learning disability with impairment in reading" in DSM-5.

Early communication intervention (ECI): An intervention approach primarily focused on a young child's speech, language, and/or feeding difficulties.

GLOSSARY

Early intervention (EI): An educational approach for young children, who have or are at risk of developing a handicapping condition or other special need that may affect their development, providing both remediation and prevention services focused on both child and family.

Echolalia: Immediate or delayed whole or partial repetition of previous utterances of others with the same intonational pattern.

Emergent literacy (EL): "Literacy-like" behaviors that are acquired prior to formal reading and writing instruction.

English language learner (ELL): Term used to refer to multilingual school-age children.

Equity: Recognizes an individual's different circumstances and allocates resources and opportunities so that all have the potential for an equal outcome.

Evaluation: Defined in Part H of the Individuals with Disabilities Education Act and must be conducted to determine a child's eligibility for services, identifying a child's level of developmental functioning in a comprehensive and nondiscriminatory manner, often structured and formal with reliance on the use of standardized instruments.

Evidence-based practice (EBP): Clinical practice based on scientific evidence, clinical experience, and client needs.

Executive function: Located in the prefrontal area of the brain and consisting of inhibition, working memory, planning, organization, and regulatory processes that enable people to engage in goal-oriented behavior.

Expansion: A response to a child's utterance that is a more mature, or more correct, version of the child's utterance which maintains the child's word order.

Explicit instruction: Teaching in which a child is made consciously aware of the underlying language pattern.

Exposition: Discourse style found in textbooks, classroom lectures, technical papers, and documentaries.

Extension: A reply to the content of the child's utterance that provides additional information on the topic.

Fast mapping: Rapid assumption of a word's meaning upon hearing it, followed by subsequent use, although the complete meaning is unknown to a child, based on phonotactic probability or predictability of the new word and previous lexical knowledge.

Focused recasting: A child's utterance is restructured in a reply to maintain its meaning while increasing its grammatical accuracy or modifying its structure.

Functional language intervention: A child-based, communication-first assessment and intervention method that employs language as it is actually used as the vehicle for change.

Generalization: Carryover of learning to new content or to a different context.

Implicit instruction: Teaching in which the underlying goal is not explicitly identified for the learner.

Inclusion: An educational philosophy that proposes one integrated educational system based on each classroom becoming a supportive environment.

Indirect reference: Typically follows direct reference and refers to entities through the use of pronouns or such terms as *that one*.

Interlanguage: A hybrid form in which an individual combines rules from two or more languages, plus ad hoc rules from neither or both.

Language disorder: A heterogeneous group of developmental and/or acquired disorders and/or delays principally characterized by deficits and/or immaturities in the use of spoken or written language for comprehension and/or production purposes that may involve the form, content, and/or function of language in any combination.

Late language emergence (LLE): Delay in early language development affecting 10% to 15% of all children and possibly the single strongest predictor of later language disorder.

Learning disability or learning disorder (DSM-5): Disorder that involves one or more of the basic psychological processes; affects the understanding or use of using spoken and/or written language; may be manifested in the imperfect ability to listen, think, speak, read, write, spell, or do mathematical calculations; and is not primarily the result of visual, hearing, motor disabilities, mental retardation, emotional disturbance, or of environmental, cultural, or economic disadvantage.

Lexical competition: An instantaneous process of comprehension consisting of all the words predicted by our brains from the phonemes we hear and the possible words that will make sense.

Lexical similarity: Neighborhood density or the number of words that differ by one phoneme from a given word.

Mass learning: Learning that occurs all at once instead of spaced over time.

Maze: Language segments that disrupt, confuse, and slow conversational movements and may consist of silent pauses, fillers, repetitions, and revisions, often indicating where a child is having difficulty.

Mental graphemic representations (MGRs): Stored mental images of specific written words or word parts, containing specific allowable sequences of graphemes or letters representing written words.

Meta-analysis: Rates all studies on a specific research question and determines the strongest data.

Metalinguistics: The ability to consider language out of context, such as making judgments of correctness or similarity and difference.

Morbidity: Illness, disorder, or disability.

Normed test: A standardized test that has been given to a sample of individuals that supposedly represents all individuals for whom the test was designed. Scores are used to determine the typical performance expected for the entire population from whom the sample was drawn.

Onsets: Initial phonemes in a syllable prior to the vowel.

Orthographic awareness: An individual's conscious attention to print.

Orthographic knowledge: The information stored in our memory that tells us how to represent spoken language in a written form, such as the regularities of print.

Otitis media: Middle ear infection.

Parallel sentence production: A structured priming approach in which the SLP provides a model of the type of utterance desired and the child is expected to provide a similar type of sentence.

Percentile: An ordinal number, a rank, a place in a series; in tests, a rank in a theoretical group of 100.

Phonics: Sound–letter correspondence used as the basis for most reading instruction.

Phonological awareness: Literacy knowledge of the sounds and the sound and syllable structure of words.

Posttraumatic stress disorder (PTSD): Found in soldiers and in children with traumatic brain injury and those who have been abused. May be manifested in personality changes and in fears and anger.

Priming: When the utterance of one person influences the structure, vocabulary selection, or sounds used by a second speaker.

Print awareness: Knowing the direction in which reading proceeds across a page and through a book; being interested in print; recognizing letters; knowing that words are discrete units; and using literacy terminology, such as *letter*, *work*, and *sentence*.

Print knowledge: A generalized concept of what print does and how it is organized, encompassing both print concept knowledge and alphabet knowledge.

Procedural memory: Learning and execution of sequential cognitive information such as language.

Recasts: Maintain the child's meaning or the relations while modifying the structure, repeating at least one of the major lexical elements while modifying other parts of the utterance.

Reformulation: Two or more utterances combined into one that includes the concepts of each.

Reliability: Repeatability of a measure, based on the accuracy or precision with which a sample, at one time, represents performance based on either a different but similar sample or the same sample at a different time.

Rimes: Includes the vowel and the remaining phonemes in a syllable, as in *-ake* or *-ack*.

Selective mutism: A relatively rare disorder in which a child does not speak in some situations, such as in school, although they may speak normally in other situations.

Semantic networking: A method of improving reading comprehension, writing cohesion, retention, and recall by teaching organization of information around a central theme or sequence.

Sensitivity: A diagnostic accuracy measure of a test's ability to identify children with a language disorder.

Social cognition: The ability to process, store, and apply information about other people and social situations.

Social communication: Speech style, perspective taking, rules for verbal and nonverbal communication, and use language to accomplish goals.

Social communication disorder (SCD): A neurodevelopmental communication disorder that affects the appropriateness of both verbal and nonverbal communication skills in speaking and writing.

Social disinhibition: Inability to inhibit "acting out" behaviors often seen with traumatic brain injury. Emotional lability refers to rapid, often exaggerated changes in mood, including strong emotions or feelings, such as uncontrollable laughing or crying, or heightened irritability or temper.

Specific learning disorder: Term used by DSM-5 to refer to learning disability.

Specificity: A diagnostic accuracy measure of a test's ability to identify children who do not have a language disorder.

Standard deviation: A statistical manipulation that describes the shape of the standard curve.

Standard error of measure (SEm): A statistical value that aids a speech-language pathologist in knowing the confidence they can have in a child's scores.

Standard score: A statistical value in which 100 is applied to the mean, and based on the distribution of the scores, other values are added below and above the mean, as in IQ.

Standardized test: Standardized means that there is a consistent or standard manner in which test items are to be presented and the adult is to respond to the child's responses.

Statistical learning: The use of frequency information or how often something occurs, such as a word, to identify underlying rules and meaning.

Structural priming: When a sentence produced by one speaker influences the structure of the sentences of a second speaker.

Taxonomic awareness: Sensitivity to the hierarchical organization of words, such as category membership, and similarity and dissimilarity.

Theory of mind (ToM): Social perception skills, such as understanding the thoughts and emotions of others.

Traumatic brain injury (TBI): Diffuse brain injury usually caused by a fall, vehicle accident, physical abuse, or gun injury.

T-units (minimal terminal units): A main clause plus any attached or embedded subordinate clause or nonclausal structure.

Utterance: A sentence or less, separated by a pause of 2 seconds or more, even if in the middle of a thought, a drop in the voice, and/or an inhalation.

Validity: Effectiveness of a test in representing, describing, or predicting an attribute. A test's ability to assess what it purports to measure.

Working memory: Memory in which information, such as incoming and outgoing language, is kept active while processed.

References

Abbeduto, L., Benson, G., Short, K., & Dolish, J. (1995). Effects of sampling context on the expressive language of children and adolescents with mental retardation. *Mental Retardation, 33*, 279–288.

Abbeduto, L., Kover, S. T., & McDuffie, A. (2012). Studying the language development of children with intellectual disabilities. In E. Hoff (Ed.), *Handbook of child language research methods* (pp. 330–346). Wiley.

Adams, C. (2002). Practitioner review: The assessment of language pragmatics. *Journal of Child Psychology and Psychiatry, 43*, 973–987.

Adams, C., Gaile, J., Freed, J., & Lockton, E. (2010). *Targeted Observation of Pragmatics in Children's Conversation (TOPICC) observation scale.* https://www.scribd.com/document/142517513/TOPICCal-applications

Adams, C., Lockton, E., Gaile, J., & Freed, J., (2011). TOPICCAL applications: Assessment of children's conversation skills. *Speech and Language Therapy in Practice*, Spring, 7– 9.

Adams, M., Foorman, B., Lundberg, I., & Beeler, T. (1998). *Phonemic awareness in young children: A classroom curriculum.* Brookes.

Adani, F., Forgiarini, M., Guasti, M. T., & van der Lely, H. K. J. (2014). Number dissimilarities facilitate the comprehension of relative clauses in children with (grammatical) specific language impairment. *Journal of Child Language, 41*, 811–841. https://doi.org/10.1017/S0305000913000184

Ad Hoc Committee on Service Delivery in Schools. (1993). American Speech-Language-Hearing Association (ASHA).

Adlof, S. M., & Hogan, T. P. (2018). Understanding dyslexia in the context of developmental language disorders. *Language, Speech, and Hearing Services in Schools, 49*, 762–773. https://doi.org/10.1044/2018_LSHSS-DYSLC-18-0049

Adlof, S. M., & Perfetti, C. (2014). Individual differences in word learning and reading ability. In C. A. Stone, E. R. Silliman, B. J. Ehren, & G. Wallach (Eds.), *Handbook of language and literacy: Development and disorders* (2nd ed., pp. 246–264). Guilford.

Adlof, S. M., Scoggins, J., Brazendale, A., Babb, S., & Petscher, Y. (2017). Identifying children at risk for language impairment or dyslexia with group-administered measures. *Journal of Speech, Language, and Hearing Research, 60*, 3507–3522.

Afacan, K., Wilkerson, K. L., & Ruppar, A. L. (2018). Multicomponent reading interventions for students with intellectual disability. *Remedial and Special Education, 39*(4), 229–242. https://doi.org/10.1177/0741932517702444

Alderete, A., Frey, S., McDaniel, N., Romero, J., Westby, C., & Roman, R. (2004, November). *Developing vocabulary in school.* Paper presented at the American Speech-Language-Hearing Association Annual Convention, Philadelphia.

Aljahlan, Y., & Spaulding, T. J. (2019). The impact of manipulating attentional shifting demands on preschool children with specific language impairment. *Journal of Speech, Language and Hearing Disorders, 62*, 324–336. https://doi.org/10.1044/2018_JSLHR-L-17-0358

Allen, J. B., & Mason, J. M. (1989). *Risk makers, risk takers, risk breakers: Reducing the risks for young literacy learners.* Heinemann.

Allor, J. H., Mathes, P. G., Roberts, J. K., Cheatham, J. P., & Champlin, T. M. (2010). Comprehensive reading instruction for students with intellectual disabilities: Findings from the first three years of a longitudinal study. *Psychology in the Schools, 47*(5), 445–466. https://doi.org/10.1002/pits.20482

Alloway, T. P., & Alloway, R. G. (2010). Investigating the predictive roles of working memory and IQ in academic attainment. *Journal of Experimental Child Psychology, 106*(1), 20–29. https://doi.org/10.1016/j.jecp.2009.11.003 http://scholar.google.com/scholar_lookup?hl=en&volume=106&publication_year=2010&pages=20-29&journal=Journal+of+Experimental+Child+Psychology&issue=1&author=T.+P.+Alloway&author=R.+G.+Alloway&title=Investigating+the+predictive+roles+of+working+memory+and+IQ+in+academic+attainment

Alloway, T. P., Gathercole, S. E., Kirkwood, H., & Elliott, J. (2009). The cognitive and behavioural characteristics of children with low working memory. *Child Development, 80*, 606–621.

Al Otaiba, S., Gillespie Rouse, A., & Baker, K. (2018). Elementary grade intervention approaches to treat specific learning disabilities, including dyslexia. *Language, Speech, and Hearing Services in Schools, 49*, 829–842. https://doi.org/10.1044/2018_LSHSS-DYSLC-18-0022

Alt, M., Figueroa, C. R., Mettler, H. M., Evans-Reitz, N., & Erikson, J. A. (2021). A Vocabulary Acquisition and Usage for Late Talkers treatment efficacy study: The effect of input utterance length and identification of responder profiles. *Journal of Speech, Language, and Hearing Research, 64*, 1235–1255. https://doi.org/10.1044/2020_JSLHR-20-00525

Alt, M., Gray, S., Hogan, T. P., Schlesinger, N., & Cowan, N. (2019). Spoken word learning differences among children with dyslexia, concomitant dyslexia and developmental language disorder, and typical development. *Language, Speech and Hearing Services in Schools, 50*, 540–561. https://doi.org/10.1044/2019_LSHSS-VOIA-18-0138

Alt, M., Hogan, T., Green, S., Gray, S., Cabbage, K., & Cowan, N. (2017). Word learning deficits in children with dyslexia. *Journal of Speech, Language, and Hearing Research, 60*, 1012–1028.

Alt, M., Meyers, C., & Ancharski, A. (2012). Using principles of learning to inform language therapy design for children with specific language impairment. *International Journal of Language & Communication Disorders, 47,* 487–498.

Alt, M., Plante, E., & Creusere, M. (2004). Semantic features in fast-mapping: Performance of preschoolers with specific language impairment versus preschoolers with normal language. *Journal of Speech, Language, and Hearing Research, 47,* 407–420.

Altmann, L., Lombardino, L. J., & Puranik, C. (2008). Sentence production in students with dyslexia. *International Journal of Language & Communication Disorders, 43*(1), 55–76.

Ambridge, B., Kidd, E., Rowland, C., & Theakston, A. (2015). The ubiquity of frequency effects in first language acquisition. *Journal of Child Language, 42,* 239–273.

Amendah, D., Grosse, S. D., Peacock, G., & Mandell, D. S. (2011). The economic costs of autism: A review. In D. Amaral, D. Geschwind, & G. Dawson (Eds.), *Autism spectrum disorders* (pp. 1347–1360). Oxford University Press.

American Academy of Pediatrics. (2022). *Fetal alcohol spectrum disorders: FAQs of parents & families.* https://www .healthychildren.org/English/health-issues/conditions/ chronic/Pages/Fetal-Alcohol-Spectrum-Disorders-FAQs-of-Parents-and-Families.aspx

American College of Obstetricians and Gynecologists. (2002, September). Perinatal care at the threshold viability. *ACOG Practice Bulletin, 38.*

American Psychiatric Association. (2013). *Diagnostic and statistical manual of mental disorders* (5th ed.).

American Psychiatric Association. (2018, November). *What is specific learning disorder.* https://www.psychiatry.org/ patients-families/specific-learning-disorder/what-is-spe cific-learning-disorder

American Speech-Language-Hearing Association. (n.d.). *Intellectual disability.* https://www.asha.org/practice-portal/ clinical-topics/intellectual-disability/

American Speech-Language-Hearing Association. (n.d.). Roles and responsibilities of speech-language pathologists with respect to reading and writing in children and adolescents. https://www.asha.org/policy/ps2001-00104/

American Speech-Language-Hearing Association. (2001). *Roles and responsibilities of speech-language pathologists with respect to reading and writing in children and adolescents.* http://www.asha.org/policy/PS2001-00104

American Speech-Language-Hearing Association. (2002). *Knowledge and skills needed by speech-language pathologists with respect to reading and writing in children and adolescents.* http://www.asha.org/policy/KS2002-00082

American Speech-Language-Hearing Association. (2004). Admission/discharge criteria in speech-language pathology. *ASHA Supplement, 24,* 65–70.

American Speech-Language-Hearing Association. (2008a). Core knowledge and skills in early intervention speech-language pathology practice. https://www.asha .org/policy

American Speech-Language-Hearing Association. (2008b). *Roles and responsibilities of speech-language pathologists in early intervention: Guidelines.* https://www.asha.org/policy

American Speech-Language-Hearing Association. (2008c). *Roles and responsibilities of speech-language pathologists in early intervention: Position statement.* https://www.asha .org/policy

American Speech-Language-Hearing Association. (2008d). *Roles and responsibilities of speech-language pathologists in early intervention: Technical report.* https://www.asha.org/ policy

American Speech-Language-Hearing Association. (2010). *Roles and responsibilities of speech-language pathologists in schools.* http://www.asha.org/policy/PI2010-00317

American Speech-Language-Hearing Association. (2013). *Cultural and linguistic competence.* http://www.asha.org/ Practice/ethics/Cultural-and-Linguistic-Competence/

American Speech-Language-Hearing Association. (2016). *Scope of practice in speech-language pathology* [Scope of practice]. www.asha.org/policy/

American Speech-Language-Hearing Association. (2017). *Issues in ethics: Cultural and linguistic competence.* http:// www.asha.org/Practice/ethics/Cultural-and-Linguistic-Competence

American Speech-Language-Hearing Association. (2019). *Social communication disorder.* http://asha.org/practice-portal/clinical-topics/social-communication-disorder/

American Speech-Language-Hearing Association. (2021). *Demographic profile of ASHA members providing bilingual services year-end 2020.* https://www.asha.org/siteassets/ surveys/demographic-profile-bilingual-spanish-service-members.pdf

Anaya, J. B., Peña, E. D., & Bedore, L. M. (2018). Conceptual scoring and classification accuracy of vocabulary testing in bilingual children. *Language, Speech, and Hearing Services in Schools, 49*(1), 85–97. https://doi.org/10.1044/ 2017_LSHSS-16-0081

Andersen Helland, W., Posserud, M., Helland, T., Heimann, M., & Lundervold, A. J. (2016a). Language impairments in children with ADHD and in children with reading disorder. *Journal of Attention Disorders, 10,* 581–589. https:// doi.org/10.1177/1087054712461530

Andersen Helland, W., Posserud, M., Helland, T., Heimann, M., & Lundervold, A. J. (2016b). Language impairments in children with ADHD and in children with reading disorder. *Journal of Attention Disorders, 20,* 581–589. https:// doi.org/10.1177/1087054712461530

Anderson, D. K., Lord, C., & Heinz, S. J. (2005, May). *Growth in language abilities among children with ASD and other developmental disabilities.* Poster presented at the International Meeting for Autism Research, Boston, MA.

Anderson, D. K., Lord, C., Risi, S., DiLavore, P. S., Shulman, C., Thurm, A., . . . Pickles, A. (2007). Patterns of growth in verbal abilities among children with autism spectrum disorder. *Journal of Consulting and Clinical Psychology, 75*(4), 594–604. https://doi.org/10.1037/0022-006X.75.4. 594

REFERENCES

Anderson, D. R., & Pempek, T. (2005). Television and very young children. *American Behavioral Scientist, 48*, 505–522. https://doi.org/10.1177/0002764204271506

Anderson, V. A., Catroppa, C., Morse, S., Haritou, F., & Rosenfeld, J. (2000). Recovery of intellectual ability following traumatic brain injury in childhood: Impact of injury severity and age at injury. *Pediatric Neurosurgery, 32*, 282–290.

Andres, E. M., Kelsey Earnest, K., Smith, S. D., Rice, M. L., & Hashim Raza, M. (2020). Pedigree-based gene mapping supports previous loci and reveals novel suggestive loci in specific language impairment. *Journal of Speech, Language, and Hearing Research, 63*, 4046–4061. https://doi.org/10.1044/2020_JSLHR-20-00102

Angelo, D. H. (2000). Impact of augmentative and alternative communication devices on families. *Augmentative and Alternative Communication, 16*, 37–47.

Anthony, J., & Lonigan, C. (2004). The nature of phonological awareness: Converging evidence from four studies of preschool and early grade school children. *Journal of Educational Psychology, 96*, 43–55.

Anthony, J., Lonigan, C., Driscoll, K., Phillips, B., & Burgess, S. (2003). Phonological sensitivity: A quasi-parallel progression of word structure units and cognitive operation. *Reading Research Quarterly, 38*, 470–487.

Apel, K. (2010). Kindergarten children's initial spoken and written word learning in a storybook context. *Scientific Studies in Reading, 14*(5), 440–463.

Apel, K. (2011). What is orthographic knowledge? *Language, Speech, and Hearing Services in Schools, 42*, 592–603.

Apel, K., & Lawrence, J. (2011). Contributions of morphological awareness skills to word-level reading and spelling in first-grade children with and without speech sound disorder. *Journal of Speech, Language, and Hearing Research, 54*, 1312–1327.

Apel, K., & Thomas-Tate, S. (2009). Morphological awareness skills of fourth-grade African American students. *Language, Speech, and Hearing Services in Schools, 40*, 312–324.

Applebee, A. N. (1978). *The child's concept of story*. University of Chicago Press.

Applequist, K. L., & Bailey, D. B. (2000). Navajo caregivers' perceptions of early intervention services. *Journal of Early Intervention, 23*, 47–61.

Archer, A. L., & Hughes, C. A. (2011). *Explicit instruction: Effective and efficient teaching*. Guilford.

Archibald, L. (2021, July 6). *DLD Toolbox*. Language and Working Memory Lab, Western University, London, Ontario, Canada. https://www.uwo.ca/fhs/lwm/news/2021/06_07_DLDUnder5.html

Archibald, L. M., & Gathercole, S. E. (2006). Short-term and working memory in specific language impairment. *International Journal of Language and Communication Disorders, 41*(6), 675–693.

Archibald, L. M., & Gathercole, S. E. (2007). The complexities of complex memory span: Storage and processing deficits in specific language impairment. *Journal of Memory and Language, 57*, 177–194.

Archibald, L. M., & Joanisse, M. (2009). On the sensitivity and specificity of nonword repetition and sentence recall to language and memory impairments in children. *Journal of Speech, Language, and Hearing Research, 52*, 899–914.

Arciuli, J., Stevens, K., Trembath, D., & Simpson, I. C. (2013). The relationship between parent report of adaptive behavior and direct assessment of reading ability in children with autism spectrum disorder. *Journal of Speech, Language, and Hearing Research, 56*, 1837–1844. https://doi.org/10.1044/1092-4388(2013/12-0034)

Arden, S. V., Gruner Gandhi, A., Zumeta Edmonds, R., & Danielson, L. (2017). Toward more effective tiered systems: Lessons from national implementation efforts. *Exceptional Children, 83*, 269–280. https://doi.org/10.1177/0014402917693565 http://scholar.google.com/scholar_lookup?hl=en&volume=83&publication_year=2017&pages=269-280&journal=Exceptional+Children&author=S.+V.+Arden&author=A.+Gruner+Gandhi&author=R.+Zumeta+Edmonds&author=L.+Danielson&title=Toward+more+effective+tiered+systems%3A+Lessons+from+national+implementation+efforts

Atchison, B. J. (2007). Sensory modulation disorders among children with a history of trauma: A frame of reference for speech-language pathologists. *Language, Speech, and Hearing Services in Schools, 38*, 109–116.

August, D., Snow, C., Carlo, M., Proctor, C. P., Rolla de San Francisco, A., Duursma, E., & Szuber, A. (2006). Literacy development in elementary school second-language learners. *Topics in Language Disorders, 26*, 351–364.

Ault, M. J., & Griffen, A. K. (2013). Teaching with the system of least prompts: An easy method for monitoring progress. *Teaching Exceptional Children, 45*, 46–53.

Autism Speaks. (n.d.). *Autism Diagnostic Criteria: DSM-5*. https://www.autismspeaks.org/autism-diagnosis-criteria-dsm-5

Bacon, E. C., Osuna, S., Courchesne, E., & Pierce, K. (2019). Naturalistic language sampling to characterize the language abilities of 3-year-olds with autism spectrum disorder. *Autism, 23*(3), 699–712. https://doi.org/10.1177/1362361318766241

Bailey, D. B. (2004). Assessing family resources, priorities, and concerns. In M. McLean, M. Wolery, & D. Bailey (Eds.), *Assessing infants and preschoolers with special needs* (3rd ed., pp. 172–203). Pearson Merrill Prentice Hall.

Balu, R., Zhu, P., Doolittle, F., Schiller, E., Jenkins, J. R., & Gersten, R. (2015). *Evaluation of response to intervention practices for elementary school reading* (NCEE 2016-4000). Institute of Education Sciences, U.S. Department of Education.http://scholar.google.com/scholar_lookup?hl=en&publication_year=2015&journal=Evaluation+of+response+to+intervention+practices+for+elementary+school+reading.+%28NCEE+2016-4000%29&author=R.+Balu&author=P.+Zhu&author=F.+Doolittle&author=E.+Schiller&author=J.+R.+Jenkins&author=R.+Gersten

Banales, E., Kohnen, S., & McArthur, G. (2015). Can verbal working memory training improve reading? *Cognitive*

Neuropsychology, 32, 104–132. https://doi.org/10.1080/02643294.2015.1014331 http://scholar.google.com/scholar_lookup?hl=en&volume=32&publication_year=2015&pages=104-132&journal=Cognitive+Neuropsychology&author=E.+Banales&author=S.+Kohnen&author=G.+McArthur&title=Can+verbal+working+memory+training+improve+reading%3F

Bangert, K. J., Halverson, D. M., & Finestack, L. H. (2019). Evaluation of an explicit instructional approach to teach grammatical forms to children with low-symptom severity autism spectrum disorder. *American Journal of Speech-Language Pathology, 28*(2), 650–663. https://doi.org/10.1044/2018_AJSLP-18-0016

Banney, R. M., Harper-Hill, K., & Arnott, W. L. (2015). The autism diagnostic observation schedule and narrative assessment: Evidence for specific narrative impairments in autism spectrum disorders. *International Journal of Speech-Language Pathology, 17*, 159–171. https://doi.org/10.3109/1 7549507.2014.977348

Barako Arndt, K., & Schiele, C. M. (2013). Multiclausal utterances aren't just for big kids: A framework for analysis of complex syntax in spoken language of preschool- and early school-age children. *Topics in Language Disorders, 33*(2), 125–139.

Baranowski, M. (2013). Ethnicity and sound change: African American English in Charleston, SC. *University of Pennsylvania Working Papers in Linguistics, 19*(2), 1–10.

Barkley, R. A. (2006). *Attention-deficit hyperactivity disorder: A handbook for diagnosis and treatment* (3rd ed.). Guilford.

Barnhill, G. P. (2001). Social attributions and depression in adolescents with Asperger's syndrome. *Focus on Autism and Other Developmental Disabilities, 16*(1), 46–53.

Barokova, M., & Tager-Flusberg, H. (2018). Commentary: Measuring language change through natural language samples. *Journal of Autism and Developmental Disorders, 50*, 2287–2306. https://doi.org/10.1007/s10803-018-3628-4

Barras, C., Geoffrois, E., Wu, Z., & Liberman, M. (1998–2008). *Transcriber* (Version 1.5) [Computer software]. DGA.

Barrouillet, P., Bernardin, S., Portrat, S., Vergauwe, E., & Camos, V. (2007). Time and cognitive load in working memory. *Journal of Experimental Psychology, Learning, Memory and Cognition, 33*, 570–585. https://doi.org/10.1037/0278-7393.33.3.570

Barrow, I. M., Holbert, D., & Rastatter, M. P. (2000). Effect of color on developmental picture vocabulary naming of 4-, 6-, and 8-year-old children. *American Journal of Speech-Language Pathology, 9*, 310–318.

Barstein, J., Martin, G. E., Lee, M., & Losh, M. (2018). A duck wearing boots?! Pragmatic language strategies for repairing communication breakdowns across genetically based neurodevelopmental disabilities. *Journal of Speech, Language, and Hearing Disorders, 61*, 1440–1454. https://doi.org/10.1044/2018_JSLHR-L-17-0064

Bashir, A. S., & Hook, P. E. (2009). Fluency: A key link between word identification and comprehension. *Language, Speech, and Hearing Services in Schools, 40*, 196–200.

Bashir, A. S., & Singer, B. D. (2006). Assisting students in becoming self-regulated writers. In T. Ukrainetz (Ed.), *Contextualized language intervention: Scaffolding preK–12 literacy achievement* (pp. 565–598). Thinking Publications.

Bean Ellawadi, A., & Ellis Weismer, S. (2015). Using spoken language benchmarks to characterize the expressive language skills of young children with autism spectrum disorders. *American Journal of Speech-Language Pathology, 24*, 696–707. https://doi.org/10.1044/2015_AJSLP-14-0190

Bear, D. R., Invernizzi, M., Templeton, S., & Johnston, F. (2016). *Words their way* (6th ed.). Pearson. http://scholar.google.com/scholar_lookup?hl=en&publication_year=2016&author=D.+R.+Bear&author=M.+Invernizzi&author=S.+Templeton&author=F.+Johnston&title=Words+their+way

Beck, A. R., & Dennis, M. (1997). Speech-language pathologists and teachers' perceptions of classroom-based interventions. *Language, Speech, and Hearing Services in Schools, 28*, 146–153.

Beck, I. L., McKeown, M. G., & Kucan, L. (2008). *Creating robust vocabulary: Frequently asked questions and extended examples*. Guilford.

Beck, I. L., McKeown, M. G., & Kucan, L. (2013). *Bringing words to life: Robust vocabulary instruction* (2nd ed.). Guilford.

Beckett, C., Bredenkamp, D., Castle, C., Groothues, C., O'Connor, T. G., & Rutter, M., & the English and Romanian Adoptees Study Team. (2002). Behavior patterns associated with institutional deprivation: A study of children adopted from Romania. *Developmental and Behavioral Pediatrics, 23*, 297–303.

Bedore, L. M., & Leonard, L. B. (2000). The effects of inflectional variation on fast mapping of verbs in English and Spanish. *Journal of Speech, Language, and Hearing Research, 43*, 21–33.

Bedore, L. M., & Leonard, L. B. (2001). Grammatical morphology deficits in Spanish-speaking children with specific language. *Journal of Speech, Language, and Hearing Research, 44*, 905–924.

Bedore, L. M., & Peña, E. D. (2008). Assessment of bilingual children for identification of language impairment: Current findings and implications for practice. *International Journal of Bilingual Education and Bilingualism, 11*(1), 1–29. https://doi.org/10.2167/beb392.0

Bedore, L. M., Peña, E. D., Anaya, J. B., Nieto, R., Lugo-Neris, M. J., & Baron, A. (2018). Understanding disorder within variation: Production of English grammatical forms by English language learners. *Language, Speech, and Hearing Services in Schools, 49*(2), 277–291. https://doi.org/10.1044/2017_LSHSS-17-0027

Bedore, L. M., Peña, E. D., Fiestas, C., & Lugo-Neris, M. J. (2020). Language and literacy together: Supporting grammatical development in dual language learners with risk for language and learning difficulties. *Language, Speech, and Hearing Services in Schools, 51*, 282–297. https://doi.org/10.1044/2020_LSHSS-19-00055

Bedore, L. M., Peria, E. D., Garcia, M., & Cortez, C. (2005). Conceptual versus monolingual scoring: When does it make a difference? *Language, Speech, and Hearing Services in Schools*, *36*, 188–200.

Beitchman, J. H., Wilson, B., Johnson, C. J., Atkinson, L., Young, A., Adlaf, E., . . . Douglas, L. (2001). Fourteen-year follow-up of speech/language-impaired and control children: Psychiatric outcome. *Journal of the American Academy of Child & Adolescent Psychiatry*, *40*, 75–82.

Bellon, M., Ogletree, B., & Harn, W. (2000). Repeated storybook reading as a language intervention for children with autism: A case study on the application of scaffolding. *Focus on Autism and Other Developmental Disabilities*, *15*(1), 52–58.

Bencini, G. M., & Valian, V. V. (2008). Abstract sentence representations in 3-year-olds: Evidence from language production and comprehension. *Journal of Memory and Language*, *59*, 97–113.

Bennett, T. A., Szatmari, P., Georgiades, K., Hanna, S., Janus, M., Georgiades, S., . . . the Pathways in ASD Study Team. (2014). Language impairment and early social competence in preschoolers with autism spectrum disorders: A comparison of DSM-5 profiles. *Journal of Autism and Developmental Disorders*, *11*, 2797–2808.

Benway, N., Owens, R. E., & Pavelko, S. L. (2021, November). *Introducing SPOON: Automated SUGAR language sample analysis*. Paper presented at the American Speech-Language-Hearing Association Convention, Washington, DC.

Berenguer, C., Miranda, A., Colomer, C., Baixauli, I., & Roselló, B. (2018). Contribution of theory of mind, executive functioning, and pragmatics to socialization behaviors of children with high-functioning autism. *Journal of Autism and Developmental Disorders*, *48*, 430–441.

Bergman, R. L., Piacentini, J., & McCracken, J. (2002). Prevalence and description of selective mutism in a school-based sample. *Journal of the American Academy of Child and Adolescent Psychiatry*, *41*, 938–946.

Berman, R. A., & Nir-Sagiv, B. (2007). Comparing narrative and expository text construction across adolescence: A developmental paradox. *Discourse Processes*, *43*, 79–120. https://doi.org/10.1080/01638530709336894

Berman, R. A., & Verhoven, L. (2002). Cross-linguistic perspectives on the development of text-production abilities: Speech and writing. *Written Language and Literacy*, *5*(1), 1–43.

Bernal, G., & Sáez-Santiago, E. (2006). Culturally centered psychosocial interventions. *Journal of Community Psychology*, *34*(2), 121–132. https://doi.org/10.1002/jcop.20096

Bernheimer, L., & Weismer, T. (2007). "Let me tell you what I do all day . . . ": The family story at the center of intervention research and practice. *Infants and Young Children*, *20*(3), 192–201.

Berninger, V. W. (2000). Development of language by hand and its connections to language by ear, mouth, and eye. *Topics in Language Disorders*, *20*, 65–84.

Berninger, V. W. (2007a). *PAL II Reading and Writing Diagnostic Test Battery*. Psychological Corporation.

Berninger, V. W. (2007b). *PAL II user guides* (2nd version). Psychological Corporation/Pearson.

Berninger, V. W. (2008). Defining and differentiating dyslexia, dysgraphia, and language learning disability within a working memory model. In E. Silliman & M. Mody (Eds.), *Language impairment and reading disability—Interactions among brain, behavior, and experience* (pp. 103–134). Guilford.

Berninger, V. W., Abbott, R. D., Swanson, H. L., Lovitt, D., Trivedi, P., Lin, S.-J., . . . Amtmann, D. (2010). Relationship of word and sentence-level working memory to reading and writing in second, fourth, and sixth grade. *Language, Speech, and Hearing Services in Schools*, *41*, 179–193.

Berninger, V. W., Nagy, W. E., Carlisle, J., Thomson, J., Hoffer, D., Abbott, S., . . . Dyslexia Foundation (2003). Effective treatment for children with dyslexia in grades 4–6: Behavioral and brain evidence. In B. R. Foorman (Ed.), *Preventing and remediating reading difficulties: Bringing science to scale* (pp. 381–417). York Press.

Berninger, V. W., Raskind, W., Richards, T., Abbott, R., & Stock, P. (2008). A multidisciplinary approach to understanding development dyslexia within working-memory architecture: Genotypes, phenotypes, brain, and instruction. *Development Neuropsychology*, *33*, 707–744.

Berninger, V. W., Vaughan, K., Abbott, R. D., Brooks, A., Begayis, K., Curtin, G., . . . Graham, S. (2000). Language-based spelling instruction: Teaching children to make multiple connections between spoken and written words. *Learning Disability Quarterly*, *23*(2), 117–135. http://scholar.google.com/scholar_lookup?hl=en&volume=23&publication_year=2000&pages=117-135&journal=Learning+Disability+Quarterly&issue=2&author=V.+W.+Berninger&author=K.+Vaughan&author=R.+D.+Abbott&author=A.+Brooks&author=K.+Begayis&author=G.+Curtin&author=S.+Graham&title=Language-based+spelling+instruction%3A+Teaching+children+to+make+multiple+connections+between+spoken+and+written+words

Berninger, V. W., Winn, W. D., Stock, P., Abbott, R. D., Eschen, K., Shi-Ju, L., . . . Nagy, W. (2008). Tier 3 specialized writing instruction for students with dyslexia. *Reading and Writing*, *21*, 95–129.

Berninger, V. W., & Wolf, B. (2009a). *Helping students with dyslexia and dysgraphia make connections: Differential instruction lesson plans in reading and writing*. Brookes.

Berninger, V. W., & Wolf, B. (2009b). *Teaching students with dyslexia and dysgraphia: Lessons from teaching and science*. Brookes.

Bernstein Ratner, N., & Brundage, S. B. (2018). *A clinician's complete guide to CLAN and PRAAT*. https://talkbank.org/manuals/Clin-CLAN.pdf

Bernstein Ratner, N., & MacWhinney, B. (2016). Your laptop to the rescue: Using the Child Language Data Exchange System archive and CLAN utilities to improve child language sample analysis. *Seminars in Speech and Language, 37*(2), 74–84. https://doi.org/10.1055/s-0036-1580742

Berry, J. R., & Oetting, J. B. (2017). Use of copula and auxiliary BE by African American children with Gullah/Geechee heritage. *Journal of Speech, Language, and Hearing Research, 60*, 2557–2568. https://doi.org/10.1044/2017_JSLHR-L-16-0120

Berry-Kravis, E., Doll, E., Sterling, A., Kover, S. T., Schroeder, S. M., Mathur, S., & Abbeduto, L. (2013). Development of an expressive language sampling procedure in fragile X syndrome: A pilot study. *Journal of Developmental Behavioral Pediatrics, 34*, 245–251. https://doi.org/10.1097/dbp.0b013e31828742fc http://scholar.google.com/scholar_lookup?hl=en&publication_year=2013&pages=245-251&title=Development+of+an+expressive+language+sampling+procedure+in+fragile+X+syndrome%3A+A+pilot+study

Beukelman, D. R., & Mirenda, P. (2005). *Augmentative and alternative communication: Supporting children and adults with complex communication needs* (3rd ed.). Brookes.

Bhasin, T. K., Brocksen, S., Avchen, R. N., & Braun, K. V. N. (2006). Prevalence of four developmental disabilities among children aged 8 years: Metropolitan Atlanta Developmental Disabilities Surveillance Program, 1996 and 2000. *Morbidity and Mortality Weekly Report, 55*(Suppl. 1), 1–9.

Bialystok, E., Craik, F. I. M., & Luk, G. (2008). Lexical access in bilinguals: Effects of vocabulary size and executive control. *Journal of Neurolinguistics, 21*, 522–538.

Bialystok, E., Luk, G., Peets, K., & Yang, S. (2010). Receptive vocabulary differences in monolingual and bilingual children. *Bilingualism, 13*, 525–531.

Bibby, P., Eikeseth, S., Martin, N., Mudford, O., & Reeves, D. (2001). Progress and outcomes for children with autism receiving parent-managed intensive interventions. *Research in Developmental Disabilities, 22*, 425–447.

Biemiller, A. (2001). Teaching vocabulary: Early, direct, and sequential. *American Educator, 25*, 24–28.

Binger, C., Kent-Walsh, J., Harrington, N., & Hollerbach, Q. C. (2020). Tracking early sentence-building progress in graphic symbol communication. *Language, Speech, and Hearing Services in Schools, 51*, 317–328. https://doi.org/10.1044/2019_LSHSS-19-00065

Binger, C., Kent-Walsh, J., & King, M. (2017). Dynamic assessment for three- and four-year old children who use augmentative and alternative communication: Evaluating expressive syntax. *Journal of Speech, Language, and Hearing Research, 60*, 1946–1958. https://doi.org/10.1044/2017_JSLHR-L-15-0269

Binger, C., & Light, J. C. (2006). Demographics of preschoolers who require augmentative and alternative communication. *Language, Speech, and Hearing Services in Schools, 37*, 200–208.

Binger, C., Ragsdale, J., & Bustos, A. (2016). Language sampling for preschoolers with severe speech impairments. *American Journal of Speech-Language Pathology, 25*, 493–507. https://doi.org/10.1044/2016_AJSLP-15-0100

Bishop, D. V. (1985). *Automated LARSP* [Computer program]. University of Manchester.

Bishop, D. V. (2003). *Children's Communication Checklist–2*. Psychological Corporation.

Bishop, D. V. (2004). *Expression, Reception, and Recall of Narrative Instrument*. Pearson.

Bishop, D. V. (2006). *Children's Communication Checklist–2* (U.S. ed.). Psychological Corporation.

Bishop, D. V. (2009). Genes, cognition and communication: Insights from neurodevelopmental disorders. *Annals of the New York Academy of Sciences, 1156*, 1–18.

Bishop, D. V. (2015). The interface between genetics and psychology: Lessons from developmental dyslexia. *Proceedings of the Royal Society B: Biological Sciences, 282*, 20143139. https://doi.org/10.1098/rspb.2014.3139 http://scholar.google.com/scholar_lookup?hl=en&volume=282&publication_year=2015&pages=20143139&journal=Proceedings+of+the+Royal+Society+B%3A+Biological+Sciences&author=D.+V.+Bishop&title=The+interface+between+genetics+and+psychology%3A+Lessons+from+developmental+dyslexia

Bishop, D. V., & Baird, G. (2001). Parent and teacher report of pragmatic aspects of communication: Use of the Children's Communication Checklist in a clinical setting. *Developmental Medicine and Child Neurology, 43*, 809–818.

Bishop, D. V., McDonald, D., Bird, S. & Hayiou-Thomas, M. E. (2009). Children who read words accurately despite language impairment: who are they and how do they do it? *Child Development, 80*, 593–605.

Bishop, D. V., Price, T. S., Dale, P. S., & Plomin, R. (2003). Outcomes of early language delay: II. Etiology of transient and persistent language difficulties. *Journal of Speech, Language, and Hearing Research, 46*, 561–575.

Bishop, D. V., Snowling, M. J., Thompson, P. A., Greenhalgh, T., & The CATALISE-2 Consortium. (2017). Phase 2 of CATALISE: A multinational and multidisciplinary Delphi consensus study of problems with language development: Terminology. *Journal of Child Psychology and Psychiatry, 58*, 1068–1080. https://doi.org/10.1111/jcpp.12721

Bitetti, D., & Scheffner Hammer, C. (2016). The home literacy environment and the English narrative development of Spanish–English bilingual children. *Journal of Speech, Language, and Hearing Research, 59*, 1159–1171. https://doi.org/10.1044/2016_JSLHR-L-15-0064

Bitetti, D., & Scheffner Hammer, C. (2021). English narrative macrostructure development of Spanish–English bilingual children from preschool to first grade. *American Journal of Speech-Language Pathology, 30*, 1100–1115. https://doi.org/10.1044/2021_AJSLP-20-00046

Bjork, E. (2004, November). *Research on learning as a foundation for curricular reform and pedagogy*. Paper presented at the Reinvention Center Conference, Washington, DC.

Bjork, R. (2011). On the symbiosis of remembering, forgetting, and learning. In A. S. Benjamin (Ed.), *Successful remembering and successful forgetting: A festschrift in honor of Robert A. Bjork* (pp. 1–22). Psychology Press.

Blachman, B. (1984). Relationship of rapid naming ability and language analysis skills in kindergarten and first grade reading achievement. *Reading Research Quarterly, 13*, 223–253.

Blachman, B., Ball, E., Black, R., & Tangel, D. (2000). *Road to the code: A phonological awareness program for young children*. Brookes.

Blackstone, S. W., & Hunt-Berg, M. (2003). *Social networks: An assessment and intervention planning inventory for individuals with complex communication needs and their communication partners*. Augmentative Communication.

Blank, M., Rose, S. A., & Berlin, L. J. (2003). *Preschool Language Assessment Instrument* (2nd ed.). Pro-Ed. http://scholar.google.com/scholar_lookup?hl=en&publication_year=2003&title=Preschool+Language+Assessment+Instrument

Bliss, L. S., McCabe, A., & Mahecha, N. R. (2001). Analyses of narratives from Spanish-speaking children. *Contemporary Issues in Communication Science and Disorders, 28*, 133–139.

Blom, E., & Paradis, J. (2013). Past tense production by English second language learners with and without language impairment. *Journal of Speech, Language, and Hearing Research, 56*, 281–294.

Bock, J. K., Dell, G. S., Chang, F., & Onishi, K. H. (2007). Persistent structural priming from language comprehension to language production. *Cognition, 104*(3), 437–458. https://doi.org/10.1016/j.cognition.2006.07.003

Bock, J. K., & Griffin, Z. M. (2000). The persistence of structural priming: Transient activation or implicit learning? *Journal of Experimental Psychology: General, 129*, 177–192.

Boland, A. M., Haden, C. A., & Ornstein, P. A. (2003). Boosting children's memory by training mothers in the use of an elaborative conversational style as an event unfolds. *Journal of Cognition and Development, 4*(1), 39–65.

Bolderson, S., Dosanjh, C., Milligan, C., Pring, T., & Chiat, S. (2011). Colourful semantics: A clinical investigation. *Child Language Teaching and Therapy, 27*(3), 344–353.

Bono, M. A., Daley, T., & Sigman, M. (2004). Relations among joint attention, amount of intervention and language gain in autism. *Journal of Autism and Developmental Disorders, 34*, 495–505.

Bopp, K. D., Mirenda, P., & Zumbo, B. D. (2009). Behavior predictors of language development over 2 years in children with autism spectrum disorders. *Journal of Speech, Language, and Hearing Research, 52*, 1106–1120.

Bora, E., & Pantelis, C. (2016). Meta-analysis of social cognition in attention-deficit/hyperactivity disorder (ADHD): Comparison with healthy controls and autistic spectrum disorder. *Psychological Medicine, 46*, 699–716.

Borovsky, A., Ellis, E. M., Evans, J. L., & Elman, J. (2016). Semantic structure in vocabulary knowledge interacts with lexical and sentence processing in infancy. *Child Development, 87*, 1893–1908. https://doi.org/10.1111/cdev.12554

Botting, N., & Conti-Ramsden, G. (2003). Autism, primary pragmatic difficulties, and specific language impairment: Can we distinguish them using psycholinguistic markers? *Developmental Medicine and Child Neurology, 45*, 515–524.

Botting, B., Rosato, M., & Wood, R. (1998). Teenage mothers and the health of their children. *Popular Trends, 93*, 19–28.

Boudreau, D. M. (2005). Use of a parent questionnaire in emergent and early literacy assessment of preschool children. *Language, Speech, and Hearing Services in Schools, 36*, 33–47.

Boudreau, D. M. (2007). Narrative abilities in children with language impairment. In R. Paul (Ed.), *Language disorders from a developmental perspective: Essays in honor of Robin S. Chapman* (pp. 331–356). Erlbaum.

Boudreau, D. M., & Costanza-Smith, A. (2011). Assessment and treatment of working memory deficits in school-age children: The role of the speech-language pathologist. *Language, Speech, and Hearing Services in Schools, 42*, 152–166.

Bourassa, D. C., & Treiman, R. (2001). Spelling development and disability: The importance of linguistic factors. *Language, Speech, and Hearing Services in Schools, 32*(3), 172–181.

Bourque Meaux, A., & Norris, J. A. (2018). Curriculum-based language interventions: What, who, why, where, and how? *Language, Speech, and Hearing Services in Schools, 49*, 165–175. https://doi.org/10.1044/2017_LSHSS-17-0057

Bowers, P. N., Kirby, J. R., & Deacon, S. H. (2010). The effects of morphological instruction on literacy skills: A systematic review of the literature. *Review of Educational Research, 80*, 144–179. https://doi.org/10.3102/0034654309359353 http://scholar.google.com/scholar_lookup?hl=en&volume=80&publication_year=2010&pages=144-179&journal=Review+of+Educational+Research&author=P.+N.+Bowers&author=J.+R.+Kirby&author=S.+H.+Deacon&title=The+effects+of+morphological+instruction+on+literacy+skills%3A+A+systematic+review+of+the+literature

Bowles, R. P., Justice, L. M., Khan, K. S., Piasta, S. B., Skibbe, L. E., & Foster, T. D. (2020). Development of the Narrative Assessment Protocol–2: A tool for examining young children's narrative skill. *Language, Speech, and Hearing Services in Schools, 51*, 390–404. https://doi.org/10.1044/2019_LSHSS-19-00038

Bowyer-Crane, C., Snowling, M. J., Duff, F. J., Fieldsend, E., Carroll, J. M., Miles, J., . . . Hulme, C. (2008). Improving early language and literacy skills: Differential effects of an oral language versus a phonology with reading intervention. *Journal of Child Psychology and Psychiatry, 49*, 422–432. https://doi.org/10.1111/j.1469-7610.2007.01849.x

Boyce, N., & Larson, V. L. (1983). *Adolescents' communication: Development and disorders*. Thinking Publications.

Boyle, C. A., Boulet, S., Schieve, L. A., Cohen, R. A., Blumberg, S. J., Yeargin-Allsopp, M., Visser, S., & Kogan, M. D. (2011). Trends in the prevalence of developmental disabilities in U.S. children 1997–2008. *Pediatrics, 127*, 1034–1042.

Boyle, S., McCoy, A., McNaughton, D., & Light, J. (2017). Using digital texts in interactive reading activities for children with language delays and disorders: A review of the research literature and pilot study. *Seminars in Speech and Language*, 38, 263–275. https://doi.org/10.1055/s-0037-1604274

Bracken, B. (1988). Rate and sequence of positive and negative poles in basic concept acquisition. *Language, Speech, and Hearing Services in Schools*, 19, 410–417.

Brackenbury, T., & Fey, M. E. (2003). Quick incidental verb learning in 4-year-olds: Identification and generalization. *Journal of Speech, Language, and Hearing Research*, 46, 313–327.

Brackenbury, T., & Pye, C. (2005). Semantic deficits in children with language impairments: Issues for clinical assessment. *Language, Speech, and Hearing Services in Schools*, 36, 5–16.

Bradshaw, M. L., Hoffman, P. R., & Norris, J. A. (1998). Efficacy of expansion and cloze procedures in the development of interpretations by preschool children exhibiting delayed language and development. *Language, Speech, and Hearing Services in Schools*, 29, 85–95.

Brady, N. C. (2000). Improved comprehension of object names following voice output communication aid use: Two case studies. *Augmentative and Alternative Communication*, 16, 197–204.

Brady, N. C., Fleming, K., Bredin-Oja, S. L., Fielding-Gebhardt, H., & Warren, S. F. (2020). Language development from early childhood to adolescence in youths with fragile X syndrome. *Journal of Speech, Language, and Hearing Research*, 63, 3727–3742. https://doi.org/10.1044/2020_JSLHR-20-00198

Brady, N. C., Warren, S. F., Fleming, K., Keller, J., & Sterling, A. (2014). Effect of sustained maternal responsivity on later vocabulary development in children with fragile X syndrome. *Journal of Speech, Language, and Hearing Research*, 57, 212–226. https://doi.org/10.1044/1092-4388(2013/12-0341)

Braillion, A., & DuBois, G. (2005). [Letter to the editor]. *Lancet*, 365, 1387.

Braten, I., & Stromso, H. (2003). A longitudinal think-aloud study of spontaneous strategic processing during the reading of multiple expository texts. *Reading and Writing*, 16, 195–218.

Breadmore, H. L., & Carroll, J. M. (2016a). Effects of orthographic, morphological and semantic overlap on short-term memory for words in typical and atypical development. *Scientific Studies of Reading*, 20, 471–489. https://doi.org/10.1080/10888438.2016.1246554 http://scholar.google.com/scholar_lookup?hl=en&volume=20&publication_year=2016a&pages=471-489&journal=Scientific+Studies+of+Reading&author=H.+L.+Breadmore&author=J.+M.+Carroll&title=Effects+of+orthographic%2C+morphological+and+semantic+overlap+on+short-term+memory+for+words+in+typical+and+atypical+development

Breadmore, H. L., & Carroll, J. M. (2016b). Morphological spelling in spite of phonological deficits: Evidence from children with dyslexia and otitis media. *Applied Psycholinguistics*, 37, 1439–1460. https://doi.org/10.1017/s0142716416000072 http://scholar.google.com/scholar_lookup?hl=en&volume=37&publication_year=2016b&pages=1439-1460&journal=Applied+Psycholinguistics&author=H.+L.+Breadmore&author=J.+M.+Carroll&title=Morphological+spelling+in+spite+of+phonological+deficits%3A+Evidence+from+children+with+dyslexia+and+otitis+media

Breadmore, H. L., & Deacon, S. H. (2019). Morphological processing before and during spelling. *Scientific Studies of Reading*, 23(2), 178–191. https://doi.org/10.1080/10888438.2018.1499745 http://scholar.google.com/scholar_lookup?hl=en&publication_year=2018&author=H.+L.+Breadmore&author=S.+H.+Deacon&title=Scientific+Studies+of+Reading

Bredin-Oja, S. L., & Fey, M. E. (2014). Children's responses to telegraphic and grammatically complete prompts to imitate. *American Journal of Speech-Language Pathology*, 23, 15–26. https://doi.org/10.1044/1058-0360(2013/12-0155)

Brice, A. E., Brice, R., & Kester, E. (2010). *Language loss in English language learners (ELLs)* [Newsletter]. Pedia Staff.

Brignell, A., Williams, K., Jachno, K., Prior, M., Reilly, S., & Morgan, A. T. (2018). Patterns and predictors of language development from 4 to 7 years in verbal children with and without autism spectrum disorder. *Journal of Autism and Developmental Disorders*, 48, 3282–3295. https://doi.org/10.1007/s10803-018-3565-2

Brinton, B., & Fujiki, M. (1989). *Conversational management with language-impaired children: Pragmatic assessment and intervention*. Aspen.

Brinton, B., & Fujiki, M. (2017). The power of stories: Facilitating social communication in children with limited language abilities. *School Psychology International*, 38, 523–540. https://doi.org/10.1177/0143034317713348

Brinton, B., Robinson, L. A., & Fujiki, M. (2004). Description of a program for social language intervention: "If you can have a conversation, you can have a relationship." *Language, Speech, and Hearing Services in Schools*, 35, 283–290.

Brinton, B., Spackman, M. P., Fujiki, M., & Ricks, J. (2007). What should Chris say? The ability of children with specific language impairment to recognize the need to dissemble emotions in social situations. *Journal of Speech, Language, and Hearing Research*, 50, 798–811.

Brock, S. E., Jimerson, S. R., & Hansen, R. L. (2009). *Identifying, assessing, and treating ADHD at school*. Springer.

Brocki, K. C., Randall, K. D., Bohlin, G., & Kerns, K. A. (2008). Working memory in school-aged children with attention-deficit/hyperactivity disorder combined type: Are deficits modality specific and are they independent of impaired inhibitory control? *Journal of Clinical and Experimental Neuropsychology*, 30, 749–759.

Bromberger, P., & Permanente, K. (2004). *Premies*. University of Michigan Health Services.

Brown, J. A., Garzarek, J. E., & Donegan, K. L. (2014). Effects of a narrative intervention on story retelling in at-risk young children. *Topics in Early Childhood Special Education*, 34(3), 154–164. https://doi.org/10.1177/0271121414536447

Brown, R. (1973). *A first language*. Harvard University Press.

Brown, T. E. (2000). *Attention-deficit disorders and comorbidities in children, adolescents, and adults*. American Psychiatric Press.

Brownlie, E. B., Bao, L., & Beitchman, J. H. (2016). Childhood language disorder and social anxiety in early adulthood. *Journal of Abnormal Child Psychology, 44*, 1061–1070.

Brownlie, E. B., Graham, E., Bao, L., Kayama, E., & Beitchman, J. H. (2017). Language disorder and retrospectively reported sexual abuse of girls: Severity and disclosure. *Journal of Child Psychology and Psychiatry, 58*, 1114–1121. https://doi.org/10.1111/jcpp.12723

Brownlie, E. B., Jabbar, A., Beitchman, J. H., Vida, R., & Atkinson, L. R. (2007). Language impairment and sexual assault of girls and women: Findings from a community sample. *Journal of Abnormal Child Psychology, 35*, 618–626.

Bruce, B., Thernlund, G., & Nettelbladt, U. (2006). ADHD and language impairment: A study of the parent questionnaire FTF (Five to Fifteen). *European Child & Adolescent Psychiatry, 15*(1), 52–60. https://doi.org/10.1007/s00787-006-0508-9

Bryant, D. P., Goodwin, M., Bryant, B. R., & Higgins, K. (2003). Vocabulary instruction for students with learning disabilities: A review of the research. *Learning Disability Quarterly, 26*, 117–128. https://doi.org/10.2307/1593594

Buysse, V., & Wesley, P. (2006). *Consultation in early childhood settings*. Brookes.

Cabell, S. Q., Justice, L. M., Piasta, S. B., Curenton, S. M., Wiggins, A., Turnbull, K. P., & Petscher, Y. (2011). The impact of teacher responsivity education on preschoolers' language and literacy skills. *American Journal of Speech-Language Pathology, 20*, 315–330.

Cabell, S. Q., Justice, L. M., Zucker, T. A., & Kilday, C. R. (2009). Validity of teacher report for assessing the emergent literacy skills of at-risk preschoolers. *Language, Speech, and Hearing Services in Schools, 40*, 161–173.

Cabell, S. Q., Justice, L. M., Kaderavek, J., Turnbull, K. P., & Breit-Smith, A. (2009). *Emergent Literacy: Lessons for Success*. Plural Publishing.

Caesar, L. G., & Kohler, P. D. (2007). The state of school-based bilingual assessment: Actual practice versus recommended guidelines. *Language, Speech, and Hearing Services in Schools, 38*, 190–200.

Cain, A. (2013). Reading comprehension difficulties in struggling readers. In B. Miller, L. E. Cutting, & P. McCardle (Eds.), *Unraveling reading comprehension: Behavioral, neurobiological, and genetic components* (pp. 54–63). Brookes.

Cain, K., & Oakhill, J. (Eds.). (2007). *Children's comprehension problems in oral and written language. A cognitive perspective*. Guilford.

Cain, K., Oakhill, J., & Bryant, P. (2004a). Children's reading comprehension ability: Concurrent prediction by working memory, verbal ability, and component skills. *Journal of Educational Psychology, 96*, 31–42.

Cain, K., Oakhill, J., & Lemmon, K. (2004b). Individual differences in the inference of word meanings from context:
The influence of reading comprehension, vocabulary knowledge, and memory capacity. *Journal of Educational Psychology, 96*, 671–681.

Calculator, S. M. (2016). Description and evaluation of a home-based, parent-administered program for teaching enhanced natural gestures to individuals with Angelman syndrome. *American Journal of Speech-Language Pathology, 25*, 1–13. https://https://doi.org/org/10.1044/2015_AJSLP-15-0017

Calder, S. D., Claessen, M., & Leitão, S. (2018). Combining implicit and explicit intervention approaches to target grammar in young children with developmental language disorder. *Child Language Teaching and Therapy, 34*(2), 171–189.

Caldera, Y. M., Velez-Gomez, P., & Lindsey, E. W. (2015). Who are Mexican Americans? An overview of history, immigration, and cultural values. In M. Caldera & E. W. Lindsay (Eds.), *Mexican American children and families: Multidisciplinary perspectives* (pp. 3–12). Routledge. https://doi.org/10.4324/9781315814612

Calkins, L. (2006). *Raising the quality of narrative writing*. Heinemann.

Callaghan, G., & Madelaine, A. (2012). Levelling the playing field for kindergarten entry: Research implications for preschool early literacy instruction. *Australasian Journal of Early Childhood, 37*, 13–23. https://doi.org/10.1177/183693911203700103

Camarata, S. M., & Nelson, K. E. (2006). Conversational recast intervention with preschool and older children. In R. J. McCauley & M. E. Fey (Eds.), *Treatment of language disorders in children* (pp. 237–264). Brookes.

Campbell, P. H., Milbourne, S. A., Dugan, L. M., & Wilcox, M. J. (2006). A review of evidence on practices for teaching young children to use assistive technology devices. *Topics in Early Childhood Special Education, 26*, 3–14.

Cannizzaro, M. S., & Coelho, C. A. (2002). Treatment of story grammar following traumatic brain injury: A pilot study. *Brain Injury, 16*, 1065–1073.

Caravolas, M., Hulme, C., & Snowling, M. J. (2001). The foundations of spelling ability: Evidence from a 3-year longitudinal study. *Journal of Memory and Language, 45*, 751–774. https://doi.org/10.1006/jmla.2000.2785 http://scholar.google.com/scholar_lookup?hl=en&volume=45&publication_year=2001&pages=751-774&journal=Journal+of+Memory+and+Language&author=M.+Caravolas&author=C.+Hulme&author=M.+J.+Snowling&title=The+foundations+of+spelling+ability%3A+Evidence+from+a+3-year+longitudinal+study

Cárdenas-Hagan, E., Carlson, C. D., & Pollard-Durodola, S. D. (2007). The cross-linguistic transfer of early literacy skills: The role of initial L1 and L2 skills and language instruction. *Language, Speech, and Hearing Services in Schools, 3*, 249–259.

Carroll, J. M., & Breadmore, H. L. (2018). Not all phonological awareness deficits are created equal: Evidence from a comparison between children with otitis media and poor readers. *Developmental Science, 21*(3), e12588.

https://doi.org/10.1111/desc.12588 http://scholar.google .com/scholar_lookup?hl=en&volume=21&publication_ year=2018&pages=e12588&journal=Developmental+ Science&issue=3&author=J.+M.+Carroll&author=H. +L.+Breadmore&title=Not+all+phonological+awareness +deficits+are+created+equal%3A+Evidence+from+a+ comparison+between+children+with+otitis+media+and +poor+readers

Carroll, J. M., Mundy, I. R., & Cunningham, A. J. (2014). The roles of family history of dyslexia, language, speech production and phonological processing in predicting literacy progress. *Developmental Science, 17,* 727–742. https:// doi.org/10.1111/desc.12153 http://scholar.google.com/ scholar_lookup?hl=en&volume=17&publication_year= 2014&pages=727-742&journal=Developmental+Science &author=J.+M.+Carroll&author=I.+R.+Mundy&author =A.+J.+Cunningham&title=The+roles+of+family+history +of+dyslexia%2C+language%2C+speech+production+ and+phonological+processing+in+predicting+literacy +progress

Carroll, J. M., Solity, J., & Shapiro, L. R. (2016). Predicting dyslexia using prereading skills: The role of sensorimotor and cognitive abilities. *Journal of Child Psychology and Psychiatry, 57,* 750–758. https://doi.org/10.1111/jcpp.12488 http:// scholar.google.com/scholar_lookup?hl=en&volume =57&publication_year=2016&pages=750-758&journal= The+Journal+of+Child+Psychology+and+Psychiatry& author=J.+M.+Carroll&author=J.+Solity&author=L.+ R.+Shapiro&title=Predicting+dyslexia+using+prereading +skills%3A+The+role+of+sensorimotor+and+cognitive+ abilities

Carter, A. S., Messinger, D. S., Stone, W. L., Celimli, S., Nahmias, A. S., & Yoder, P. J. (2011). A randomized controlled trial of Hanen's "More Than Words" in toddlers with early autism symptoms. *Journal of Child Psychology and Psychiatry, 52*(7), 741–752. https://doi.org/10.1111/j.14 69-7610.2011.02395.x

Casenhiser, D. M., Binns, A., McGill, F., Morderer, O., & Shanker, S. G. (2015). Measuring and supporting language function for children with autism: Evidence from a randomized control trial of a social-interaction-based therapy. *Journal of Autism and Developmental Disorders, 45,* 846–857.

Castilla-Earls, A., Francis, D., Iglesias, A., & Davidson, K. (2019). The impact of the Spanish-to-English proficiency shift on the grammaticality of English learners. *Journal of Speech, Language, and Hearing Research, 62,* 1739–1754. https://doi.org/10.1044/2018_JSLHR-L-18-0324

Castilla-Earls, A., & Fulcher-Rood, K. (2018). Convergent and divergent validity of the Grammaticality and Utterance Length Instrument. *Journal of Speech, Language, and Hearing Disorders, 61,* 120–129. https://doi.org/10 .1044/2017_JSLHR-L-17-0152

Castilla-Earls, A., Pérez-Leroux, A. T., Fulcher-Rood, K., & Barr, C. (2021). Morphological errors in Spanish-speaking bilingual children with and without developmental language disorders. *Language, Speech, and Hearing Services in Schools, 52,* 497–511.https://doi.org/10.1044/2020_LS HSS-20-00017

Castilla-Earls, A. P., Restrepo, M. A., Perez-Leroux, A. T., Gray, S., Holmes, P., Gail, D., & Chen, Z. (2016). Interactions between bilingual effects and language impairment: Exploring grammatical markers in Spanish-speaking bilingual children. *Applied Psycholinguistics, 37,* 1147–1173.

Catts, H. W. (1997). The early identification of language-based reading disabilities. *Language, Speech, and Hearing Services in Schools, 28,* 86–89.

Catts, H. W. (2004). Language impairments and reading disabilities. In R. D. Kent (Ed.), *The MIT encyclopedia of communication disorders* (pp. 329–331). MIT Press.

Catts, H. W. (2017). Early identification of reading disabilities. In K. Cain, D. L. Compton, & R. Parrila (Eds.), *Theories of reading development* (15th ed., pp. 311–332). Benjamins. http://scholar.google.com/scholar_lookup?hl=en&pub lication_year=2017&pages=311-332&author=H.+W.+ Catts&title=Theories+of+reading+development

Catts, H. W., Adlof, S. M., & Ellis Weismer, S. (2006). Language deficits in poor comprehenders: A case for the simple view of reading. *Journal of Speech, Language, and Hearing Research, 49,* 278–293.

Catts, H. W., Adlof, S. M., Hogan, T. P., & Weismer, S. E. (2005). Are specific language impairment and dyslexia distinct disorders? *Journal of Speech, Language, and Hearing Research, 48,* 1378–1396.

Catts, H. W., Compton, D., Tomblin, J. B., & Bridges, M. S. (2012). Prevalence and nature of late-emerging poor readers. *Journal of Educational Psychology, 104*(1), 166–181. https://doi.org/10.1037/a0025323

Catts, H. W., Fey, M. E., Tomblin, J. B., & Zhang, X. (2002). A longitudinal investigation of reading outcomes in children with language impairments. *Journal of Speech, Language, and Hearing Research, 45,* 1142–1157. https:// doi.org/10.1044/1092-4388(2002/093) http://scholar .google.com/scholar_lookup?hl=en&volume=45&publi cation_year=2002&pages=1142-1157&journal=Journal+ of+Speech%2C+Language%2C+and+Hearing+Research &author=H.+W.+Catts&author=M.+E.+Fey&author= J.+B.+Tomblin&author=X.+Xhang&title=A+longitudi nal+investigation+of+reading+outcomes+in+children+ with+language+impairments

Catts, H. W., Fey, M. E., Weismer, S. E., & Bridges, M. S. (2014). The relationship between language and reading abilities. In J. B. Tomblin & M. A. Nippold (Eds.), *Understanding individual differences in language development across the school years* (pp. 144–165). Psychological Press.

Catts, H. W., & Hogan, T. P. (2003). Language basis of reading disabilities and implications for early identification and remediation. *Reading Psychology, 24,* 223–246. https:// doi.org/10.1080/02702710390227314

Catts, H. W., Hogan, T. P., & Adlof, S. M. (2005). Developmental changes in reading and reading disabilities. In H. W. Catts & A. Kamhi (Eds.), *The connections between language and reading disabilities* (pp. 25–40). Erlbaum.

REFERENCES

Catts, H. W., Hogan, T. P., & Fey, M. E. (2003). Subgrouping poor readers on the basis of individual differences in reading-related abilities. *Journal of Learning Disabilities*, 6(2), 151–164.

Catts, H. W., & Kamhi, A. G. (2017). Prologue: Reading comprehension is not a single ability. *Language, Speech, and Hearing Services in Schools*, 48, 73–76. https://doi.org/10.1044/2017_LSHSS-16-0033

Catts, H. W., Nielsen, D. C., Bridges, M. S., Liu, Y. S., & Bontempo, D. E. (2015). Early identification of reading disabilities within an RTI framework. *Journal of Learning Disabilities*, 48, 281–297. https://doi.org/10.1177/0022219413498115 http://scholar.google.com/scholar_lookup?hl=en&volume=48&publication_year=2015&pages=281-297&journal=Journal+of+Learning+Disabilities&author=H.+W.+Catts&author=D.+C.+Nielsen&author=M.+S.+Bridges&author=Y.+S.+Liu&author=D.+E.+Bontempo&title=Early+identification+of+reading+disabilities+within+an+RTI+framework

Centers for Disease Control and Prevention. (2016). *Community report on autism.* https://www.cdc.gov/features/new-autism-data/community-report-autism-key-findings.pdf

Centers for Disease Control and Prevention. (2018a, February 14). *Attention-deficit/hyperactivity disorder (ADHD): Data and statistics.* https://www.cdc.gov/NCBDDD/adhd/data.html

Centers for Disease Control and Prevention. (2018b, April 17). *Facts about developmental disabilities.* https://www.cdc.gov/ncbddd/developmentaldisabilities/facts.html

Centers for Disease Control and Prevention. (2018c, April 26). *Signs and symptoms of autism spectrum disorder.* https://www.cdc.gov/ncbddd/autism/signs.html

Centers for Disease Control and Prevention. (2020, November 25). *Polysubstance use in pregnancy.* https://www.cdc.gov/pregnancy/polysubstance-use-in-pregnancy.html#:~:text=Substance%20use%20during%20pregnancy%20can,alcohol%20spectrum%20disorders%20(FASDs).

Centers for Disease Control and Prevention. (2021a, February 4). *Fetal alcohol spectrum disorder: Data and statistics.* http://www.cdc.gov/ncbddd/fasd/data.html

Centers for Disease Control and Prevention. (2021b, June 10). *Hearing loss in children: Data and statistics.* https://www.cdc.gov/ncbddd/hearingloss/data.html

Centers for Disease Control and Prevention. (2021c, November 1). *Reproductive health: Preterm birth.* https://www.cdc.gov/reproductivehealth/maternalinfanthealth/pretermbirth.htm

Centers for Disease Control and Prevention. (2021d, December 9). *Traumatic brain injury & concussion.* https://www.cdc.gov/TraumaticBrainInjury/index.html

Cermak, C. A., Scratch, S. E., Reed, N. P., Bradley, K., Quinn de Launay, K. L., & Beal, D. S. (2019). Cognitive communication impairments in children with traumatic brain injury. *Journal of Head Trauma Rehabilitation*, 34(2), E13–E20. https://doi.org/10.1097/HTR.0000000000000419

Champion, T. B., Hyter, Y. D., McCabe, A., & Bland-Stewart, L. M. (2003). A matter of vocabulary: Performances of low-income African American Head Start children on the Peabody Picture Vocabulary Test–III. *Communication Disorders Quarterly*, 24(3), 121–127.

Chaney, C. (1992). Language development, metalinguistic skills, and print awareness in 3-year-old children. *Applied Psycholinguistics*, 13, 485–514.

Chang, F., Early, D., & Winton, P. (2005). Early childhood teacher preparation in special education at 2- and 4-year institutions of higher education. *Journal of Early Intervention*, 27, 110–124.

Chao, P., Bryan, T., Burstein, K., & Cevriye, E. (2006). Family-centered intervention for young children at-risk for language and behavior problems. *Early Childhood Education Journal*, 34, 147–153.

Chapman, R. S. (1981). Exploring children's communicative intents. In J. Miller (Ed.), *Assessing language production in children* (pp. 22–25). University Park Press.

Chapman, R. S., Sindberg, H., Bridge, C., Gigstead, K., & Hasketh, L. (2006). Effect of memory support and elicited production on fast mapping of new words by adolescents with Down syndrome. *Journal of Speech, Language, and Hearing Research*, 49, 3–15.

Charest, M., Skoczylas, M. J., & Schneider, P. (2020). Properties of lexical diversity in the narratives of children with typical language development and developmental language disorder. *American Journal of Speech-Language Pathology*, 29, 1866–1882. https://doi.org/10.1044/2020_AJSLP-19-00176

Charman, T. R., Baron-Cohen, S., Swettenham, J., Baird, G., Drew, A., & Cox, A. (2003). Predicting language outcome in infants with autism and pervasive developmental disorder. *International Journal of Language and Communication Disorders*, 38, 265–285.

Chiat, S., & Roy, P. (2007). The Preschool Repetition Test: An evaluation of performance in typically developing and clinically referred children. *Journal of Speech, Language, and Hearing Research*, 50, 429–443.

Cholemkery, H., Medda, J., Lempp, T., & Freitag, C. M. (2016). Classifying autism spectrum disorders by ADI-R: Subtypes or severity gradient? *Journal of Autism and Developmental Disorders*, 46, 2327–2339.

Choudhury, N., & Benasich, A. A. (2003). A family aggregation study: The influence of family history and other risk factors on language development. *Journal of Speech, Language, and Hearing Research*, 46, 261–272.

Christensen, R. V., & Hansson, K. (2012). The use and productivity of past tense morphology in specific language impairment: An examination of Danish. *Journal of Speech, Language, and Hearing Research*, 55, 1671–1689.

Ciccia, A., Lundine, J. P., O'Brien, K. H., Salley, J., Krusen, S., Wilson, B., . . . Haarbauer-Krupa, J. (2021). Understanding cognitive communication needs in pediatric traumatic brain injury: Issues identified at the 2020 International Cognitive-Communication Disorders Conference. *American Journal of Speech-Language Pathology*, 30(Suppl. 2), 853–862. https://doi.org/10.1044/2020_AJSLP-20-00077

Cirrin, F. M., Schooling, T. L., Nelson, N. W., Diehl, S. F., Flynn, P. F., Staskowski, M., . . . Adamczyk, D. F. (2010). Evidence-based systematic review: Effects of different service delivery models on communication outcomes for elementary school-age children. *Language, Speech, and Hearing Services in Schools*, *41*, 233–264.

Clark, A., O'Hare, A., Watson, J., Cohen, W., Cowie, H., Elton, R., . . . Seckl, J. (2007). Severe receptive language disorder in childhood-familial aspects and long-term outcomes: Results from a Scottish study. *Archives of Disease in Childhood*, *92*, 614–619.

Clarke, K. A., & Williams, D. L. (2020). Instruction using augmentative and alternative communication supports: Description of current practices by speech-language pathologists who work with children with autism spectrum disorder. *American Journal of Speech-Language Pathology*, *29*, 586–596. https://doi.org/10.1044/2019_AJSLP-19-00045

Clarke, P., Snowling, M. J., Truelove, E., & Hulme, C. (2010). Ameliorating children's reading comprehension difficulties: A randomised controlled trial. *Psychological Science*, *21*, 1106–1116.

Clay, M. M. (1979). *The early detection of reading difficulties: A diagnostic survey with recovery procedures*. Heinemann.

Cleave, P. L., Becker, S. D., Curran, M. K., Owen Van Horne, A. J., & Fey, M. E. (2015). The efficacy of recasts in language intervention: A systematic review and meta-analysis. *American Journal of Speech-Language Pathology*, *24*, 237–255. https://doi.org/10.1044/2015_AJSLP-14-0105

Clegg, J., Hollis, C., Mawhood, L., & Rutter, M. (2005). Developmental language disorders—A follow-up in later adult life: Cognitive, language and psychosocial outcomes. *Journal of Child Psychology and Psychiatry*, *46*, 128–149.

Clendon, S., Paynter, J., Walker, S., Bowen, R., & Westerveld, M. F. (2021). Emergent literacy assessment in children with autism spectrum disorder who have limited verbal communication skills: A tutorial. *Language, Speech, and Hearing Services in Schools*, *52*, 165–180. https://doi.org/10.1044/2020_LSHSS-20-00030

Cleveland, E., & Morris, A. (2014). Autonomy support and structure enhance children's memory and motivation to reminisce: A parental training study. *Journal of Cognition and Development*, *15*, 414–436.

Cleveland, L. H., & Oetting, J. B. (2013). Children's marking of verbal –s by nonmainstream English dialect and clinical status. *American Journal of Speech-Language Pathology*, *22*, 604–614. https://doi.org/10.1044/1058-0360(2013/12-0122)

Cochrane, R. (1983). Language and the atmosphere of delight. In H. Winitz (Ed.), *Treating language disorders: For clinicians by clinicians* (pp. 143–162). University Park Press.

Coggins, T. (1991). Bringing context back into assessment. *Topics in Language Disorders*, *11*(4), 43–54.

Coggins, T., Olswang, L., Carmichael Olson, H., & Timler, G. (2003). On becoming socially competent communicators: The challenge for children with fetal alcohol expo-

sure. *International Review of Research in Mental Retardation*, *27*, 121–150.

Coggins, T., Timler, G. R., & Olswang, L. B. (2007). A state of double jeopardy: Impact of prenatal alcohol exposure and adverse environments on the social communicative abilities of school-age children with fetal alcohol spectrum disorder. *Language, Speech, and Hearing Services in Schools*, *38*, 117–127.

Cohen, N., Vallance, D., Barwick, M., Im, N., Menna, R., Horodezky, N., & Isaacson, L. (2000).The interface between ADHD and language impairment: An examination of language, achievement, and cognitive processing. *Journal of Child Psychology and Psychiatry*, *41*, 353–362.

Cohen, W., Hodson, A., O'Hare, A., Boyle, J., Durrani, T., McCartney, E., & Watson, J. (2005). Effects of computer-based intervention through acoustically modified speech (Fast ForWord) in severe mixed receptive–expressive language impairment: Outcomes from a randomized controlled trial. *Journal of Speech, Language, and Hearing Research*, *48*, 715–729.

Colenbrander, D., Pace Miles, K., & Ricketts, J. (2019). To see or not to see: How does seeing spellings support vocabulary learning? *Language, Speech and Hearing Services in Schools*, *50*, 609–628. https://doi.org/10.1044/2019_LSHSS-VOIA-18-0135

Colenbrander, D., Ricketts, J., & Breadmore, H. L. (2018). Early identification of dyslexia: Understanding the issues. *Language, Speech, and Hearing Services in Schools*, *49*, 817–828. https://doi.org/10.1044/2018_LSHSS-DYSLC-18-0007

Colmar, S. H. (2014). A parent-based book-reading intervention for disadvantaged children with language difficulties. *Child Language Teaching and Therapy*, *30*, 79–90. https://doi.org/10.1177/0265659013507296

Colozzo, P., Garcia, R., Megan, C., Gillam, R., & Johnson, J. (2006, June). *Narrative assessment in SLI: Exploring interactions between content and form*. Poster session presented at the annual meeting of the Symposium on Research in Child Language Disorders, Madison, WI.

Colozzo, P., Gillam, R. B., Wood, M., Schnell, R. D., & Johnston, J. R. (2011). Content and form in the narratives of children with specific language impairment. *Journal of Speech, Language, and Hearing Research*, *54*, 1609–1627.

Common Core State Standards Initiative. (2010). *Common Core State Standards (CCSS)*. http://www.corestandards.org/read-the-standards

Common Sense Media. (2013). *Zero to eight: Children's media use in America*. https://www.commonsensemedia.org/zero-to-eight-2013-infographic

Compton, D. L., Fuchs, D., Fuchs, L. S., Bouton, B., Gilbert, J. K., Barquero, L. A., . . . Crouch, C. (2010). Selecting at-risk first graders for early intervention: Eliminating false positives and exploring the promise of a two-stage gated screening process. *Journal of Educational Psychology*, *102*, 327–340. https://doi.org/10.1037/a0018448 http://scholar.google.com/scholar_lookup?hl=en&volume=102&publication_year=2010&pages=327-340&journal=Journal+of+Educational+Psychology&author=D.+L.+

Compton&author=D.+Fuchs&author=L.+S.+Fuchs&author=B.+Bouton&author=J.+K.+Gilbert&author=L.+A.+Barquero&author=C.+Crouch&title=Selecting+at-risk+first+graders+for+early+intervention%3A+Eliminating+false+positives+and+exploring+the+promise+of+a+two-stage+gated+screening+process

Condouris, K., Meyer, E., & Tager-Flusberg, H. (2003). The relationship between standardized measures of language and measures of spontaneous speech in children with autism. *American Journal of Speech-Language Pathology, 12*, 349–358.

Conti-Ramsden, G. (2003). Processing and linguistic markers in young children with specific language impairment (SLI). *Journal of Speech, Language, and Hearing Research, 46*, 1029–1037.

Conti-Ramsden, G., & Botting, N. (2008). Emotional health in adolescents with and without a history of specific language impairment (SLI). *Journal of Child Psychology and Psychiatry, 49*, 516–525. https://doi.org/10.1111/j.1469-7610.2007.01858.x

Conti-Ramsden, G., Botting, N., & Durkin, K. (2008). Parental perspectives during the transition to adulthood of adolescents with a history of specific language impairment (SLI). *Journal of Speech, Language, and Hearing Research, 51*, 84–96.

Conti-Ramsden, G., & Durkin, K. (2008). Language and independence in adolescents with and without a history of specific language impairment (SLI). *Journal of Speech, Language, and Hearing Research, 51*, 70–83.

Conti-Ramsden, G., Simkin, Z., & Pickles, A. (2006). Estimating familial loading in SLI: A comparison of direct assessment versus parental interview. *Journal of Speech, Language, and Hearing Research, 49*(1), 88–101.

Cornish, H., Dale, R., Kirby, S., & Christiansen, M. (2017). Sequence memory constraints give rise to language-like structure through iterated learning. *PLoS One, 12*(1), e0168532. https://doi.org/10.1371/journal.pone.0168532

Corriveau, K., Posquine, E., & Goswami, U. (2007). Basic auditory processing skills and specific language impairment: A new look at an old hypothesis. *Journal of Speech, Language, and Hearing Research, 50*, 647–666.

Cortiella, C., & Horowitz, S. H. (2014). *The state of learning disabilities: Facts, trends, and emerging issues* (3rd ed.). National Center for Learning Disabilities. http://www.ncld.org/wp-content/uploads/2014/11/2014-State-of-LD.pdf

Cowan, N., Nugent, L., Elliott, E., Ponomarev, I., & Saults, S. (2005). The role of attention in the development of short-term memory: Age differences in the verbal span of apprehension. *Child Development, 70*, 1082–1097.

Coxhead, A. (2000). A new academic word list. *TESOL Quarterly, 34*(2), 213–238.

Craig, H. K., Kolenic, G. E., & Hensel, S. L. (2014). African American English-speaking students: A longitudinal examination of style shifting from kindergarten through second grade. *Journal of Speech, Language, and Hearing Research, 57*, 143–157. https://doi.org/10.1044/1092-4388(2013/12-0157)

Craig, H. K., Zhang, L., Hensel, S. L., & Quinn, E. J. (2009). African American English-speaking students: An examination of the relationship between dialect shifting and reading outcomes. *Journal of Speech, Language, and Hearing Research, 52*, 839–855.

Crais, E. R., & Roberts, J. (1991). Decision making in assessment and early intervention planning. *Language, Speech, and Hearing Services in Schools, 22*, 19–30.

Crais, E. R., & Roberts, J. (2004). Assessing communication skills. In M. McLean, M. Wolery, & D. Bailey (Eds.), *Assessing infants and preschoolers with special needs* (3rd ed., pp. 345–411). Pearson Merrill Prentice Hall.

Creaghead, N. A. (1992). Classroom interactional analysis/script analysis. *Best Practices in School Speech Language Pathology, 2*, 65–72.

Cress, C. J. (2003). Responding to a common early AAC question: "Will my child talk?" *Perspectives on Augmentative and Alternative Communication, 12*, 10–11.

Cress, C. J., & Marvin, C. A. (2003). Common questions about AAC services in early intervention. *Augmentative and Alternative Communication, 19*, 254–272.

Crick Software. (2022a). *Clicker 8.* https://www.cricksoft.com/us/clicker/8

Crick Software. (2022b). *Clicker Writer.* https://www.cricksoft.com/us/clicker/apps

Crooke, P. J., Winner, M. G., & Olswang, L. B. (2016). Thinking socially: Teaching social knowledge to foster social behavior change. *Topics in Language Disorders, 36*, 284–298.

Crosson, A. C., McKeown, M. G., Robbins, K. P., & Brown, K. J. (2019). Key elements of robust vocabulary instruction for emergent bilingual adolescents. *Language, Speech, and Hearing Services in Schools, 50*, 493–505. https://doi.org/10.1044/2019_LSHSS-VOIA-18-0127

Crowe, L. K. (2003). Comparison of two reading feedback strategies in improving the oral and written language performance of children with language learning disabilities. *American Journal of Speech-Language Pathology, 12*, 16–27.

Crowhurst, M., & Piche, G. L. (1979). Audience and mode of discourse effects on syntactic complexity in writing at two grade levels. *Research in the Teaching of English, 13*, 101–109.

Crystal, D. (1982). *Profiling linguistic disability.* Arnold.

Crystal, D., Fletcher, P., & Garman, R. (1976). *The grammatical analysis of language disability.* Elsevier.

Culatta, B., Hall-Kenyon, K. M., & Black, S. (2010). Teaching expository comprehension skills in early childhood classrooms. *Topics in Language Disorders, 30*(4), 323–338. https://doi.org/10.1097/TLD.0b013e3181ff5a65

Cummins, J. (2014). Beyond language: Academic communication and student success. *Linguistics and Education, 26*, 145–154. http://scholar.google.com/scholar_lookup?hl=en&publication_year=2014&pages=145-154&title=Beyond+language%3A+Academic+communication+and+student+success

Cunningham, A., Perry, K., Stanovich, K., & Stanovich, P. (2004). Disciplinary knowledge of K–3 teachers and their knowledge calibration in the domain of early literacy. *Annals of Dyslexia*, *54*, 139–167.

Cunningham, B. J., Hanna, S. E., Rosenbaum, P., Thomas-Stonell, N., & Oddson, B. (2018). Factors contributing to preschoolers' communicative participation outcomes: Findings from a population-based longitudinal cohort study in Ontario, Canada. *American Journal of Speech-Language Pathology*, *27*, 737–750. https://doi.org/10.1044/2017_AJSLP-17-0079

Cunningham, M., & Cox, E. O. (2003, February). Hearing assessment in infants and children: Recommendations beyond neonatal screening. *Pediatrics*, *111*(2), 436–440.

Curenton, S. M., & Justice, L. M. (2004). African American and Caucasian preschoolers' use of decontextualized language: Literate language features in oral narratives. *Language, Speech, and Hearing Services in Schools*, *35*(3), 240–253. https://doi.org/10.1044/0161-1461(2004/023)

Curtis, M. E. (2006). The role of vocabulary instruction in adult basic education. In J. Comings, B. Garner, & C. Smith (Eds.), *Review of adult learning and literacy* (Vol. 6, pp. 43–69). Erlbaum.

Cycyk, L. M., De Anda, S., Moore, H., & Huerta, L. (2021). Cultural and linguistic adaptations of early language interventions: Recommendations for advancing research and practice. *American Journal of Speech-Language Pathology*, *30*, 1224–1246. https://doi.org/10.1044/2020_AJSLP-20-00101

Cycyk, L. M., & Huerta, L. (2020). Exploring the cultural validity of parent-implemented naturalistic language intervention procedures for families from Spanish-speaking Latinx homes. *American Journal of Speech-Language Pathology*, *29*, 1241–1259. https://doi.org/10.1044/2020_AJSLP-19-00038

Dale, P. S., Price, T. S., Bishop, D. V. M., & Plomin, R. (2003). Outcomes of early language delay: I. Predicating persistent and transient language difficulties at 3 and 4 years. *Journal of Speech, Language, and Hearing Research*, *46*, 544–560.

Dale, P. S., Tosto, M. G., Hayiou-Thomas, M., & Plomin, R. (2015). Why does parental language input style predict child language development? A twin study of gene–environment correlation. *Journal of Communication Disorders*, *57*, 106–117.

Dam, Q., Pham, G., Potapova, I., & Pruitt-Lord, S. (2020). Grammatical characteristics of Vietnamese and English in developing bilingual children. *American Journal of Speech-Language Pathology*, *29*, 1212–1225. https://doi.org/10.1044/2019_AJSLP-19-00146

Damico, J. S. (1991). Clinical discourse analysis: A functional language assessment technique. In C. S. Simon (Ed.), *Communication skills and classroom success: Assessment and therapy methodologies for language and learning disabled students* (pp. 125–150). Thinking Publications.

Danahy Ebert, K., & Kohnert, K. (2011). Sustained attention in children with primary language impairment: A meta-analysis. *Journal of Speech, Language, and Hearing Research*, *54*, 1372–1384.

Danahy Ebert, K., & Pham, G. (2017). Synthesizing information from language samples and standardized tests in school-age bilingual assessment. *Language, Speech and Hearing Services in Schools*, *48*, 42–55. https://doi.org/10.1044/2016_LSHSS-16-0007

Danahy Ebert, K., & Scott, C. M. (2014). Relationships between narrative language samples and norm-referenced test scores in language assessments of school-age children. *Language, Speech and Hearing Services in Schools*, *45*, 337–350. https://doi.org/10.1044/2014_LSHSS-14-0034

Daniels, A. M., & Mandell, D. S. (2014). Explaining differences in age at autism spectrum disorder diagnosis: A critical review. *Autism*, *18*, 583–597. https://doi.org/10.1177/1362361313480277

Danzak, R. L. (2011). The integration of lexical, syntactic, and discourse features in bilingual adolescents' writing: An exploratory approach. *Language, Speech, and Hearing Services in Schools*, *42*, 491–505.

Datchuk, S. M., & Kubina, R. M. (2013). A review of teaching sentence-level writing skills to students with writing difficulties and learning disabilities. *Remedial and Special Education*, *34*(3), 180–192. http://scholar.google.com/scholar_lookup?hl=en&volume=34&publication_year=2013&pages=180-192&journal=Remedial+and+Special+Education&issue=3&author=S.+M.+Datchuk&author=R.+M.+Kubina&title=A+review+of+teaching+sentence-level+writing+skills+to+students+with+writing+difficulties+and+learning+disabilities

Davidovitch, M., Stein, N., Koren, G., & Chen Friedman, B. (2018). Deviations from typical developmental trajectories detectable at 9 months of age in low risk children later diagnosed with autism spectrum disorder. *Journal of Autism and Developmental Disorders*, *48*, 2854–2869. https://doi.org/10.1007/s10803-018-3549-2

Davidson, M. M. (2021). Reading comprehension in school-age children with autism spectrum disorder: Examining the many components that may contribute. *Language, Speech and Hearing Services in Schools*, *52*, 181–196. https://doi.org/10.1044/2020_LSHSS-20-00010

Davidson, M. M., & Ellis Weismer, S. (2014). Characterization and prediction of early reading abilities in children on the autism spectrum. *Journal of Autism and Developmental Disorders*, *24*, 828–845. https://doi.org/10.1007/s10803-013-1936-2

Davison, D. M., & Qi, C. H. (2017). Language teaching strategies for preschool English learners. *ASHA Perspectives, SIG 1 Language Learning and Education*, *2*, 170–178. https://doi.org/10.1044/persp2.SIG1.170

Deacon, S. H., Benere, J., & Pasquarella, A. (2013). Reciprocal relationship: Children's morphological awareness and their reading accuracy across grades 2 to 3. *Developmental Psychology*, *49*, 1113–1126. https://doi.org/10.1037/a0029474 http://scholar.google.com/scholar_lookup?hl=en&volume=49&publication_year=2013&pages=1113-1126&journal=Developmental+Psychology&author=S.+H.+Deacon&author=J.+Benere&author=A.+Pasquarella&title=Reciprocal+relationship%3A+Children%27s+

morphological+awareness+and+their+reading+accuracy+across+grades+2+to+3

Deacon, S. H., Tong, X., & Francis, K. (2017). The relationship of morphological analysis and morphological decoding to reading comprehension. *Journal of Research in Reading, 40*, 1–16. https://doi.org/10.1111/1467-9817.12056 http://scholar.google.com/scholar_lookup?hl=en&volume=40&publication_year=2017&pages=1-16&journal=Journal+of+Research+in+Reading&author=S.+H.+Deacon&author=X.+Tong&author=K.+Francis&title=The+relationship+of+morphological+analysis+and+morphological+decoding+to+reading+comprehension

De Anda, S., Bosch, L., Poulin-Dubois, D., Zesiger, P., & Friend, M. (2016). The Language Exposure Assessment Tool: Quantifying language exposure in infants and children. *Journal of Speech, Language, and Hearing Research, 59*, 1346–1356. https://doi.org/10.1044/2016_JSLHR-L-15-0234

DeBose, C. E. (2015). The systematic marking of tense, modality, and aspect in African American language. In J. Bloomquist, L. J. Green, & S. J. Lanehart (Eds.), *The Oxford handbook of African American English* (pp. 371–385). Oxford University Press.

Deckers, S., Van Zaalen, Y., Van Balkom, H., & Verhoeven, L. (2017). Predictors of receptive and expressive vocabulary development in children with Down syndrome. *International Journal of Speech-Language Pathology, 21*, 10–22. https://doi.org/10.1080/17549507.2017.1363290

Deevy, P., Wisman Weil, L., Leonard, L. B., & Goffman, L. (2010). Extending use of the NRT to preschool-age children with and without specific language impairment. *Language, Speech, and Hearing Services in Schools, 41*, 277–288.

De Groot, B. J., Van den Bos, K. P., Van der Meulen, B. F., & Minnaert, A. E. (2015). Rapid naming and phonemic awareness in children with reading disabilities and/or specific language impairment: Differentiating processes? *Journal of Speech, Language, and Hearing Research, 58*, 1538–1548. https://doi.org/10.1044/2015_JSLHR-L-14-0019

DeKroon, D. M. A., Kyte, C. S., & Johnson, C. J. (2002). Partner influences on the social pretend play of children with language impairments. *Language, Speech, and Hearing Services in Schools, 33*, 253–267.

de Marchena, A., & Eigsti, I. (2016). The art of common ground: Emergence of a complex pragmatic language skill in adolescents with autism spectrum disorders. *Journal of Child Language, 43*, 43–80. https://doi.org/10.1017/S0305000915000070

Demmert, W. G., McCardle, P., & Leos, K. (2006). Conclusions and commentary. *Journal of American Indian Education, 45*(2), 77–88.

Dempsey, L., Jacques, J., Skarakis-Doyle, E., & Lee, C. (2002, November). *The relationship between preschoolers' comprehension monitoring ability and their knowledge of truth conditions.* Paper presented at the annual convention of the American Speech-Language-Hearing Association, Atlanta, GA.

Denham, S. A., & Burton, R. (1996). Social–emotional intervention for at-risk 4-year-olds. *Journal of School Psychology, 34*, 223–245.

Dennis, M., Lazenby, A. L., & Lockyer, L. (2001). Inferential language in high-functioning children with autism. *Journal of Autism and Developmental Disorders, 31*(1), 47–54.

Denton, C., Cirino, P., Barth, A., Romain, M., Vaughn, S., Wexler, J., . . . Fletcher, J. M. (2011). An experimental study of scheduling and duration of "Tier 2" first-grade reading intervention. *Journal of Research on Educational Effectiveness, 4*, 208–230.

Derewianka, B., & Jones, P. (2016). *Teaching language in context* (2nd ed.). Oxford University Press.

de Rivera, C, Girolametto, L., Greenberg, J., & Weitzman, E. (2005). Children's responses to educators' questions in day care play groups. *American Journal of Speech-Language Pathology, 14*, 14–26.

DeThorne, L. S., Petrill, S. A., Hart, S. A., Channell, R. W., Campbell, R. J., Deater-Deckard, K., . . . Vandenbergh, D. J. (2008). Genetic effects on children's conversational language use. *Journal of Speech, Language, and Hearing Research, 51*, 423–435.

de Valenzuela, J. S., Copeland, S. R., Qi, C. H., & Park, M. (2006). Examining educational equity: Revisiting the disproportionate representation of minority students in special education. *Exceptional Children, 72*, 425–441.

de Zeeuw, P., Zwart, F., Schrama, R., van Engeland, H., & Durston, S. (2012). Prenatal exposure to cigarette smoke or alcohol and cerebellum volume in attention-deficit/hyperactivity disorder and typical development. *Translational Psychiatry, 2*, e84. https://doi.org/10.1038/tp.2012.12

Diana v. California State Board of Education, No. C-70, RFT. (1970). U.S. District Court, N. D. California.

DiCecco, V. M., & Gleason, M. M. (2002). Using graphic organizers to attain relational knowledge from expository text. *Journal of Learning Disabilities, 35*, 306–320.

Dickinson, D. K., Darrow, C. L., & Tinubu, T. A. (2008). Patterns of teacher–child conversations in Head Start classrooms: Implications for an empirically grounded approach to professional development. *Early Education and Development, 19*, 396–429.

Dickinson, D. K., & DeTemple, J. (1998). Putting parents in the picture: Maternal reports of preschoolers' literacy as a predictor of early reading. *Early Childhood Research Quarterly, 13*, 241–261.

Dickinson, D. K., & Tabors, P. O. (2001). *Beginning literacy with language: Young children learning at home and school.* Brookes.

Diehl, S. F., Ford, C., & Federico, J. (2005). The communication journey of a fully included child with an autism spectrum disorder. *Topics in Language Disorders, 25*(4), 375–387.

Diemand-Vauman, C., Oppenheimer, D., & Vaughn, E. (2011). Fortune favors the bold (and the italicized): Effects of disfluency on educational outcomes. *Cognition, 118*, 111–115.

Diessel, H. (2004). *The acquisition of complex sentences.* Cambridge University Press.

Diessel, H., & Tomasello, M. (2000). The development of relative clauses in spontaneous child speech. *Cognitive*

Linguistics, 11(1–2), 131–151. https://doi.org/10.1515/cogl.2001.006 http://scholar.google.com/scholar_lookup?hl=en&publication_year=2000&pages=131-151&issue=1-2&title=The+development+of+relative+clauses+in+spontaneous+child+speech

Diessel, H., & Tomasello, M. (2001). The acquisition of finite complement clauses in English: A corpus-based analysis. *Cognitive Linguistics, 12,* 97–142.

Diessel, H., & Tomasello, M. (2005). A new look at the acquisition of relative clauses. *Language, 81*(4), 1–25. http://scholar.google.com/scholar_lookup?hl=en&publication_year=2005&pages=1-25&issue=4&title=A+new+look+at+the+acquisition+of+relative+clauses

DiGuiseppi, C., Hepburn, S., Davis, J. M., Fidler, D. J., Hartway, S., Raitano Lee, N., . . . Robinson, C. (2010). Screening for autism spectrum disorders in children with Down syndrome: Population prevalence and screening test characteristics. *Journal of Developmental Behavioral Pediatrics, 31,* 181–191. https://doi.org/10.1097/DBP.0b013e3181d5aa6d

Dijkhuis, R. R., Ziermans, T. B., Van Rijy, S., Stall, W. G., & Swaab, H. (2016). Self-regulation and quality of life in high-functioning young adults with autism. *Autism, 21,* 896–906.

Dinnebeil, L. A., Pretti-Frontczak, K., & McInemey, W. (2009). A consultative itinerant approach to service delivery: Considerations for the early childhood community. *Language, Speech, and Hearing Services in Schools, 40,* 435–445.

Dion, E., Brodeur, M., Gosselin, C., Campeau, M., & Fuchs, D. (2010). Implementing research-based instruction to prevent reading problems among low-income students: Is earlier better? *Learning Disabilities Research & Practice, 25,* 87–96. https://doi.org/10.1111/j.1540-5826.2010.00306.x http://scholar.google.com/scholar_lookup?hl=en&volume=25&publication_year=2010&pages=87-96&journal=Learning+Disabilities+Research+%26+Practice&author=E.+Dion&author=M.+Brodeur&author=C.+Gosselin&author=M.+Campeau&author=D.+Fuchs&title=Implementing+research-based+instruction+to+prevent+reading+problems+among+low-income+students%3A+Is+earlier+better%3F

Dockrell, J. E., Lindsay, G., Connelly, V., & Mackie, C. (2007). Constraints in the production of written text in children with specific language impairments. *Exceptional Children, 73,* 147–164. https://doi.org/10.1177/001440290707300202

Dockrell, J. E., & Marshall, C. R. (2015). Measurement issues: Assessing language skills in young children. *Child and Adolescent Mental Health, 20,* 116–125. https://doi.org/10.1111/camh.12072

Dodd, B., & Carr, A. (2003). Young children's letter-sound knowledge. *Language, Speech, and Hearing Services in Schools, 34,* 128–137.

Dollaghan, C. A., & Campbell, T. (1998). Nonword repetition and child language impairment. *Journal of Speech, Language, and Hearing Research, 41,* 1136–1146.

Donovan, C. A., & Smolkin, L. B. (2002). Children's genre knowledge: An examination of K–5 students' performance on multiple tasks providing differing levels of scaffolding. *Reading Research Quarterly, 37,* 428–465. https://doi.org/10.1598/RRQ.37.4.5

Dore, J. (1974). A pragmatic description of early language development. *Journal of Psycholinguistic Research, 3,* 343–350.

Dore, J. (1986). The development of conversational competence. In R. Schiefelbusch (Ed.), *Language competence: Assessment and intervention* (pp. 3–60). College-Hill.

Douglas, J. M. (2010). Relation of executive functioning to pragmatic outcome following severe traumatic brain injury. *Journal of Speech, Language, and Hearing Research, 53,* 365–382.

Douglas, S. P., & Craig, C. S. (2007). Collaborative and iterative translation: An alternative approach to back translation. *Journal of International Marketing, 15*(1), 30–43.

Drager, K. D., Light, J. C., Carlson, R., D'Silva, K., Larsson, B., Pitkin, L., & Stopper, G. (2004). Learning of dynamic display AAC technologies by typically developing 3-year-olds: Effect of different layouts and menu approaches. *Journal of Speech, Language, and Hearing Research, 47,* 1133–1148.

Drager, K. D., Light, J. C., Curran Speltz, J., Fallon, K. A., & Jeffries, L. Z. (2003). The performance of typically developing 2½-year-olds on dynamic display AAC technologies with different system layouts and language organizations. *Journal of Speech, Language, and Hearing Research, 46,* 298–312.

Dragoo, K. E. (2017, July 10). *Students with disabilities graduating from high school and entering postsecondary education: In brief* (Congressional Research Service Report R44887, Version 2: Updated). https://www.everycrsreport.com/files/20170710_R44887_44f9ad63208ab839433a798210d3a3e1c6980425.pdf

Drysdale, H., van der Meer, L., & Kagohara, D. (2015). Children with autism spectrum disorder from bilingual families: A systematic review. *Review Journal of Autism and Developmental Disorders, 2,* 26–38.

Duchan, J. F. (1997). A situated pragmatics approach for supporting children with severe communication disorders. *Topics in Language Disorders, 17*(2), 1–18.

Duff, D. (2019). The effect of vocabulary intervention on text comprehension: Who benefits? *Language, Speech, and Hearing Services in Schools, 50,* 562–578. https://doi.org/10.1044/2019_LSHSS-VOIA-18-0001

Duff, D., Tomblin, J. B., & Catts, H. (2015). The influence of reading on vocabulary growth: A case for a Matthew effect. *Journal of Speech, Language, and Hearing Research, 58,* 853–864. https://doi.org/10.1044/2015_JSLHR-L-13-0310

Duncan, M., Cunningham, A., & Eyre, E. (2019). A combined movement and story-telling intervention enhances motor competence and language ability in pre-schoolers to a greater extent than movement or story-telling alone. *European Physical Education Review, 25,* 221–235. https://doi.org/10.1177/1356336X17715772

REFERENCES

Dunst, C. J. (2002). Family-centered practices: Birth through high school. *Journal of Special Education, 36,* 139–147.

Dunst, C. J., Hamby, D., Trivette, C. M., Raab, M., & Bruder, M. B. (2000). Everyday family and community life and children's naturally occurring learning opportunities. *Journal of Early Intervention, 23*(3), 151–164.

Dunst, C. J., & Trivette, C. M. (2009). Let's be PALS: An evidence-based approach to professional development. *Infants and Young Children, 22,* 164–176.

Dunst, C. J., Trivette, C. M., & Hamby, D. W. (2007). Meta-analysis of family-centered help-giving practices research. *Mental Retardation and Developmental Disabilities Research Reviews, 13,* 370–378. https://doi.org/10.1002/mrdd.20176

Durán, L. K., Hartzheim, D., Lund, E. M., Simonsmeier, V., & Kohlmeier, T. L. (2016). Bilingual and home language interventions with young dual language learners: A research synthesis. *Language, Speech, and Hearing Services in Schools, 47,* 347–371. https://doi.org/10.1044/2016_LSHSS-15-0030

Durham, R. E., Farkas, G., Scheffner Hammer, C., Tomblin, J. B., & Catts, H. W. (2007). Kindergarten oral language skill: A key variable in the intergenerational transmission of socioeconomic status. *Research in Social Stratification and Mobility, 25,* 294–305. http://scholar.google.com/scholar_lookup?hl=en&publication_year=2007&pages=294-305&title=Kindergarten+oral+language+skill%3A+A+key+variable+in+the+intergenerational+transmission+of+socioeconomic+status

Durkin, K., & Conti-Ramsden, G. (2007). Language, social behavior, and the quality of friendships in adolescents with and without a history of specific language impairment. *Child Development, 78,* 1441–1457. https://doi.org/10.1111/j.1447-8624.2007.01076.x

Durkin, K., Mok, P. L. H., & Conti-Ramsden, G. (2015). Core subjects at the end of primary school: Identifying and explaining relative strengths of children with specific language impairment (SLI). *International Journal of Language & Communication Disorders, 50,* 226–240. https://doi.org/10.1111/1460-6984.12137

Durkin, K., Toseeb, U., Botting, N., Pickles, A., & Conti-Ramsden, G. (2017). Social confidence in early adulthood among young people with and without a history of language impairment. *Journal of Speech, Language, and Hearing Disorders, 60,* 1635–1647. https://doi.org/10.1044/2017_JSLHR-L-16-0256

Dyson, H., Best, W., Solity, J., & Hulme, C. (2017). Training mispronunciation correction and word meanings improves children's ability to learn to read words. *Scientific Studies of Reading, 21,* 392–407. https://doi.org/10.1080/10888438.2017.1315424 http://scholar.google.com/scholar_lookup?hl=en&volume=21&publication_year=2017&pages=392-407&journal=Scientific+Studies+of+Reading&author=H.+Dyson&author=W.+Best&author=J.+Solity&author=C.+Hulme&title=Training+mispronunciation+correction+and+word+meanings+improves+children%27s+ability+to+learn+to+read+words

Dzwilewski, K. L. C., & Schantz, S. L. (2015). Prenatal chemical exposures and child language development. *Journal of Communication Disorders, 57,* 41–65.

Ebbels, S. (2007). Teaching grammar to school-aged children with specific language impairment using Shape Coding. *Child Language Teaching and Therapy, 23*(1), 67–93.

Ebbels, S. H., McCartney, E., Slonims, V., Dockrell, J. E., & Frazier Norbury, C. (2019). Evidence-based pathways to intervention for children with language disorders. *International Journal of Language and Communication Disorders, 54*(1), 3–19. https://doi.org/10.1111/1460-6984.12387

Ebbers, S. M., & Denton, C. A. (2008). A root awakening: Vocabulary instruction for older students with reading difficulties. *Learning Disabilities Research & Practice, 23,* 90–102. https://doi.org/10.1111/j.1540-5826.2008.00267.x

Eberhardt, M. (2008). The low-back merger in the Steel City: African American English in Pittsburgh. *American Speech, 83,* 284–311. https://doi.org/10.1215/00031283-2008-021

Edmonston, N. K., & Thane, N. L. (1990, April). *Children's concept comprehension: Acquisition, assessment, intervention.* Paper presented at the Annual Convention of the New York State Speech-Language-Hearing Association, Kiamesha Lake, NY.

Education Northwest. (2018). *6 + 1 Trait writing rubric.* https://educationnorthwest.org/traits/traits-rubrics

Ehren, B. J. (2000). Maintaining a therapeutic focus and sharing responsibility for student success: Keys to in-classroom speech-language services. *Language, Speech, and Hearing Services in Schools, 31,* 219–229.

Ehren, B. J. (2005). Looking for evidence-based practice in reading comprehension instruction. *Topics in Language Disorders, 25,* 310–321.

Ehren, B. J. (2006). Partnerships to support reading comprehension for students with language impairments. *Topics in Language Disorders, 26*(1), 42–54.

Ehren, B. J. (2009). Looking through an adolescent literacy lens at the narrow view of reading. *Language, Speech, and Hearing Services in Schools, 40,* 192–295. https://doi.org/10.1044/0161-1461(2009/08-0036)

Ehren, B. J. (2012, September). *Language underpinnings and curriculum standards for older students: Important work for SLPs.* Paper presented at the meeting of the Kentucky Speech-Language Hearing Association, Lexington, KY.

Ehren, B. J., Lenz, B. K., & Deshler, D. D. (2014). Adolescents who struggle and 21st-century literacy. In C. A. Stone, E. R. Silliman, B. J. Ehren, & G. P. Wallach (Eds.), *Handbook of language and literacy: Development and disorders* (2nd ed., pp. 619–636). Guilford.

Ehri, L. C. (2000). Learning to read and learning to spell: Two sides of a coin. *Topics in Language Disorders, 20*(3), 19–36.

Ehri, L. C., Nunes, S. R., Stahl, S. A., & Willows, D. M. (2001). Systematic phonics instruction helps students learn to read: Evidence from the National Reading Panel's meta-analysis. *Review of Educational Research, 71*(3), 393–447. http://scholar.google.com/scholar_lookup?hl=en&volume=71&publication_year=2001&pages=393-447

&journal=Review+of+Educational+Research&issue=3&author=L.+C.+Ehri&author=S.+R.+Nunes&author=S.+A.+Stahl&author=D.+M.+Willows&title=Systematic+phonics+instruction+helps+students+learn+to+read%3A+Evidence+from+the+National+Reading+Panel%27s+meta-analysis

Eigsti, L., & Cicchetti, D. (2004). The impact of child maltreatment on the expressive syntax at 60 months. *Developmental Science, 7,* 88–102.

Eisel Hendricks, A., & Adlof, S. M. (2017). Language assessment with children who speak nonmainstream dialects: Examining the effects of scoring modifications in norm-referenced assessment. *Language, Speech, and Hearing Services in Schools, 48,* 168–182. https://doi.org/10.1044/2017_LSHSS-16-0060

Eisel Hendricks, A., & Adlof, S. M. (2020). Production of morphosyntax within and across different dialects of American English. *Journal of Speech, Language, and Hearing Research, 63,* 2322–2233. https://doi.org/10.1044/2020_JSLHR-19-00244

Eisenberg, S. (2004). Production of infinitives by 5-year-old children with language-impairment on an elicitation task. *First Language, 24,* 305–321.

Eisenberg, S. (2005). When conversation is not enough: Assessing infinitival complements through elicitation. *American Journal of Speech-Language Pathology, 14,* 92–106.

Eisenberg, S. L., Bredin-Oja, S. L., & Crumrine, K. (2020). Use of imitation training for targeting grammar: A narrative review. *Language, Speech, and Hearing Services in Schools, 51,* 205–225. https://doi.org/10.1044/2019_LSHSS-19-00024

Eisenberg, S. L., & Guo, L.-Y. (2013). Differentiating children with and without language impairment based on grammaticality. *Language, Speech, and Hearing Services in Schools, 44,* 20–31. https://doi.org/10.1044/0161-1461 (2012/11-0089)

Eisenberg, S. L., McGovern Fersko, T., & Lundgren, C. (2001). The use of MLU for identifying language impairment in preschool children: A review. *American Journal of Speech-Language Pathology, 10,* 323–342.

Elleman, A. M., Lindo, E. J., Morphy, P., & Compton, D. L. (2009). The impact of vocabulary instruction on passage-level comprehension of school-age children: A meta-analysis. *Journal of Research on Educational Effectiveness, 2,* 1–44. https://doi.org/10.1080/19345740802 539200

Elleman, A. M., Oslund, E. L., Griffin, N. M., & Myers, K. E. (2019). A review of middle school vocabulary interventions: Five research-based recommendations for practice. *Language, Speech, and Hearing Services in Schools, 50,* 477–492. https://doi.org/10.1044/2019_LSHSS-VOIA-18-0145

Ellis, E. M., & Thal, D. J. (2008). Early language delay and risk for language impairment. *Perspectives on Language Learning and Education, 15,* 93–100.

Ellis Weismer, S., & Evans, J. L. (2002). The role of processing limitations in early identification of specific language impairment. *Topics in Language Disorders, 22*(3), 15–29.

Ellis Weismer, S., & Hesketh, L. J. (1998). The impact of emphatic stress on novel word learning by children with specific language impairment. *Journal of Speech, Language, and Hearing Research, 41,* 1444–1458.

Ellis Weismer, S., Lord, C., & Esler, A. (2010). Early language patterns of toddlers on the autism spectrum compared to toddlers with developmental delay. *Journal of Autism and Developmental Disorders, 40*(10), 1259–1273. https://doi.org/10.1007/s10803-010-0983-1

Ellis Weismer, S., Plante, E., Jones, M., & Tomblin, J. B. (2005). A functional magnetic resonance imaging investigation of verbal working memory in adolescents with specific language impairment. *Journal of Speech, Language, and Hearing Research, 48,* 405–425.

Ellis Weismer, S., Tomblin, J. B., Zhang, X., Buckwalter, P., Chynoweth, J. G., & Jones, M. (2000). Non-word repetition performance in school-age children with and without language impairment. *Journal of Speech, Language, and Hearing Research, 43,* 865–878.

Elwer, S., Keenan, J. M., Olson, R. K., Byrne, B., & Samuelsson, S. (2013). Longitudinal stability and predictors of poor oral comprehenders and poor decoders. *Journal of Experimental Child Psychology, 115,* 497–516. https://doi.org/10.1016/j.jecp.2012.12.001 http://scholar.google.com/scholar_lookup?hl=en&volume=115&publication_year=2013&pages=497-516&journal=Journal+of+Experimental+Child+Psychology&author=S.+Elwer&author=J.+M.+Keenan&author=R.+K.+Olson&author=B.+Byrne&author=S.+Samuelsson&title=Longitudinal+stability+and+predictors+of+poor+oral+comprehenders+and+poor+decoders

Engel de Abreu, P. M. J., Baldassi, M., Puglisi, M. L., & Befi-Lopes, D. M. (2013). Cross-linguistic and cross-cultural effects on verbal working memory and vocabulary: Testing language minority children with an immigrant background. *Journal of Speech, Language, and Hearing Research, 56,* 630–642.

Ertmer, D. J., Strong, L. M., & Sadagopan, N. (2003). Beginning to communicate after cochlear implantation: Oral language development in a young child. *Journal of Speech, Language, and Hearing Research, 46,* 328–340.

Ervin-Tripp, S. (1977). Wait for me roller skate. In S. Ervin-Tripp & C. Mitchell-Kerner (Eds.), *Child discourse* (pp. 165–188). Academic Press.

Evans, J. L., & Craig, H. K. (1992). Language sample collection and analysis: Interview compared to freeplay assessment contexts. *Journal of Speech and Hearing Research, 35,* 343–353.

Evans, J. L., Gillam, R. B., & Montgomery. J. M. (2018). Cognitive predictors of spoken word recognition in children with and without developmental language disorders. *Journal of Speech, Language, and Hearing Research, 61,* 1409–1425. https://doi.org/10.1044/2018_JSLHR-L-17-0150

Evans, J. L., Saffran, J. R., & Robe-Torres, K. (2009). Statistical learning in children with specific language impairment. *Journal of Speech, Language, and Hearing Research, 52*(2), 321–335. https://doi.org/10.1044/1092-4388(2009/07-0189)

Everitt, A., Hannaford, P., & Conti-Ramsden, G. (2013). Markers for persistent specific expressive language delay in 3–4-year-olds. *International Journal of Language and Communication Disorders, 48*, 534–553.

Ezell, H. K., Justice, L. M., & Parsons, D. (2000). Enhancing the emergent literacy skills of preschoolers with communication disorders: A pilot investigation. *Child Language Teaching and Therapy, 16*, 121–160.

Fallon, K. A., & Katz, L. A. (2011). Providing written language services in the schools: The time is now. *Language, Speech, and Hearing Services in Schools, 42*, 3–17.

Fallon, K. A., Light, J. C., & Kramer Paige, T. (2001). Enhancing vocabulary selection for preschoolers who require augmentative and alternative communication (AAC). *American Journal of Speech-Language Pathology, 10*, 81–94.

Fang, Z. (2008). Going beyond the fab five: Helping students cope with the unique linguistic challenges of expository reading in intermediate grades. *Journal of Adolescent & Adult Literacy, 51*, 476–487. https://doi.org/10.1598/JAAL.51.6.4

Fang, Z., & Schleppegrel, M. J. (2008). *Reading in secondary content areas: A language-based pedagogy.* University of Michigan Press.

Fang, Z., Schleppegrell, M. J., & Cox, B. E. (2006). Understanding the language demands of schooling: Nouns in academic registers. *Journal of Literacy Research, 38*(3), 247–273. https://doi.org/10.1207/s15548430jlr3803_1

Faul, M., Xu, L., Wald, M. M., Coronado, V., & Dellinger, A. M. (2010). Traumatic brain injury in the United States: National estimates of prevalence and incidence, 2002–2006. *Injury Prevention, 16*, A268. https://doi.org/10.1136/ip.2010.029215.951

Favot, K., Carter, M., & Stephenson, J. (2018). The effects of an oral narrative intervention on the fictional narrative retells of children with ASD and severe language impairment: A pilot study. *Journal of Developmental and Physical Disabilities, 30*, 615–637. https://doi.org/10.1007/s10882-018-9608-y

Fayol, M. (2016). From language to text: The development and learning of translation. In C. MacArthur, S. Graham, & J. Fitzgerald (Eds.), *Handbook of writing research* (2nd ed., pp. 130–143). Guilford. http://scholar.google.com/scholar_lookup?hl=en&publication_year=2016&pages=130-143&author=M.+Fayol&title=Handbook+of+writing+research

Feimster, Y., Jacewicz, E., & Fox, R. A. (2015). Variation in vowel duration among Southern African American English speakers. *American Journal of Speech-Language Pathology, 24*, 460–469.

Feldman, H. M., Dollaghan, C. A., Campbell, T. F., Colborn, D. K., Janosky, J., Kurs-Lasky, M., . . . Paradise, J. L. (2003). Parent-reported language skills in relation to otitis media during the first 3 years of life. *Journal of Speech, Language, and Hearing Research, 46*, 273–287.

Fenson, L., Marchman, V. A., Thal, D. J., Dale, P. S., Reznick, J. S., & Bates, E. (2006). *MacArthur–Bates Communicative Development Inventories (CDI), second edition.* Brookes.

Fey, M. E., Catts, H., Proctor-Williams, K., Tomblin, B., & Zhang, X. (2004). Oral and written story composition skills of children with language impairment. *Journal of Speech, Language, and Hearing Research, 47*, 1301–1318.

Fey, M. E., Finestack, L. H., Gajewski, B. J., Popescu, M., & Lewine, J. D. (2010). A preliminary evaluation of Fast ForWord-Language as an adjuvant treatment in language intervention. *Journal of Speech, Language, and Hearing Research, 53*, 430–449.

Fey, M. E., & Frome Loeb, D. (2002). An evaluation of the facilitative effects of inverted yes–no questions on the acquisition of auxiliary verbs. *Journal of Speech, Language, and Hearing Research, 45*, 160–174.

Fey, M. E., Leonard, L. B., Bredin-Oja, S. L., & Deevy, P. (2017). A clinical evaluation of the competing sources of input hypothesis. *Journal of Speech, Language, and Hearing Disorders, 60*, 104–120. https://doi.org/10.1044/2016_JSLHR-L-15-0448

Fey, M. E., Long, S. H., & Finestack, L. H. (2003). Ten principles of grammar facilitation for children with specific language impairments. *American Journal of Speech-Language Pathology, 12*, 3–15.

Fey, M. E., Yoder, O., Warren, S., & Bredin-Oja, S. (2013). Is more better? Milieu communication teaching in toddlers with intellectual disabilities. *Journal of Speech, Language, and Hearing Research, 56*, 679–693.

Fichman, S., & Altman, C. (2019). Referential cohesion in the narratives of bilingual and monolingual children with typically developing language and with specific language impairment. *Journal of Speech, Language, and Hearing Research, 62*, 123–142. https://doi.org/10.1044/2018_JSLHR-L-18-0054

Filiatrault-Veilleux, P., Bouchard, C., Trudeau, N., & Desmarais, C. (2016). Comprehension of inferences in a narrative in 3- to 6-year-old children. *Journal of Speech, Language, and Hearing Research, 59*, 1099–1110. https://doi.org/10.1044/2016_JSLHR-L-15-0252

Finestack, L. H. (2018). Evaluation of an explicit intervention to teach novel grammatical forms to children with developmental language disorder. *Journal of Speech, Language, and Hearing Disorders, 61*, 2065–2075. https://doi.org/10.1044/2018_JSLHR-L-17-0339

Finestack, L. H., & Abbeduto, L. (2010). Expressive language profiles of verbally expressive adolescents and young adults with Down syndrome or fragile X syndrome. *Journal of Speech, Language, and Hearing Research, 53*, 1334–1348.

Finestack, L. H., Engman, J., Huang, T., Bangert, K. J., & Bader, K. (2020). Evaluation of a combined explicit–implicit approach to teach grammatical forms to children with grammatical weaknesses. *American Journal of Speech-Language Pathology, 29*, 63–79. https://doi.org/10.1044/2019_AJSLP-19-0056

Finestack, L. H., & Fey, M. E. (2009). Evaluation of a deductive procedure to teach grammatical inflections to children with language impairment. *American Journal of Speech-Language Pathology, 18*, 289–302.

Finestack, L. H., Rohwer, B., Hilliard, L., & Abbeduto, L. (2020). Using computerized language analysis to evaluate grammatical skills. *Language, Speech, and Hearing Services in Schools, 51*, 184–204. https://doi.org/10.1044/2019_LSHSS-19-00032

Finke, E. H., Davis, J. M., Benedict, M., Goga, L., Kelly, J., Palumbo, L., . . . Waters, S. (2016). Effects of a least-to-most prompting procedure on multisymbol message production in children with autism spectrum disorder who use augmentative and alternative communication. *American Journal of Speech-Language Pathology, 26*, 81–98. https://doi.org/10.1044/2016_AJSLP-14-0187

Finneran, D. A., & Leonard, L. B. (2010). The role of linguistic input in third person singular *–s* use in the speech of young children. *Journal of Speech, Language, and Hearing Research, 53*, 1065–1074.

Finneran, D. A., Leonard, L. B., & Miller, C. (2010). Speech disruptions in the sentence formulation of school-age children with specific language impairment. *International Journal of Language and Communication Disorders, 46*, 271–286.

Finney, M., Montgomery, J., Gillam, R., & Evans, J. (2014). Role of working memory storage and attention focus switching in children's comprehension of spoken object relative sentences. *Child Development Research, 54*, 1–11. https://doi.org/10.1155/2014/450734

Fitton, L., Hoge, R., Petscher, Y., & Wood, C. (2019). Psychometric evaluation of the Bilingual English–Spanish Assessment Sentence Repetition Task for clinical decision making. *Journal of Speech, Language, and Hearing Research, 62*, 1906–1922. https://doi.org/10.1044/2019_JSLHR-L-18-0354

Flax, J. F., Realpe-Bonilla, T., Hirsch, L. S., Brzustowicz, L. M., Bartlett, C. W., & Tallal, P. (2003). Specific language impairment in families: Evidence for co-occurrence with reading impairments. *Journal of Speech, Language, and Hearing Research, 46*, 530–543.

Flenthrope, J. L., & Brady, N. C. (2010). Relationships between early gestures and later language in children with fragile X syndrome. *American Journal of Speech-Language Pathology, 19*, 135–142.

Fletcher, J., Coulter, W. A., Reschly, D. J., & Vaughn, S. (2004). Alternative approaches to the definition and identification of learning disabilities: Some questions and answers. *Annals of Dyslexia, 54*, 305–331. https://doi.org/10.1007/s11881-004-0015-y http://scholar.google.com/scholar_lookup?hl=en&volume=54&publication_year=2004&pages=305-331&journal=Annals+of+Dyslexia&author=J.+Fletcher&author=W.+A.+Coulter&author=D.+J.+Reschly&author=S.+Vaughn&title=Alternative+approaches+to+the+definition+and+identification+of+learning+disabilities%3A+Some+questions+and+answers

Fletcher, J., & Vaughn, S. (2009). Response to intervention: Preventing and remediating academic difficulties. *Child Development Perspective, 3*, 30–37. https://doi.org/10.1111/j.1750-8606.2008.00072.x http://scholar.google.com/scholar_lookup?hl=en&volume=3&publication_year=2009&pages=30-37&journal=Child+Development+Perspective&author=J.+Fletcher&author=S.+Vaughn&title=Response+to+intervention%3A+Preventing+and+remediating+academic+difficulties

Flippin, M., Reszka, S., & Watson, L. R. (2010). Effectiveness of the Picture Exchange Communication System (PECS) on communication and speech for children with autism spectrum disorders: A meta-analysis. *American Journal of Speech-Language Pathology, 19*, 178–195.

Fluharty N. (2001). *Fluharty Preschool Speech and Language Screening Test–Second Edition (FLUHARTY-2)*. Pro-Ed.

Folger, J., & Chapman, R. (1978). A pragmatic analysis of spontaneous imitations. *Journal of Child Language, 5*, 25–38.

Fombonne, E. (2003). Epidemiological surveys of autism and other pervasive developmental disorders: An update. *Journal of Autism and Developmental Disorders, 33*, 365–382.

Foorman, B., & Torgesen, J. (2001). Critical elements of classroom and small-group instruction promote reading success in all children. *Learning Disabilities Research & Practice, 16*, 203–212. https://doi.org/10.1111/0938-8982.00020

Ford, J. A., & Milosky, L. M. (2003). Inferring emotional reactions in social situations: Differences in children with language impairment. *Journal of Speech, Language, and Hearing Research, 46*, 21–30.

Ford, J. A., & Milosky, L. M. (2008). Inference generation during discourse and its relation to social competence: An online investigation of abilities of children with and without language impairment. *Journal of Speech, Language, and Hearing Research, 51*, 367–380.

Ford-Connors, E., & Paratore, J. R. (2015). Vocabulary instruction in fifth grade and beyond: Sources of word learning and productive contexts for development. *Review of Educational Research, 85*, 50–91. https://doi.org/10.3102/0034654314540943

Fortunato-Tavares, T., de Andrade, C. R. F., Befi-Lopes, D. M., Hestvik, A., Epstein, B., Tornyova, L., & Schwartz, R. G. (2012). Syntactic structural assignment in Brazilian Portuguese-speaking children with specific language impairment. *Journal of Speech, Language, and Hearing Research, 55*, 1097–1111.

Foster, W. A., & Miller, M. (2007). Development of the literacy achievement gap: A longitudinal study of kindergarten through third grade. *Language, Speech, and Hearing Services in Schools, 38*, 173–181.

Fox, C. B., Israelsen-Augenstein, M., Jones, S., & Laing Gillam, S. (2021). An evaluation of expedited transcription methods for school-age children's narrative language: Automatic speech recognition and real-time transcription. *Journal of Speech, Language, and Hearing Research, 63*, 3533–3548. https://doi.org/10.1044/2021_JSLHR-21-00096

Frazier, J., Goswami, U., & Conti-Ramsden, G. (2010). Dyslexia and specific language impairment: The role of phonology and auditory processing. *Scientific Studies of Reading, 14*, 8–29. https://doi.org/10.1080/10888430903242068

Frazier Norbury, C., Gooch, D., Wray, C., Baird, G., Charman, T., Simonoff, E., . . . Pickles, A. (2016). The impact of nonverbal ability on prevalence and clinical presentation of language disorder: Evidence from a population study. *Journal of Child Psychology and Psychiatry, 57*, 1247–1257. https://doi.org/10.1111/jcpp.12573

Fried-Oken, M. (1987). Qualitative examination of children's naming skills through test adaptations. *Language, Speech, and Hearing Services in Schools, 18*, 206–216.

Frizelle, P., & Fletcher, P. (2014a). Profiling relative clause constructions in children with specific language impairment. *Clinical Linguistics & Phonetics, 28*, 437–449. https://doi.org/10.3109/02699206.2014.882991 http://scholar.google.com/scholar_lookup?hl=en&publication_year=2014a&pages=437-449&title=Profiling+relative+clause+constructions+in+children+with+specific+language+impairment

Frizelle P., & Fletcher P. (2014b). Relative clause constructions in children with specific language impairment. *International Journal of Language & Communication Disorders, 49*, 255–264. https://doi.org/10.1111/1460-6984.12070 http://scholar.google.com/scholar_lookup?hl=en&publication_year=2014b&pages=255-264&title=Relative+clause+constructions+in+children+with+specific+language+impairment

Frizelle, P., & Fletcher, P. (2015). The role of memory in processing relative clauses in children with specific language impairment. *American Journal of Speech-Language Pathology, 24*, 47–59. https://doi.org/10.1044/2014_AJSLP-13-0153

Frome Loeb, D., Imgrund, C. M., Lee, J., & Barlow, S. M. (2020). Language, motor, and cognitive outcomes of toddlers who were born preterm. *American Journal of Speech-Language Pathology, 19*, 625–637. https://doi.org/10.1044/2019_AJSLP-19-00049

Fry, R. (2007). *The changing racial and ethnic composition of U.S. public schools.* Pew Hispanic Center.

Fuchs, D., & Fuchs, L. S. (2006). Introduction to response to intervention: What, why, and how valid is it? *Reading Research Quarterly, 41*, 93–99. https://doi.org/10.1598/rrq.41.1.4 http://scholar.google.com/scholar_lookup?hl=en&volume=41&publication_year=2006&pages=93-99&journal=Reading+Research+Quarterly&author=D.+Fuchs&author=L.+S.+Fuchs&title=Introduction+to+response+to+intervention%3A+What%2C+why%2C+and+how+valid+is+it%3F

Fuchs, D., Fuchs, L. S., & Compton, D. L. (2012). Smart RTI: A next-generation approach to multilevel prevention. *Exceptional Children, 78*, 263–279. https://doi.org/10.1177/001440291207800301 http://scholar.google.com/scholar_lookup?hl=en&volume=78&publication_year=2012&pages=263-279&journal=Exceptional+Children&author=D.+Fuchs&author=L.+S.+Fuchs&author=D.+L.+Compton&title=Smart+RTI%3A+A+next-generation+approach+to+multilevel+prevention

Fujiki, M., Brinton, B., Isaacson, T., & Summers, C. (2001). Social behavior of children with language impairment on the playground: A pilot study. *Language, Speech, and Hearing Services in Schools, 32*, 101–113.

Galaburda, A. L. (2005). Neurology of learning disabilities: What will the future bring? The answer comes from the successes of the recent past. *Journal of Learning Disabilities, 28*, 107–109.

Gallagher, A., Frith, U., & Snowling, M. J. (2000). Precursors of literacy delay among children at genetic risk of dyslexia. *Journal of Child Psychology and Psychiatry and Allied Disciplines, 41*, 202–213.

Gallagher, A. L., Murphy, C., Conway, P., & Perry, A. (2019). Consequential differences in perspectives and practices concerning children with developmental language disorders: An integrative review. *International Journal of Language and Communication Disorders, 54*, 529–552. https://doi.org/10.1111/1460-6984.12469

Gallinat, E., & Spaulding, T. J. (2014). Differences in the performance of children with specific language impairment and their typically developing peers on nonverbal cognitive tests: A meta-analysis. *Journal of Speech, Language, and Hearing Research, 57*, 1363–1382. https://doi.org/10.1044/2014_JSLHR-L-12-0363

Ganz, J. B., Earles-Vollrath, T. L., Heath, A. K., Parker, R. I., Rispoli, M. J., & Duran, J. B. (2012). A meta-analysis of single case research studies on aided augmentative and alternative communication systems with individuals with autism spectrum disorders. *Journal of Autism and Developmental Disorders, 42*(1), 60–74. https://doi.org/10.1007/s10803-011-1212-2

Garcia, S. B., Mendez-Perez, A., & Ortiz, A. A. (2000). Mexican American mothers' beliefs about disabilities: Implications for early childhood intervention. *Remedial and Special Education, 21*, 90–100.

García Coll, C., Akiba, D., Palacios, N., Bailey, B., Silver, R., DiMartino, L., & Chin, C. (2002). Parental involvement in children's education: Lessons from three immigrant groups. *Parenting: Science and Practice, 2*(3), 303–324. https://doi.org/10.1207/S15327922PAR0203_05

Gardner, C., & Spencer, T. D. (2016, November). *Oral narrative intervention improves inferential word learning.* Paper presented at the American Speech-Language-Hearing Association Annual Convention, Philadelphia, PA.

Gardner, D., & Davies, M. (2013). A new academic vocabulary list. *Applied Linguistics, 35*(3), 305–327.

Garnett, K. (1986). Telling tales: Narratives and learning disabled children. *Topics in Language Disorders, 6*(2), 44–56.

Garraffa, M., Coco, M. I., & Branigan, H. P. (2012, March). *Processing of subject relatives in SLI children during structural priming and sentence repetition.* Poster session presented at the annual CUNY Conference on Human Sentence Processing, New York, NY.

Gary, K. W., Sima, A., Wehman, P., & Johnson, K. R. (2019). Transitioning racial/ethnic minorities with intellectual developmental disabilities: Influence of socioeconomic status on related services. *Career Development and Transition for Exceptional Individuals, 42*(3), 158–167.

Gathercole, S. E. (2006). Nonword repetition and word learning: The nature of the relationship. *Applied Psycholinguistics, 27*, 513–543.

Gathercole, S. E., & Alloway, T. (2006). Short-term and working memory impairments in neurodevelopmental disorders: Diagnosis and remedial support. *Journal of Child Psychology and Psychiatry*, *47*, 4–15.

Gathercole, S. E., & Alloway, T. P. (2008). Working memory and classroom learning. In S. K. Thurman & C. A. Fiorello (Eds.), *Applied cognitive research in K–3 classrooms* (pp. 17–40). Routledge.

Gathercole, S. E., Alloway, T. P., Willis, C., & Adams, A. M. (2006). Working memory in children with reading disabilities. *Journal of Experimental Child Psychology*, *93*, 256–281. https://doi.org/10.1016/j.jecp.2005.08.003 http://scholar.google.com/scholar_lookup?hl=en&volume=93&publication_year=2006&pages=256-281&journal=Journal+of+Experimental+Child+Psychology&author=S.+E.+Gathercole&author=T.+P.+Alloway&author=C.+Willis&author=A.+M.+Adams&title=Working+memory+in+children+with+reading+disabilities

Gathercole, S. E., & Baddeley, A. (1996). *The Children's Test of Nonword Repetition*. Psychological Corporation.

Gatlin, B., & Wanzek, J. (2015). Relations among children's use of dialect and literacy skills: A meta-analysis. *Journal of Speech, Language, and Hearing Research*, *58*, 1306–1310. https://doi.org/10.1044/2015_JSLHR-L-14-0311

Gaulin, C. A., & Campbell, T. F. (1994). Procedure for assessing verbal working memory in normal school-age children: Some preliminary data. *Perceptual & Motor Skills*, *79*, 55–64.

Gellert, A. S., & Arnbak, E. (2020). Predicting response to vocabulary intervention using dynamic assessment. *Language, Speech, and Hearing Services in Schools*, *51*, 1112–1123. https://doi.org/10.1044/2020_LSHSS-20-00045

Gengoux, G. W., Schapp, S., Burton, S., Ardel, C. M., Libove, R. A., Baldi, G., . . . Hardan, A. Y. (2019). Effects of a parent-implemented Developmental Reciprocity Treatment Program for children with autism spectrum disorder. *Autism*, *23*, 713–725. https://doi.org/10.1177/1362361318775538

Gerken, L., Wilson, R., & Lewis, W. (2005). Infants can use distributional cues to form syntactic categories. *Journal of Child Language*, *32*, 249–268.

German, D. J. (1992). Word-finding intervention for children and adolescents. *Topics in Language Disorders*, *13*(1), 33–50.

German, D. J. (2014). *Test of Word Finding, Third Edition (TOWF-3)*. Pro-Ed.

German, D. J., & Newman, R. S. (2004). The impact of lexical factors on children's word-finding errors. *Journal of Speech, Language, and Hearing Research*, *47*, 624–636.

Gersten, R., & Baker, S. (2001). Teaching expressive writing to students with learning disabilities: A meta-analysis. *Elementary School Journal*, *101*(3), 251–272. http://scholar.google.com/scholar_lookup?hl=en&volume=101&publication_year=2001&pages=251-272&journal=Elementary+School+Journal&issue=3&author=R.+Gersten&author=S.+Baker&title=Teaching+expressive+writing+to+students+with+learning+disabilities%3A+A+meta-analysis

Gersten, R., Compton, D., Connor, C. M., Dimino, J., Santoro, L., Linan-Thompson, S., & Tilly, W. D. (2009). *Assisting students struggling with reading: Response to intervention and multi-tier intervention for reading in the primary grades. A practice guide* (NCEE 2009–4045). National Center for Education Evaluation and Regional Assistance, Institute of Education Sciences, U.S. Department of Education.

Gersten, R., & Geva, E. (2003). Teaching reading to early language learners. *Educational Leadership*, *60*, 44–49.

Gersten, R., Jayanthi, M., & Dimino, J. A. (2017). Too much, too soon? Unanswered questions from national response to intervention evaluation. *Exceptional Children*, *83*, 244–254. https://doi.org/10.1177/0014402917692847 http://scholar.google.com/scholar_lookup?hl=en&volume=83&publication_year=2017&pages=244-254&journal=Exceptional+Children&author=R.+Gersten&author=M.+Jayanthi&author=J.+A.+Dimino&title=Too+much%2C+too+soon%3F+Unanswered+questions+from+national+response+to+intervention+evaluation

Gettinger, M., & Stoiber, K. (2008). Applying a response-to-intervention model for early literacy development in low-income children. *Topics in Early Childhood Special Education*, *27*, 198–213.

Geurts, H., & Embrechts, M. (2008). Language profiles in ASD, SLI, and ADHD. *Journal of Autism and Developmental Disorders*, *38*, 1931–1943. https://doi.org/10.1007/s10803-008-0587-1

Geurts, H. M., Verte, S., Oosterlaan, J., Roeyers, H., & Sergeant, J. A. (2004). How specific are executive functioning deficits in attention deficit hyperactivity disorder and autism. *Journal of Child Psychology and Psychiatry*, *45*(4), 836–854. https://doi.org/10.1111/j.1469-7610.2004.00276.x

Gevarter, C., & Zamora, C. (2018). Naturalistic speech-generating device interventions for children with complex communication needs: A systematic review of single-subject studies. *American Journal of Speech-Language Pathology*, *27*, 1073–1090. https://doi.org/10.1044/2018_AJSLP-17-0128 http://scholar.google.com/scholar_lookup?hl=en&volume=46&publication_year=2016&pages=2327-2339&journal=Journal+of+Autism+and+Developmental+Disorders&author=H.+Cholemkery&author=J.+Medda&author=T.+Lempp&author=C.+M.+Freitag&title=Classifying+Autism+Spectrum+Disorders+by+ADI-R%3A+Subtypes+or+severity+gradient%3F

Gibson, J., Adams, C., Lockton, E., & Green, J. (2013). Social communication disorder outside autism? A diagnostic classification approach to delineating pragmatic language impairment, high functioning autism and specific language impairment. *Journal of Child Psychology and Psychiatry*, *54*, 1186–1197.

Gibson, T. A., Peña, E. D., & Bedore, L. M. (2014). The receptive–expressive gap in bilingual children with and without primary language impairment. *American Journal of Speech-Language Pathology*, *23*, 655–6667. https://doi.org/10.1044/2014_AJSLP-12-0119

Gibson, T. A., Peña, E. D., & Bedore, L. M. (2018). The receptive–expressive gap in English narratives of Spanish–English bilingual children with and without language impairment. *Journal of Speech, Language, and Hearing Disorders, 61*, 1381–1392. https://doi.org/10.1044/2018_JSLHR-L-16-0432

Gilbert, J. K., Goodwin, A. P., Compton, D. L., & Kearns, D. M. (2014). Multisyllabic word reading as a moderator of morphological awareness and reading comprehension. *Journal of Learning Disabilities, 47*, 34–43. https://https://doi.org/10.1177/0022219413509966

Gilchrist, A., Green, J., Cox, A., Burton, D., Rutter, M., & Le Couteur, A. (2001). Development and current functioning in adolescents with Asperger syndrome: A comparative study. *Journal of Child Psychology and Psychiatry and Allied Disciplines, 42*, 227–240.

Gill, C., Klecan-Aker, J., Roberts, T., & Fredenburg, K. (2003). Following directions: Rehearsal and visualization strategies for children with specific language impairment. *Child Language Teaching and Therapy, 19*, 85–103.

Gillam, R. B., & Bedore, L. M. (2000). Communication across the lifespan. In R. B. Gillam, T. P. Marquart, & F. N. Martin (Eds.), *Communication sciences and disorders: From science to clinical practice*. Singular Publishing.

Gillam, R. B., Frome Loeb, D., Hoffman, L. M., Bohman, T., Champlin, C. A., Thibodeau, L., . . . Friel-Patti, S. (2008). The efficacy of Fast ForWord language intervention in school-age children with language impairment: A randomized controlled trial. *Journal of Speech, Language, and Hearing Research, 51*, 97–119.

Gillam, R. B., Hoffman, L. M., Marler, J. A., & Wynn-Dancy, M. L. (2002). Sensitivity to increased task demands: Contributions from data-driven and conceptually driven information processing deficits. *Topics in Language Disorders, 22*(3), 30–48.

Gillam, R. B., & Johnston, J. R. (1985). Development of print awareness in language-disordered preschoolers. *Journal of Speech and Hearing Research, 28*, 521–526.

Gillam, R. B., Montgomery, J. W., Evans, J. L., & Gillam, S. L. (2019). Cognitive predictors of sentence comprehension in children with and without developmental language disorder: Implications for assessment and treatment. *International Journal of Language & Communication Disorders, 21*(3), 240–251.

Gillam, R. B., & Pearson, N. A. (2004). *Test of Narrative Language*. Pro-Ed.

Gillam, R. B., & Pearson, N. A. (2017). *Test of Narrative Language–Second Edition (TNL-2)*. Pro-Ed.

Gillam, R. B., & Ukrainetz, T. A. (2006). Language intervention through literature-based units. In T. A. Ukrainetz (Ed.), *Contextualized language intervention* (pp. 59–94). Thinking Publications.

Gillam, S. L., & Gillam, R. B. (2006). Making evidence-based decisions about child language intervention in schools. *Language, Speech, and Hearing Services in Schools, 37*, 304–315.

Gillam, S. L., & Gillam, R. B. (2016). Narrative discourse intervention for school-aged children with language impairment. *Topics in Language Disorders, 36*(1), 20–34. https://doi.org/10.1097/TLD.0000000000000081

Gillam, S. L., & Gillam, R. B. (2018). *Supporting Knowledge in Language and Literacy (SKILL)*. Utah State University.

Gillam, S. L., Gillam, R. B., Fargo, J. D., Olszewski, A., & Segura, H. (2017). Monitoring indicators of scholarly language: A progress-monitoring instrument for measuring narrative discourse skills. *Communication Disorders Quarterly, 38*(2), 96–106. https://https://doi.org/org/10.1177/1525740116651442

Gillam, S. L., Gillam, R. B., & Laing, C. E. (2014). *Supporting Knowledge in Language and Literacy*. Utah State University.

Gillam, S. L., Gillam, R. B., & Laing, C. E. (2018). *Supporting Knowledge in Language and Literacy* (3rd ed.). Utah State University.

Gillam, S. L., Gillam, R. B., & Reece, K. (2012). Language outcomes of contextualized and decontextualized language intervention: Results of an early efficacy study. *Language, Speech, and Hearing Services in Schools, 43*, 276–291. https://doi.org/10.1044/0161-1461(2011/11-0022)

Gillam, S. L., Hartzheim, D., Studenka, B., Simonsmeier, V., & Gillam, R. (2015). Narrative intervention for children with autism spectrum disorder (ASD). *Journal of Speech, Language, and Hearing Research, 58*, 920–933. https://doi.org/10.1044/2015_JSLHR-L-14-0295

Gillespie, A., & Graham, S. (2014). A meta-analysis of writing interventions for students with learning disabilities. *Exceptional Children, 80*(4), 454–473. http://scholar.google.com/scholar_lookup?hl=en&volume=80&publication_year=2014&pages=454-473&journal=Exceptional+Children&issue=4&author=A.+Gillespie&author=S.+Graham&title=A+meta-analysis+of+writing+interventions+for+students+with+learning+disabilities

Gillespie-Lynch, K., Khalulyan, A., del Rosario, M., McCarthy, B., Gomez, L., Sigman, M., & Hutman, T. (2015). Is early joint attention associated with school-age pragmatic language? *Autism, 19*, 168–177. https://doi.org/10.1177/1362361313515094

Gillon, G. T. (2005). Facilitating phoneme awareness development in 3- and 4-year-old children with speech impairment. *Language, Speech, and Hearing Services in Schools, 36*, 308–324.

Girolametto, L., & Weitzman, E. (2002). Responsiveness of child care providers in interactions with toddlers and preschoolers. *Language, Speech, and Hearing Services in Schools, 33*, 268–281.

Girolametto, L., Weitzman, E., & Greenberg, J. (2003). Training day care staff to facilitate children's language. *American Journal of Speech-Language Pathology, 12*, 299–311.

Gladfelter, A., & Leonard, L. (2013). Alternative tense and agreement morpheme measures for assessing grammatical deficits during the preschool period. *Journal of Speech, Language, and Hearing Research, 56*, 542–552.

Gladfelter, A., & VanZuiden, C. (2020). The influence of language context on repetitive speech use in children with autism spectrum disorder. *American Journal of Speech-Language Pathology, 29*, 327–334. https://doi.org/10.1044/2019_AJSLP-19-00003

Glenberg, A. M., Brown, M., & Levin, J. R. (2007). Enhancing comprehension in small reading groups using a manipulation strategy. *Contemporary Educational Psychology, 32,* 389–399.

Glenberg, A. M., Jaworski, B., & Rischal, M. (2005). *Improving reading improves math.* Unpublished manuscript, University of Wisconsin–Madison.

Glenn, C. G., & Stein, N. L. (1980). *Syntactic structures and real world themes in stories generated by children.* University of Illinois, Center for the Study of Reading.

Glennen, S. (2014). A longitudinal study of language and speech in children who were internationally adopted at different ages. *Language, Speech, and Hearing Services in Schools, 45,* 185–203. https://doi.org/10.1044/2014_LSHSS-13-0035

Glennen, S. L., & Masters, M. G. (2002). Typical and atypical language development in infants and toddlers adopted from Eastern Europe. *American Journal of Speech-Language Pathology, 11,* 417–433.

Goffman, L., & Leonard, J. (2000). Growth of language skills in preschool children with specific language impairment. *American Journal of Speech-Language Pathology, 9,* 151–161.

Goldbart, J., & Marshall, J. (2004). "Pushes and pulls" on the parents of children who use AAC. *Augmentative and Alternative Communication, 20,* 194–208.

Goldenberg, R. L., Culhane, J. F., Iams, J. D., & Romero, R. (2008). Epidemiology and causes of preterm birth. *Lancet, 5*(371), 75–84.

Goldstein, B. (2012). *Bilingual language development and disorders in Spanish-English speakers* (2nd ed.). Brookes.

Goldstein, B. A. (2006). Clinical implications of research on language development and disorders in bilingual children. *Topics in Language Disorders, 26,* 305–321.

Goldstein, H. (2016). *Path to literacy.* Brookes.

Goldstein, H., English, K., Shafer, K., & Kaczmarek, L. (1997). Interaction among preschoolers with and without disabilities: Effects of across-the-day peer intervention. *Journal of Speech, Language, and Hearing Research, 40,* 33–48.

Goldstein, H., Kelley, E., Greenwood, C., McCune, L., Carta, J., Atwater, J., . . . Spencer, T. (2016). Embedded instruction improves vocabulary learning during automated storybook reading among high-risk preschoolers. *Journal of Speech, Language, and Hearing Research, 59,* 484–500. https://doi.org/10.1044/2015_JSLHR-L-15-0227

Goldstein, H., Olszewski, A., Haring, C., Greenwood, C. R., McCune, L., Carta, J., . . . Kelley, E. S. (2017). Efficacy of a supplemental phonemic awareness curriculum to instruct preschoolers with delays in early literacy development. *Journal of Speech, Language, and Hearing Disorders, 60,* 89–103. https://doi.org/10.1044/2016_JSLHR-L-15-0451

Goldstein, H., & Strain, P. S. (1988). Peers as communication intervention agents: Some new strategies and research findings. *Topics in Language Disorders, 9*(1), 44–59.

Goldstein, H., Walker, D., & Fey, M. (2005, November). *Comparing strategies for promoting communication of infants and toddlers.* Seminar presented at the Association for Speech and Hearing Conference, San Diego, CA.

Gómez, R. L. (2002). Variability and detection of invariant structure. *Psychological Science, 13,* 431–436.

Goodrich, J. M., Lonigan, C. J., & Farver, J. M. (2013). Do early literacy skills in children's first language promoted development of skills in their second language? An experimental evaluation of transfer. *Journal of Educational Psychology, 105,* 414–426.

Gorman, B. K. (2012). Relationships between vocabulary size, working memory, and phonological awareness in Spanish-speaking English language learners. *American Journal of Speech-Language Pathology, 21,* 109–123.

Gorman, B. K., Fiestas, C. E., Peña, E. D., & Reynolds Clark, M. (2011). Creative and stylistic devices employed by children during a storybook narrative task: A cross-cultural study. *Language, Speech, and Hearing Services in Schools, 42,* 167–181.

Gough Kenyon, S. M., Palikara, O., & Lucas, R. M. (2018). Explaining reading comprehension in children with developmental language disorder: The importance of elaborative inferencing. *Journal of Speech, Language, and Hearing Disorders, 61,* 2517–2531. https://doi.org/10.1044/2018_JSLHR-L-17-0416

Govindarajan, K., & Paradis, J. (2019). Narrative abilities of bilingual children with and without developmental language disorder (SLI): Differentiation and the role of age and input factors. *Journal of Communication Disorders, 77,* 1–16. https://doi.org/10.1016/j.jcomdis.2018.10.001

Graham, H. (2015). Intellectual disabilities and socioeconomic inequalities in health: An overview of research. *Journal of Applied Research in Intellectual Disabilities, 18*(2), 101–111. https://doi.org/10.1111/j.1468-3148.2005.00239.x

Graham, L., Graham, A., & West, C. (2015). From research to practice: The effect of multi-component vocabulary instruction on increasing vocabulary and comprehension performance in social studies. *International Electronic Journal of Elementary Education, 8,* 615–628.

Graham, S. (1999). Handwriting and spelling instruction for students with learning disabilities: A review. *Learning Disability Quarterly, 22,* 78–98.

Graham, S. (2006). Writing. In E. Anderman, P. H. Winne, P. A. Alexander, & L. Corno (Eds.), *Handbook of educational psychology* (pp. 457–478). Routledge. http://scholar.google.com/scholar_lookup?hl=en&publication_year=2006&pages=457-478&author=S.+Graham&title=Handbook+of+educational+psychology

Graham, S., & Harris, K. R. (1999). Assessment and intervention in overcoming writing difficulties: An illustration from the self-regulation strategy development model. *Language, Speech, and Hearing Services in Schools, 30,* 255–264.

Graham, S., & Hebert, M. (2010). *Writing to read: Evidence for how writing can improve* (Carnegie Corporation Time to Act Report). Alliance for Excellent Education.

Graham, S., & Perin, D. (2007). A meta-analysis of writing instruction for adolescent students. *Journal of Educational Psychology, 99,* 445–476. https://doi.org/10.1037/0022-0663.99.3.445

Graham, S., & Sandmel, K. (2011). The process writing approach: A meta-analysis. *Journal of Educational Research, 104*(6), 396–407. http://scholar.google.com/scholar_lookup?hl=en&volume=104&publication_year=2011&pages=396-407&journal=Journal+of+Educational+Research&issue=6&author=S.+Graham&author=K.+Sandmel&title=The+process+writing+approach%3A+A+meta-analysis

Granlund, M., Bjorck-Åkesson, E., Wilder, J., & Ylven, R. (2008). AAC interventions for children in a family environment: Implementing evidence in practice. *Augmentative and Alternative Communication, 24*, 207–219.

Gray, S. (2003). Word learning by preschoolers with specific language impairment: What predicts success? *Journal of Speech, Language, and Hearing Research, 46*, 56–67.

Gray, S. (2005). Word learning by preschoolers with specific language impairment: Effect of phonological or semantic cues. *Journal of Speech, Language, and Hearing Research, 48*, 1452–1467.

Gray, S., & Brinkley, S. (2011). Fast mapping and word learning by preschoolers with specific language impairment in a supported learning context: Effect of encoding cues, phonotactic probability, and object familiarity. *Journal of Speech, Language, and Hearing Research, 54*, 870–884.

Gray, S., Fox, A. B., Green, S., Alt, M., Hogan, T. P., Petscher, Y., & Cowan, N. (2019). Working memory profiles of children with dyslexia, developmental language disorder, or both. *Journal of Speech, Language, and Hearing Research, 62*, 1839–1858. https://doi.org/10.1044/2019_JSLHR-L-18-0148 http://scholar.google.com/scholar_lookup?hl=en&volume=54&publication_year=2013&pages=1186-1197&journal=Journal+of+Child+Psychology+and+Psychiatry&author=J.+Gibson&author=C.+Adams&author=E.+Lockton&author=J.+Green&title=Social+communication+disorder+outside+autism%3F+A+diagnostic+classification+approach+to+delineating+pragmatic+language+impairment%2C+high+functioning+autism+and+specific+language+impairment

Greaves-Lord, K., Eussen, M. L., Verhulst, F. C., Minderaa, R. B., Mandy, W., Hudziak, J. J., . . . Hartman, C. A. (2013). Empirically based phenotypic profiles of children with pervasive developmental disorders: Interpretation in the light of the DSM-5. *Journal of Autism and Developmental Disorders, 43*, 1784–1797.

Grech, H., & McLeod, S. (2012). Multilingual speech and language development and disorders. In D. E. Battle (Ed.), *Communication disorders in multicultural and international populations* (4th ed., pp. 120–147). Mosby.

Green, B. C., Johnson, K. A., & Bretherton, L. (2014). Pragmatic language difficulties in children with hyperactivity and attention problems: An integrated review. *International Journal of Language & Communication Disorders, 49*, 15–29. https://doi.org/10.1111/1460-6984.12056

Green, J., Charman, T., McConachie, H., Aldred, C., Slonims, V., Howlin, P., . . . the PACT Consortium. (2010). Parent-mediated communication-focused treatment in children with autism (PACT): A randomised controlled trial.

Lancet, 375(9732), 2152–2160. https://doi.org/10.1016/S0140-6736(10)60587-9

Green, L. (2004, November). *Morphology and literacy: Implications for students with reading disabilities*. Paper presented at the American Speech-Language-Hearing Annual Convention, Philadelphia, PA.

Green, L., Chance, P., & Stockholm, M. (2019). Implementation and perceptions of classroom-based service delivery: A survey of public school clinicians. *Language Speech and Hearing Services in Schools, 50*, 1–17. https://doi.org/10.1044/2019_LSHSS-18-0101

Greenhalgh, K. S., & Strong, C. J. (2001). Literate language features in spoken narratives of children with typical language and children with language impairments. *Language, Speech, and Hearing Services in Schools, 32*, 114–126.

Greenwood, C. R., Carta, J. J., Kelley, E. S., Guerrero, G., Kong, N. Y., Atwater, J., & Goldstein, H. (2016). Systematic replication of the effects of a supplementary, technology-assisted, storybook intervention for preschool children with weak vocabulary and comprehension skills. *Elementary School Journal, 116*, 574–599.

Griffin, T. M., Hemphill, L., Camp, L., & Wolf, D. P. (2004). Oral discourse in the preschool years and later literacy skills. *First Language, 24*, 123–147.

Grigorenko, E. L. (2005). A conservative meta-analysis of linkage and linkage-association studies of developmental dyslexia. *Scientific Studies of Reading, 9*, 285–316.

Grimm, A., & Schulz, P. (2014). Specific language impairment and early second language acquisition: The risk of over- and underdiagnosis. *Child Indicators Research, 7*(4), 821–841. https://doi.org/10.1007/s12187-013-9230-6

Griner, D., & Smith, T. B. (2006). Culturally adapted mental health intervention: A meta-analytic review. *Psychotherapy, 43*(4), 531–548. https://doi.org/10.1037/0033-3204.43.4.531

Grinstead, J., Baron, A., Vega-Mendoza, M., De La Mora, J., Canti-Sanchez, M., & Flores, B. (2013). Tense marking and spontaneous speech measures in Spanish specific language impairment: A discriminant function analysis. *Journal of Speech, Language, and Hearing Research, 56*, 352–363.

Grisham-Brown, J. L., Hemmeter, M. L., & Pretti-Frontczak, K. L. (2005). *Blended practices for teaching young children in inclusive settings*. Brookes.

Griswold, K. E., Barnhill, G. P., Smith-Myles, B., Hagiwara, T., & Simpson, R. L. (2002). Asperger syndrome and academic achievement. *Focus on Autism and Other Developmental Disabilities, 77*(2), 94–102.

Gross, M., Buac, M., & Kaushanskay, M. (2014). Conceptual scoring of receptive and expressive vocabulary measures in simultaneous and sequential bilingual children. *American Journal of Speech-Language Pathology, 23*, 574–586. https://doi.org/10.1044/2014_AJSLP-13-0026

Grossman, R. B., Bemis, R. H., Plesa Skwerer, D., & Tager Flusberg, H. (2010). Lexical and affective prosody in children with high-functioning autism. *Journal of Speech, Language, and Hearing Research, 53*, 778–793.

Gruenewald, L., & Pollack, S. (1984). *Language interaction in teaching and learning*. University Park Press.

Grunow, H., Spaulding, T., Gómez, R., & Plante, E. (2006). The effects of variation on learning word order rules by adults with and without language-based learning disabilities. *Journal of Communication Disorders, 39*, 158–170.

Grysman, A., & Hudson, J. A. (2010). Abstracting and extracting: Causal coherence and the development of the life story. *Memory, 18*, 565–580.

Guiberson, M. (2016). Telehealth measures screening for developmental language disorders in Spanish-speaking toddlers. *Telemedicine and e-Health, 22*, 739–745. https://doi.org/10.1089/tmj.2015.0247

Guiberson, M. M., & Ferris, K. P. (2019). Identifying culturally consistent early interventions for Latino caregivers. *Communication Disorders Quarterly, 40*(4), 239–249. https://doi.org/10.1177/1525740118793858

Guiberson, M. M., & Rodriguez, B. L. (2013). Classification accuracy of nonword repetition when used with preschool-age Spanish-speaking children. *Language, Speech, and Hearing Services in Schools, 44*, 121–132.

Guiberson, M. M., & Rodriguez, B. L. (2020). Working memory and linguistic performance of dual language learners with and without developmental language disorders. *American Journal of Speech-Language Pathology, 29*, 1301–1306. https://doi.org/10.1044/2019_AJSLP-19-00109

Guo, L. Y., & Eisenberg, S. (2015). Sample length affects the reliability of language sample measures in 3-year-olds: Evidence from parent-elicited conversational samples. *Language, Speech, and Hearing Services in Schools, 46*, 141–153. https://doi.org/10.1044/2015_LSHSS-14-0052

Guo, L. Y., & Schneider, P. (2016). Differentiating school-aged children with and without language impairment using tense and grammaticality measures from a narrative task. *Journal of Speech, Language, and Hearing Research, 59*, 317–329.

Guo, L. Y., Tomblin, J. B., & Samelson, V. (2008). Speech disruptions in the narratives of English-speaking children with specific language impairment. *Journal of Speech, Language, and Hearing Research, 51*, 722–738.

Guo, Y.-U., Schneider, P., & Harrison, W. (2021). Clausal density between ages 4 and 9 years for the Edmonton Narrative Norms Instrument: Reference data and psychometric properties. *Language, Speech, and Hearing Services in Schools, 52*, 354–368. https://doi.org/10.1044/2020_LSHSS-20-00043

Gutierrez-Clellan, V., & Peña, E. D. (2001). Dynamic assessment of diverse children: A tutorial. *Language, Speech, and Hearing Services in Schools, 32*, 212–224.

Gutiérrez-Clellen, V., & Simon-Cereijido, G. (2007). The discriminant accuracy of a grammatical measure with Latino English-speaking children. *Journal of Speech, Language, and Hearing Research, 50*, 968–981. https://doi.org/10.1044/1092-4388(2007/068)

Gutierrez-Clellen, V., Simon-Cerejido, G., & Restrepo, M. (2014). *Improving the vocabulary and oral language skills of bilingual Latino preschoolers: An intervention for speech-language pathologists*. Plural Publishing.

Gutiérrez-Clellen, V., Simon-Cereijido, G., & Sweet, M. (2012). Predictors of second language acquisition in Latino children with specific language impairment. *American Journal of Speech-Language Pathology, 21*, 64–77. https://doi.org/10.1044/1058-0360(2011/10-0090)

Gutierrez-Clellen, V., Simon-Cereijido, G., & Wagner, C. (2008). Bilingual children with language impairment: A comparison with monolingual and second language learners. *Applied Linguistics, 29*, 3–20.

Haarbauer-Krupa, J., Heggs Lee, A., Bitsko, R. H., Zhang, X., & Kresnow-Sedacca, M. (2018). Prevalence of parent-reported traumatic brain injury in children and associated health conditions. *JAMA Pediatrics, 172*, 1078–1086. https://doi.org/10.1001/jamapediatrics.2018.2740

Habermas, T., & de Silveira, C. (2008). The development of global coherence in life narratives across adolescence: Temporal, causal, and thematic aspects. *Developmental Psychology, 44*, 707–721.

Hadley, P. A. (1998). Language sampling protocols for eliciting text-level discourse. *Language, Speech, and Hearing Services in Schools, 29*, 132–147. https://doi.org/10.1044/0161-1461.2903.132

Hadley, P. A. (2014). Approaching early grammatical intervention from a sentence-focused framework. *Language, Speech, and Hearing Services in Schools, 45*, 110–116. https://doi.org/10.1044/2014_LSHSS-14-0017

Hadley, P. A., & Holt, J. (2006). Individual differences in the onset of tense marking: A growth curve analysis. *Journal of Speech, Hearing, and Language Research, 49*, 984–1000.

Hadley, P. A., McKenna, M. M., & Rispoli, M. (2018). Sentence diversity in early language development: Recommendations for target selection and progress monitoring. *American Journal of Speech-Language Pathology, 27*, 553–565. https://doi.org/10.1044/2017_AJSLP-17-0098

Hadley, P. A., Rispoli, M., Fitzgerald, C., & Bahnsen, A. (2011). Predictors of morphosyntactic growth in typically developing toddlers: Contribution of parent input and child sex. *Journal of Speech, Language, and Hearing Research, 54*, 549–566.

Hadley, P. A., Rispoli, M., & Holt, J. K. (2017). Input subject diversity accelerates the growth of tense and agreement: Indirect benefits from a parent-implemented intervention. *Journal of Speech, Language, and Hearing Disorders, 60*, 2619–2635. https://doi.org/10.1044/2017_JSLHR-L-17-0008

Hadley, P. A., Rispoli, M., & Hsu, N. (2016). Toddlers' verb lexicon diversity and grammatical outcomes. *Language, Speech, and Hearing Services in Schools, 47*, 44–58. https://doi.org/10.1044/2015_LSHSS-15-0018

Hadley, P. A., & Short, H. (2005). The onset of tense marking in children at risk for specific language impairment. *Journal of Speech, Language, and Hearing Research, 48*, 1344–1362.

Hadley, P. A., & Walsh, K. (2014). Toy talk: Simple strategies to create richer grammatical input. *Language, Speech, and Hearing Services in Schools, 45*, 159–172.

Haebig, E., Leonard, L. B., Deevy, P., Schumaker, J., Karpicke, J. D., & Weber, C. (2021). The neural underpinnings of processing newly taught semantic information: The role of retrieval practice. *Journal of Speech, Language, and Hearing Research, 64*, 3195–3211. https://doi.org/10.1044/2021_JSLHR-20-00485

Haebig, E., Saffran, J. R., & Ellis Weismer, S. (2017). Statistical word learning in children with autism spectrum disorder and specific language impairment. *Journal of Child Psychology and Psychiatry, 58*, 1251–1263. https://doi.org/10.1111/jcpp.12734

Hahn, L. J., Brady, N. C., Fleming, K. K., & Warren, S. F. (2016). Joint engagement and early language in young children with fragile X syndrome. *Journal of Speech, Language, and Hearing Research, 59*, 1087–1098. https://doi.org/10.1044/2016_JSLHR-L-15-0005

Hall, J., McGregor, K. K., & Oleson, J. (2017). Weaknesses in lexical–semantic knowledge among college students with specific learning disabilities: Evidence from a semantic fluency task. *Journal of Speech, Language, and Hearing Disorders, 60*, 640–653. https://doi.org/10.1044/2016_JSLHR-L-15-0440

Hall-Mills, S., & Apel, K. (2013). Narrative and expository writing of adolescents with language-learning disabilities: A pilot study. *Communication Disorders Quarterly, 34*, 135–143. https://doi.org/10.1177/1525740112465001

Halpern, R. (2000). Early childhood intervention for low-income children and families. In J. P. Shonkoff & S. J. Meisels (Eds.), *Handbook of early childhood intervention* (2nd ed., pp. 361–386). Cambridge University Press.

Halpin, E., Prishker, N., & Melzi, G. (2021). The bilingual language diversity of Latino preschoolers: A latent profile analysis. *Language, Speech, and Hearing Services in Schools, 52*, 877–888. https://doi.org/10.1044/2021_LSHSS-21-00015

Hambly, C., & Fombonne, E. (2012). The impact of bilingual environments on language development in children with autism spectrum disorders. *Journal of Autism and Developmental Disorders, 42*, 1342–1352. https://doi.org/10.1007/s10803-011-1365-z

Hambly, C., & Riddle, L. (2002, April). *Phonological awareness training for school-age children*. Paper presented at the annual convention of the New York State Speech-Language-Hearing Association, Rochester, NY.

Hamm, B., & Mirenda, P. (2006). Post-school quality of life for individuals with developmental disabilities who use AAC. *Augmentative and Alternative Communication, 22*, 134–146.

Hammer, C. S. (2012). More than just talk. *American Journal of Speech-Language Pathology, 21*, 1–2.

Hammer, C. S., Komaroff, E., Rodriguez, B. L. Lopez, L. M., Scarpino, S. E., & Goldstein, B. (2012). Predicting Spanish-English bilingual children's language abilities. *Journal of Speech Language and Hearing Research, 55*, 1251–1264. https://doi.org/10.1044/1092-4388(2012/11-0016)

Hammer, C. S., Lawrence, F. R., & Miccio, A. W. (2007). Bilingual children's language abilities and early reading outcomes in Head Start and kindergarten. *Language, Speech, and Hearing Services in Schools, 38*, 237–248.

Hammer, C. S., & Miccio, A. W. (2006). Early language and reading development of bilingual preschoolers from low-income families. *Topics in Language Disorders, 26*, 322–337.

Hammer, C. S., Miccio, A. W., & Wagstaff, D. A. (2003). Home literacy experiences and their relationship to bilingual preschoolers' developing English literacy abilities: An initial investigation. *Language, Speech, and Hearing Services in Schools, 34*, 20–30.

Hammer, C. S., & Rodriguez, B. (2012). Bilingual language acquisition and the child socialization process. In B. A. Goldstein (Ed.), *Bilingual language development and disorders in Spanish–English speakers* (2nd ed., pp. 31–46). Brookes.

Hammer, C. S., Rodriguez, B. L., Lawrence, F. R., & Miccio, A. W. (2007). Puerto Rican mothers' beliefs on home literacy practices. *Language, Speech, and Hearing Services in Schools, 38*, 216–224.

Hammill, D. D., & Larson, S. C. (2009). *Test of Written Language, Fourth Edition (TOWL-4)*. Pro-Ed.

Hancock, T. B., & Kaiser, A. P. (2006). Enhanced milieu teaching. In R. J. McCauley & M. E. Fey (Eds.), *Treatment of language disorders in children* (pp. 203–236). Brookes.

Hand, L. (2011). Working bilingually with language disordered children: What is the evidence? *Acquiring Knowledge in Speech, Language, and Hearing, 13*, 148–154.

Hanft, B. E., Miller, L. J., & Lane, S. J. (2000). Towards a consensus in terminology in sensory integration theory and practice: Part I. Taxonomy of neurophysiologic processes. *Sensory Integration Special Interest Section Quarterly, 23*, 1–4.

Hanft, B. E., Rush, D. D., & Shelden, M. L. (2004). *Coaching families and colleagues in early childhood*. Brookes.

Hardan, A. Y., Gengoux, G. W., Berquist, K. L., Libove, R. A., Ardel, C. M., Phillips, J., . . . Minjarez, M. B. (2015). A randomized controlled trial of pivotal response treatment group for parents of children with autism. *Journal of Child Psychology and Psychiatry, 56*(8), 884–892. https://doi.org/10.1111/jcpp.12354

Hardin, K. Y., & Kelly, J. P. (2019). The role of speech-language pathology in an interdisciplinary care model for persistent symptomatology of mild traumatic brain injury. *Seminars in Speech and Language, 40*(1), 65–78. https://doi.org/10.1055/s-0038-1676452

Harlaar, N., Segebart DeThorne, L., Mahurin Smith, J., Aparicio Betancourt, M., & Petrill, S. A. (2016). Longitudinal effects on early adolescent language: A twin study. *Journal of Speech, Language, and Hearing Research, 59*, 1059–1073. https://doi.org/10.1044/2016_JSLHR-L-15-0257

Harris, A. W., & Waugh, R. M. (2002). Dyadic synchrony: Its structure and function in children's development. *Developmental Review, 22*, 555–592.

Harris, K. R., Graham, S., Mason, L. H., & Friedlander, B. (2008). *Powerful writing strategies for all students*. Brookes. http://scholar.google.com/scholar_lookup?hl=en&publication_year=2008&author=K.+R.+Harris&author=S.+Graham&author=L.+H.+Mason&author=B.+Friedlander&title=Powerful+writing+strategies+for+all+students

Harrison, L. J., & McLeod, S. (2010). Risk and protective factors associated with speech and language impairment in a nationally representative sample of 4- to 5-year-old children. *Journal of Speech, Language, and Hearing Research*, *53*, 508–529. https://doi.org/10.1044/1092-4388(2009/08-0086)

Harris Wright, H., & Newhoff, M. (2001). Narration abilities of children with language-learning disabilities in response to oral and written stimuli. *American Journal of Speech-Language Pathology*, *10*, 308–319.

Hart, K. I., Fujiki, M., Brinton, B., & Hart, C. H. (2004). The relationship between social behavior and severity of language impairment. *Journal of Speech, Language, and Hearing Research*, *47*, 647–662.

Hartsuiker, R. J., Bernolet, S., Schoonbaert, S., Speybroeck, S., & Vanderelst, D. (2008). Syntactic priming persists while the lexical boost decays: Evidence from written and spoken dialogue. *Journal of Memory and Language*, *58*, 214–238.

Hashimoto, N., McGregor, K. K., & Graham, A. (2007). Conceptual organization at 6 and 8 years of age: Evidence from the semantic priming of object decisions. *Journal of Speech, Language, and Hearing Research*, *50*, 161–176.

Hasson, N., Camilleri, B., Jones, C., Smith, J., & Dodd, B. (2013). Discriminating disorder from difference using dynamic assessment with bilingual children. *Child Language Teaching and Therapy*, *29*, 57–75.

Hayiou-Thomas, M. E., Carroll, J. M., Leavett, R., Hulme, C., & Snowling, M. J. (2017). When does speech sound disorder matter for literacy? The role of disordered speech errors, co-occurring language impairment and family risk of dyslexia. *Journal of Child Psychology and Psychiatry*, *58*, 197–205. https://doi.org/10.1111/jcpp.12648 http://scholar.google.com/scholar_lookup?hl=en&volume=58&publication_year=2017&pages=197-205&journal=The+Journal+of+Child+Psychology+and+Psychiatry&author=M.+E.+Hayiou-Thomas&author=J.+M.+Carroll&author=R.+Leavett&author=C.+Hulme&author=M.+J.+Snowling&title=When+does+speech+sound+disorder+matter+for+literacy%3F+The+role+of+disordered+speech+errors%2C+co-occurring+language+impairment+and+family+risk+of+dyslexia

Hayiou-Thomas, M. E., Harlaar, N., Dale, P. S., & Plomin, R. (2010). Preschool speech, language skills, and reading at 7, 9, and 10 years: Etiology of the relationship. *Journal of Speech, Language, and Hearing Research*, *53*, 311–332.

Haynes, W. O., & Pindzola, R. H. (2012). *Diagnosis and evaluation in speech pathology* (8th ed.). Pearson.

Hayward, D., Gillam, R. B., & Lien, P. (2007). Retelling a script-based story: Do children with and without language impairments focus on script or story element? *Journal of Speech-Language Pathology*, *16*, 235–245.

Hedberg, N. L., & Stoel-Gammon, C. (1986). Narrative analysis: Clinical procedures. *Topics in Language Disorders*, *7*, 58–69.

Heilmann, J. J., Miller, J., Iglesias, A., Fabiano-Smith, L., Nockerts, A., & Digney-Andriacchi, K. (2008). Narrative transcription accuracy and reliability in two languages. *Topics in Language Disorders*, *28*, 178–188.

Heilmann, J. J., Nockerts, A., & Miller, J. F. (2010). Language sampling: Does the length of the transcript matter? *Language, Speech, and Hearing Services in Schools*, *41*, 393–404.

Helder, A., van den Broek, P., Van Leijenhorst, L., & Beker, K. (2013). Sources of comprehension problems during reading. In B. Miller, L. E. Cutting, & P. McCardle (Eds.), *Unraveling reading comprehension: Behavioral, neurobiological, and genetic components* (pp. 43–53). Brookes.

Helland, W. A., Biringer, E., Helland, T., & Heimann, M. (2012). Exploring language profiles for children with ADHD and children with Asperger syndrome. *Journal of Attention Disorders*, *16*, 34–43. https://doi.org/10.1177/1087054710378233

Helland, W. A., & Heimann, M. (2007). Assessment of pragmatic language impairment in children referred to psychiatric services: A pilot study of the Children's Communication Checklist in a Norwegian sample. *Logopedics Phoniatrics Vocology*, *32*, 22–30.

Hemphill, L., Uccelli, P., Winner, K., Chang, C., & Bellinger, D. (2002). Narrative discourse in young children with histories of early corrective heart surgery. *Journal of Speech, Language, and Hearing Research*, *45*, 318–331.

Henry, L. A., & Botting, N. (2017). Working memory and developmental language impairments. *Child Language Teaching and Therapy*, *33*, 19–32. https://doi.org/10.1177/0265659016655378

Hernandez, D. J. (2004). *Demographic change and the life circumstances of immigrant families*. State University of New York Press.

Hesketh, A. (2006). The use of relative clauses by children with language impairment. *Clinical Linguistics & Phonetics*, *20*(7–8), 539–546. https://doi.org/10.1080/02699200500266398

Hickmann, M., & Schneider, P. (2000). Cohesion and coherence anomalies and their effects on children's referent introduction in narrative retell. In M. Perkins & S. Howard (Eds.), *New directions in language development and disorders* (pp. 251–260). Plenum.

Hicks, S. C., Rivera, C. J., & Wood, C. L. (2015). Using direct instruction: Teaching preposition use to students with intellectual disability. *Language, Speech, and Hearing Services in Schools*, *46*, 194–206. https://doi.org/10.1044/2015_LSHSS-14-0088

Hilvert, E., Davidson, D., & Gamez, P. (2016). Examination of script and non-script based narrative retellings in children with autism spectrum disorders. *Research in Autism Spectrum Disorders*, *29–30*, 79–92. https://doi.org/10.1016/j.rasd.2016.06.002

Hixson, P. K. (1983). *DSS computer program* [Computer program]. Computer Language Analysis.

Hoff, E., Core, C., Place, S., Rumiche, R., Señor, M., & Parra, M. (2012). Dual language exposure and early bilingual development. *Journal of Child Language*, *39*(1), 1–27. https://doi.org/10.1017/S0305000910000759

Hoffman, L. M. (2013). An exploratory study of real-time morphosyntactic judgments with preschool children. *International Journal of Speech-Language Pathology*, *15*(2), 198–208

Hoffman, L. M., & Gillam, R. B. (2004). Verbal and spatial information processing constraints in children with specific language impairment. *Journal of Speech-Language-Hearing Research, 47,* 114–125.

Hofstede, G. (2001). *Culture's consequences: Comparing values, behaviors, institutions and organizations across nations* (2nd ed.). SAGE.

Hollo, A., Wehby, J. H., & Oliver, R. M. (2014). Unidentified language deficits in children with emotional and behavioral disorders: A meta-analysis. *Exceptional Children, 80,* 169–186. https://doi.org/10.1177/001440291408000203

Honna, N. (2005). English as a multilingual language in Asia. *Intercultural Communication Studies, 14,* 73–89.

Hood, J., & Rankin, P. M. (2005). How do specific memory disorders present in the school classroom? *Pediatric Rehabilitation, 8,* 272–282.

Hooper, S. J., Roberts, J. E., Zeisel, S. A., & Poe, M. (2003). Core language predictors of behavioral functioning in early elementary school children: Concurrent and longitudinal findings. *Behavioral Disorders, 29*(1), 10–21.

Horohov, J. E., & Oetting, J. B. (2004). Effects of input manipulations on the word learning abilities of children with and without specific language impairment. *Applied Psycholinguistics, 25,* 43–65.

Horton, R., & Apel, K. (2014). Examining the use of spoken dialect indices with African American children in the southern United States. *American Journal of Speech-Language Pathology, 23,* 448–460. https://doi.org/10.1044/2014_AJSLP-13-0028

Horton-Ikard, R., & Weismer, S. E. (2007). A preliminary examination of vocabulary and word learning in African American toddlers from middle and low socioeconomic status homes. *American Journal of Speech-Language Pathology, 16*(4), 381–392.

Horvath, S., & Arunachalam, S. (2021). Repetition versus variability in verb learning: Sometimes less is more. *Journal of Speech, Language, and Hearing Research, 64,* 4235–4249. https://doi.org/10.1044/2021_JSLHR-21-00091

Horwitz, S. M., Irwin, J. R., Briggs-Gowan, M. J., Heenan, J. M. B., Mendoza, J., & Carter, A. S. (2003). Language delay in a community cohort of young children. *Journal of the American Academy of Child & Adolescent Psychiatry, 42,* 932–940.

Howes, C., Burchinal, M., Pianta, R. C., Bryant, D., Early, D., Clifford, R., & Barbarin, O. (2008). Ready to learn? Children's pre-academic achievement in pre-kindergarten programs. *Early Childhood Research Quarterly, 23,* 27–50. http://scholar.google.com/scholar_lookup?hl=en&publi cation_year=2008&pages=27-50&title=Ready+to+learn %3F+Children%27s+pre-academic+achievement+in+pre-kindergarten+programs

Howlin, P., Mawhood, L., & Rutter, M. (2000). Autism and developmental receptive language disorder—A follow-up comparison in early adult life. II: Social, behavioural, and psychiatric outcomes. *Journal of Child Psychology and Psychiatry, 41,* 561–578.

Howlin, P., Moss, P., Savage, S., & Rutter, M. (2013). Social outcomes in mid- to later adulthood among individuals diagnosed with autism and average nonverbal IQ as children. *Journal of the American Academy of Child & Adolescent Psychiatry, 52,* 572–581.e1. https://doi.org/10.1016/j.jaac.2013.02.017

Hsu, H. J., & Bishop, D. V. M. (2014). Sequence-specific procedural learning deficits in children with specific language impairment. *Developmental Science, 17,* 352–365. https://doi.org/10.1111/desc.12125

Huang, T., & Finestack, L. (2020). Comparing morphosyntactic profiles of children with developmental language disorder or language disorder associated with autism spectrum disorder. *American Journal of Speech-Language Pathology, 29,* 714–731. https://doi.org/10.1044/2019_AJSLP-19-00207

Hubbs-Tait, L., Culp, A. M., Huey, E., Culp, R., Starost, H., & Hare, C. (2002). Relation of Head Start attendance to children's cognitive and social outcomes: Moderation by family risk. *Early Childhood Research Quarterly, 17,* 539–558.

Hudson, R., Lane, H., & Mercer, C. (2005). Writing prompts: The role of various priming conditions on the compositional fluency of developing writers. *Reading and Writing, 18,* 473–495.

Hugdahl, K., Gundersen, H., Brekke, C., Thomsen, T., Rimol, L. M., Ersland, L., & Niemi, J. (2004). fMRI brain activation in a Finnish family with specific language impairment compared with a normal control group. *Journal of Speech, Language, and Hearing Research, 47,* 162–172.

Hughes, K. R., Hogan, A. L., Roberts, J. E., & Klusek, J. (2019). Gesture frequency and function in infants with fragile X syndrome and infant siblings of children with autism spectrum disorder. *Journal of Speech, Language, and Hearing Research, 62,* 2386–2399. https://doi.org/10.1044/2019_JSLHR-L-17-0491

Hulme, C., & Snowling, M. J. (2014). The interface between spoken and written language: Developmental disorders. *Philosophical Transactions of the Royal Society of London B: Biological Sciences, 369,* 20120395. https://doi.org/10.1098/rstb.2012.0395 http://scholar.google.com/scholar_lookup?hl=en&volume=369&publication_year=2014 &pages=20120395&journal=Philosophical+Transactions +of+the+Royal+Society+of+London+B%3A+Biological+ Sciences&author=C.+Hulme&author=M.+J.+Snowling &title=The+interface+between+spoken+and+written+ language%3A+Developmental+disorders

Humphries, T., Cardy, J. O., Worling, D. E., & Peets, K. (2004). Narrative comprehension and retelling abilities of children with nonverbal learning disabilities. *Brain and Cognition, 56,* 77–88.

Hunt, K. W. (1970). Syntactic maturity in schoolchildren and adults. *Monographs of the Society for Research in Child Development, 35*(1), 1–67.

Hustad, K. C., Morehouse, T. B., & Gutmann, M. (2002). AAC strategies for enhancing the usefulness of natural speech in children with severe intelligibility challenges. In J. Reichle, D. Beukelman, & J. Light (Eds.), *Implementing an augmentative communication system: Exemplary strategies for beginning communicators* (pp. 433–452). Brookes.

Hutchins, T. L., Prelock, P. A., Morris, H., Benner, J., LaVigne, T., & Hoza, B. (2016). Explicit vs applied theory of mind competence: A comparison of typically developing males, males with ASD, and males with ADHD. *Research in Autism Spectrum Disorder, 21,* 94–108.

Hwa-Froelich, D. A., & Matsuo, H. (2005). Vietnamese children and language-based processing tasks. *Language, Speech, and Hearing Services in Schools, 36,* 230–243.

Hwa-Froelich, D. A., & Westby, C. E. (2003). Frameworks of education: Perspectives of Southeast Asian parents and Head Start staff. *Language, Speech, and Hearing Services in Schools, 34,* 299–319.

Hyter, Y. D., Atchinson, B., & Blashill, M. (2006). *A model of supporting children at risk: The School Intervention Program (SIP).* Unpublished manuscript.

Iams, J. (2003). Prediction and early detection of preterm labor. *Obstetrics & Gynecology, 101,* 402–412.

Ijalba, E. (2016). Hispanic immigrant mothers of young children with autism spectrum disorders: How do they understand and cope with autism? *American Journal of Speech–Language Pathology, 25,* 200–213. https://doi.org/10.1044/2015_AJSLP-13-0017

Imgrund, C. M., Loeb, D. F., & Barlow, S. M. (2019). Expressive language in preschoolers born preterm: Results of language sample analysis and standardized assessment. *Journal of Speech, Language, and Hearing Research, 62,* 884–895. https://doi.org/10.1044/2018_JSLHR-L-18-0224

Individuals with Disabilities Education Act (IDEA), P.L. 101–476 (2004).

Individuals with Disabilities Education Improvement Act of 2004, P. L. 108–446, 118 Stat. 2647 (2004).

Individuals with Disabilities Education Act (IDEA, 2006, Part B.) (2019, November 7). Subchapter II. https://sites.ed.gov/idea/statute-chapter-33#

Ingersoll, B., & Schreibman, L. (2006). Teaching reciprocal imitation skills to young children with autism using a naturalistic behavioral approach: Effects on language, pretend play, and joint attention. *Journal of Autism and Developmental Disorders, 36*(4), 487–505.

Inglebret, E., Jones, C., & Pavel, D. M. (2008). Integrating American Indian/Alaska Native culture into shared storybook intervention. *Language, Speech, and Hearing Services in Schools, 39,* 521–527.

Institute of Medicine. (2006). *Preterm birth: Causes, consequences, and prevention.*

International Dyslexia Association. (2002, November 12). *Definition of dyslexia.* https://dyslexiaida.org/definition-of-dyslexia/

International Expert Panel on Multilingual Children's Speech. (2012). *Multilingual children with speech sound disorders: Position paper.* Research Institute for Professional Practice, Learning and Education, Charles Sturt University, Bathurst, Australia. http://www.csu.edu.au/research/multilingual-speech/position-paper

Irwin, J., Carter, A., & Briggs-Gowan, M. (2002). The social-emotional development of late-talking toddlers.

Journal of the American Academy of Child & Adolescent Psychiatry, 41, 1324–1332.

Isaacs, G. J. (1996). Persistence of non-standard dialect in school-age children. *Journal of Speech and Hearing Research, 39,* 434–441.

Isaki, E., Spauiding, T. J., & Plante, E. (2008). Contributions of language and memory demands to verbal memory performance in language-learning disabilities. *Journal of Communication Disorders, 41,* 512–530.

Iverson, J. M., & Braddock, B. A. (2011). Gesture and motor skill in relation to language in children with language impairment. *Journal of Speech, Language, and Hearing Research, 54,* 72–86.

Ivy, L. J., & Masterson, J. J. (2011). A comparison of oral and written English styles in African American students at different stages of writing development. *Language, Speech, and Hearing Services in Schools, 42,* 31–40.

Jackson, S., Pretti-Frontczak, K., Harjusola-Webb, S., Grisham-Brown, J., & Romani, J. M. (2009). Response to intervention: Implications for early childhood professionals. *Language, Speech, and Hearing Services in Schools, 40,* 424–434.

Jackson-Maldonado, D., Thal, D., Marchman, V., Newton, T., Fenson, L., & Conboy, B. (2003). *MacArthur Inventarios del Desarrollo de Habilidades Comunicativas: User's guide and technical manual.* Brookes.

Jacob, R., & Parkinson, J. (2015). The potential for school-based interventions that target executive function to improve academic achievement. *Review of Educational Research, 85,* 512–552. https://doi.org/10.3102/0034654314561338 http://scholar.google.com/scholar_lookup?hl=en&volume=85&publication_year=2015&pages=512-552&journal=Review+of+Educational+Research&author=R.+Jacob&author=J.+Parkinson&title=The+potential+for+school-based+interventions+that+target+executive+function+to+improve+academic+achievement

Jacobson, P. F., & Schwartz, R. G. (2005). English past tense use in bilingual children with language impairment. *American Journal of Speech-Language Pathology, 14,* 313–323.

Jacobson, P. F., & Walden, P. R. (2013). Lexical diversity and omission errors as predictors of language ability in the narratives of sequential bilingual Spanish–English bilinguals: A crosslanguage comparison. *American Journal of Speech-Language Pathology, 22,* 554–565.

Jacobson, S., & Jacobson, J. (2000). Teratogenic insult and neurobehavioral function in infancy and childhood. In C. Nelson (Ed.), *Minnesota symposia on child psychology* (pp. 61–112). Erlbaum.

Jacoby, G. P., Lee, L., & Kummer, A. W. (2002). The number of individual treatment units necessary to facilitate functional communication improvements in the speech and language of young children. *American Journal of Speech-Language Pathology, 11,* 370–380.

Jahromi, L. B., Bryce, C. I., & Swanson, J. (2013). The importance of self-regulation for the school and peer engagement of children with high-functioning autism. *Research in Autism Spectrum Disorder, 7*, 235–246.

Janes, H., & Kermani, H. (2001). Caregivers' story reading to young children in family literacy programs: Pleasure or punishment? *Journal of Adolescent & Adult Literacy, 44*, 458–466.

Jankovic, J. (2001). Tourette's syndrome. *New England Journal of Medicine, 345*, 1184–1192.

Jasso, J., McMillen, S., Anaya, J. B., Bedore, L. M., & Peña, E. D. (2020). The utility of an English semantics measure for identifying developmental language disorder in Spanish–English bilinguals. *American Journal of Speech-Language Pathology, 29*, 776–788. https://doi.org/10.1044/2020_AJSLP-19-00202

Jerome, A. C., Fujiki, M., Brinton, B., & James, S. L. (2002). Self-esteem in children with specific language impairment. *Journal of Speech, Language, and Hearing Research, 45*, 700–714.

Jin, F., Schjølberg, S., Vaage Wang, M., Eadie, P. Bang Nes, R., Røysamb, E., & Tambs, K. (2020). Predicting literacy skills at 8 years from preschool language trajectories: A population-based cohort study. *Journal of Speech, Language, and Hearing Research, 63*, 2752–2762. https://doi.org/10.1044/2020_JSLHR-19-00286

Johnson, C. J., Beitchman, J. H., & Brownlie, E. B. (2010). Twenty-year follow-up of children with and without speech-language impairments: Family, educational, occupational, and quality of life outcomes. *American Journal of Speech-Language Pathology, 19*, 51–65.

Johnson, D. E. (2000). Medical and developmental sequelae of early childhood institutionalization in Eastern European adoptees. In C. A. Nelson (Ed.), *The Minnesota Symposia on Child Psychology: The effects of early adversity on neurobiological development* (Vol. 31, pp. 113–162). Erlbaum.

Johnston, D. (2022). *Co:Writer.* https://learningtools.donjohnston.com/product/cowriter

Johnston, J. R., & Kamhi, A. (1984). The same can be less: Syntactic and semantic aspects of the utterances of language impaired children. *Merrill-Palmer Quarterly, 30*, 65–86.

Johnston, J. R., & Wong, M. Y. A. (2002). Cultural differences in beliefs and practices concerning talk to children. *Journal of Speech, Language, and Hearing Research, 45*, 916–926.

Johnston, S. S., Reichle, J., & Evans, J. (2004). Supporting augmentative and alternative communication use by beginning communicators with severe disabilities. *American Journal of Speech Language Pathology, 13*, 20–30.

John Thurman, A., Kover, S. T., Brown, W. T., Harvey, D. J., & Abbeduto, L. (2017). Noncomprehension signaling in males and females with fragile X syndrome. *Journal of Speech, Language, and Hearing Disorders, 60*, 1606–1621. https://doi.org/10.1044/2016_JSLHR-L-15-0358

Jones, C. R. G., Happé, F., Golden, H., Marsden, A. J. S., Tregay, J., Simonoff, E., . . . Charman, T. (2009). Reading and arithmetic in adolescents with autism spectrum disorders: Peaks and dips in attainment. *Neuropsychology, 23*, 718–728. https://doi.org/10.1037/a0016360

Jongman, S. R., Roelofs, A., Scheper, A. R., & Meyer, A. S. (2017). Picture naming in typically developing and language-impaired children: The role of sustained attention. *International Journal of Language & Communication Disorders, 52*, 323–333. https://doi.org/10.1111/1460-6984.12275

Jonsdottir, S., Bouma, A., Sergeant, J., & Scherder, E. (2005). The impact of specific language impairment on working memory in children with ADHD combined subtype. *Archives of Clinical Neuropsychology, 20*, 443–456. https://doi.org/2005-06391-00410.1016/j.acn.2004.10.004

Juel, C. (1988). Learning to read and write: A longitudinal study of 54 children from first through fourth grades. *Journal of Educational Psychology, 80*, 437–447.

Justice, L. M. (2006). Evidence-based practice, response to intervention, and the prevention of reading difficulties. *Language, Speech, and Hearing Services in Schools, 37*, 284–297. https://doi.org/10.1044/0161-1461(2006/033) http://scholar.google.com/scholar_lookup?hl=en&volume=37&publication_year=2006&pages=284-297&journal=Language%2C+Speech%2C+and+Hearing+Services+in+Schools&author=L.+M.+Justice&title=Evidence-based+practice%2C+response+to+intervention%2C+and+the+prevention+of+reading+difficulties

Justice, L. M. (2013, October 1). From my perspective: A+ speech-language goals. *The ASHA Leader.* http://www.asha.org/Publications/leader/2013/131001/FromMy-Perspective-A-Speech-Language-Goals.htm

Justice, L. M., Bowles, R. P., Kaderavek, J. N., Ukrainetz, T. A., Eisenberg, S. L., & Gillam, R. B. (2006). The Index of Narrative Microstructure: A clinical tool for analyzing school-age children's narrative performances. *American Journal of Speech-Language Pathology, 15*, 177–191.

Justice, L. M., Chow, S., Capellini, C., Flanigan, K., & Colton, S. (2003). Emergent literacy intervention for vulnerable preschoolers: Relative effects of two approaches. *American Journal of Speech-Language Pathology, 12*, 320–332.

Justice, L. M., & Ezell, H. K. (2000). Enhancing children's print and word awareness through home-based parent intervention. *American Journal of Speech-Language Pathology, 9*, 257–269.

Justice, L. M., & Ezell, H. K. (2002). Use of storybook reading to increase print awareness in at-risk children. *American Journal of Speech-Language Pathology, 11*, 17–29.

Justice, L. M., & Ezell, H. K. (2004). Print referencing: An emergent literacy enhancement strategy and its clinical applications. *Language, Speech, and Hearing Services in Schools, 35*, 185–193.

Justice, L. M., Invernizzi, M. A., & Meier, J. D. (2002). Designing and implementing an early literacy screening protocol: Suggestions for the speech-language pathologist. *Language, Speech, and Hearing Services in Schools, 33*, 84–101.

Justice, L. M., Jiang, H., Logan, J. A., & Schmitt, M. B. (2017). Predictors of language gains among school-age children with language impairment in the public schools. *Journal of Speech, Language, and Hearing Disorders, 60*, 1590–1605. https://doi.org/10.1044/2016_JSLHR-L-16-0026

Justice, L. M., Jiang, H., Purtwell, K. M., Schneer, K., Boone, K., Bates, R., & Salsberry, P. (2019). Conditions of poverty, parent–child interactions, and toddlers' early language skills in low-income families. *Maternal and Child Health Journal, 23*, 971–978.

Justice, L. M., & Kaderavek, J. (2004). Embedded-explicit emergent literacy intervention I: Background and description of approach. *Language, Speech, and Hearing Services in Schools, 35*, 201–211.

Justice, L. M., Mashburn, A., Hamre, B., & Pianta, R. C. (2008). Quality of language instruction in preschool classrooms serving at-risk pupils. *Early Childhood Research Quarterly, 23*, 51–68.

Justice, L. M., & McGinty, A. S. (2016). *Read It Again!* (RIA). https://crane.osu.edu/our-work/read-it-again

Justice, L. M., McGinty, A. S., Cabell, S. Q., Kilday, C. R., Knighton, K., & Huffman, G. (2010). Literacy curriculum supplement for preschoolers who are academically at risk: A feasibility study. *Language, Speech, and Hearing Services in Schools, 41*, 161–178.

Justice, L. M., Meier, J., & Walpole, S. (2005). Learning new words from storybooks: An efficacy study with at-risk kindergartners. *Language, Speech, and Hearing Services in Schools, 36*, 17–33.

Justice, L. M., & Schuele, C. M. (2004). Phonological awareness: Description, assessment, and intervention. In J. Bernthal & N. Bankson (Eds.), *Articulation and phonological disorders* (5th ed., pp. 376–405). Allyn & Bacon.

Kaderavek, J. N., Pentimonti, J. M., & Justice, L. M. (2013). Children with communication impairments: Caregivers' and teachers' shared book-reading quality and children's level of engagement. *Child Language Teaching & Therapy, 30*, 289–302.

Kaderavek, J. N., & Sulzby, E. (1998, November). *Low versus high orientation towards literacy in children*. Paper presented at the annual convention of the American Speech-Language-Hearing Association, San Antonio, TX.

Kaiser, A. P., Hancock, T., & Neitfield, J. P. (2000). The effects of parent-implemented enhanced milieu teaching on social communication of children who have autism [Special issue]. *Journal of Early Education and Development, 4*, 423–446.

Kame'enui, E. J., Simmons, D. C., & Coyne, M. D. (2000). Schools as host environments: Towards a schoolwide reading improvement model. *Annals of Dyslexia, 50*, 33–51.

Kamhi, A. G. (2011). What speech-language pathologists need to know about auditory processing disorder. *Language, Speech, and Hearing Services in Schools, 42*, 265–273.

Kamhi, A. G. (2014). Improving clinical practices for children with language and learning disorders. *Language, Speech, and Hearing Services in Schools, 45*, 92–103. https://doi.org/10.1044/2014_LSHSS-13-0063

Kamhi, A. G., & Hinton, L. N. (2000). Explaining individual differences in spelling ability. *Topics in Language Disorders, 20*(3), 37.

Kamhi, A. G., & Johnston, J. (1992). Semantic assessment: Determining propositional complexity. *Best Practices in School Speech-Language Pathology, 2*, 99–107.

Kamil, M. L., Borman, G. D., Dole, J., Kral, C. C., Salinger, T., & Torgesen, J. (2008). *Improving adolescent literacy: Effective classroom and intervention practices: A practice guide* (NCEE 208–4027). National Center for Education Evaluation and Regional Assistance, Institute of Education Sciences, U.S. Department of Education. http://ies.ed.gov/ncee/wwc

Kamps, D., Thiemann-Bourque, K., Heitzman-Powell, L., Schwartz, I., Rosenberg, N., Mason, R., & Cox, S. (2015). A comprehensive peer network intervention to improve social communication of children with autism spectrum disorders: A randomized trial in kindergarten and first grade. *Journal of Autism and Developmental Disorders, 45*, 1809–1824.

Kan, P. F., & Windsor, J. (2010). Word learning in children with primary language impairment: A meta-analysis. *Journal of Speech, Language, and Hearing Research, 53*(3), 739–756. https://doi.org/10.1044/1092-4388(2009/08-0248)

Kapa, L. L., & Erikson, J. A. (2020). The relationship between word learning and executive function in preschoolers with and without developmental language disorder. *Journal of Speech, Language, and Hearing Research, 63*, 2293–2307. https://doi.org/10.1044/2020_JSLHR-19-00342

Kapa, L. L., Plante, E., & Doubleday, K. (2017). Applying an integrative framework of executive function to preschoolers with specific language impairment. *Journal of Speech, Language, and Hearing Disorders, 60*, 2170–2184. https://doi.org/10.1044/2017_JSLHR-L-16-0027

Kapp, S. A., McDonald, T. P., & Diamond, K. L. (2001). The path to adoption for children of color. *Child Abuse & Neglect, 21*, 215–229.

Kasambira Fannin, D., Barbarin, O. A., & Crais, E. R. (2018). Communicative function use of preschoolers and mothers from differing racial and socioeconomic groups. *Language, Speech, and Hearing Services in Schools, 49*, 306–319. https://doi.org/10.1044/2017_LSHSS-17-0004

Kasari, C., Freeman, S., & Paparella, T. (2006). Joint attention and symbolic play in young children with autism: A randomized controlled intervention study. *Journal of Child Psychology and Psychiatry, 47*(6), 611–620. https://doi.org/10.1111/j.1469-7610.2005.01567.x

Kasari, C., Gulsrud, A. C., Wong, C., Kwon, S., & Locke, J. (2010). Randomized controlled caregiver mediated joint engagement intervention for toddlers with autism. *Journal of Autism and Developmental Disorders, 40*(9), 1045–1056. https://doi.org/10.1007/s10803-010-0955-5

Kasari, C., Kaiser, A., Goods, K., Nietfeld, J., Mathy, P., Landa, R., . . . Almirall, D. (2014). Communication interventions for minimally verbal children with autism: A sequential multiple assignment randomized trial. *Journal of the*

American Academy of Child & Adolescent Psychiatry, *53*, 635–646. https://doi.org/10.1016/j.jaac.2014.01.019

Kashinath, S., Woods, J., & Goldstein, H. (2006). Enhancing generalized teaching strategy use in daily routines by parents of children with autism. *Journal of Speech, Language, and Hearing Research*, *49*, 466–485.

Katzir, T., Kim, Y., Wolf, M., O'Brien, B., Kennedy, B., Lovett, M., & Morris, R. (2006). Reading fluency: The whole is more than the parts. *Annals of Dyslexia*, *56*, 51–82.

Kaufman, A. S., & Kaufman, N. L. (2014). *Kaufman Brief Intelligence Test (K-Bit), 2nd edition*. Pearson.

Kay-Raining Bird, E., Cleave, P. L., Trudeau, N., Thordardottir, E., Sutton, A., & Thorpe, A. (2005). The language abilities of bilingual children with Down syndrome. *American Journal of Speech-Language Pathology*, *14*, 187–199. https://doi.org/10.1044/1058-0360(2005/019)

Kay-Raining Bird, E., Cleave, P. L., White, D., Pike, H., & Helmkay, A. (2008). Written and oral narratives of children and adolescents with Down syndrome. *Journal of Speech, Language, and Hearing Research*, *51*, 436–450.

Kay-Raining Bird, E., & Trudeau, N. (2009). *Questions and answers about bilingualism and developmental disabilities*. Paper presented at the American Speech-Language-Hearing Association Conference, New Orleans, LA.

Keenan, J. M., & Meenan, C. E. (2014). Test differences in diagnosing reading comprehension deficits. *Journal of Learning Disabilities*, *47*(2), 125–135. https://doi.org/10.1177/0022219412439326

Kelley, E. S., Barker, R. M., Peters-Sanders, L., Madsen, K., Seven, Y., Soto, X., . . . Goldstein, H. (2020). Feasible implementation strategies for improving vocabulary knowledge of high-risk preschoolers: Results from a cluster-randomized trial. *Journal of Speech, Language, and Hearing Research*, *63*, 4000–4017. https://doi.org/10.1044/2020_JSLHR-20-00316

Kelley, E. S., & Goldstein, H. (2014). Building a Tier 2 intervention: A glimpse behind the data. *Journal of Early Intervention*, *36*(4), 292–312. https://doi.org/10.1177/1053815115581657

Kelley, E. S., Goldstein, H., Spencer, T., & Sherman, A. (2015). Effects of automated Tier 2 storybook intervention on vocabulary and comprehension learning in preschool children with limited oral language skills. *Early Childhood Research Quarterly*, *31*, 47–61. https://doi.org/10.1016/j.ecresq.2014.12.004

Kelly, R., O'Malley, M., & Antonijevic, S. (2018). "Just trying to talk to people . . . It's the hardest": Perspectives of adolescents with high-functioning autism spectrum disorder on their social communication skills. *Child Language Teaching and Therapy*, *34*, 319–334. https://doi.org/10.1177/0265659018806754

Kemp, N., Lieven, E., & Tomasello, M. (2005). Young children's knowledge of the "determiner" and "adjective" categories. *Journal of Speech, Language, and Hearing Research*, *48*, 592–609.

Kemper, A. R., & Downs, S. M. (2000, May). A cost-effectiveness analysis of newborn hearing screening strategies. *Archives of Pediatric and Adolescent Medicine*, *154*(5), 484–488.

Kent-Walsh, J., Binger, C., & Buchanan, C. (2015). Teaching children who use augmentative and alternative communication to ask inverted yes–no questions using aided modeling. *American Journal of Speech-Language Pathology*, *24*, 222–236. https://doi.org/10.1044/2015_AJSLP-14-0066

Kent-Walsh, J., & Light, J. (2003). *Communication partner training in AAC: A literature review*. Paper presented at the Pennsylvania Speech-Language-Hearing Association annual convention, Harrisburg, PA.

Ketelaars, M. P., Alphonsus Hermans, T. S. L., Cuperus, J., Jansonius, K., & Verhoeven, L. (2011). Semantic abilities in children with pragmatic language impairment: The case of picture naming skills. *Journal of Speech, Language, and Hearing Research*, *54*, 87–98.

Ketelaars, M. P., Cuperus, J., van Daal, J., Jansonius, K., & Verhoeven, L. (2009). Screening for pragmatic language impairment: The potential of the Children's Communication Checklist. *Research in Developmental Disabilities*, *30*, 952–60. https://doi.org/10.1016/j.ridd.2009.01.006

Kibby, M., Marks, W., Morgan, S., & Long, C. (2004). Specific impairment in developmental reading disabilities: A working memory approach. *Journal of Learning Disabilities*, *37*, 349–363.

Kidd, E. (2013). The role of working memory in children's sentence comprehension. *Topics in Language Disorders*, *33*(3), 208–223.

Kieffer, M. J. (2014). Morphological awareness and reading difficulties in adolescent Spanish-speaking language minority learners and their classmates. *Journal of Learning Disability*, *47*, 44–53. https://doi.org/10.1177/0022219413509968

Kim, J.-H. (2016). *Understanding narrative inquiry: The crafting and analysis of stories as research*. SAGE.

Kim, S., & Lombardino, L. J. (2013). What do diagnostic test data tell us about differences in the profiles of children diagnosed with reading disability or language impairments? *Journal of Communication Disorders*, *46*(5–6), 465–474.

Kim, Y., Al Otaiba, S., Puranik, C., Folsom, J., Greulich, L., & Wagner, R. K. (2011). Componential skills of beginning writing: An exploratory study. *Learning and Individual Differences*, *21*(5), 517–525. https://https://doi.org/org/10.1016/j.lindif.2011.06.004

Kimble, C. (2013). Speech-language pathologists' comfort levels in English language learner service delivery. *Communication Disorders Quarterly*, *35*(1), 21–27.

King, D., Dockrell, J., & Stuart, M. (2014). Constructing fictional stories: A study of story narratives by children with autistic spectrum disorder. *Research in Developmental Disabilities*, *35*, 2438–2449. https://doi.org/10.1016/j.ridd.2014.06.015

Kintsch, W. (2013). Revisiting the Construction-Integration Model of Text Comprehension and its implications for instruction. In D. Alvermann, N. J. Unrau, & R. B. Ruddell

(Eds.), *Theoretical models and processes of reading* (6th ed., pp. 807–839). International Reading Association. https://doi.org/10.1598/0710.32

Kirby, J. R., Georgiou, G. K., Martinussen, R., Parrila, R., Bowers, P., & Landerl, K. (2010). Naming speed and reading: From prediction to instruction. *Reading Research Quarterly*, *45*, 341–362. https://doi.org/10.1598/RRQ.45.3.4 http://scholar.google.com/scholar_lookup?hl=en&volume=45&publication_year=2010&pages=341-362&journal=Reading+Research+Quarterly&author=J.+R.+Kirby&author=G.+K.+Georgiou&author=R.+Martinussen&author=R.+Parrila&author=P.+Bowers&author=K.+Landerl&title=Naming+speed+and+reading%3A+From+prediction+to+instruction

Kirjavainen, M., Theakston, A., & Lieven, E. (2009). Can input explain children's me-for-I errors? *Journal of Child Language*, *36*, 1091–1114.

Kirk, C., & Gillon, G. T. (2007). Longitudinal effects of phonological awareness intervention on morphological awareness in children with speech impairment. *Language, Speech, and Hearing Services in Schools*, *38*, 342–352.

Kirk, C., & Gillon, G. T. (2009). Integrated morphological awareness intervention as a tool for improving literacy. *Language, Speech, and Hearing Services in Schools*, *40*, 341–351.

Kirkorian, H., Choi. K., & Pempek, T. (2016). Toddlers' word learning from contingent and noncontingent video on touch screens. *Child Development*, *87*, 405–413. https://doi.org/10.1111/cdev.12508

Klee, T. (1992). Developmental and diagnostic characteristics of quantitative measures of children's language production. *Topics in Language Disorders*, *12*(2), 28–41.

Klee, T., Schaffer, M., Mays, S., Membrino, I., & Mougey, K. (1989). A comparison of the age–MLU relationship in normal and specifically language impaired preschool children. *Journal of Speech and Hearing Disorders*, *54*, 226–233.

Klein, H. B., Moses, N., & Jean-Baptiste, R. (2010). Influence of context on the production of complex sentences by typically developing children. *Language, Speech, and Hearing Services in Schools*, *41*, 289–302.

Klem, M., Melby-Lervåg, M., Hagtvet, B., Halaas Lyster, S., Gustafsson, J., & Hulme, C. (2015). Sentence repetition is a measure of children's language skills rather than working memory limitations. *Developmental Science*, *18*, 146–154.

Kline, A., & Volkmar, F. R. (2000). Treatment and intervention guidelines for individuals with Asperger's syndrome. In A. Kline, F. R. Volkmar, & S. S. Sparrow (Eds.), *Asperger's syndrome* (pp. 340–366). Guilford.

Klingberg, T., Fernell, W., Oelson, P., Johnson, M., Gustafsson, P., Dahltrom, K., . . . Westerberg, H. (2005). Computerized training of working memory in children with. ADHD: A randomized, controlled trial. *Journal of the American Academy of Child and Adolescent Psychiatry*, *44*, 177–186.

Klusek, J., Martin, G. E., & Losh, M. (2014). A comparison of pragmatic language in boys with autism and fragile X syndrome. *Journal of Speech, Language, and Hearing Research*, *57*, 1692–1707. https://doi.org/10.1044/2014_JSLHR-L-13-0064

Knapp, F. A., & Desrochers, M. N. (2009). An experimental evaluation of the instructional effectiveness of a student response system: A comparison with constructed overt responding. *International Journal of Teaching and Learning in Higher Education*, *21*, 36–46.

Knutsen, J., Crossman, M., Perrin, J., Shui, A., & Kuhlthau, K. (2019). Sex differences in restricted repetitive behaviors and interests in children with autism spectrum disorder: An Autism Treatment Network study. *Autism*, *23*, 858–868. https://doi.org/10.1177/1362361318786490

Koegel, L. K., Bryan, K. M., Su, P. L., Vaidya, M., & Camarata, S. (2020). Parent education in studies with nonverbal and minimally verbal participants with autism spectrum disorder: A systematic review. *American Journal of Speech-Language Pathology*, *29*, 890–902. https://doi.org/10.1044/2019_AJSLP-19-00007

Koegel, L. K., Koegel, J. K., Harrower, J. K., & Carter, C. M. (1999). Pivotal response intervention I: Overview of approach. *Journal of the Association for Persons with Severe Handicaps*, *24*(3), 174–185.

Koegel, R .L., Bradshaw, J. L., Ashbaugh, K., & Koegel, L. K. (2014). Improving question-asking initiations in young children with autism using pivotal response treatment. *Journal of Autism and Developmental Disorders*, *44*, 816–827.

Koegel, R. L., & Koegel, L. K. (2006). *Pivotal response treatments for autism*. Brookes.

Koegel, R. L., & Koegel, L. K. (2012). *The PRT pocket guide: Pivotal response treatment for autism spectrum disorders*. Brookes.

Kohnert, K. J. (2008). *Language disorders in bilingual children and adults*. Plural Publishing.

Kohnert, K. J. (2013). *Language disorders in bilingual children and adults* (2nd ed.). Plural Publishing.

Kohnert, K. J., & Bates, E. (2002). Balancing bilinguals II: Lexical comprehension and cognitive processing in children learning Spanish and English. *Journal of Speech, Language, and Hearing Research*, *45*, 347–359.

Kohnert, K. J., Yim, D., Nett, K., Kan, P. F., & Duran, L. (2005). Intervention with linguistically diverse preschool children: A focus on developing home languages. *Language, Speech, and Hearing Services in Schools*, *36*, 251–263.

Komesidou, R., Brady, N. C., Fleming, K., Esplund, A., & Warren, S. F. (2017). Growth of expressive syntax in children with fragile X syndrome. *Journal of Speech, Language, and Hearing Disorders*, *60*, 422–434. https://doi.org/10.1044/2016_JSLHR-L-15-0360

Konopka, A., & Bock, K. (2005, March). *Helping syntax out: How much do words do?* Paper presented at the CUNY Conference on Human Sentence Processing, Tucson, AZ.

Koppenhaver, D., & Erickson, K. (2003). Natural emergent literacy supports for preschoolers with autism and severe communication impairments. *Topics in Language Disorders*, *23*(4), 283–292.

Kouri, T. A., Selle, C. A., & Riley, S. A. (2006). Comparison of meaning and graphophonemic feedback strategies for guided reading instruction of children with language delays. *American Journal of Speech-Language Pathology, 15,* 236–246.

Kovacs, T., & Hill, K. (2017). Language samples from children who use speech-generating devices: Making sense of small samples and utterance length. *American Journal of Speech-Language Pathology, 26,* 939–950. https://doi.org/10.1044/2017_AJSLP-16-0114

Kover, S. T., Davidson, M. M., Sindberg, H. A., & Ellis Weismer, S. (2014). Use of the ADOS for assessing spontaneous expressive language in young children with ASD: A comparison of sampling contexts. *Journal of Speech, Language, and Hearing Research, 57,* 2221–2233. https://doi.org/10.1044/2014_JSLHR-L-13-0330

Kover, S. T., McDuffie, A., Abbeduto, L., & Brown, W. T. (2012). Effects of sampling context on spontaneous expressive language in males with fragile X syndrome or Down syndrome. *Journal of Speech, Language, and Hearing Research, 55,* 1022–1038.

Kraemer, R., & Fabiano-Smith, L. (2017). Language assessment of Latino English learning children: A records abstraction study. *Journal of Latinos and Education, 16*(4), 349–358. https://https://doi.org/10.1080/15348431.2016.1257429

Krantz, L. R., & Leonard, L. B. (2007). The effect of temporal adverbials on past tense production by children with specific language impairment. *Journal of Speech, Language, and Hearing Research, 50,* 137–148.

Krashen, S., & Brown, C. L. (2005). The ameliorating effects of high socioeconomic status: A secondary analysis. *Bilingual Research Journal, 29,* 185–196.

Krcmar, M., Grela, B., & Lin, K. (2007). Can toddlers learn vocabulary from television? An experimental approach. *Media Psychology, 10,* 41–61.

Kristensen, H. (2000). Selective mutism and comorbidity wih developmental disorder/delay, anxiety disorder, and elimination disorder. *Journal of the American Academy of Child and Adolescent Psychiatry, 39,* 249–256.

Kroecker, J., Lyle, K., Allen, K., Filippini, E., Galvin, M., Johnson, M., . . . Owens, R. E. (2010, Spring). Effects of student training on child language sample quality. *Contemporary Issues in Communication Science and Disorders, 36,* 4–13.

Kuder, S. J. (2013). *Teaching students with language and communication disabilities* (4th ed.). Pearson.

Kulkarni, A., Pring, T., & Ebbels, S. (2014). Evaluating the effectiveness of therapy based around Shape Coding to develop the use of regular past tense morphemes in two children with language impairments. *Child Language Teaching and Therapy, 30*(3), 245–254.

Kummerer, S. E., Lopez-Reyna, N. A., & Hughes, M. T. (2007). Mexican immigrant mothers' perceptions of their children's communication disabilities, emergent literacy development, and speech-language therapy program. *American Journal of Speech-Language Pathology, 16,* 271–282.

Kyle, F. E., Campbell, R., & MacSweeney, M. (2016). The relative contributions of speechreading and vocabulary to deaf and hearing children's reading ability. *Research in Developmental Disabilities, 48*(Suppl. C), 13–24. https://doi.org/10.1016/j.ridd.2015.10.004 http://scholar.google.com/scholar_lookup?hl=en&volume=48&publication_year=2016&pages=13-24&journal=Research+in+Developmental+Disabilities&author=F.+E.+Kyle&author=R.+Campbell&author=M.+MacSweeney&title=The+relative+contributions+of+speechreading+and+vocabulary+to+deaf+and+hearing+children%27s+reading+ability

Ladd, G. W., Kochenderfer-Ladd, B., Visconti, K. J., & Ettekal, I. (2012). Classroom peer relations and children's social and scholastic development: Risk factors and resources. In A. M. Ryan & G. W. Ladd (Eds.), *Adolescence and education: Peer relationships and adjustment at school* (pp. 11–49). Information Age Publishing.

Lahey, M. (1988). *Language disorders and language development.* Macmillan.

Laing Gillam, S., Fargo, J. D., & St. Clair Robertson, K. (2009). Comprehension of expository text: Insights gained from think-aloud data. *American Journal of Speech-Language Pathology, 18,* 82–94.

Lainhart, J. E. (2015). Brain imaging research in autism spectrum disorders: In search of neuropathology and health across the lifespan. *Current Opinion in Psychiatry, 28,* 76–82. https://doi.org/10.1097/YCO.0000000000000130

Lam, B. P. W., & Sheng, L. (2016). The development of morphological awareness in young bilinguals: Effects of age and L1 background. *Journal of Speech, Language, and Hearing Research, 59*(4), 732–744.

Lammertink, I., Boersma, P., Wijnen, F., & Rispens, J. (2017). Statistical learning in specific language impairment: A meta-analysis. *Journal of Speech, Language, and Hearing Disorders, 60,* 3474–3486. https://doi.org/10.1044/2017_JSLHR-L-16-0439

Landa, R. (2000). Social language use in Asperger syndrome and high-functioning autism. In A. Klin, F. Volkmar, & S. Sparrow (Eds.), *Asperger syndrome* (pp. 125–158). Guilford.

Landa, R., Piven, J., Wzorek, M., Gayle, J., Chase, G., & Folstein, S. (1992). Social language use in parents of autistic individuals. *Psychological Medicine, 22,* 245–254. https://doi.org/10.1017/S0033291700032918

Lane, S. J. (2002). Sensory modulation. In A. Bundy, S. Lane, & E. Murray (Eds.), *Sensory integration: Theory and practice* (pp. 101–122). Davis.

Language and Reading Research Consortium. (2015). The dimensionality of language ability in young children. *Child Development, 86,* 1948–1965. https://doi.org/10.1111/cdev.12450

Language and Reading Research Consortium, Jiang, H., & Davis, D. (2017). Let's Know! Proximal impacts on pre-kindergarten through grade 3 students' comprehension-related skills. *Elementary School Journal, 118*(2), 177–206.

Language and Reading Research Consortium, Jiang, H., & Logan, J. (2019). Improving reading comprehension in the primary grades: Mediated effects of a language-focused classroom intervention. *Journal of Speech, Language, and Hearing Research, 62*, 2812–2828. https://doi.org/10.1044/2019_JSLHR-L-19-0015

Language ENvironment Analysis (2015–2021). LENA ProSystem. https://www.lena.org/

La Paro, K. M., Justice, L., Skibbe, L. E., & Planta, R. C. (2004). Relations among maternal, child, and demographic factors and the persistence of preschool language impairment. *American Journal of Speech-Language Pathology, 13*, 291–303.

Larney, R. (2002). The relationship between early language delay and later difficulties in literacy. *Early Child Development and Care, 172*, 183–193.

Larroque, B., Ancel, P. Y., Marret, S., Marchand, L., Andre, M., Arnaud, C., . . . Kaminski, M. (2008). Neurodevelopmental disabilities and special care of 5-year-old children born before 33 weeks of gestation (the EPIPAGE study): A longitudinal cohort study. *Lancet, 371*(9615), 813–820.

Larry P. vs. Riles, Superintendent of Public Instruction for the State of California, No. C-71–22270 RFP. (1979). United States District Court, N. D. California.

Larson, A. L., Cycyk, L. M., Carta, J., Hammer, C. S., Baralth, M., Uchikoshi, Y., . . . Wood, C. (2020). A systematic review of language-focused interventions for children from culturally and linguistically diverse backgrounds. *Early Childhood Research Quarterly, 50*(Pt. 1), 157–178.

Larson, S. C., Hammill, D. D., & Moats, L. (2013). *Test of Written Spelling (TWS-5)*. Pro-Ed.

Larson, V. L., & McKinley, N. L. (1987). *Communication assessment and intervention strategies for adolescents*. Thinking Publications.

Lau v. Nichols, 414 U.S. 563. (1974). United States Supreme Court, 414 U.S.

Lavelli, M., & Majorano, M. (2016). Spontaneous gesture production and lexical abilities in children with specific language impairment in a naming task. *Journal of Speech, Language, and Hearing Research, 59*, 784–796. https://doi.org/10.1044/2016_JSLHR-L-14-0356

Law, J. (2004). The implications of different approaches to evaluating intervention: Evidence from the study of language delay/disorders. *Folia Phoniatrica et Logopaedica, 56*, 199–219.

Law, J., Garrett, Z., & Nye, C. (2004). The efficacy of treatment for children with developmental speech and language delay/disorder: A meta-analysis. *Journal of Speech, Language, and Hearing Research, 47*, 924–943.

Law, J., Rush, R., Schoon, I., & Parsons, S. (2009). Modeling developmental language difficulties from school entry into adulthood: Literacy, mental health, and employment outcomes. *Journal of Speech, Language, and Hearing Research, 52*, 1401–1416.

Laws, G., & Bishop, D. V. M. (2003). A comparison of language abilities in adolescents with Down syndrome and children with specific language impairment. *Journal of Speech, Language, and Hearing Research, 46*, 1324–1339.

Lazewnik, R., Creaghead, N. A., Breit Smith, A., Prendeville, J., Raisor-Becker, L., & Silbert, N. (2019). Identifiers of language impairment for Spanish–English dual language learners. *Journal of Speech, Language, and Hearing Services in Schools, 50*, 126–137. https://doi.org/10.1044/2018_LSHSS-17-0046

Lee, L. (1974). *Developmental sentence analysis*. Northwestern University Press.

Lenz, B. K., Adams, G. L., Bulgren, J. A., Pouliot, N., & Laraux, M. (2007). Effects of curriculum maps and guiding questions on the test performance of adolescents with learning disabilities. *Learning Disabilities Quarterly, 30*, 1–10.

Leonard, L. B. (2009). Is expressive language disorder an accurate diagnostic category? *American Journal of Speech-Language Pathology, 18*, 115–123.

Leonard, L. B. (2014). *Children with specific language impairment*. MIT Press.

Leonard, L. B., Camarata, S. M., Brown, B., & Camarata, M. N. (2004). Tense and agreement in the speech of children with specific language impairment: Patterns of generalization through intervention. *Journal of Speech, Language, and Hearing Research, 47*, 1363–1379.

Leonard, L. B., Camarata, S. M., Pawlowska, M., Brown, B., & Camarata, M. N. (2006). Tense and agreement morphemes in the speech of children with specific language impairment during intervention: Phase 2. *Journal of Speech, Language, and Hearing Research, 49*, 749–770.

Leonard, L. B., & Deevy, P. (2017). The changing view of input in the treatment of children with grammatical deficits. *American Journal of Speech-Language Pathology, 26*, 1031–1041. https://doi.org/10.1044/2017_AJSLP-16-0095

Leonard, L. B., Deevy, P., Fey, M. E., & Bredin-Oja, S. L. (2013). Sentence comprehension in specific language impairment: A task designed to distinguish between cognitive capacity and syntactic complexity. *Journal of Speech, Language, and Hearing Research, 56*, 577–589. https://doi.org/10.1044/1092-4388(2012/11-0254)

Leonard, L. B., Deevy, P., Karpicke, J. D., Christ, S. L., & Kueser, J. B. (2020). After initial retrieval practice, more retrieval produces better retention than more study in the word learning of children with developmental language disorder. *Journal of Speech, Language, and Hearing Research, 63*, 2763–2776. https://doi.org/10.1044/2020_JSLHR-20-00105

Leonard, L. B., Ellis Weismer, S., Miller, C. A., Francis, D. J., Tomblin, J. B., & Kail, R. V. (2007). Speed of processing, working memory, and language impairment in children. *Journal of Speech, Language, and Hearing Research, 50*, 408–428. https://doi.org/10.1044/1092-4388(2007/029)

Leonard, L. B., Fey, M., Deevy, P., & Bredin-Oja, S. (2015). Input sources of third person singular –s inconsistency in children with and without specific language impairment. *Journal of Child Language, 42*, 786–820.

Leonard, L. B., Miller, C. A., Deevy, P., Rauf, L., Gerber, E., & Charest, M. (2002). Production operations and the use of nonfinite verbs by children with specific language impairment. *Journal of Speech, Language, and Hearing Research, 45*, 744–758.

Leonard, L. B., Miller, C. A., Grela, B., Holland, A. L., Gerber, E., & Petucci, M. (2000). Production operations contribute to the grammatical morpheme limitations of children with specific language impairment. *Journal of Memory and Language*, *43*, 362–378.

Leonard, M. A., Milich, R., & Lorch, E. P. (2011). Pragmatic language use in mediating the relation between hyperactivity and inattention and social skills problems. *Journal of Speech, Language, and Hearing Research*, *54*, 567–579.

Lerna, A., Esposito, D., Conson, M., & Massagli, A. (2014). Long-term effects of PECS on social-communicative skills of children with autism spectrum disorders: A follow-up study. *International Journal of Language & Communication Disorders*, *49*, 478–485. https://doi.org/10.1111/1460-6984.12079

Leslie, L., & Caldwell, J. S. (2021). *Qualitative Reading Inventory, Seventh Edition (QRI-7)*. Pearson.

Lewis, B. A., Freebairn, L., & Taylor, H. G. (2000). Follow-up of children with early expressive phonology disorders. *Journal of Learning Disabilities*, *25*, 586–597.

Lewis, B. A., Freebairn, L., & Taylor, H. G. (2002). Correlates of spelling abilities in children with early speech sound disorders. *Reading and Writing*, *15*, 389–407.

Lewis, N., Castilleja, N., Moore, B. J., & Rodriguez, B. (2010). Assessment 360°: A panoramic framework for assessing English language learners. *Perspectives on Communication Disorders and Sciences in Culturally and Linguistically Diverse Populations*, *17*(2), 37. https://doi.org/ 10.1044/cds17.2.37

Liang, J., & Wilkinson, K. (2018). Gaze toward naturalistic social scenes by individuals with intellectual and developmental disabilities: Implications for augmentative and alternative communication designs. *Journal of Speech, Language, and Hearing Disorders*, *61*, 1157–1170. https://doi.org/10.1044/2018_JSLHR-L-17-0331

Liégeois, F., Mayes, A., & Morgan, A. (2014). Neural correlates of developmental speech and language disorders: Evidence from neuroimaging. *Current Developmental Disorders Reports*, *1*, 215–227. https://doi.org/10.1007/s40474-014-0019-1

Lienemann, T. O., & Reid, R. (2008). Using self-regulated strategy development to improve expository writing with students with attention deficit hyperactivity disorder. *Exceptional Children*, *74*(4), 471–486. http://scholar .google.com/scholar_lookup?hl=en&volume=74&publi cation_year=2008&pages=471-486&journal=Exceptional +Children&issue=4&author=T.+O.+Lienemann&author= R.+Reid&title=Using+self-regulated+strategy+development+ to+improve+expository+writing+with+students+with +attention+deficit+hyperactivity+disorder

Light, J. C., & Drager, K. D. (2005). *Maximizing language development with young children who require AAC*. Paper presented at the annual convention of the American Speech-Language-Hearing Association, San Diego, CA.

Light, J. C., & Drager, K. D. (2007). AAC technologies for young children with complex communication needs: State of the science and future research directions. *Augmentative and Alternative Communication*, *23*, 204–216.

Light, J. C., Drager, K., & Nemser, J. (2004). Enhancing the appeal of AAC technologies for young children: Lessons from the toy manufacturers. *Augmentative and Alternative Communication*, *20*, 137–149.

Light, J. C., McNaughton, D., Weyer, M., & Karg, L. (2008). Evidence-based literacy instruction for individuals who require augmentative and alternative communication: A case study of a student with multiple disabilities. *Seminars in Speech and Language*, *29*, 120–132. https://doi.org/ 10.1055/s-2008-1079126

Liiva, C. A., & Cleave, P. L. (2005). Roles of initiation and responsiveness in access and participation for children with specific language impairment. *Journal of Speech, Language, and Hearing Research*, *48*, 868–883. https://doi .org/10.1044/1092-4388(2005/060)

Lim, N., O'Reilly, M. F., Sigafoos, J., Ledbetter-Cho, K., & Lancioni, G. E. (2019). Should heritage languages be incorporated into interventions for bilingual individuals with neurodevelopmental disorders? A systematic review. *Journal of Autism and Developmental Disorders*, *49*, 1–26.

Lindell, A. K. (2016). Atypical hemispheric asymmetry in fetal alcohol spectrum disorders: A review of the effects of prenatal alcohol exposure on language lateralization. *Acta Neuropsychologica*, *14*, 367–380.

Linderholm, T., Everson, M. G., van den Broek, P., Mischinski, M., Crittenden, A., & Samuels, J. (2000). Effects of causal text revisions on more and less skilled readers: Comprehension of easy and difficult text. *Cognition and Instruction*, *18*, 525–556.

Lindsey, D. (2003). *The welfare of children* (2nd ed.). Oxford University Press.

Liss, M., Harel, B., Fein, D., Allen, D., Dunn, M., Feinstein, C., . . . Rapin, I. (2001). Predictors and correlates of adaptive functioning in children with developmental disorders. *Journal of Autism and Developmental Disorders*, *31*, 219–230.

LoCasale-Crouch, J., Konold, T., Pianta, R. C., Howes, C., Burchinal, M., Bryant, D., . . . Barbarin, O. A. (2007). Observed classroom quality profiles in state-funded pre-kindergarten programs and associations with teacher, program, and classroom characteristics. *Early Childhood Research Quarterly*, *22*, 3–17. http://scholar.google.com/ scholar_lookup?hl=en&publication_year=2007&pages =3-17&title=Observed+classroom+quality+profiles+in +state-funded+pre-kindergarten+programs+and+associa tions+with+teacher%2C+program%2C+and+classroom +characteristics

Lohmann, H., & Tomasello, M. (2003). The role of language in the development of false belief understanding: A training study. *Child Development*, *74*, 1130–1144.

Lomax, R. G., & McGee, L. M. (1987). Young children's concepts about print and reading: Toward a model of word acquisition. *Reading Research Quarterly*, *22*, 237–256.

Long, E. (2012, April 3). Integrating dynamic assessment and response-to-intervention in reading instruction. *The*

ASHA Leader. http://www.asha.org/Publications/leader/2012/120403/Integrating-Dynamic-Assessment-and-Response-to-Intervention-in-Reading-Instruction.htm

Long, S. H. (2001). About time: A comparison of computerized and manual procedures for grammatical and phonological analysis. *Clinical Linguistics & Phonetics, 15*(5), 399–426.

Long, S. H., & Fey, M. E. (1988). *Computerized Profiling Version 6.1 (Apple II series)* [Computer program]. Ithaca College.

Long, S. H., & Fey, M. E. (1989). *Computerized Profiling Version 6.2 (Macintosh and MS-DOS series)* [Computer program]. Ithaca College.

Lonigan, C. J., Burgess, S. R., Anthony, J. S., & Barker, T. A. (1998). Development of phonological sensitivity in 2- to 5-year-old children. *Journal of Educational Psychology, 90,* 294–311.

Loomes, C., Rasmussen, C., Pei, J., Manji, S., & Andrew, G. (2008). The effect of rehearsal training on working memory span of children with fetal alcohol spectrum disorder. *Research in Developmental Disabilities, 29,* 113–124.

Loosli, S., Buschkuehl, M., Perrig, W., & Jaeggi, S. (2008, July). *Working memory training enhances reading in 9–11 year old healthy children.* Poster presented at the Jean Piaget Archives 18th Advanced Course, Geneva, Switzerland.

Lopez, L. (2012). Language and the educational setting. In B. A. Goldstein (Ed.), *Bilingual language development and disorders in Spanish–English speakers* (2nd ed., pp. 267–284). Brookes.

Lorang, E., Sterling, A., & Schroeder, B. (2018). Maternal responsiveness to gestures in children with Down syndrome. *American Journal of Speech-Language Pathology, 27,* 1018–1029. https://doi.org/10.1044/2018_AJSLP-17-0138

Lord, C., Risi, S., & Pickles, A. (2004). Trajectory of language development in autistic spectrum disorders. In M. L. Rice & S. F. Warren (Eds.), *Developmental language disorders: From phenotypes to etiologies* (pp. 1–38). Erlbaum.

Lord, C., Rutter, M., DiLavore, P. C., Risi, S., Gotham, K., & Bishop, S. (2012). *Autism diagnostic observation schedule* (2nd ed.). Western Psychological Services.

Losh, M., & Capps, L. (2003). Narrative ability in high-functioning children with autism or Asperger's syndrome. *Journal of Autism and Developmental Disorders, 33,* 239–251.

Loukusa, S., Mäkinen, L., Kuusikko-Gauffin, S., Ebeling, H., & Moilanen, I. (2014). Theory of mind and emotion recognition skills in children with specific language impairment, autism spectrum disorder and typical development: Group differences and connection to knowledge of grammatical morphology, word-finding abilities and verbal working memory. *International Journal of Language & Communication, 48,* 498–507. https://doi.org/10.1111/1460-6984.12091

Lovelace, L., & Stewart, S. R. (2007). Increasing print awareness in preschoolers with language impairment using non-evocative print referencing. *Language, Speech, and Hearing Services in Schools, 38,* 16–30. https://doi.org/10.1044/0161-1461(2007/003)

Lowe, E., Slater, A., Wefley, J., & Hardie, D. (2002). *A status report on hunger and homelessness in America's cities 2002: A 25-city survey.* U.S. Conference of Mayors.

Lucas, R., & Frazier Norbury, C. (2015). Making inferences from text: It's vocabulary that matters. *Journal of Speech, Language, and Hearing Research, 58,* 1224–1232. https://doi.org/10.1044/2015_JSLHR-L-14-0330

Luckasson, R., Borthwick-Duffy, S., Buntinx, W. H., Coulter, D. L., Craig, E. M., Reeve, A., . . . Tasse, M. J. (2002). *Mental retardation: Definition, classification, and systems of supports* (10th ed.). American Association on Mental Retardation.

Lugo-Neris, M. J., Jackson, C., & Goldstein, H. (2010). Facilitating vocabulary acquisition of young English language learners. *Language, Speech, and Hearing Services in Schools, 41,* 314–327.

Lum, J., Conti-Ramsden, G., Morgan, A., & Ullman, M. (2014). Procedural learning deficits in specific language impairment (SLI): A meta-analysis of serial reaction time task performance. *Cortex, 51,* 1–10. https://doi.org/10.1016/j.cortex.2013.10.011

Lund, N. J., & Duchan, J. F. (1993). *Assessing children's language in naturalistic contexts.* Prentice-Hall.

Lund, S., & Light, J. (2006). Long term outcomes for individuals who use augmentative and alternative communication: Part I. What is a good outcome? *Augmentative and Alternative Communication, 22,* 284–299.

Lundine, J. P., Harnish, S. H., McCauley, R. J., Schwen Blackett, D., Zezinka, A., Chen, W., & Fox, R. A. (2018). Adolescent summaries of narrative and expository discourse: Differences and predictors. *Language, Speech, and Hearing Services in Schools, 49,* 551–568. https://doi.org/10.1044/2018_LSHSS-17-0105

Lundine, J. P., & McCauley, R. J. (2016). A tutorial on expository discourse: Structure, development, and disorders in children and adolescents. *American Journal of Speech-Language Pathology, 25,* 306–320. https://doi.org/10.1044/2016_AJSLP-14-0130

Luyster, R. J., Kadlec, M. B., Carter, A., & Tager-Flusberg, H. (2008). Language assessment and development in toddlers with autism spectrum disorders. *Journal of Autism and Developmental Disorders, 38*(8), 1426–1438. https://doi.org/10.1007/s10803-007-0510-1

Lynch, E. W., & Hanson, M. J. (Eds.). (2004). *Developing cross-cultural competence: A guide for working with children and their families* (3rd ed.). Brookes.

Lyon, G. R., Shaywitz, S. E., & Shaywitz, B. A. (2003). A definition of dyslexia. *Annals of Dyslexia, 53*(1), 1–14.

Lyytinen, P., Poikkeus, A., Laakso, M., Eklund, K., & Lyytinen, H. (2001). Language development and symbolic play in children with and without familial risk of dyslexia. *Journal of Speech, Language, and Hearing Research, 44,* 873–885.

Määttä, S., Laakso, M., Tolvanen, A., Westerholm, J., & Aro, T. (2016). Continuity from prelinguistic communication to later language ability: A follow-up study from infancy to early school age. *Journal of Speech, Language, and Hearing Research, 59*, 1357–1372. https://doi.org/10.1044/2016_JSLHR-L-15-0209

MacArthur, C. A., & Graham, S. (2016). Writing research from a cognitive perspective. In C. MacArthur, S. Graham, & J. Fitzgerald (Eds.), *Handbook of writing research* (2nd ed., pp. 24–40). Guilford. http://scholar.google.com/scholar_lookup?hl=en&publication_year=2016&pages=24-40&author=C.+A.+MacArthur&author=S.+Graham&title=Handbook+of+writing+research

MacArthur, C. A., Graham, S., Haynes, J. A., & DeLaPaz, S. (1996). Spelling checkers and students with learning disabilities: Performance comparisons and impact on spelling. *Journal of Special Education, 30*, 35–57.

MacDuff, G. S., Krantz, P. J., & McClannahan, L. E. (2001). Prompts and prompt-fading strategies for people with autism. In C. Maurice, G. Green, & R. M. Foxx (Eds.), *Making a difference: Behavioral intervention for autism* (pp. 37–50). Pro-Ed.

Mackie, C., & Dockrell, J. E. (2004). The nature of written language deficits in children with SLI. *Journal of Speech, Language, and Hearing Research, 47*, 1469–1483.

Maclean, M., Bryant, P., & Bradley, L. (1987). Rhymes, nursery rhymes, and reading in early childhood. *Merrill–Palmer Quarterly, 33*, 255–282.

MacWhinney, B. (2000). *CLAN* [Computer software]. Carnegie Mellon University.

MacWhinney, B. (2022). *Tools for analyzing talk Part 2: The CLAN program* [Computerized Language Analysis (CLAN) program of the Child Language Data Exchange System (CHILDES)]. Retrieved March 18, 2022, from https://talkbank.org/manuals/CLAN.pdf

Magill, J. (1986). *The nature of social deficits of children with autism*. Unpublished doctoral dissertation, University of Alberta, Edmonton, Alberta, Canada.

Maher, Z. K., Erskine, M. E., Byrd, A. S., Harring, J. R., & Edwards, J. R. (2021). African American English and early literacy: A comparison of approaches to quantifying nonmainstream dialect use. *Language, Speech, and Hearing Services in Schools, 52*, 118–130. https://doi.org/10.1044/2020_LSHSS-19-00115

Mahurin-Smith, J., DeThorne, L. S., & Petrill, S. A. (2017). Longitudinal associations across prematurity, attention, and language in school-age children. *Journal of Speech, Language, and Hearing Disorders, 60*, 3601–3608. https://doi.org/10.1044/2017_JSLHR-L-17-0015

Mahurin-Smith, J., Segebart DeThorne, L., Logan, J. A. R., Channell, R. W., & Petrill, S. A. (2014). Impact of prematurity on language skills at school age. *Journal of Speech, Language, and Hearing Research, 57*, 901–916. https://doi.org/10.1044/1092-4388(2013/12-0347)

Mainela-Arnold, E., Evans, J. J., & Alibali, M. W. (2006). Understanding conservation delays in children with specific language impairment: Task representations revealed in speech and gesture. *Journal of Speech, Language, and Hearing Research, 49*, 1267–1279.

Mainela-Arnold, E., Evans, J. L., & Coady, J. A. (2008). Lexical representations in children with SLI: Evidence from a frequency-manipulated gating task. *Journal of Speech, Language, and Hearing Research, 51*, 381–393.

Mainela-Arnold, E., Evans, J. L., & Coady, L. A. (2010). Explaining lexical–semantic deficits in specific language impairment: The role of phonological similarity, phonological working memory, and lexical competition. *Journal of Speech, Language, and Hearing Research, 53*, 1742–1756.

Manhardt, J., & Rescorla, L. (2002). Oral narrative skills of late talkers at ages 8 and 9. *Applied Psycholinguistics, 23*, 1–21.

Manly, T., Anderson, V., Crawford, J., George, M., & Robertson, I. H. (2016). *Test of Everyday Attention for Children*. Pearson.

Mann, V., & Singson, M. (2003). Linking morphological knowledge to English decoding ability: Large effects of little suffixes. In E. Assink & D. Sandra (Eds.), *Reading complex words: Cross-language studies* (pp. 1–25). Kluwer.

Månsson, J., & Stjernqvist, K. (2014). Children born extremely preterm show significant lower cognitive, language and motor function levels compared with children born at term, as measured by the Bayley-III at 2.5 years. *Acta Pediatrica, 103*, 504–511. https://doi.org/10.1111/apa.12585

March of Dimes. (2007). *Premature birth*. Updated February 2007. http://www.marchofdimes.com/prematurity/21326_115 7.asp

Maridaki-Kassotaki, K. (2002). The relation between phonological memory skills and reading ability in Greek-speaking children: Can training of phonological memory contribute to reading development? *European Journal of Psychology of Education, 17*, 63–73.

Markowitz, J., Carlson, E., Frey, W., Riley, J., Shimshak, A., Heinzen, H., . . . Lee, H. (2006). *Preschoolers with disabilities: Characteristics, services, and results: Wave 1 overview report from the Pre-Elementary Education Longitudinal Study (PEELS)*.

Martin, G. E., Bush, L., Klusek, J., Patel, S., & Losh, M. (2018). A multimethod analysis of pragmatic skills in children and adolescents with fragile X syndrome, autism spectrum disorder, and Down syndrome. *Journal of Speech, Language, and Hearing Disorders, 61*, 3023–3037. https://doi.org/10.1044/2018_JSLHR-L-18-0008

Martin, J. A., Hamilton, B. E., Sutton, P. D., Ventura, S. J., Menacker, F., & Kirmeyer, S. (2006, September 29). Births: Final data for 2004. *National Vital Statistics Reports, 55*(1).

Marton, K., Campanelli, L., Eichorn, N., Scheuer, J., & Yoon, J. (2014). Information processing and proactive interference in children with and without specific language impairment. *Journal of Speech, Language, and Hearing Research, 57*, 106–119. https://doi.org/10.1044/1092-4388(2013/12-0306)

Marton, K., Kelmenson, L., & Pinkhasova, M. (2007). Inhibition control and working memory capacity in children with SLI. *Psychologia, 50*, 110–121.

Marton, K., Schwartz, R., Farkas, L., & Katsnelson, V. (2006). Effect of sentence length and complexity on working memory performance in Hungarian children with specific language impairment (SLI): A cross-linguistic comparison. *International Journal of Language & Communication Disorders, 41*, 653–673. http://scholar.google.com/scholar_lookup?hl=en&publication_year=2006&pages=653-673&title=Effect+of+sentence+length+and+complexity+on+working+memory+performance+in+Hungarian+children+with+specific+language+impairment+%28SLI%29%3A+A+cross%E2%80%90linguistic+comparison

Mashburn, A. J., Pianta, R. C., Hamre, B. K., Downer, J. T., Barbarin, O. A., Bryant, D., . . . Howes, C. (2008). Measures of classroom quality in prekindergarten and children's development of academic, language, and social skills. *Child Development, 3*, 732–749. http://scholar.google.com/scholar_lookup?hl=en&publication_year=2008&pages=732-749&title=Measures+of+classroom+quality+in+prekindergarten+and+children%27s+development+of+academic%2C+language%2C+and+social+skills

Massachusetts Department of Education. (2006). *Massachusetts Comprehensive Assessment System.* https://www.doe.mass.edu/mcas

Masterson, J. J., & Apel, K. (2000). Spelling assessment: Charting a path to optimal intervention. *Topics in Language Disorders, 20*(3), 50–65.

Masterson, J. J., & Crede, L. A. (1999). Learning to spell: Implications for assessment and intervention. *Language, Speech, and Hearing Services in Schools, 30*, 243–354.

Mathrick, R., Meagher, T., & Frazier Norbury, C. (2017). Evaluation of an interview skills training package for adolescents with speech, language and communication needs. *International Journal of Language & Communication Disorders, 52*, 786–799. https://doi.org/10.1111/1460-6984.12315

Maul, C. A., & Ambler, K. L. (2014). Embedding language therapy in dialogic reading to teach morphologic structures to children with language disorders. *Communication Disorders Quarterly, 35*, 237–247.

Mayberry, R. I., del Giudice, A. A., & Lieberman, A. M. (2011). Reading achievement in relation to phonological coding and awareness in deaf readers: A meta-analysis. *Journal of Deaf Studies and Deaf Education, 16*, 164–188. https://doi.org/10.1093/deafed/enq049 http://scholar.google.com/scholar_lookup?hl=en&volume=16&publication_year=2011&pages=164-188&journal=The+Journal+of+Deaf+Studies+and+Deaf+Education&author=R.+I.+Mayberry&author=A.+A.+del+Giudice&author=A.+M.+Lieberman&title=Reading+achievement+in+relation+to+phonological+coding+and+awareness+in+deaf+readers%3A+A+meta-analysis

Mayer, M. (1969). *Frog, where are you?* Dial Books.

Mayer, M. (1973). *Frog on his own.* Penguin.

Mayer, M. (1974). *Frog goes to dinner.* Penguin.

Mayer, M., & Mayer, M. (1975). *One frog too many.* Penguin Putnam.

Mayes, S. D., Lockridge, R., & Tierney, C. D. (2017). Tantrums are not associated with speech or language deficits in preschool children with autism. *Journal of Developmental and Physical Disabilities, 29*, 587–596.

McArthur, G. M., Hogben, J. H., Edwards, V. T., Heath, S. M., & Mengler, E. D. (2000). On the "specifics" of specific reading disability and specific language impairment. *Journal of Child Psychology and Psychiatry, and Allied Disciplines, 41*(7), 869–874.

McCabe, A., & Bliss, L. S. (2004–2005). Narratives from Spanish-speaking children with impaired and typical language development. *Imagination, Cognition and Personality, 24*, 331–346.

McCabe, A., & Rollins, P. R. (1994). Assessment of preschool narrative skills. *American Journal of Speech-Language Pathology, 3*(1), 45–56.

McCardle, P., Scarborough, H. S., & Catts, H. W. (2001). Predicting, explaining, and preventing children's reading difficulties. *Learning Disabilities Research & Practice, 16*(4), 230–239.

McCathren, R. B., Yoder, P. J., & Warren, S. F. (2000). Testing predictive validity of the Communication Composite of the Communication and Symbolic Behavior Scales. *Journal of Early Intervention, 23*, 36–46.

McCauley, S., & Christiansen, M. (2015). Individual differences in chunking ability predict on-line sentence processing. In *Proceedings of the 37th Annual Conference of the Cognitive Science Society* (pp. 1553–1558). https://cogsci.mindmodeling.org/2015/papers/0271/paper0271.pdf

McCormack, J., Harrison, L. J., McLeod, S., & McAllister, L. (2011). A nationally representative study of the association between communication impairment at 4–5 years and children's life activities at 7–9 years. *Journal of Speech, Language, and Hearing Research, 54*, 1328–1348.

McDaniel, J., D'Ambrose Slaboch, K., & Yoder, P. J. (2018). A meta-analysis of the association between vocalizations and expressive language in children with autism spectrum disorder. *Research in Developmental Disabilities, 72*, 202–213. https://doi.org/10.1016/j.ridd.2017.11.010

McDaniel, J., & Schuele, C. M. (2021). When will he talk? An evidence-based tutorial for measuring progress toward use of spoken words in preverbal children with autism spectrum disorder. *American Journal of Speech-Language Pathology, 30*, 1–18. https://doi.org/10.1044/2020_AJSLP-20-00206

McDaniel, J., Yoder, P. J., & Watson, L. R. (2017). A path model of expressive vocabulary skills in initially preverbal preschool children with autism spectrum disorder. *Journal of Autism and Developmental Disorders, 47*(4), 947–960. https://doi.org/10.1007/s10803-016-3016-x

McDuffie, A., Oakes, A., Machalicek, W., Ma, M., Bullard, L., Nelson, S., & Abbeduto, L. (2016). Early language intervention using distance video-teleconferencing: A pilot study of young boys with fragile X syndrome and their mothers. *American Journal of Speech-Language Pathology, 25*, 46–66. https://doi.org/10.1044/2015_AJSLP-14-0137

McDuffie, A., & Yoder, P. (2010). Types of parent verbal responsiveness that predict language in young children with autism spectrum disorder. *Journal of Speech, Language, and Hearing Research, 53*, 1026–1039. https://doi.org/10.1044/1092-4388(2009/09-0023)

McGee, G. G. (2005). Incidental teaching. In M. Hersen, G. Sugai, & R. H. Horner (Eds.), *Encyclopedia of behavior modification and cognitive behavior therapy: Educational applications* (Vol. 3, pp. 1359–1362). SAGE.

McGill-Franzen, A., & Smith, K. (2013). RTI and the Common Core. In S. B. Neuman & L. B. Gambrell (Eds.), *Quality reading instruction in the age of Common Core standards* (pp. 107–120). International Reading Association.

McGinty, A. S., & Justice, L. M. (2009). Predictors of print knowledge in children with specific language impairment: Experiential and developmental factors. *Journal of Speech, Language, and Hearing Research, 52*, 81–97.

McGregor, K. K. (2000). The development and enhancement of narrative skills in a preschool classroom: Towards a solution to clinician–client mismatch. *American Journal of Speech-Language Pathology, 9*, 55–71.

McGregor, K. K. (2019). How we fail children with developmental language disorder. *Language, Speech, and Hearing Services in Schools, 50*, 981–992. https://doi.org/10.1044/2020_LSHSS-20-00003

McGregor, K. K., Goffman, L., Owen Van Horne, A., Hogan, T. P., & Finestack, L. (2020). Developmental language disorder: Applications for advocacy, research, and clinical service. *Perspectives, 5*(1), 38–46.

McGregor, K. K., Newman, R. M., Reilly, R. M., & Capone, N. C. (2002). Semantic representation and naming in children with specific language impairment. *Journal of Speech, Language, and Hearing Research, 45*, 998–1014.

McGregor, K. K., Oleson, J., Bahnsen, A., & Duff, D. (2013). Children with developmental language impairment have vocabulary deficits characterized by limited breadth and depth. *International Journal of Language and Communication Disorders, 48*, 307–319. https://doi.org/10.1111/1460-6984.12008

McKeown, M. G. (2019). Effective vocabulary instruction fosters knowing words, using words, and understanding how words work. *Language, Speech, and Hearing Services in Schools, 50*, 466–476. https://doi.org/10.1044/2019_LSHSS-VOIA-18-0126

McLaughlin, T. F., Weber, K. P., & Derby, M. (2013). Classroom spelling interventions for students with learning disabilities. In H. L. Swanson, K. R. Harris, & S. Graham (Eds.), *Handbook of learning disabilities* (2nd ed., pp. 439–447). Guilford. http://scholar.google.com/scholar_lookup?hl=en&publication_year=2013&pages=439-447&author=T.+F.+McLaughlin&author=K.+P.+Weber&author=M.+Derby&title=Handbook+of+learning+disabilities

McLeod, S,, & Threats, T. (2008). The ICF-CY and children with communication disabilities. *International Journal of Speech-Language Pathology, 10*, 92–109.

McMaster, K. L., Fuchs, D., Fuchs, L. S., & Compton, D. L. (2005). Responding to nonresponders: An experimental field trial of identification and intervention methods. *Exceptional Children, 71*, 445–463. https://doi.org/10.1111/1467-9817.12075 http://scholar.google.com/scholar_lookup?hl=en&volume=71&publication_year=2005&pages=445-463&journal=Exceptional+Child ren&author=K.+L.+McMaster&author=D.+Fuchs&author=L.+S.+Fuchs&author=D.+L.+Compton&title=Responding+to+nonresponders%3A+An+experimental+-field+trial+of+identification+and+intervention+methods

McMaster, K. L., Kunkel, A., Shin, J., Jung, P. G., & Lembke, E. (2017). Early writing intervention: A best evidence synthesis. *Journal of Learning Disabilities, 51*(4), 363–380. http://scholar.google.com/scholar_lookup?hl=en&volume=51&publication_year=2017&pages=363-380&journal=Journal+of+Learning+Disabilities&issue=4&author=K.+L.+McMaster&author=A.+Kunkel&author=J.+Shin&author=P.+G.+Jung&author=E.+Lembke&title=Early+writing+intervention%3A+A+best+evidence+synthesis

McNeilly, L. (2016, March). Rise in speech-language disorders in SSI-supported children reflects national trends: A new national report reviews the prevalence and implications of speech-language disorders for children living in poverty. *The ASHA Leader, 21* [online only]. https://doi.org/10.1044/leader.PA2.21032016.np

Mealings, K. T., & Demuth, K. (2014). The role of utterance length and position in 3-year-olds' production of third person singular –*s*. *Journal of Speech, Language, and Hearing Research, 57*, 484–494. https://doi.org/10.1044/2013_JSLHR-L-12-0354

Meilijson, S. R., Kasher, A., & Elizur, A. (2004). Language performance in chronic schizophrenia: A pragmatic approach. *Journal of Speech, Language, and Hearing Research, 47*, 695–713.

Melby-Lervåg, M., & Hulme, C. (2013). Is working memory training effective? A meta-analytic review. *Developmental Psychology, 49*, 270–291. https://doi.org/10.1037/a0028228 http://scholar.google.com/scholar_lookup?hl=en&volume=49&publication_year=2013&pages=270-291&journal=Developmental+Psychology&author=M.+Melby-Lervag&author=C.+Hulme&title=Is+working+memory+training+effective%3F+A+meta-analytic+review

Melby-Lervåg, M., Lyster, S. A., & Hulme, C. (2012). Phonological skills and their role in learning to read: A meta-analytic review. *Psychological Bulletin, 138*, 322–352. https://doi.org/10.1037/a0026744.supp http://scholar.google.com/scholar_lookup?hl=en&volume=138&publication_year=2012&pages=322-352&journal=Psychological+Bulletin&author=M.+Melby-Lervag&author=S.+A.+Lyster&author=C.+Hulme&title=Phonological+skills+and+their+role+in+learning+to+read%3A+A+meta-analytic+review

Merritt, D. H., & Klein, S. (2015). Do early care and education services improve language development for maltreated children? Evidence from a national child welfare sample. *Child Abuse & Neglect, 39*, 185–196. https://doi.org/10.1016/j.chiabu.2014.10.011

Mesibov, G. B., & Shea, V. (2010). The TEACCH program in the area of evidence-based practice. *Journal of Autism and Developmental Disorders, 40*, 570–579.

Messenger, K., Branigan, H. P., McLean, J. F., & Sorace, A. (2012). Is young children's passive syntax semantically constrained? Evidence from syntactic priming. *Journal of Memory and Language, 66*(4), 568–587. https://doi.org/10.1016/j.jml.2012.03.008

Mihai, A., Butera, G., & Friesen, A. (2017). Examining the use of curriculum to support early literacy instruction: A multiple case study of Head Start teachers. *Early Education and Development, 28*, 323–342. https://doi.org/10.10 80/10409289.2016.1218729

Miles, S., & Chapman, R. S. (2002). Narrative content as described by individuals with Down syndrome and typically developing children. *Journal of Speech, Language, and Hearing Research, 45*, 175–189.

Miles, S., Chapman, R., & Sindberg, H. (2006). Sampling context affects MLU in the language of adolescents with Down syndrome. *Journal of Speech, Language, and Hearing Research, 49*, 325–337.

Millar, D. C., Light, J. C., & Schlosser, R. W. (2000). The impact of AAC on natural speech development: A meta-analysis. In *Proceedings of the 9th Biennial Conference of the International Society for Augmentative and Alternative Communication* (pp. 740–741). International Society for Augmentative and Alternative Communication.

Millar, D. C., Light, J. C., & Schlosser, R. W. (2006). The impact of augmentative and alternative communication intervention on the speech production of individuals with developmental disabilities: A research review. *Journal of Speech, Language, and Hearing Research, 49*, 248–264.

Miller, A. C., & Keenan J. M. (2009). How word decoding skill impacts text memory: The centrality deficit and how domain knowledge can compensate. *Annals of Dyslexia, 59*, 99–113. https://doi.org/10.1007/s11881-009-0025-x

Miller, C. A., & Deevy, P. (2006). Structural priming in children with and without specific language impairment. *Clinical Linguistics & Phonetics, 20*, 387–399.

Miller, C. A., Kail, R., Leonard, L. B., & Tomblin, J. B. (2001). Speed of processing in children with specific language impairment. *Journal of Speech, Language, and Hearing Research, 44*, 416–433.

Miller, J. F. (1981). *Assessing language production in children: Experimental procedures*. University Park Press.

Miller, J. F., Andriacchi, K., & Nockerts, A. (2016). Using language sample analysis to assess spoken language production in adolescents. *Language, Speech, and Hearing Services in Schools, 47*, 99–112. https://doi.org/10.1044/2015_LSH SS-15-0051

Miller, J. F., & Iglesias, A. (2006). *Systematic Analysis of Language Transcripts (SALT), English & Spanish (Version 9)* [Computer software]. Language Analysis Lab, University of Wisconsin–Madison.

Miller, J. F., & Iglesias, A. (2015). *Systematic Analysis of Language Transcripts (SALT; Research Version 2012)* [Computer software]. SALT Software.

Miller, L. (1999a). *Two friends*. Smart Alternatives.

Miller, L. (1999b). *Bird and his ring*. Smart Alternatives.

Miller, L., & Hendric, N. (2000). Health of children adopted from China. *Pediatrics, 105*(6).

Mills, M. T. (2015). Narrative performance of gifted African American school-aged children from low-income backgrounds. *American Journal of Speech-Language Pathology, 24*, 36–46.

Mills, M.T., Moore, L.C., Chang, R., Kim, S., & Frink, B. (2021). Perceptions of Black children's narrative language: A mixed-methods study. *Language Speech and Hearing Services in Schools* 52, 84–99. https://doi.org/10.1044/2020_LSHSS-20-00014

Minear, M., & Shah, P. (2006). Sources of working memory deficits in children and possibilities for remediation. In S. E. Pickering & G. D. Phye (Eds.), *Working memory and education* (pp. 273–297). Erlbaum.

Miniscalco, C., Fernell, E., Thompson, L., Sandberg, E., Kadesjö, B., & Gillberg, C. (2018). Development problems were common five years after positive screening for language disorders and/or, autism at 2.5 years of age. *Acta Paediatrica, 107*, 1739–1749. https://doi.org/10.1111/apa .14358

Miolo, G., Chapman, R. S., & Sindberg, H. A. (2005). Sentence comprehension in children with Down syndrome and typically developing children: Role of sentence voice, visual context, and auditory–verbal short-term memory. *Journal of Speech, Language, and Hearing Research, 48*, 172–188.

Mirenda, P. (2003). "He's not really a reader . . . ": Perspectives on supporting literacy development in individuals with autism. *Topics in Language Disorders, 23*(4), 271–282. https://doi.org/10.1097/00011363-200310000-00003

Mirenda, P., Smith, V., Fawcett, S., & Johnston, J. (2003, November). *Language and communication intervention outcomes for young children with autism*. Paper presented at the American Speech-Language-Hearing Association Annual Meeting.

Mirrett, P. L., Roberts, J. E., & Price, J. (2003). Early intervention practices and communication intervention strategies for young males with fragile X syndrome. *Language, Speech, and Hearing Services in Schools, 34*, 320–331.

Moats, L. (1995). *Spelling development, disability, and instruction*. York Press.

Moats, L., & Foorman, B. (2003). Measuring teacher's content knowledge of language and reading. *Annals of Dyslexia, 53*, 23–45.

Mohammadzaheri, F., Koegel, L. K., Rezaee, M., & Majid Rafiee, S. (2014). A randomized clinical trial comparison between Pivotal Response Treatment (PRT) and Structured Applied Behavior Analysis (ABA) intervention for children with autism. *Journal of Autism and Developmental Disorders, 44*, 2769–2777.

Mohr Jensen, C., & Steinhausen, H. (2015). Comorbid mental disorders in children and adolescents with attention-deficit/hyperactivity disorder in a large nationwide study. *Attention Deficit and Hyperactivity Disorders, 7*, 27–38.

Mol, S. E., & Bus, A. G. (2011). To read or not to read: A meta-analysis of print exposure from infancy to early adulthood. *Psychological Bulletin, 137*, 267–296. https://doi.org/10.1037/a0021890 http://scholar.google.com/scholar_lookup?hl=en&volume=137&publication_year=2011&pages=267-296&journal=Psychological+Bulletin&author=S.+E.+Mol&author=A.+G.+Bus&title=To

+read+or+not+to+read%3A+A+meta-analysis+of+print+exposure+from+infancy+to+early+adulthood

Mol, S. E., Bus, A. G., de Jong, M. T., & Smeets, D. J. H. (2008). Added value of dialogic parent–child book readings: A meta-analysis. *Early Education & Development, 19*, 7–26.

Moncrieff, D., Miller, E., & Hill, E. (2018). Screening tests reveal high risk among adjudicated adolescents of auditory processing and language disorders. *Journal of Speech, Language, and Hearing Research, 61*, 924–935. https://doi.org/10.1044/2017_JSLHR-H-17-0098

Montgomery, J. W. (2000). Relation of working memory to off-line and real-time sentence processing in children with specific language impairment. *Applied Psycholinguistics, 21*, 117–148.

Montgomery, J. W. (2002). Understanding the language difficulty of children with specific language impairments: Does verbal working memory matter? *American Journal of Speech-Language Pathology, 11*, 77–91.

Montgomery, J. W. (2005). Effects of input rate and age on the real-time language processing of children with specific language impairment. *International Journal of Language and Communication Disorders, 40*, 171–188.

Montgomery J. W., & Evans, J. L. (2009). Complex sentence comprehension and working memory in children with specific language impairment. *Journal of Speech, Language, and Hearing Research, 52*, 269–288. https://doi.org/10.1044/1092-4388(2008/07-0116)

Montgomery, J. W., Evans, J. L., Fargo, J., Schwartz, S., & Gillam, R. (2018). Structural relationship between cognitive processing and syntactic sentence comprehension in children with and without developmental language disorder. *Journal of Speech, Language, and Hearing Research, 61*(12), 2950–2976. https://doi.org/10.1044/2018_JSLHR-L-17-0421

Montgomery, J. W., Gillam, R. B., & Evans, J. L. (2016). Syntactic versus memory accounts of the sentence comprehension deficits of specific language impairment: Looking back, looking ahead. *Journal of Speech, Language, and Hearing Research, 59*, 1491–1504. https://doi.org/10.1044/2016_JSLHR-L-15-0325

Montgomery, J. W., Gillam, R. B., & Evans, J. L. (2021). A new memory perspective on the sentence comprehension deficits of school-age children with developmental language disorder: Implications for theory, assessment, and intervention. *Language, Speech, and Hearing Services in Schools, 52*, 449–466. https://doi.org/10.1044/2021_LSHSS-20-00128

Montgomery, J. W., Gillam, R. B., Evans, J. L., & Sergeev, A. (2017). Whatdunit? Sentence comprehension abilities of children with SLI: Sensitivity to word order in canonical and noncanonical sentences. *Journal of Speech, Language, and Hearing Research, 60*(9), 2603–2618. https://doi.org/10.1044/2017_JSLHR-L-17-0025

Montgomery, J. W., Magimairaj, B. M., & Finney, M. C. (2010). Working memory and specific language impairment: An update on the relation and perspectives on assessment and treatment. *American Journal of Speech-Language Pathology, 19*, 78–94.

Montgomery, J. W., & Windsor, J. (2007). Examining the language performances of children with and without specific language impairment: Contributions of phonological short-term memory and processing speed. *Journal of Speech, Language, and Hearing Research, 50*, 778–797.

Moore, S. M., & Perez-Mendez, C. (2006). Working with linguistically diverse families in early intervention: Misconceptions and missed opportunities. *Seminars in Speech and Language, 27*, 187–198.

Moore Channell, M., Loveall, S. J., Conners, F. A., Harvey, D. J., & Leonard Abbeduto, L. (2018). Narrative language sampling in typical development: Implications for clinical trials. *American Journal of Speech-Language Pathology, 27*, 123–135. https://doi.org/10.1044/2017_AJSLP-17-0046

Moran, C., & Gillon, G. (2005). Inference comprehension of adolescents with traumatic brain injury: A working memory hypothesis. *Brain Injury, 19*, 743–751.

Moran, C., & Gillon, G. T. (2010). Expository discourse in older children and adolescents with traumatic brain injury. In M. A. Nippold & C. M. Scott (Eds.), *Expository discourse in children, adolescents, and adults: Development and disorders* (pp. 275–301). Psychology Press.

Moran, T. P. (2016). Anxiety and working memory capacity: A meta-analysis and narrative review. *Psychological Bulletin, 831*, 1–34.

Mordecai, D. R., Palin, M. W., & Palmer, C. B. (1985). *Lingquest 1* [Computer program]. Macmillan.

Moreau, M., & Fidrych, H. (2008). *The Story Grammar Marker teachers manual*. MindWing Concepts.

Morgan, A., Bonthrone, A., & Liégeois, F. (2016). Brain basis of childhood speech and language disorders: Are we closer to clinically meaningful MRI markers? *Current Opinion in Pediatrics, 28*, 725–730. https://doi.org/10.1097/MOP.0000000000000420

Morgan, P. L., Hammer, C. S., Farkas, G., Hillemeir, M. M., Maczuga, S., Cook, M., & Morano, S. (2016). Who receives speech/language services by 5 years of age in the United States? *American Journal of Speech-Language Pathology, 25*(2), 183–199. https://doi.org/10.1044/2015_AJSLP-14-0201

Morrier, M. J., McGee, G. G., & Daly, T. (2009). Effects of toy selection and arrangement on the social behaviors of an inclusive group of preschool-aged children. *Early Childhood Services, 3*, 157–177.

Mosse, E. K., & Jarrold, C. (2011). Evidence for preserved novel word learning in Down syndrome suggests multiple routes to vocabulary acquisition. *Journal of Speech, Language, and Hearing Research, 54*(4), 1137–1152.

Motallebzadeh, K., & Yazdi, M. (2016). The relationship between EFL learners' reading comprehension ability and their fluid intelligence, crystallized intelligence, and processing speed. *Cogent Education, 3*(1), 1–8. https://doi.org/10.1080/2331186X.2016.1228733

Motsch, H.-J., & Riehemann, S. (2008). Effects of "context-optimization" on the acquisition of grammatical case in children with specific language impairment: An experimental evaluation in the classroom. *International Journal of Language & Communication Disorders*, *43*(6), 683–698.

Moxam, C. (2019). The link between language and spelling: What speech-language pathologists and teachers need to know. *Language, Speech, and Hearing Services in Schools*, *50*, 939–954. https://doi.org/10.1044/2020_LSHSS-19-00009

Mueller, K. L., & Tomblin, J. B. (2012) Examining the comorbidity of language disorders and ADHD. *Topics in Language Disorders*, *32*(3), 229–246. https://doi.org/ 10.1097/TLD.0b013e318262010d

Mueller, T. G., Milian, M., & Lopez, M. I. (2009). Latina mothers' views of a parent-to-parent support group in the special education system. *Research and Practice for Persons with Severe Disabilities*, *34*(3–4), 113–122. https://doi.org/10.2511/rpsd.34.3-4.113

Mufwene, S., Rickford, J. R., Bailey, G., & Baugh, J. (Eds.). (1998). *African-American English: Structure, history, and use.* Routledge.

Müller, E., Cannon, L. R., Kornblum, C., Clark, J., & Powers, M. (2016). Description and preliminary evaluation of a curriculum for teaching conversational skills to children with high-functioning autism and other social cognition challenges. *Language, Speech, and Hearing Services in Schools*, *47*, 191–208. https://doi.org/10.1044/2016_LSHSS-15-0042

Mundy, P., Block, J., Delgado, C., Pomaes, Y., Van Hecke, A. V., & Parlade, M. V. (2007). Individual differences and the development of joint attention in infancy. *Child Development*, *78*, 938–954.

Muñoz, M. L., Gillam, R. B., Peña, E. D., & Gulley-Faehnle, A. (2003). Measures of language development in fictional narratives of Latino children. *Language, Speech, and Hearing Services in Schools*, *34*, 332–342.

Munson, B., Kurtz, B. A., & Windsor, J. (2005). The influence of vocabulary size, phonotactic probability, and word likeness on nonword repetitions of children with and without specific language impairment. *Journal of Speech, Language, and Hearing Research*, *48*, 1033–1047.

Murphy, K. A., & Diehm, E. (2020). Collecting words: A clinical example of a morphology-focused orthographic intervention. *Language, Speech, and Hearing Services in Schools*, *51*, 544–560. https://doi.org/10.1044/2020_LSHSS-19-00050

Murphy, K. A., Justice, L. M., O'Connell, A. A., Pentimonti, J. M., & Kaderavek, J. N. (2016). Understanding risk for reading difficulties in children with language impairment. *Journal of Speech, Language, and Hearing Research*, *59*, 1436–1447. https://doi.org/10.1044/2016_JSLHR-L-15-0110

Murray, D. S., Ruble, L. A., Willis, H., & Molloy, C. A. (2009). Parent and teacher report of social skills in children with autism spectrum disorders. *Language, Speech, and Hearing Services in Schools*, *40*, 109–115.

Muter, V., Hulme, C., Snowling, M. J., & Stevenson, J. (2004). Phonemes, rimes, vocabulary, and grammatical skills as foundations of early reading development: Evidence from a longitudinal study. *Developmental Psychology*, *40*, 665–681. https://doi.org/10.1037/0012-1649.40.5.665 http://scholar.google.com/scholar_lookup?hl=en&volume=40&publication_year=2004&pages=665-681&journal=Developmental+Psychology&author=V.+Muter&author=C.+Hulme&author=M.+J.+Snowling&author=J.+Stevenson&title=Phonemes%2C+rimes%2C+vocabulary%2C+and+grammatical+skills+as+foundations+of+early+reading+development%3A+Evidence+from+a+longitudinal+study

Nagele, D., Hooper, S. R., Hildebrant, K., Mccart, M., Dettmer, J., & Glang, A. (2019). Under-identification of students with long term disability from moderate to severe TBI. *Physical Disabilities Education and Related Services*, *38*, 10–25. https://doi.org/10.14434/pders.v38i1.26850

Nagy, W., Berninger, V. W., & Abbott, R. D. (2006). Contributions of morphology beyond phonology to literacy outcomes of upper elementary and middle-school students. *Journal of Educational Psychology*, *98*(1), 134–147. https://doi.org/10.1037/0022-0663.98.1.134

Nagy, W., & Townsend, D. (2012). Words as tools: Learning academic vocabulary as language acquisition. *Reading Research Quarterly*, *47*, 91–108. https://doi.org/10.1002/RRQ.011

Naigles, L. R., Hoff, E., & Vear, D. (2009). Flexibility in early verb use: Evidence from a multiple-*n* diary study. *Monographs of the Society for Research in Child Development*, *74*(2), Serial No. 293.

Nail-Chiwetula, B. J., & Bernstein Ratner, N. (2006). Information literacy for speech-language pathologists: A key to evidence-based practice. *Language, Speech, and Hearing Services in Schools*, *37*, 157–167.

Naremore, R. C. (2001, April). *Narrative frameworks and early literacy.* Seminar presentation by Rochester Hearing and Speech Center and Nazareth College, Rochester, NY.

Nash, M., & Donaldson, M. L. (2005). Word learning in children with vocabulary deficits. *Journal of Speech, Language, and Hearing Research*, *48*, 439–458.

Nathan, L., Stackhouse, J., Goulandris, N., & Snowling, M. J. (2004). The development of early literacy skills among children with speech difficulties: A test of the "critical age hypothesis." *Journal of Speech, Language, and Hearing Research*, *47*, 377–391.

Nation, K., Clarke, P., Marshall, C. M., & Durand, M. (2004). Hidden language impairments in children: Parallels between poor reading comprehension and specific language impairment? *Journal of Speech, Language, and Hearing Research*, *47*(1), 199–211.

Nation, K., Clarke, P., Wright, B., & Williams, C. (2006). Patterns of reading ability in children with autism spectrum disorder. *Journal of Autism and Developmental Disorders*, *36*, 911–919. https://doi.org/10.1007/s10803-006-0130-1

Nation, K., Cocksey, J., Taylor, J. S. H., & Bishop, D. V. M. (2010). A longitudinal investigation of early reading and language skills in children with poor reading comprehension. *Journal of Child Psychology and Psychiatry*, *51*, 1031–1039. https://doi.org/10.1111/j.1469-7610.2010.02254.x

Nation, K., & Frazier Norbury, C. (2005). Why reading comprehension fails. *Topics in Language Disorders*, *25*, 21–32.

Nation, K., & Snowling, M. J. (2004). Beyond phonological skills: Broader language skills contribute to the development of reading. *Journal of Research in Reading*, *27*, 342–356. https://doi.org/10.1111/j.1467-9817.2004.00238.x http://scholar.google.com/scholar_lookup?hl=en&volume=27&publication_year=2004&pages=342-356&journal=Journal+of+Research+in+Reading&author=K.+Nation&author=M.+J.+Snowling&title=Beyond+phonological+skills%3A+Broader+language+skills+contribute+to+the+development+of+reading

Nation, K., Snowling, M. J., & Clarke, P. J. (2007). Dissecting the relationship between language skills and learning to read: Semantic and phonological contributions to new vocabulary learning in children with poor reading comprehension. *Advances in Speech-Language Pathology*, *9*, 131–139. https://doi.org/10.1080/14417040601145166 http://scholar.google.com/scholar_lookup?hl=en&volume=9&publication_year=2007&pages=131-139&journal=Advances+in+Speech-Language+Pathology&author=K.+Nation&author=M.+J.+Snowling&author=P.+J.+Clarke&title=Dissecting+the+relationship+between+language+skills+and+learning+to+read%3A+Semantic+and+phonological+contributions+to+new+vocabulary+learning+in+children+with+poor+reading+comprehension

National Academies of Sciences, Engineering, and Medicine. (2017). *Promoting the educational success of children and youth learning English: Promising futures*. National Academies Press.

National Assessment of Educational Progress. (2021). *Reading*. National Center for Educational Statistics, U.S. Department of Education. https://nces.ed.gov/nationsreportcard/reading

National Center for Education Statistics. (2021). *Enrollment rates of young children*. https://nces.ed.gov/programs/coe/indicator/cfa

National Clearinghouse for English Language Acquisition. (2018, April). *Fast facts: English learner (EL) populations by local educational agency*. https://ncela.ed.gov/files/fast_facts/LEAs_Fact_Sheet_2018_Final.pdf

National Early Literacy Panel. (2008). *Developing early literacy*. National Institute for Literacy. https://lincs.ed.gov/publications/pdf/NELPReport09.pdf

National Governors Association Center for Best Practices and Council of Chief State School Officers. (2010). *Common Core State Standards for English language arts and literacy in history/social studies, science, and technical subjects*. http://www.corestandards.org/assets/CCSSI_ELA%20Standards.pdf

National Institute of Child Health and Human Development. (2000). *Teaching children to read*. National Reading Panel, U.S. National Institutes of Health. https://www.nichd.nih.gov/sites/default/files/publications/pubs/nrp/Documents/report.pdf

National Institute of Child Health and Human Development Early Child Care Research Network. (2005). Pathways to reading: The role of oral language in the transition to reading. *Developmental Psychology*, *41*(2), 428–442.

National Institute of Deafness and Other Communication Disorders. (2017, September 13). *Specific language impairment*. https://www.nidcd.nih.gov/health/specific-language-impairment

National Institute of Neurological Disorders and Stroke. (2017). *Dyslexia information page*. https://www.ninds.nih.gov/Disorders/All-Disorders/Dyslexia-Information-Page

Neitzel, J., & Wolery, M. (2009). *Steps for implementation: Least-to-most prompts*. National Professional Development Center on Autism Spectrum Disorders, Frank Porter Graham Child Development Institute, University of North Carolina.

Nelson, D. L., & Zhang, N. (2000). The ties that bind what is known to the recall of what is new. *Psychonomic Bulletin & Review*, *7*, 604–617.

Nelson, K. E., Camarata, S. M., Welsh, J., Butkovsky, L., & Camarata, M. (1996). Effects of imitative and conversational recasting treatment on the acquisition of grammar in children with specific language impairment and younger language-normal children. *Journal of Speech, Language, and Hearing Research*, *39*(4), 850–859. https://doi.org/10.1044/jshr.3904.850

Nelson, N. W. (1992). Targets of curriculum-based language assessment. *Best Practices in School Speech-Language Pathology*, *2*, 73–86.

Nelson, N. W. (1994). Curriculum-based language assessment and intervention across grades. In G. P. Wallach & K. G. Butler (Eds.), *Language learning disabilities in school-age children and adolescents* (pp. 104–131). Allyn & Bacon.

Nelson, N. W. (2010). *Language and literacy disorders: Infancy through adolescence*. Pearson.

Nelson, N. W., Bahr, C. M., & Van Meter, A. M. (2004). *The writing lab approach to language instruction and intervention*. Brookes.

Nelson, N. W., & Van Meter, A. M. (2002). Assessing curriculum-based reading and writing samples. *Topics in Language Disorders*, *22*(2), 35–59.

Nelson, N. W., & Van Meter, A. (2003, June). *Measuring written language abilities and change through the elementary years*. Poster session presented at the annual meeting of the Symposium for Research in Child Language Disorders, Madison, WI.

NeuroDevelopmental Center. (2013). *Cogmed working memory training*.

Newbury, D. F., Gibson, J. L., Conti-Ramsden, G., Pickles, A., Durkin, K., & Toseeb, U. (2019). Using polygenic profiles to predict variation in language and psychosocial outcomes in early and middle childhood. *Journal of Speech, Language, and Hearing Research*, *62*, 3381–3396. https://doi.org/10.1044/2019_JSLHR-L-19-0001

Newkirk-Turner, B. L., Oetting, J. B., & Stockman, I. J. (2014). BE, DO, and modal auxiliaries of three-year-old African American English speakers. *Journal of Speech, Language, and Hearing Research*, *57*, 1383–1393. https://doi.org/10.1044/2014_JSLHR-L-13-0063

Newkirk-Turner, B. L., Oetting, J. B., & Stockman, I. J. (2016). Development of auxiliaries by young children learning African American English. *Language, Speech, and Hearing Services in Schools, 47*, 209–224. https://doi.org/10.1044/2016_LSHSS-15-0063

Newman, R. S., & German, D. J. (2002). Effects of lexical factors on lexical access among typical language-learning children and children with word-finding difficulties. *Language and Speech, 45*, 285–317.

Nicholas, J. G., & Geers, A. E. (2007, August). Will they catch up? The role of age at cochlear implantation in the spoken language development of children with severe to profound hearing loss. *Journal of Speech, Language, Hearing Research, 50*, 1048–1062.

Nicolson, R., Lenane, M., Singaracharlu, S., Malaspina, D., Giedd, J. N., Hamburger, S. D., . . . Rapoport, J. L. (2000). Premorbid speech and language impairments in childhood-onset schizophrenia: Association with risk factors. *American Journal of Psychiatry, 157*, 794–800.

Nippold, M. A. (2000). Language development during the adolescent years: Aspects of pragmatics, syntax, and semantics. *Topics in Language Disorders, 20*(2), 15–28.

Nippold, M. A. (2004). Research on later language development: International perspectives. In R. A. Berman (Ed.), *Language development across childhood and adolescence: Volume 3. Trends in language acquisition research* (pp. 1–8). Benjamins.

Nippold, M. A. (2007). *Later language development: School-age children, adolescents, and young adults* (3rd ed.). Pro-Ed.

Nippold, M. A. (2009). School-age children talk about chess: Does knowledge drive syntactic complexity? *Journal of Speech, Language, and Hearing Research, 52*, 856–871. https://doi.org/10.1044/1092-4388(2009/08-0094)

Nippold, M. A. (2010). Explaining complex matters: How knowledge of a domain drives language. In M. A. Nippold & C. M. Scott (Eds.), *Expository discourse in children, adolescents, and adults: Development and disorders* (pp. 41–61).Psychology Press.

Nippold, M. A. (2011). Language intervention in the classroom: What it looks like. *Language, Speech, and Hearing Services in Schools, 42*, 393–394.

Nippold, M. A. (2014). *Language sampling with adolescents: Implications for intervention* (2nd ed.). Plural Publishing.

Nippold, M. A. (2017). Reading comprehension deficits in adolescents: Addressing underlying language abilities. *Language, Speech, and Hearing Services in Schools, 48*(2), 125–131. https://doi.org/10.1044/2016_LSHSS-16-0048

Nippold, M. A., Frantz-Kaspar, M. W., Cramond, P. M., Kirk, C., Hayward-Mayhew, C., & MacKinnon, M. (2014). Conversational and narrative speaking in adolescents: Examining the use of complex syntax. *Journal of Speech, Language, and Hearing Research, 57*, 876–886. https://doi.org/10.1044/1092-4388(2013/13-0097)

Nippold, M. A., Frantz-Kaspar, M. W., Cramond, P. M., Kirk, C., Hayward-Mayhew, C., & MacKinnon, M. (2015). Critical thinking about fables: Examining language production and comprehension in adolescents. *Journal of Speech,*

Language, and Hearing Research, 58, 325–335. https://doi.org/10.1044/2015_JSLHR-L-14-0129

Nippold, M. A., Hesketh, L. J., Duthie, J. K., & Mansfield, T. C. (2005). Conversational versus expository discourse: A study of syntactic development in children, adolescents, and adults. *Journal of Speech, Language, and Hearing Research, 48*, 1048–1064. https://doi.org/10.1044/1092-4388(2005/073)

Nippold, M. A., Mansfield, T. C., & Billow, J. L. (2007). Peer conflict explanations in children, adolescents, and adults: Examining the development of complex syntax. *American Journal of Speech-Language Pathology, 16*, 179–186.

Nippold, M. A., Mansfield, T. C., Billow, J. L., & Tomblin, J. B. (2008). Expository discourse in adolescents with language impairments: Examining syntactic development. *American Journal of Speech-Language Pathology, 17*, 356–366. https://doi.org/10.1044/1058-0360(2008/07-0049)

Nippold, M. A., Mansfield, T. C., Billow, J. L., & Tomblin, J. B. (2009). Syntactic development in adolescents with a history of language impairments: A follow-up investigation. *American Journal of Speech-Language Pathology, 18*, 241–251. https://doi.org/10.1044/1058-0360(2008/08-0022)

Nippold, M. A., & Sun, L. (2008). Knowledge of morphologically complex words: A developmental study of older children and young adolescents. *Language, Speech, and Hearing Services in Schools, 39*, 365–373. https://doi.org/10.1044/0161-1461(2008/034)

Nippold, M. A., Vigeland, L. M., Frantz-Kaspar, M. W., & Ward-Lonergan, J. M. (2017). Language sampling with adolescents: Building a normative database with fables. *American Journal of Speech-Language Pathology, 26*, 908–920. https://doi.org/10.1044/2017_AJSLP-16-0181

Noel, K., & Westby, C. E. (2014). Applying theory of mind concepts when designing interventions targeting social cognition among youth offenders. *Topic in Language Disorders, 34*, 344–361.

Nogueira Peredo, T., Zelaya, M. I., & Kaiser, A. P. (2018). Teaching low-income Spanish-speaking caregivers to implement EMT en Español with their young children with language impairment: A pilot study. *American Journal of Speech-Language Pathology, 27*, 136–153. https://doi.org/10.1044/2017_AJSLP-16-0228

Norbury, C. F. (2014). Practitioner review: Social (pragmatic) communication disorder conceptualization, evidence, and clinical implications. *Journal of Child Psychology and Psychiatry, 55*(3), 204–216. https://doi.org/10.111/jcpp.12154

Norbury, C. F., & Bishop, D. V. (2003). Narrative skills of children with communication impairments. *International Journal of Language and Communication Disorders, 38*, 287–313.

Norbury, C. F., Gemmell, T. & Paul, R. (2013). Pragmatics abilities in narrative production: A cross-disorder comparison. *Journal of Child Language, 41*(3), 485–510. https://doi.org/ 10.1017/S030500091300007X

Novogrodsky, R., & Edelson, L. R. (2016). Ambiguous pronoun use in narratives of children with autism spectrum disorders. *Child Language Teaching and Therapy, 32*, 241–252. https://doi.org/10.1177%2F0265659015602935

Novogrodsky, R., & Friedmann, N. (2006). The production of relative clauses in syntactic SLI: A window to the nature of the impairment. *Advances in Speech-Language Pathology, 8*(4), 364–375. https://doi.org/10.1080/14417040600919496

Nowell, S. W., Watson, L. R., Boyd, B., & Klinger, L. G. (2019). Efficacy study of a social communication and self-regulation intervention for school-age children with autism spectrum disorder: A randomized controlled trial. *Language, Speech, and Hearing Services in Schools, 50*, 416–433. https://doi.org/10.1044/2019_LSHSS-18-0093

Nystrand, M. (2006). Research on the role of classroom discourse as it affects reading comprehension. *Research in the Teaching of English, 40*, 392–412. http://scholar.google .com/scholar_lookup?hl=en&publication_year=2006 &pages=392-412&title=Research+on+the+role+of+classroom+discourse+as+it+affects+reading+comprehension

Odom, S. L. (2000). What do we know and where do we go from here? *Topics in Early Childhood Special Education, 20*, 20–27.

Oetting, J. B. (2019). Variability within varieties of English profiles of typicality and impairment. In T. Ionin & M. Rispoli (Eds.), *Three streams of generative language acquisition research: Selected papers from the 7th Meeting of Generative Approaches to Language Acquisition–North America, University of Illinois at Urbana-Champaign.* Benjamins.

Oetting, J. B., Berry, J. R., Gregory, K. D., Rivière, A. M., & McDonald, J. (2019). Specific language impairment in African American English and Southern White English: Measures of tense and agreement with dialect-informed probes and strategic scoring. *Journal of Speech, Language, and Hearing Research, 62*, 3443–3461. https://doi.org/10 .1044/2019_JSLHR-L-19-0089

Oetting, J. B., & Garrity, A. W. (2006). Variation within dialects: A case of Cajun/Creole influence within child SAAE and SWE. *Journal of Speech, Language, and Hearing Research, 49*, 16–26. https://doi.org/10.1044/1092-4388(2006/002)

Oetting, J. B., & McDonald, J. L. (2001). Nonmainstream dialect use and specific language impairment. *Journal of Speech, Language, and Hearing Research, 44*(1), 207–223. https:// https://doi.org/org/10.1044/1092-4388(2001/018)

Oetting, J. B., McDonald, J. L., Seidel, C. M., & Hegarty, M. (2016). Sentence recall by children with SLI across two nonmainstream dialects of English. *Journal of Speech, Language, and Hearing Research, 59*, 183–194. https://doi. org/10.1044/2015_JSLHR-L-15-0036

Oetting, J. B., & Newkirk, B. L. (2008). Subject relatives by children with and without SLI across different dialects of English. *Clinical Linguistics and Phonetics, 22*, 111–125. https://doi.org/10.1080/02699200701731414

Office of Head Start. (2016). *Services snapshot (2015–2016). National all programs.* https://eclkc.ohs.acf.hhs.gov/sites/ default/files/pdf/service-snapshot-all-programs-2015-2016.pdf

Ogle, D., Blachowicz, C., Fisher, P., & Lang, L. (2016). *Academic vocabulary in middle and high school: Effective practices across the disciplines.* Guilford. https://www.guilford.com/ books/Academic-Vocabulary-in-Middle-and-HighSchool/ Ogle-Blachowicz-Fisher-Lang/9781462522583

Ohashi, J. K., Mirenda, P., Marinova-Todd, S., Hambly, C., Fombonne, E., Szatmari, P., . . . the Pathways in ASD Study Team. (2012). Comparing early language development in monolingual- and bilingual-exposed young children with autism spectrum disorders. *Research in Autism Spectrum Disorders, 6*, 890–897. https://doi.org/10.1016/j .rasd.2011.12.002

Olinghouse, N. G., & Wilson, J. (2013). The relationship between vocabulary and writing quality in three genres. *Reading and Writing, 26*(1), 45–65. https://doi.org/10.10 07/s11145-008-9124-z

Olswang, L. B., Coggins, T. E., & Timler, G. R. (2001). Outcome measures of school-age children with social communication. *Topics in Language Disorders, 22*(1), 50–73.

Olswang, L. B., Svensson, L., & Astley, S. (2010). Observation of classroom social communication: Do children with fetal alcohol spectrum disorders spend their time differently than their typically developing peers? *Journal of Speech, Language, and Hearing Research, 53*, 1687–1703.

Olswang, L. B., Svensson, L., Coggins, T. E., Beilinson, J., & Donaldson, A. L. (2006). Reliability issues and solutions for coding social communication performance in classroom settings. *Journal of Speech, Language, and Hearing Research, 49*, 1058–1071.

O'Neill, T., Light, J., & Pope, L. (2018). Effects of interventions that include aided augmentative and alternative communication input on the communication of individuals with complex communication needs: A meta-analysis. *Journal of Speech, Language, and Hearing Disorders, 61*, 1743–1765. https://doi.org/10.1044/2018_JSLHR-L-17-0132

O'Neil-Pirozzi, T. M. (2003). Language functioning of residents in family homeless shelters. *American Journal of Speech-Language Pathology, 12*, 229–242.

O'Neil-Pirozzi, T. M. (2009). Feasibility and benefit of parent participation in a program emphasizing preschool child language development while homeless. *American Journal of Speech-Language Pathology, 18*, 252–263.

O'Shaughnessy, T. E., & Swanson, H. L. (2000). A comparison of two reading interventions for children with reading disabilities. *Journal of Learning Disabilities, 33*, 257–277.

Ouellette, G. P. (2006). What's meaning got to do with it: The role of vocabulary in word reading and reading comprehension. *Journal of Educational Psychology, 98*(3), 554–566. https://doi.org/10.1037/0022-0663.98.3.554

Owen Van Horne, A. J., Curran, M., Larson, C., & Fey, M. E. (2018). Effects of a complexity-based approach on generalization of past tense –ed and related morphemes. *Language, Speech, and Hearing Services in Schools, 49*, 681–693. https://doi.org/10.1044/2018_LSHSS-STLT1-17-0142

Owen Van Horne, A. J., & Lin, S. (2011). Cognitive state verbs and complement clauses in children with SLI and their typically developing peers. *Clinical Linguistics & Phonetics, 25*, 881–898.

Owens, R. (1978). *Speech acts in the early language of nondelayed and retarded children: A taxonomy and distributional study.* Unpublished doctoral dissertation, Ohio State University, Columbus.

Owens, R. E. (2018). *Early communication intervention.* Pearson.

Owens, R. E. (2020). *Language development: An introduction.* Pearson.

Owens, R. E., & Kim, K. (2007, November). *Holistic reading and semantic investigation intervention with struggling readers.* Paper presented at the Annual Convention of the American Speech-Language-Hearing Association, Boston, MA.

Owens, R. E., & Pavelko, S. L. (2017). Relationships among conversational language samples and norm-referenced test scores. *Clinical Archives of Communication Disorders, 2*(1), 1–8. https://doi.org/10.21849/cacd.2017.00052

Owens, R. E., & Pavelko, S. L. (2020). Sampling Utterances and Grammatical Analysis Revised (SUGAR): New normative values for language sample analysis measures in 7- to 11-year-old children. *Language, Speech, and Hearing Services in Schools, 51*, 734–744.

Owens, R. E., & Pavelko, S. L. (2021). *SUGAR: Sampling Utterances and Grammatical Analysis Revised.* https://www.sugarlanguage.org

Owens, R. E, Pavelko, S. L., & Bambinell, D. (2018). Moving beyond mean length of utterance: Analyzing language samples to identify intervention targets. *Perspectives, 3,* 5–22. https://doi.org/10.1044/persp3.SIG1.5

Pacton, S., & Deacon, S. H. (2008). The timing and mechanisms of children's use of morphological information in spelling: A review of evidence from English and French. *Cognitive Development, 23,* 339–359. https://doi.org/10.1016/j.cogdev.2007.09.004 http://scholar.google.com/scholar_lookup?hl=en&volume=23&publication_year=2008&pages=339-359&journal=Cognitive+Development&author=S.+Pacton&author=S.+H.+Deacon&title=The+timing+and+mechanisms+of+children%27s+use+of+morphological+information+in+spelling%3A+A+review+of+evidence+from+English+and+French

Paez, M., & Rinaldi, C. (2006). Predicting English word reading skills for Spanish-speaking students in first grade. *Topics in Language Disorders, 26,* 338–350.

Papaeliou, C. F., Maniadaki, K., & Kakouros, E. (2015). Association between story recall and other language abilities in schoolchildren with ADHD. *Journal of Attention Disorders, 19,* 53–62. https://doi.org/10.1177/1087054712446812

Paradis, J. (2005). Grammatical morphology in children learning English as a second language: Implications of similarities with specific language impairment. *Language, Speech, and Hearing Services in Schools, 36,* 172–187.

Paradis, J. (2007). Bilingual children with specific language impairment: Theoretical and applied issues. *Applied Psycholinguistics, 28,* 551–564.

Paradis, J. (2016). The development of English as a second language with and without specific language impairment: Clinical implications. *Journal of Speech, Language, and Hearing Research, 59,* 171–182. https://doi.org/10.1044/2015_JSLHR-L-15-0008

Paradis, J., Crago, M., Genesee, F., & Rice, M. (2003). French–English bilingual children with specific language impairment: How do they compare with their monolingual peers? *Journal of Speech, Language, and Hearing Research, 46,* 1–15. https://doi.org/10.1044/1092-4388(2003/009)

Paradis, J., Genesee, F., & Crago, M. (2011). *Dual language development and disorders: A handbook on bilingualism and language learning* (2nd ed.). Brookes.

Paradis, J., Schneider, P., & Sorenson Duncan, T. (2013). Discriminating children with language impairment among English-language learners from divers first-language backgrounds. *Journal of Speech, Language, and Hearing Research, 565,* 571–581.

Parente, R., & Hermann, D. (1996). Retraining memory strategies. *Topics in Language Disorders, 17*(1), 45–57.

Parsons, S., & Branagan, A. (2014). *Word Aware: Teaching vocabulary across the day, across the curriculum.* Routledge. http://scholar.google.com/scholar_lookup?hl=en&publication_year=2014&author=S.+Parsons&author=A.+Branagan&title=Word+Aware%3A+Teaching+vocabulary+across+the+day%2C+across+the+curriculum

Patterson, J. L. (2000). Observed and reported expressive vocabulary and word combinations in bilingual toddlers. *Journal of Speech, Language, and Hearing Research, 43,* 121–128.

Patterson, J. L., & Pearson, B. Z. (2012). Bilingual lexical development, assessment, and intervention. In B. A. Goldstein (Ed.), *Bilingual language development and disorders in Spanish–English speakers* (2nd ed., pp. 113–130). Brookes.

Patton Terry, N., McDonald Connor, C., Thomas-Tate, S., & Love, M. (2010). Examining relationships among dialect variation, literacy skills, and school context in first grade. *Journal of Speech, Language, and Hearing Research, 53,* 126–145.

Paul, R., & Norbury, C. (2011). *Language disorders from infancy through adolescence* (4th ed.). Elsevier.

Paul, R., & Norbury, C. (2012). *Language disorders from infancy through adolescence: Listening, speaking, writing, and communicating* (4th ed.). Mosby.

Paul, R., Norbury, C., & Gosse, C. (2018). *Language disorders from infancy through adolescence: Listening, speaking, reading, writing, and communicating* (5th ed.). Elsevier.

Pauls, L. J., & Archibald, L. M. D. (2016). Executive functions in children with specific language impairment: A meta-analysis. *Journal of Speech, Language, and Hearing Research, 59,* 1074–1086. https://doi.org/10.1044/2016_JSLHR-L-15-0174

Pavelko, S. L., & Owens, R. E. (2017). Sampling Utterances and Grammatical Analysis Revised (SUGAR): New normative values for language sample analysis measures. *Language, Speech and Hearing Services in Schools, 48,* 197–215. https://doi.org/10.1044/2017_LSHSS-17-0022

Pavelko, S. L., & Owens, R. E. (2019a). Diagnostic accuracy of the SUGAR measures for identifying children with language impairment. *Language, Speech, and Hearing Services in Schools, 50*(2), 211–223. https://https://doi.org/org/10.1044/2018_LSHSS-18-0050

Pavelko, S. L., & Owens, R. E. (2019b). SUGAR (Sampling Utterances and Grammatical Analysis Revised): Breaking tradition. *Language, Speech, and Hearing Services in Schools, 50*, 452–456.

Pavelko, S. L., Owens, R. E., Ireland, M., & Hahs-Vaughn, D. L. (2016). Use of language sample analysis by school-based SLPs: Results of a nationwide survey. *Language, Speech, and Hearing Services in Schools, 47*, 246–258. https://doi.org/10.1044/2016_LSHSS-15-0044

Pavelko, S. L., Price, L. R., & Owens, R. E. (2020). Revisiting reliability: Using Sampling Utterances and Grammatical Analysis Revised (SUGAR) to compare 25- and 50-utterance language samples. *Language, Speech, and Hearing Services in Schools, 51*(3), 778–794.

Pawlowska, M. (2014). Evaluation of three proposed markers for language impairment in English: A meta-analysis of diagnostic accuracy studies. *Journal of Speech, Language, and Hearing Research, 57*, 2261–2273. https://doi.org/10.1044/2014_JSLHR-L-13-0189

Pearce, W., McCormack, P., & James, D. (2003). Exploring the boundaries of SLI: Findings from morphosyntactic and story grammar analyses. *Clinical Linguistics & Phonetics, 17*, 325–334.

Peets, K. F. (2009). The effects of context on the classroom discourse skills of children with language impairment. *Language, Speech, and Hearing Services in Schools, 40*, 5–16.

Peña, E. D. (2002, April). *Solving the problems of biased speech and language assessment with bilingual children.* Paper presented at the Annual Convention of the New York State Speech-Language-Hearing Association, Rochester, NY.

Peña, E. D., Bedore, L. M., & Kester, E. S. (2015). Discriminant accuracy of a semantics measure with Latino English-speaking, Spanish-speaking, and English–Spanish bilingual children. *Journal of Communication Disorders, 53*, 30–41. https://doi.org/10.1016/j.jcomdis.2014.11.001

Peña, E. D., Bedore, L. M., & Kester, E. S. (2016). Assessment of language impairment in bilingual children using semantic tasks: Two languages classify better than one. *International Journal of Language & Communication Disorders, 51*, 192–202. https://https://doi.org/org/10.1111/1460-6984.12199

Peña, E. D., Bedore, L. M., & Zlatic-Giunta, R. (2002). Category-generation performance of bilingual children: The influence of condition, category, and language. *Journal of Speech, Language, and Hearing Research, 45*(5), 938–947. https://doi.org/10.1044/1092-4388(2002/076)

Peña, E. D., Gillam, R. B., & Bedore, L. M. (2014). Dynamic assessment of narrative ability in English accurately identifies language impairment in English language learners. *Journal of Speech, Language, and Hearing Research, 57*, 2208–2220. https://doi.org/10.1044/2014_JSLHR-L-13-0151

Peña, E. D., Gillam, R. B., Malek, M., Felter, R., Resendiz, M., Fiestas, C., & Sabel, T. (2006). Dynamic assessment of children from culturally diverse backgrounds: Applica-

tions to narrative assessment. *Journal of Speech, Language, and Hearing Research, 49*, 1037–1057.

Peña, E. D., Gutiérrez-Clellen, V. F., Iglesias, A., Goldstein, B. A., & Bedore, L. M. (2018). *Bilingual English–Spanish Assessment (BESA).* Brookes.

Peña, E. D., & Halle, T. G. (2011). Assessing preschool dual language learners: Traveling a multiforked road. *Child Development Perspectives, 5*, 28–32. https://doi.org/10.1111/j.1750-8606.2010.00143.x

Peña, E. D., Iglesias, A., & Lidz, C. S. (2001). Reducing test bias through dynamic assessment of children's word learning ability. *American Journal of Speech-Language Pathology, 10*, 138–154.

Peña, E. D., Kester, S. K., & Sheng, L. (2012). Semantic development in Spanish–English bilinguals: Theory, assessment, and intervention. In B. A. Goldstein (Ed.), *Bilingual language development and disorders in Spanish–English speakers* (2nd ed., pp. 131–152). Brookes.

Pence, K. L., Justice, L. M., & Wiggins, A. K. (2008). Preschool teachers' fidelity in implementing a comprehensive language-rich curriculum. *Language, Speech, and Hearing Services in Schools, 39*, 329–341.

Pennington, B. F., & Lefly, D. L. (2001). Early reading development in children at family risk for dyslexia. *Child Development, 72*, 816–833. https://doi.org/10.1111/1467-8624.00317 http://scholar.google.com/scholar_lookup?hl=en&volume=72&publication_year=2001&pages=816-833&journal=Child+Development&author=B.+F.+Pennington&author=D.+L.+Lefly&title=Early+reading+development+in+children+at+family+risk+for+dyslexia

Pennington, B. F., Santerre-Lemmon, L., Rosenberg, J., MacDonald, B., Boada, R., Friend, A., . . . Olson, R. K. (2012). Individual prediction of dyslexia by single versus multiple deficit models. *Journal of Abnormal Psychology, 121*, 212–224. https://doi.org/10.1037/a0025823 http://scholar.google.com/scholar_lookup?hl=en&volume=121&publication_year=2012&pages=212-224&journal=Journal+of+Abnormal+Psychology&author=B.+F.+Pennington&author=L.+Santerre-Lemmon&author=J.+Rosenberg&author=B.+MacDonald&author=R.+Boada&author=A.+Friend&author=R.+K.+Olson&title=Individual+prediction+of+dyslexia+by+single+versus+multiple+deficit+models

Peredo, T. N., Zelaya, M. I., & Kaiser, A. P. (2017). Teaching low-income Spanish-speaking caregivers to implement EMT en Español with their young children with language impairment: A pilot study. *American Journal of Speech-Language Pathology, 27*, 136–153. https://doi.org/10.1044/2017_AJSLP-16-0228

Perfetti, C., & Stafura, J. (2014). Word knowledge in a theory of reading comprehension. *Scientific Studies of Reading, 18*, 22–37. https://doi.org/10.1080/10888438.2013.827687

Perrault, A., Chaby, L. Bigouret, F., Oppetit, A., Cohen, D., Plaza, M., & Xavier, J. (2018). Comprehension of conventional gestures in typical children, children with autism spectrum disorders and children with language disorders.

Neuropsychiatrie de l'Enfance et de l'Adolescence, 67, 1–9. https://doi.org/10.1016/j.neurenf.2018.03.002

Petersen, D. B. (2011). A systematic review of narrative-based language intervention with children who have language impairment. *Communication Disorders Quarterly, 32*, 207–220.

Petersen, D. B., Brown, C., Ukrainetz, T. A., Wise, C., Spencer, T. D., & Zebre, J. (2014). Systematic individualized narrative language intervention on the personal narratives of children with autism. *Language, Speech, and Hearing Services in Schools, 45*, 67–86.

Petersen, D. B., Chanthongthip, H., Ukrainetz, T. A., Spencer, T. D., & Steeve, R. W. (2017). Dynamic assessment of narratives: Efficient, accurate identification of language impairment in bilingual students. *Journal of Speech, Language, and Hearing Disorders, 60*, 983–998. https://doi.org/10.1044/2016_JSLHR-L-15-0426

Petersen, D. B., Gillam, S. L., Spencer, T. D., & Gillam, R. B. (2010). The effects of literate narrative intervention on children with neurologically based language impairments: An early stage study. *Journal of Speech, Language, and Hearing Research, 53*, 961–981.

Petersen, D. B., & Spencer, T. D. (2012). The narrative language measures: Tools for language screening, progress monitoring, and intervention planning. *Perspectives on Language Learning and Education, 19*, 119–129.

Petersen, D. B., & Spencer, T. D. (2016). *CUBED narrative language measures (NLM)*. https://www.languagedynamicsgroup.com/cubed/cubed_download

Petersen, E. A. (2003). *A practical guide to early childhood curriculum: Linking thematic, emergent, and skill-based planning to children's outcomes* (2nd ed.). Allyn & Bacon.

Pezold, M. J., Imgrund, C. M., & Storkel, C. M. (2020). Using computer programs for language sample analysis. *Language, Speech, and Hearing Services in Schools, 51*, 103–114. https://doi.org/10.1044/2019_LSHSS-18-0148

Pham, G., Kohnert, K., & Mann, D. (2011). Addressing clinician–client mismatch: A preliminary intervention study with a bilingual Vietnamese–English preschooler. *Language, Speech, and Hearing Services in Schools, 42*, 408–422.

Pham, G., & Tipton, T. (2018). Internal and external factors that support children's minority first language and English. *Language, Speech, and Hearing Services in Schools, 49*, 595–606. https://doi.org/10.1044/2018_LSHSS-17-0086

Phelps-Terasaki, D., & Phelps-Gunn, T. (2007). *Test of Pragmatic Language–Second Edition* (TOPL-2). Psychological Corporation.

Phillips, B. M., Tabulda, G., Ingrole, S. A., Webb Burris, P., Sedgwick, T. K., & Chen, S. (2016). Literate language intervention with high-need prekindergarten children: A randomized trial. *Journal of Speech, Language, and Hearing Research, 59*, 1409–1420. https://doi.org/10.1044/2016_JSLHR-L-15-0155

Philofsky, A., Hepburn, S. L., Hayes, A., Hagerman, R., & Rogers, S. J. (2004). Language and cognitive functioning and autism symptoms in young children with fragile X syndrome. *American Journal on Mental Retardation, 109*, 208–218.

Pianta, R. C., Howes, C., Burchinal, M., Bryant, D., Clifford, R., Early, D. M., & Barbarin, O. A. (2005). Features of pre-kindergarten programs, classrooms, and teachers: Do they predict observed classroom quality and child–teacher interactions? *Applied Developmental Science, 9*, 144–159. http://scholar.google.com/scholar_lookup?hl=en&publication_year=2005&pages=144-159&title=Features+of+pre-kindergarten+programs%2C+classrooms%2C+and+teachers%3A+Do+they+predict+observed+classroom+quality+and+child-teacher+interactions%3F

Pickering, M. J., & Ferreira, V. S. (2008). Structural priming: A critical review. *Psychological Bulletin, 134*, 427–459.

Pickett, E., Pullara, O., O'Grady, J., & Gordon, B. (2009). Speech acquisition in older nonverbal individuals with autism: A review of features, methods, and prognosis. *Cognitive and Behavioral Neurology, 22*(1), 1–21. https://doi.org/10.1097/WNN.0b013e318190d185

Pieretti, R. A. (2011). *Response to intervention and literacy: A bright spot for Hmong-speaking English language learners?* Available from ProQuest Dissertations and Theses database (UMI No. 3474448), Proposition 227—Full Text of the Proposed Law (1998). https://www.semanticscholar.org/paper/Response-to-Intervention-and-Literacy%3A-A-Bright-for-Pieretti/d464ea0fdf7df2eaa94010d6ef64e1ed61f17a0e

Pieretti, R. A., & Roseberry-McKibbin, C. (2016). Assessment and intervention for English language learners with primary language impairment: Research-based best practices. *Communication Disorders Quarterly, 37*, 117–128.

Plakas, A., van Zuijen, T., van Leeuwen, T., Thomson, J. M., & van der Leij, A. (2013). Impaired non-speech auditory processing at a pre-reading age is a risk-factor for dyslexia but not a predictor: An ERP study. *Cortex, 49*(4), 1034–1045.

Plante, E., Ogilvie, T., Vance, R., Aguilar, J. M., Dailey, N. S., Meyers, C., . . . Burton, R. (2014). Variability in the language input to children enhances learning in a treatment context. *American Journal of Speech-Language Pathology, 23*, 530–545. https://doi.org/10.1044/2014_AJSLP-13-0038

Plante, E., Vance, R., Moody, A., & Gerken, L. (2013). What influences children's conceptualizations of language input? *Journal of Speech, Language, and Hearing Research, 56*, 1613–1624.

Pokorni, J. L., Worthington, C. K., & Jamison, P. J. (2004). Phonological awareness intervention: Comparison of Fast For Word, Earobics, and LiPS. *Journal of Educational Research, 97*, 147–157.

Popova, S., Lange, S., Shield, K., Mihic, A., Chudley, A. E., Mukherjee, R.A.S., . . . Rehm, J. (2016). Comorbidity of fetal alcohol spectrum disorder: A systematic review and meta-analysis. *Lancet, 387*(10022), 978–987. https://doi.org/10.1016/S0140-6736(15)01345-8

Porzsolt, F., Ohletz, A., Gardner, D., Ruatti, H., Meier, H., Schlotz-Gorton, N., & Schrott, L. (2003). Evidence-based decision making: The 6-step approach. *American College of Physicians Journal Club, 139*(3), 1–6.

REFERENCES

Potocki, A., & Laval, V. (2019). Comprehension and inference: Relationships between oral and written modalities in good and poor comprehenders during adolescence. *Journal of Speech, Language, and Hearing Research, 62*, 3431–3442. https://doi.org/10.1044/2019_JSLHR-L-18-0400

Prelock, P. A., Beatson, J., Bitner, B., Broder, C., & Ducker, A. (2003). Interdisciplinary assessment of young children with autism spectrum disorder. *Language, Speech, and Hearing Services in Schools, 34*, 194–202.

Prelock, P. A., Miller, B. L., & Reed, N. L. (1995). Collaborative partnerships in a language in the classroom program. *Language, Speech, and Hearing Services in Schools, 26*, 286–292.

Prendeville, J., & Ross-Allen, J. (2002). The transition process in the early years: Enhancing speech-language pathologists' perspective. *Language, Speech, and Hearing Services in Schools, 33*, 130–136.

Price, J. R., & Jackson, S. C. (2015). Procedures for obtaining and analyzing writing samples of school-age children and adolescents. *Language, Speech, and Hearing Services in Schools, 46*, 277–293. https://doi.org/10.1044/2015_LSHSS-14-0057

Price, J. R., Roberts, J. E., Hennon, E. A., Berni, M. C., Anderson, K. L., & Sideris, J. (2008). Syntactic complexity during conversation of boys with fragile X syndrome and Down syndrome. *Journal of Speech, Language, and Hearing Research, 51*, 3–15.

Proctor-Williams, K., Fey, M. E., & Frome Loeb, D. (2001). Parental recasts and production of copulas and articles by children with specific language impairment and typical language. *American Journal of Speech-Language Pathology, 10*, 155–168.

Pruitt, S. L., & Oetting, J. B. (2009). Past tense marking by African American English-speaking children reared in poverty. *Journal of Speech, Language, and Hearing Research, 52*, 2–15. https://doi.org/10.1044/1092-4388(2008/07-0176)

Pruitt, S. L., Oetting, J. B., & Hegarty, M. (2011). Passive participle marking by African American English-speaking children reared in poverty. *Journal of Speech, Language, and Hearing Research, 54*, 598–607.

Prutting, C. A., & Kirchner, D. M. (1983). Applied pragmatics. In T. M. Gallagher & C. A. Prutting (Eds.), *Pragmatic assessment and intervention issues in language* (pp. 29– 64). Pro-Ed.

Prutting, C. A., & Kirchner, D. M. (1987). A clinical appraisal of the pragmatic aspects of language. *Journal of Speech and Hearing Disorders, 52*, 105–119.

Pry, R., Petersen, A., & Baghdadli, A. (2005). The relationship between expressive language level and psychological development in children with autism 5 years of age. *Autism, 9*, 179–189.

Pua, E. P. K., Lee, L. C. M., & Rickard Liow, S. J. (2013). *Bilingual Language Assessment Battery (BLAB): Preschool Parent and Teacher Report*. Unpublished measure, National University of Singapore.

Puranik, C. S., Lombardino, L. J., & Altmann, L. J. (2007). Writing through retellings: An exploratory study of language impaired and dyslexic populations. *Reading and Writing, 20*, 251–272.

Puranik, C. S., Lombardino, L. J., & Altmann, L. J. P. (2008). Assessing the microstructure of written language using a retelling paradigm. *American Journal of Speech-Language Pathology, 17*, 107–120. https://doi.org/10.1044/1058-0360(2008/012)

Pye, C. (1987). *Pye Analysis of Language (PAL)* [Computer program]. University of Kansas.

Qi, C. H., & Kaiser, A. P. (2004). Problem behaviors of low-income children with language delays: An observational study. *Journal of Speech, Language, and Hearing Research, 47*, 595–609.

Qi, C. H., Kaiser, A. P., Milan, S. E., Yzquierdo, Z., & Hancock, T. B. (2003). The performance of low-income African American children on the Preschool Language Scale–3. *Journal of Speech, Language, and Hearing Research, 46*, 576–590.

Quail, M., Williams, C., & Leitao, S. (2009). Verbal working memory in specific language impairment: The effect of providing visual support. *International Journal of Speech-Language Pathology, 11*, 220–233.

Quinn, J. M., Wagner, R. K., Petscher, Y., & Lopez, D. (2015). Developmental relations between vocabulary knowledge and reading comprehension: A latent change score modeling study. *Child Development, 86*, 159–175. https://doi.org/10.1111/cdev.12292.

Raghavan, R., Camarata, S., White, K., Barbaresi, W., Parish, S., & Krahn, G. (2018). Population health in pediatric speech and language disorders: Available data sources and a research agenda for the field. *Journal of Speech, Language, and Hearing Research, 61*, 1279–1291. https://doi.org/10.1044/2018_JSLHR-L-16-0459

Rajesh, V., & Venkatesh, L. (2019). Preliminary evaluation of a low-intensity parent training program on speech-language stimulation for children with language delay. *International Journal of Pediatric Otorhinolaryngology, 22*, 99–104. https://doi.org/10.1016/j.ijporl.2019.03.034

Ramchand, G. (2008). *Verb meaning and the lexicon: A first phase syntax*. Cambridge University Press.

Ramus, F., Marshall, C. R., Rosen, S., & van der Lely, H. K. (2013). Phonological deficits in specific language impairment and developmental dyslexia: Towards a multidimensional model. *Brain, 136*(2), 630–645.

Randall, L., & Tyldesley, K. (2016). Evaluating the impact of working memory training programmes on children—A systematic review. *Educational & Child Psychology, 33*, 34–50.

Rankin, P. M., & Hood, J. (2005). Designing clinical interventions for children with specific memory disorders. *Pediatric Rehabilitation, 8*, 283–297.

Rao, P. A., Beidel, D. C., & Murray, M. J. (2008). Social skills interventions for children with Asperger's syndrome or high-functioning autism: A review and recommendations. *Journal of the American Academy of Child & Adolescent Psychiatry, 38*, 353–361. https://doi.org/10.1007/s10803-007-0402-4

Redmond, S. M. (2002). The use of rating scales with children who have language impairments: A tutorial. *American Journal of Speech-Language Pathology, 11,* 124–138.

Redmond, S. M. (2004). Conversational profiles of children with ADHD, SLI and typical development. *Clinical Linguistics & Phonetics, 18,* 107–125.

Redmond, S. M. (2011). Peer victimization among students with specific language impairment, attention-deficit/hyperactivity disorder, and typical development. *Language, Speech, and Hearing Services in Schools, 42,* 520–535.

Redmond, S. M. (2016). Language impairment in attention-deficit/hyperactive disorder context. *Journal of Speech, Language and Hearing Research, 59,* 133–142. https://doi.org/ 10.1044/2015_JSLHR-L-15-0038.

Redmond, S. M., Ash, A. C., & Hogan, T. P. (2015). Consequences of co-occurring attention-deficit/hyperactive disorder on children's language impairments. *Language, Speech and Hearing Services in Schools, 46,* 68–80. https://doi.org/ 10.1044/2014_LSHSS-14-0045

Redmond, S. M., & Rice, M. L. (2001). Detection of irregular verb violations by children with and without SLI. *Journal of Speech, Language, and Hearing Research, 44,* 655–669.

Redmond, S. M., & Rice, M. L. (2002). Stability of behavioral ratings of children with SLI. *Journal of Speech, Language, and Hearing Research, 45,* 190–201.

Redmond, S. M., Thompson, H. L., & Goldstein, S. (2011). Psycholinguistic profiling differentiates specific language impairment from typical development and from attention deficit/hyperactivity disorder. *Journal of Speech, Language, and Hearing Research, 41,* 688–700.

Reed, V. (2012). *An introduction to children with language disorders* (4th ed.). Pearson.

Reed, V. A., & Spicer, L. (2003). The relative importance of selected communication skills for adolescents' interactions with their teachers: High school teachers' opinions. *Language, Speech, and Hearing Services in Schools, 34,* 343–357.

Reese, E., Yan, C., Jack, F., & Hayne, H. (2010). Emerging identities: Narrative and self from early childhood to early adolescence. In K. C. McLean & M. Pasupathi (Eds.), *Narrative development in adolescence* (pp. 23–43). Springer.

Reichle, J., Beukelman, D., & Light, J. (2002). *Implementing an augmentative communication system: Exemplary strategies for beginning communicators.* Brookes.

Reichle, J., Dropik, P. L., Alden-Anderson, E., & Haley, T. (2008). Teaching a young child with autism to request assistance conditionally: A preliminary study. *American Journal of Speech-Language Pathology, 17,* 231–240.

Reichle, J., & McComas, J. (2004). Conditional use of a request for assistance. *Disability and Rehabilitation, 26,* 1255–1262.

Reid, D. K., Hresko, W. P., & Hammill, D. H. (2017). *Test of Early Reading Ability, Fourth Edition (TERA-4).* Western Psychological Services.

Reilly, J., Losh, M., Bellugi, U., & Wulfeck, B. (2004). Frog, where are you? Narratives in children with specific language impairment, early focal brain injury and Williams syndrome. *Brain & Language, 88,* 229–247.

Reilly, S., Bishop, D. V. M., & Tomblin, B. (2014). Terminological debate over language impairment in children: Forward movement and sticking points. *International Journal of Language & Communication Disorders, 49,* 452–462. https://doi.org/10.1111/1460-6984.12111

Reilly, S., Wake, M., Ukoumunne, O. C., Bavin, E., Prior, M., Cini, E., . . . Bretherton, L. (2010). Predicting language outcomes at 4 years of age: Findings from Early Language in Victoria Study. *Pediatrics, 126,* e1530–e1537. https://doi.org/10.1542/peds.2010-0254

Rescorla, L. A. (2005). Age 13 language and reading outcomes in late talking toddlers. *Journal of Speech, Language, and Hearing Research, 48,* 459–473.

Rescorla, L. A. (2009). Age 17 language and reading outcomes in late-talking toddlers: Support for a dimensional perspective on language delay. *Journal of Speech, Language, and Hearing Research, 52,* 16–30.

Rescorla, L. A., Ross, G. S., & McClure, S. (2007). Language delay and behavioral/emotional problems in toddlers: Findings from two developmental clinics. *Journal of Speech, Language, and Hearing Research, 50,* 1063–1078.

Restrepo, M. A. (1998). Identifiers of predominantly Spanish-speaking children with language impairment. *Journal of Speech, Language, and Hearing Research, 41,* 1398–1411.

Restrepo, M. A., Castilla, A. P., Schwanenflugel, P. J., Neuharth-Pritchett, S., Hamilton, C. E., & Arboleda, A. (2010). Supplemental oral language program in sentence length, complexity, and grammaticality in Spanish-speaking children attending English-only preschools. *Language, Speech, and Hearing Services in Schools, 41,* 3–13.

Restrepo, M. A., & Gutiérrez-Clellen, V. F. (2012). Grammatical impairments in Spanish–English bilingual children. In B. A. Goldstein (Ed.), *Bilingual language development and disorders in Spanish–English speakers* (2nd ed., pp. 213–232). Brookes.

Restrepo, M. A., & Kruth, K. (2000). Grammatical characteristics of a Spanish–English bilingual child with specific language impairment. *Communication Disorders Quarterly, 21,* 66–76. https://doi.org/10.1177/152574010002100201

Restrepo, M. A., Morgan, G. P., & Thompson, M. S. (2013). The efficacy of a vocabulary intervention for dual-language learners with language impairment. *Journal of Speech, Language, and Hearing Research, 56,* 748–765.

Rezzonico, S., Goldberg, A., Mak, K. K., Yap, S., Milburn, T., Belletti, A., & Girolametto, L. (2016). Narratives in two languages: Storytelling of bilingual Cantonese–English preschoolers. *Journal of Speech, Language, and Hearing Research, 59,* 521–532. https://doi.org/10.1044/2015_JSLHR-L-15-0052

Riccio, C. A., Cash, D. L., & Cohen, M. J. (2007). Learning and memory performance of children with specific language impairment (SLI). *Applied Neuropsychology, 14,* 255–261.

Rice, M. L. (2012). Toward epigenetic and gene regulation models of specific language impairment: Looking for links among growth, genes, and impairments. *Journal of Neurodevelopmental Disorders, 4,* 27. https://doi.org/10.1186/1866-1955-4-27

Rice, M. L. (2017). *Specific language impairment in children.* https://www.openaccessgovernment.org/specific-language-impairment-in-children/40152/

Rice, M. L., Cleave, P. L., & Oetting, J. B. (2000). The use of syntactic cues in lexical acquisition by children with SLI. *Journal of Speech, Language, and Hearing Research, 43,* 582–594.

Rice, M. L., & Hoffman, L. (2015). Predicting vocabulary growth in children with and without specific language impairment: A longitudinal study from 2;6 to 21 years of age. *Journal of Speech, Language, and Hearing Research, 58,* 345–359. https://doi.org/10.1044/2015_JSLHR-L-14-0150

Rice, M. L., Hoffman, L., & Wexler, K. (2009). Judgments of omitted BE and DO in questions as extended finiteness clinical markers of specific language impairment (SLI) to 15 years: A study of growth and asymptote. *Journal of Speech, Language, and Hearing Research, 52,* 1417–1433.

Rice, M. L., Redmont, S. M., & Hoffman, L. (2006). Mean length of utterance in children with specific language impairment and in younger control children shows concurrent validity and stable and parallel growth trajectories. *Journal of Speech, Language, and Hearing Research, 49,* 793–808.

Rice, M. L., Smolik, F., Perpich, D., Thompson, T., Rytting, N., & Blossom, M. (2010). Mean length of utterance levels in 6-month intervals for children 3 to 9 years with and without language impairments. *Journal of Speech, Language, and Hearing Research, 53,* 333–349.

Rice, M. L., Taylor, C. L., & Zubrick, S. R. (2008). Language outcomes of 7-year-old children with or without a history of late language emergence at 24 months. *Journal of Speech, Language, and Hearing Research, 51,* 394–407. https://doi.org/10.1044/1092-4388(2008/029)

Rice, M. L., Taylor, C. L., Zubrick, S. R., Hoffman, L., & Earnest, K. K. (2020). Heritability of specific language impairment and nonspecific language impairment at ages 4 and 6 years across phenotypes of speech, language, and nonverbal cognition. *Journal of Speech, Language, and Hearing Research, 63,* 793–813.

Riches, N. G., Loucas, T., Baird, G., Charman, T., & Simonoff, E. (2010). Sentence repetition in adolescents with specific language impairments and autism: An investigation of complex syntax. *International Journal of Language & Communication Disorders, 45,* 47–60.

Riches, N. G., Tomasello, M., & Conti-Ramsden, G. (2005). Verb learning in children with SLI: Frequency and spacing effects. *Journal of Speech, Language, and Hearing Research, 48,* 1397–1411.

Richman, D. M., Wacker, D. P., & Winborn, L. (2001). Response efficiency during functional communication training: Effects of effort and response allocation. *Journal of Applied Behavior Analysis, 34,* 73–36.

Ricketts, J., Bishop, D. V. M., & Nation, K.(2009). Orthographic facilitation in oral vocabulary acquisition. *Quarterly Journal of Experimental Psychology, 62,* 1948–1966. https://doi.org/10.1080/17470210802696104 http://scholar.google.com/scholar_lookup?hl=en&volume=62&publication_year=2009&pages=1948-1966&journal=Quarterly+Journal+of+Experimental+Psychology&author=J.+Ricketts&author=D.+V.+M.+Bishop&author=K.+Nation&title=Orthographic+facilitation+in+oral+vocabulary+acquisition

Ricketts, J., Davies, R., Masterson, J., Stuart, M., & Duff, F. J. (2016). Evidence for semantic involvement in regular and exception word reading in emergent readers of English. *Journal of Experimental Child Psychology, 150,* 330–345. https://doi.org/10.1016/j.jecp.2016.05.013 http://scholar.google.com/scholar_lookup?hl=en&volume=150&publication_year=2016&pages=330-345&journal=Journal+of+Experimental+Child+Psychology&author=J.+Ricketts&author=R.+Davies&author=J.+Masterson&author=M.+Stuart&author=F.+J.+Duff&title=Evidence+for+semantic+involvement+in+regular+and+exception+word+reading+in+emergent+readers+of+English

Ricketts, J., Dockrell, J. E., Patel, N., Charman, T., & Lindsay, G. (2015). Do children with specific language impairment and autism spectrum disorders benefit from the presence of orthography when learning new spoken words? *Journal of Experimental Child Psychology, 134,* 43–61. https://doi.org/10.1016/j.jecp.2015.01.015

Ricketts, J., Nation, K., & Bishop, D. V. M. (2007). Vocabulary is important for some, but not all reading skills. *Scientific Studies of Reading, 11,* 235–257. https://doi.org/10.1080/10888430701344306 http://scholar.google.com/scholar_lookup?hl=en&volume=11&publication_year=2007&pages=235-257&journal=Scientific+Studies+of+Reading&author=J.+Ricketts&author=K.+Nation&author=D.+V.+M.+Bishop&title=Vocabulary+is+important+for+some%2C+but+not+all+reading+skills

Rimm-Kaufman, S. E., Pianta, R. C., & Cox, M. J. (2000). Teachers' judgments of problems in the transition to kindergarten. *Early Childhood Research Quarterly, 15,* 147–166.

Riquelme, L. F., & Rosas, J. (2014). Multicultural perspectives: The road to cultural competence. In N. C. Singleton & B. B. Shulman (Eds.), *Language development: Foundations, processes, and clinical applications* (2nd ed., pp. 231–249). Jones & Bartlett.

Rispens, J., & Baker, A. (2012). Nonword repetition: The relative contributions of phonological short-term memory and phonological representations in children with language and reading impairment. *Journal of Speech, Language, and Hearing Research, 55,* 683–694.

Rispoli, M. (2019). The sequential unfolding of first phase syntax: Tutorial and applications to development. *Journal of Speech, Language, and Hearing Research, 62,* 693–705. https://doi.org/10.1044/2018_JSLHR-L-18-0227

Rispoli, M., & Hadley, P. (2001). The leading-edge: The significance of sentence disruption in the development of grammar. *Journal of Speech, Language, and Hearing Research, 44,* 1131–1143.

Rivière, A. M., Oetting, J. B., & Roy, J. (2018). Effects of specific language impairment on a contrastive dialect structure: The case of infinitival TO across various nonmainstream dialects of English. *Journal of Speech, Language,* and Hearing Disorders, 61, 1989–2001. https://doi.org/10.1044/2018_JSLHR-L-17-0209

Roberts, J. A., Altenberg, E. P., & Hunter, M. (2020). Machine-scored syntax: Comparison of the CLAN automatic scoring program to manual scoring. Language, Speech, and Hearing Services in Schools, 51, 479–493. https://doi.org/10.1044/2019_LSHSS-19-00056

Roberts, J. A., Altenberg, E. P., Hunter, H., & Lang, M. (2020). Machine-scored syntax: Comparison of the CLAN automatic scoring program to manual scoring. Language, Speech, and Hearing Services in Schools, 51, 479–493. https://doi.org/10.1044/2019_LSHSS-19-00056

Roberts, J. E., Long, S. H., Malkin, C., Barnes, E., Skinner, M., Hennon, E. A., & Anderson, K. (2005). A comparison of phonological skills with fragile X syndrome and Down syndrome. Journal of Speech, Language, and Hearing Research, 48, 980–995.

Roberts, J. E., Martin, G. E., Maskowitz, L., Harris, A. A., Foreman, J., & Nelson, L. (2007). Discourse skills of boys with fragile X syndrome in comparison to boys with Down syndrome. Journal of Speech, Language, and Hearing Research, 50, 475–492.

Roberts, J. E., Mirrett, P., & Burchinal, M. (2001). Receptive and expressive communication development in young males with fragile X syndrome. American Journal of Mental Retardation, 106, 216–231.

Roberts, M. Y., & Kaiser, A. P. (2011). The effectiveness of parent-implemented language interventions: A meta-analysis. American Journal of Speech-Language Pathology, 20, 180–199.

Roberts, M. Y., & Kaiser, A. P. (2015). Early intervention for toddlers with language delays: A randomized controlled trial. Pediatrics, 135, 686–693. https://doi.org/10.1542/peds.2014-2134

Roberts, M. Y., Kaiser, A. P., Wolfe, C. E., Bryant, J. D., & Spidalieri, A. M. (2014). Effects of the teach–model–coach–review instructional approach on caregiver use of language support strategies and children's expressive language skills. Journal of Speech, Language, and Hearing Research, 57, 1851–1869. https://doi.org/10.1044/2014_JSLHR-L-13-0113

Roberts, M. Y., Kaiser, A. P., & Wright, C. (2010). Parent training: Specific strategies beyond "Try this at home." Paper presented at the annual convention of the American Speech-Language-Hearing Association, Philadelphia, PA.

Robertson, C., & Salter, W. (2017). Phonological Awareness Test (PAT). Linguisystems.

Rodekohr, R., & Haynes, W. O. (2001). Differentiating dialect from disorder: A comparison of two processing tasks and a standardized language test. Journal of Communication Disorders, 34, 255–272.

Rodriguez, B. L., Hines, R., & Montiel, M. (2009). Mexican American mothers of low and middle socioeconomic status: Communication behaviors and interactive strategies during shared book reading. Language, Speech, and Hearing Services in Schools, 40, 271–282.

Rodriguez, B. L., & Olswang, L. B. (2003). Mexican American and Anglo-American mothers' beliefs and values about child rearing, education, and language impairment. American Journal of Speech-Language Pathology, 12, 452–462.

Rollins, P. R., McCabe, A., & Bliss, L. (2000). Culturally sensitive assessment of narrative in children. Seminars in Speech and Language, 21, 223–234.

Rolstad, K., Mahoney, K., & Glass, G. V. (2005). The big picture: A meta-analysis of program effectiveness research on English language learners. Educational Policy, 19, 572–594. https://doi.org/10.1177/0895904805278067

Romano, M., Eugenio, J., & Kiratzis, E. (2021). Coaching childcare providers to support toddlers' gesture use with children experiencing early childhood poverty. Language, Speech, and Hearing Services in Schools, 52, 686–701. https://doi.org/10.1044/2020_LSHSS-20-00112

Romski, M. A., & Sevcik, R. A. (2005). Augmentative communication and early intervention: Myths and realities. Infants and Young Children, 18, 174–185.

Romski, M. A., Sevcik, R. A., Cheslock, M. B., & Hyatt, A. (2002). Enhancing communication competence in beginning communicators: Identifying a continuum of AAC language intervention strategies. In J. Reichle, D. Beukelman, & J. Light (Eds.), Implementing an augmentative communication system: Exemplary strategies for beginning communicators (pp. 1–23). Brookes.

Romski, M. A., Sevcik, R. A., & Forrest, S. (2001). Assistive technology and augmentative communication in early childhood inclusion. In M. J. Guralnick (Ed.), Early childhood inclusion: Focus on change (pp. 465–479). Brookes.

Roper, N., & Dunst, C. J. (2003). Communication intervention in natural environments. Infants & Young Children, 16, 215–225.

Rosa-Lugo, L. I., Mihai, F. M., & Nutta, J. W. (2012). Language and literacy development: An interdisciplinary focus on English learners with communication disorders. Plural Publishing.

Roseberry-McKibbin, C. (2014). Increasing oral and literate language skills of children in poverty. Professional development continuing education program. American Speech-Language-Hearing Association.

Roseberry-McKibbin, C., Brice, A. E., & O'Hanlon, L. (2005). Serving English language learners in public school settings: A national survey. Language, Speech, and Hearing Services in Schools, 36, 48–61.

Ross, G., Demaria, R., & Yap, V. (2018). The relationship between motor delays and language development in very low birthweight premature children at 18 months corrected age. Journal of Speech, Language, and Hearing Disorders, 61, 114–119. https://doi.org/10.1044/2017_JSLHR-L-17-0056

Roth, F. P. (1986). Oral narrative abilities of learning-disabled students. Topics in Language Disorders, 7(1), 1–30.

Roth, F. P. (2000). Narrative writing: Development and teaching with children with writing difficulties. Topics in Language Disorders, 20(4), 15–28.

REFERENCES

Roth, F. P., Dixon, D. A., Paul, D. R., & Bellini, P. I. (2013). *RtI in action grades 3–5: Oral and written language activities for the Common Core State Standards*. American Speech-Language-Hearing Association.

Rouse, C. E., & Krueger, A. B. (2004). Putting computerized instruction to the test: A randomized evaluation of a "scientifically based" reading program. *Economics of Education Review*, *23*, 323–338.

Rowland, C., & Schweigert, P. D. (2000). Tangible symbols, tangible outcomes. *Augmentative and Alternative Communication*, *16*, 61–78.

Roy, J., Oetting, J. B., & Moland, C. W. (2013). Linguistic constraints on children's overt marking of BE by dialect and age. *Journal of Speech, Language, and Hearing Research*, *56*, 933–944.

Rubin, K. H., Begle, A. S., & McDonald, K. L. (2012). Peer relations and social competence in childhood. In V. Anderson & M. H. Beauchamp (Eds.), *Developmental social neuroscience and childhood brain insult: Theory and practice* (pp. 23–44). Guilford.

Rudolph, J. M. (2017). Case history risk factors for specific language impairment: A systematic review and meta-analysis. *American Journal of Speech-Language Pathology*, *26*, 991–1010. https://doi.org/10.1044/2016_AJSLP-15-0181

Rudolph, J. M., & Leonard, L. B. (2016). Early language milestones and specific language impairment. *Journal of Early Intervention*, *38*, 41–58.

Rush, D. D., & Shelden, M. L. (2011). *The early childhood coaching handbook*. Brookes.

Rutter, M., Caspi, A., Fergusson, D., Horwood, L. J., Goodman, R., Maughan, B., . . . Carroll, J. (2004). Sex differences in developmental reading disability: New findings from 4 epidemiological studies. *Journal of the American Medical Association*, *291*, 2007–2012.

Rutter, M. L., Kreppner, J. M., & O'Connor, T. G. (2001). Specificity and heterogeneity in children's responses to profound institutional privation. *British Journal of Psychiatry*, *179*(2), 97–103.

Rvachew, S., Ohberg, A., Grawburg, M., & Heyding, J. (2003). Phonological awareness and phonemic perception in 4-year-old children with delayed expressive phonological skills. *American Journal of Speech-Language Pathology*, *12*, 463–471.

Saddler, B. (2013). Best practices in sentence construction skills. In S. Graham, C. A. MacArthur, & J. Fitzgerald (Eds.), *Best practices in writing instruction* (2nd ed., pp. 238–256). Guilford. http://scholar.google.com/scholar_lookup?hl=en&publication_year=2013&pages=238-256&author=B.+Saddler&title=Best+practices+in+writing+instruction

Saddler, B., Behforooz, B., & Asaro, K. (2008). The effects of sentence-combining instruction on the writing of fourth-grade students with writing difficulties. *Journal of Special Education*, *42*(2), 79–90. http://scholar.google.com/scholar_lookup?hl=en&volume=42&publication_year=2008&pages=79-90&journal=Journal+of+Special+Education&issue=2&author=B.+Saddler&author=B.+Behfor ooz&author=K.+Asaro&title=The+effects+of+sentence-combining+instruction+on+the+writing+of+fourth-grade+students+with+writing+difficulties

Saddler, B., & Graham, S. (2005). The effects of peer-assisted sentence-combining instruction on the writing performance of more and less skilled young writers. *Journal of Educational Psychology*, *97*(1), 43–54. https://https://doi.org/org/10.1037/0022-0663.97.1.43

Salameh, E., Håkansson, G., & Nettelbladt, U. (2004). Developmental perspectives on bilingual Swedish-Arabic children with and without language impairment: A longitudinal study. *International Journal of Language and Communication Disorders*, *39*, 65–91. https://doi.org/10.1080/13682820310001595628

Salas-Provance, M. B., Erickson, J. G., & Reed, J. (2002). Disabilities as viewed by four generations of one Hispanic family. *American Journal of Speech-Language Pathology*, *11*, 151–162.

Samuel, A. (2001). Knowing a word affects the fundamental perception of the sounds within it. *Psychological Science*, *12*, 348–351.

Sanchez, K., Spittle, A. J., Boyce, J. O., Leembruggen. L., Mantelos, A., Mills, S., . . . Morgan, A. T. (2020). Conversational language in 3-year-old children born very preterm and at term. *Journal of Speech, Language, and Hearing Research*, *63*, 206–215. https://doi.org/10.1044/2019_JSLHR-19-00153

Sandall, S. R., McLean, M., & Smith, B. (2001). *DEC recommended practices in early intervention/early childhood special education*. Sopris West.

Sandbank, M., & Yoder, P. (2016). The association between parental mean length of utterance and language outcomes in children with disabilities: A correlational meta-analysis. *American Journal of Speech-Language Pathology*, *25*, 240–251. https://doi.org/10.1044/2015_AJSLP-15-0003

Savage, C., Lieven, E., Theakston, A., & Tomasello, M. (2003). Testing the abstractness of children's linguistic representations: Lexical and structural priming of syntactic constructions in young children. *Developmental Science*, *6*, 557–567.

Sawyer, D. J. (2006). Dyslexia: A generation of inquiry. *Topics in Language Disorders*, *26*, 95–109.

Scally, C. (2001). Visual design: Implications for developing dynamic display systems. *Perspectives on Augmentative and Alternative Communication*, *10*(4), 16–19.

Scanlon, D. M., Vellutino, F. R., Small, S. G., Fanuele, D. P., & Sweeney, J. M. (2005). Severe reading difficulties—Can they be prevented? A comparison of prevention and intervention approaches. *Exceptionality*, *13*, 209–227. https://doi.org/10.1207/s15327035ex1304_3 http://scholar.google.com/scholar_lookup?hl=en&volume=13&publication_year=2005&pages=209-227&journal=Exceptionality&author=D.+M.+Scanlon&author=F.+R.+Vellutino&author=S.+G.+Small&author=D.+P.+Fanuele&author=J.+M.+Sweeney&title=Severe+reading+difficulties%E2%80%94can+they+be+prevented%3F+A+comparison+of+prevention+and+intervention+approaches

Scarborough, H. S. (1990). Index of productive syntax. *Applied Psycholinguistics*, *11*, 1–22. https://doi.org/10.1017/S0142716400008262

Scarborough, H. S., Wyckoff, J., & Davidson, R. (1986). A reconsideration of the relationship between age and mean utterance length. *Journal of Speech and Hearing Research*, *29*, 394–399.

Scarcella, R. (2003). *Academic English: A conceptual framework*. University of California Linguistic Minority Research Institute. http://escholarship.org/uc/item/6pd082d4 http://scholar.google.com/scholar_lookup?hl=en&publication_year=2003&title=Academic+English%3A+A+conceptual+framework

Scheepers, C. (2003). Syntactic priming of relative clause attachments: Persistence of structural configuration in sentence production. *Cognition*, *89*(3), 179–205. https://doi.org/10.1016/S0010-0277(03)00119-7

Scheffner Hammer, C., Farkas, G., & Maczuga, S. (2010). The language and literacy development of Head Start children: A study using the Family and Child Experiences Survey database. *Language, Speech, and Hearing Services in Schools*, *41*, 70–83.

Scheule, C. M., & Ehren, T. C. (2016). *No more flippin' cards: Linking speech sound intervention to curriculum for preschoolers & school-age children*. Paper presented at the American Speech-Language-Hearing Association Convention, Philadelphia, PA.

Schleppegrell, M. J. (2001). Linguistic features of the language of schooling. *Linguistics and Education*, *12*, 431–459. https://doi.org/10.1016/S0898-5898(01)00073-0

Schleppegrell, M. J. (2004). *The language of schooling: A functional linguistics perspective*. Routledge. https://doi.org/10.4324/9781410610317

Schlesinger, N. W., & Gray, S. (2017). The impact of multisensory instruction on learning letter names and sounds, word reading, and spelling. *Annals of Dyslexia*, *67*, 219–258. http://scholar.google.com/scholar_lookup?hl=en&volume=67&publication_year=2017&pages=219-258&journal=Annals+of+Dyslexia&author=N.+W.+Schlesinger&author=S.+Gray&title=The+impact+of+multisensory+instruction+on+learning+letter+names+and+sounds%2C+word+reading%2C+and+spelling

Schlosser, R. W., & Lee, D. L. (2000). Promoting generalization and maintenance in augmentative and alternative communication: A meta-analysis of 20 years of effectiveness research. *Augmentative and Alternative Communication*, *16*, 208–226.

Schmitt, M. B. (2020). Children's active engagement in public school language therapy relates to greater gains. *American Journal of Speech-Language Pathology*, *29*, 1505–1513. https://doi.org/10.1044/2020_AJSLP-19-00157

Schmitt, M. B., Justice, L. M., & O'Connell, A. (2014). Vocabulary gain among children with language disorders: Contributions of children's behavior regulation and emotionally supportive environments. *American Journal of Speech-Language Pathology*, *23*, 373–384. https://doi.org/10.1044/2014_AJSLP-12-0148

Schmitt, M. B., Logan, J. A. R., Tambyraja, S. R., Farquharson, K., & Justice, L. M. (2017). Establishing language benchmarks for children with typically developing language and children with language impairment. *Journal of Speech, Language, and Hearing Disorders*, *60*, 364–378. https://doi.org/10.1044/2016_JSLHR-L-15-0273

Schneider, P. (2008, June). *Referent introduction in stories by children and adults*. Poster presented at the Triennial Meeting of the International Association for the Study of Child Language, Edinburgh, Scotland.

Schneider, P., & Dubé, R. (2005). Story presentation effects on children's retell content. *American Journal of Speech-Language Pathology*, *14*, 52–60.

Schneider, P., Dubé, R. V., & Hayward, D. (2005). *The Edmonton Narrative Norms Instrument*. University of Alberta Faculty of Rehabilitation Medicine [website]. http://www.rehabresearch.ualberta.ca/enni

Schneider, P., Dubé, R. V., & Hayward, D. (2009). *The Edmonton Narrative Norms Instrument*. http://www.rehabmed.ualberta.ca/spa/enni

Schneider, P., & Hayward, D. (2010). Who does what to whom: Introduction of referents in children's storytelling from pictures. *Language, Speech, and Hearing Services in Schools*, *41*, 459–473.

Schoon, I., Parsons, S., Rush, R., & Law, J. (2010). Childhood language skills and adult literacy: A 29-year follow-up study. *Pediatrics*, *125*, e459–e466.

Schore, A. N. (2001). The effects of early relational trauma on right brain development, affect regulation, and infant mental health. *Infant Mental Health Journal*, *22*, 201–269.

Schreibman, L., Dawson, G., Stahmer, A. C., Landa, R., Rogers, S. J., McGee, G. G., . . . Halladay, A. (2015). Naturalistic developmental behavioral interventions: Empirically validated treatments for autism spectrum disorder. *Journal of Autism and Developmental Disorders*, *45*, 2411–2428.

Schreibman, L., & Koegel, R. L. (2005). Training for parents of children with autism: Pivotal responses, generalization, and individualization of interventions. In E. D. Hibbs & P. S. Jensen (Eds.), *Psychosocial treatment for child and adolescent disorders: Empirically based strategies for clinical practice* (2nd ed., pp. 605–631). American Psychological Association.

Schuele, C. M. (2001). Socioeconomic influences on children's language acquisition. *Journal of Speech-Language Pathology and Audiology*, *25*(2), 77–88.

Schuele, C. M., & Boudreau, D. (2008). Phonological awareness intervention: Beyond the basics. *Language, Speech, and Hearing Services in Schools*, *39*, 3–20.

Schuele, C. M., & Dayton, N. D. (2000). *Intensive Phonological Awareness Program*.

Schwaighofer, M., Fischer, F., & Buhner, M. (2015). Does working memory training transfer? A meta-analysis including training conditions as moderators. *Educational Psychologist*, *50*, 138–166. https://doi.org/10.1080/00461520.2015.1036274

Schwichtenberg, A. J., Kellerman, A. M., Young, G. S., Miller, M., & Ozonoff, S. (2019). Mothers of children with autism spectrum disorders: Play behaviors with infant siblings and social responsiveness. *Autism*, *23*, 821–833. https://doi.org/10.1177/1362361318782220

Schwob, S., Eddé, L., Jacquin, L., Leboulanger, M., Picard, M., Ramos Oliveira, P., & Skoruppa, K. (2021). Using nonword repetition to identify developmental language disorder in monolingual and bilingual children: A systematic review and meta-analysis. *Journal of Speech, Language, and Hearing Research*, *64*, 3578–3593. https://doi.org/10.1044/2021_JSLHR-20-00552

Sciberras, E., Mueller, K., Efron, D., Bisset, M., Anderson, V., Schilpzand, E. J., . . . Nicholson, J. M. (2014). Language problems in children with ADHD: A community-based study. *Pediatrics*, *133*, 793–800.

Scientific Learning Corporation. (2021). *Fast ForWord Language*.

Scott, C. M. (2000). Principles and methods of spelling instruction: Applications for poor spellers. *Topics in Language Disorders*, *20*(3), 66–82.

Scott, C. M. (2005). Learning to write. In H. W. Catts & A. G. Kamhi (Eds.), *Language and reading disabilities* (2nd ed., pp. 233–273). Pearson.

Scott, C. M. (2014). One size does not fit all: Improving clinical practice in older children and adolescents with language and learning disorders. *Language, Speech, and Hearing Services in Schools*, *45*, 145–152. https://doi.org/10.1044/2014_LSHSS-14-0014

Scott, C. M., & Balthazar, C. H. (2010). The grammar of information: Challenges for older students with language impairments. *Topics in Language Disorders*, *30*(4), 288–307. https://doi.org/10.1097/TLD.0b013e3181f90878

Scott, C. M., & Erwin, D. L. (1992). Descriptive assessment of writing: Process and products. *Best Practices in School Speech-Language Pathology*, *2*, 87–98.

Scott, C. M., Nippold, M. A., Norris, J. A., & Johnson, C. J. (1992, November). *School-age children and adolescents: Establishing language norms*. Paper presented at the Annual Convention of the American Speech-Language-Hearing Association, San Antonio, TX.

Scott, C. M., & Windsor, J. (2000). General language performance measures in spoken and written narrative and expository discourse of school-age children with language learning disabilities. *Journal of Speech, Language, and Hearing Research*, *43*, 324–339.

Segebart DeThorne, L., Hart, S. A., Petrill, S. A., Deater Deckard, K., Thompson, L. A., Schatschneider, C., & Dunn Davison, M. (2006). Children's history of speech-language difficulties: Genetic influences and association with reading-related measures. *Journal of Speech, Language, and Hearing Research*, *49*, 1280–1293.

Segebart DeThorne, L., Petrill, S. A., Schatschneider, C., & Cutting, L. (2010). Conversational language use as a predictor of early reading development: Language history as a moderating variable. *Journal of Speech, Language, and Hearing Research*, *53*, 209–223.

Segebert DeThorne, L., & Watkins, R. V. (2001). Listeners' perceptions of language use in children. *Language, Speech, and Hearing Services in Schools*, *32*, 142–148.

Segers, E., & Verhoeven, L. (2004). Computer-supported phonological awareness intervention for kindergarten children with specific language impairment. *Language, Speech, and Hearing Services in Schools*, *35*, 229–239.

Selber Beilinson, J., & Olswang, L. B. (2003). Facilitating peer-group entry in kindergartners with impairments in social communication. *Language, Speech, and Hearing Services in Schools*, *34*, 154–166.

Self, T. L., Hale, L. S., & Crumrine, D. (2010). Pharmacotherapy and children with autism spectrum disorder: A tutorial for speech-language pathologists. *Language, Speech, and Hearing Services in Schools*, *41*, 367–375.

Sénéchal, M., LeFevre, J., Smith-Chant, B. L., & Colton, K. V. (2001). On refining theoretical models of emergent literacy: The role of empirical evidence. *Journal of School Psychology*, *39*(5), 439–460.

Seven, Y., Ferron, J., & Goldstein, H. (2020). Effects of embedding decontextualized language through book-sharing delivered by mothers and fathers in coparenting environments. *Journal of Speech, Language, and Hearing Research*, *63*, 4062–4081. https://doi.org/10.1044/2020_JSLHR-20-00206

Seymour, H. N., Roeper, T. W., & deVilliers, J. (2003). *Diagnostic Evaluation of Language Variance (DELV)*. Psychological Corporation.

Seymour, H. N., Roeper, T. W., & de Villiers, J. (2018). *Diagnostic Evaluation of Language Variance–Norm Referenced (DELV-NR)*. Psychological Corporation.

Shahar-Yames, D., & Share, D. (2008). Spelling as a self-teaching mechanism in orthographic learning. *Journal of Research in Reading*, *31*, 22–39.

Shanahan, T., Callison, K., Carriere, C., Duke, N. K., Pearson, P. D., Schatschneider, C., & Torgesen, J. (2010). *Improving reading comprehension in kindergarten through 3rd grade: IES practice guide* (NCEE 2010–4038). National Center for Education Evaluation and Regional Assistance, Institute of Education Sciences, U.S. Department of Education. http://scholar.google.com/scholar_lookup?hl=en&publication_year=2010&author=T.+Shanahan&author=K.+Callison&author=C.+Carriere&author=N.+K.+Duke&author=P.+D.+Pearson&author=C.+Schatschneider&author=J.+Torgesen&title=Improving+reading+comprehension+in+kindergarten+through+3rd+grade%3A+IES+practice+guide+%28NCEE+2010-4038%29

Shane, H. C. (2006). Using visual scene displays to improve communication and communication instruction in persons with autism spectrum disorders. *Perspectives in Augmentative and Alternative Communication*, *15*(1), 8–13.

Shaywitz, S. E., & Shaywitz, B. A. (2003). Neurobiological indices of dyslexia. In H. L. Swanson, K. R. Harris, & S. Graham (Eds.), *Handbook of learning disabilities* (pp. 514–531). Guilford.

Sheng, L., Bedore, L. M., Peña, E. D., & Fiestas, C. (2013). Semantic development in Spanish–English bilingual children: Effects of age and language experience. *Child Development*, *84*(3), 1034–1045. https://doi.org/10.1111/cdev.12015

Sheng, L., & McGregor, K. A. (2010). Object and action naming in children with specific language impairment. *Journal of Speech, Language, and Hearing Research, 53*, 1704–1719.

Shimpi, P. M., Gámez, P. B., Huttenlocher, J., & Vasilyeva, M. (2007). Syntactic priming in 3- and 4-year-old children: Evidence for abstract representations of transitive and dative forms. *Developmental Psychology, 43*, 1334–1346.

Shipley, K., Maddox, M., & Driver, J. (1991). Children's development of irregular past tense verb forms. *Language, Speech, and Hearing Services in Schools, 22*, 115–122.

Shipstead, Z., Harrison, T., & Engle, R. (2016). Working memory capacity and fluid intelligence: Maintenance and disengagement. *Perspectives on Psychological Science, 11*, 771–779. https://doi.org/10.1177/1745691616650647

Shire, S. Y., & Jones, N. (2015). Communication partners supporting children with complex communication needs who use AAC: A systematic review. *Communication Disorders Quarterly, 37*, 3–15. https://doi.org/10.1177/1525740114558254

Shriberg, L. D., Tomblin, J. B., & Mcsweeny, J. L. (1999). Prevalence of speech delay in 6-year-old children and comorbidity with language impairment. *Journal of Speech, Language, and Hearing Research, 42*, 1461–1481. https://doi.org/10.1044/jslhr.4206.1461

Shumway, S., & Wetherby, A. M. (2009). Communicative acts of children with autism spectrum disorders in the second year of life. *Journal of Speech, Language, and Hearing Research, 52*, 1139–1156.

Sigafoos, J., & Drasgow, E. (2001). Conditional use of aided and unaided AAC: A review and clinical case demonstration. *Focus on Autism and Other Developmental Disabilities, 16*, 152–161.

Sigafoos, J., O'Reilly, E., Drasgow, E., & Reichle, J. (2002). Strategies to achieve socially acceptable escape and avoidance. In J. Reichle, D. Beukelman, & J. Light (Eds.), *Exemplary practices for beginning communicators: Implications for AAC* (pp. 157–186). Brookes.

Silliman, E. R., Bahr, R., Beasman, J., & Wilkinson, L. C. (2000). Scaffolds for learning to read in an inclusion classroom. *Language, Speech, and Hearing Services in Schools, 31*, 265–279.

Silliman, E. R., & Scott, C. (2009). Research-based oral language intervention routes to the academic language of literacy: Finding the right road. In S. Rosenfield & V. Berninger (Eds.), *Implementing evidence-based interventions in school settings* (pp. 107–145). Oxford University Press.

Silverman, R., & Doyle, B. (2013). Vocabulary and comprehension instruction for ELLs in the era of Common Core State Standards. In S. B. Neuman & L. B. Gambrell (Eds.), *Quality reading instruction in the age of Common Core standards* (pp. 121–135). International Reading Association.

Simon, C. S. (1984). *Evaluating communicative competence: A functional-pragmatic procedure*. Communication Skill Builders.

Simon-Cereijido, G., Gutiérrez-Clellen, V. F., & Sweet, M. (2013). Predictors of language development or attrition in Latino children with specific language impairment. *Applied Psycholinguistics, 34(6)*, 1219–1243. https://doi.org/10.1017/S0142716412000215.

Simon-Cereijido, G., & Méndez, L. I. (2018). Using language-specific and bilingual measures to explore lexical–grammatical links in young latino dual-language learners. *Language, Speech, and Hearing Services in Schools, 49*, 537–550. https://doi.org/10.1044/2018_LSHSS-17-0058

Singer, B. (2007). Assessment of reading comprehension and written expression in adolescents and adults. In A. G. Kamhi, J. J. Masterson, & K. Apel (Eds.), *Clinical decision making in developmental language disorders* (pp. 77–98). Brookes.

Singer, B. D., & Bashir, A. S. (2018). Wait . . . what??? Guiding intervention principles for students with verbal working memory limitations. *Language Speech, and Hearing Services in Schools, 49*, 449–462. https://doi.org/10.1044/2018_LSHSS-17-0101

Singer, B. D., & Bashir, A. S. (2000). *Teachers guide to Brain Frames: Graphic strategies for language, literacy, teaching, and learning*. Architects for Learning.

Singer, B. D., & Tamborella, A. (2018). *What does this chunk do? A meaning-based approach for teaching complex syntax to school-age students*. Invited webinar for the American Speech-Language-Hearing Association, Rockville, MD.

Singleton, N., & Shulman, B. B. (2014). *Language development: Foundations, processes, and clinical applications* (2nd ed.). Jones & Bartlett.

Skarakis-Doyle, E. (2002). Young children's detection of violations in familiar stories and emerging comprehension monitoring. *Discourse Processes, 33(2)*, 175–197.

Skarakis-Doyle, E., & Dempsey, L. (2008). The detection and monitoring of comprehension errors by preschool children with and without language impairment. *Journal of Speech, Language, and Hearing Research, 51*, 1227–1243.

Skarakis-Doyle, E., Dempsey, L., Campbell, W., Lee, C., & Jaques, J. (2005, June). *Constructs underlying emerging comprehension monitoring: A preliminary study*. Poster session presented at the 26th Annual Symposium on Research in Child Language Disorders, Madison, WI.

Skarakis-Doyle, E., Dempsey, L., & Lee, C. (2008). Language comprehension impairment in preschool children. *Language, Speech, and Hearing Services in Schools, 39*, 54–65.

Smeets, D. J. H., van Dijken, M. J., & Bus, A. G. (2014). Using electronic storybooks to support word learning in children with severe language impairments. *Journal of Learning Disabilities, 47*, 435–449. https://doi.org/10.1177/0022219412467069

Smith, T., Scahill, L., Dawson, G., Guthrie, D., Lord, C., Odom, S. L., . . . Wagner, A. (2007). Designing research studies on psychosocial interventions in autism. *Journal of Autism and Developmental Disorders, 37*, 354–366. https://doi.org/10.1007/s10803-006-0173-3

Smith, V., Mirenda, P., & Zaidman-Zait, A. (2007). Predictors of expressive vocabulary growth in children with autism. *Journal of Speech, Language, and Hearing Research, 50*, 149–160.

Smith-Lock, K. M., Leitão, S., Lambert, L., & Nickels, L. (2013). Effective intervention for expressive grammar in children with specific language impairment. *International Journal of Language & Communication Disorders, 48*(3), 265–282. https://doi.org/10.1111/1460-6984.12003

Smith-Lock, K. M., Leitão, S., Prior, P., & Nickels, L. (2015). The effectiveness of two grammar treatment procedures for children with SLI: A randomized clinical trial. *Language, Speech, and Hearing Services in Schools, 46*, 312–324. https://doi.org/10.1044/2015_LSHSS-14-0041

Smith-Myles, B., Hilgenfeld, T., Barnhill, G., Griswold, D., Hagiwara, T., & Simpson, R. (2002). Analysis of reading skills in individuals with Asperger syndrome. *Focus on Autism and Other Developmental Disabilities, 17*(1), 44–47.

Smolak, E., McGregor, K. K., Arbisi-Kelm, T., & Eden, N. (2020). Sustained attention in developmental language disorder and its relation to working memory and language. *Journal of Speech, Language, and Hearing Research, 63*, 4096–4108. https://doi.org/10.1044/2020_JSLHR-20-00265

Snow, C. E., Scarborough, H. S., & Burns, M. S. (1999). What speech-language pathologists need to know about early reading. *Topics in Language Disorders, 20*(1), 48–58.

Snow, C. E., & Uccelli P. (2009). The challenge of academic language. In D. R. Olson & N. Torrance (Eds.), *The Cambridge handbook of literacy* (pp. 112–133). Cambridge University Press. http://scholar.google.com/scholar_lookup ?hl=en&publication_year=2009&pages=112-133&title= The+Cambridge+handbook+of+literacy

Snowling, M. J. (2008). Specific disorders and broader phenotypes: The case of dyslexia. *Quarterly Journal of Experimental Psychology, 61*, 142–156. https://doi.org/10.1080/ 17470210701508830 http://scholar.google.com/scholar_ lookup?hl=en&volume=61&publication_year=2008 &pages=142-156&journal=Quarterly+Journal+of+Experi mental+Psychology&author=M.+J.+Snowling&title= Specific+disorders+and+broader+phenotypes%3A+The+ case+of+dyslexia

Snowling, M. J. (2013). Early identification and interventions for dyslexia: A contemporary view. *Journal of Research in Special Education Needs, 13*, 7–14. https://doi .org/10.1111/j.1471-3802.2012.01262.x http://scholar .google.com/scholar_lookup?hl=en&volume=13&publi cation_year=2013&pages=7-14&journal=Journal+of+ Research+in+Special+Education+Needs&author=M.+J.+ Snowling&title=Early+identification+and+interventions +for+dyslexia%3A+A+contemporary+view

Snowling, M. J. (2014). Dyslexia: A language learning impairment. *Journal of the British Academy, 2*, 43–58. https:// doi.org/10.5871/jba/002.043 http://scholar.google .com/scholar_lookup?hl=en&volume=2&publication_ year=2014&pages=43-58&journal=Journal+of+the+Brit ish+Academy&author=M.+J.+Snowling&title=Dyslexia %3A+A+language+learning+impairment

Snowling, M. J., Bishop, D. V. M., & Stothard, S. E. (2000). Is preschool language impairment a risk factor for dyslexia in adolescence? *Journal of Child Psychology and Psychiatry, 41*, 587–600.

Snowling, M. J., Duff, F. J., Nash, H. M., & Hulme, C. (2016). Language profiles and literacy outcomes of children with resolving, emerging, or persisting language impairments. *Journal of Child Psychology and Psychiatry, 57*, 1360–1369. https://doi.org/10.1111/jcpp.12497 http://scholar .google.com/scholar_lookup?hl=en&volume=57&pub lication_year=2016&pages=1360-1369&journal=The+ Journal+of+Child+Psychology+and+Psychiatry& author=M.+J.+Snowling&author=F.+J.+Duff&author=H. +M.+Nash&author=C.+Hulme&title=Language+profiles +and+literacy+outcomes+of+children+with+resolving% 2C+emerging%2C+or+persisting+language+impairments

Snowling, M. J., Gallagher, A., & Frith, U. (2003). Family risk of dyslexia is continuous: Individual differences in the precursors of reading skill. *Child Development, 74*, 358–373. https://doi.org/10.1111/1467-8624.7402003 http://scholar.google.com/scholar_lookup?hl=en&vol ume=74&publication_year=2003&pages=358-373&jour nal=Child+Development&author=M.+J.+Snowling& author=A.+Gallagher&author=U.+Frith&title=Family +risk+of+dyslexia+is+continuous%3A+Individual+differ ences+in+the+precursors+of+reading+skill

Snowling, M. J., & Melby-Lervåg, M. (2016). Oral language deficits in familial dyslexia: A meta-analysis and review. *Psychological Bulletin, 142*(5), 498–545. https://doi.org/ 10.1037/bul0000037

Snowling, M. J., Muter, V., & Carroll, J. M. (2007). Children at family risk of dyslexia: A follow-up in adolescence. *Journal of Child Psychology and Psychiatry and Allied Disciplines, 48*, 609–618.

Snyder, L., & Caccamise, D. (2010). Comprehension processes for expository text: Building meaning and making sense. In M. A. Nippold & C. M. Scott (Eds.), *Expository discourse in children, adolescents, and adults: Development and disorders* (pp. 13–39). Psychology Press.

Snyder, L., Caccamise, D., & Wise, B. (2005). The assessment of reading comprehension. *Topics in Language Disorders, 25*, 33–50.

Snyder, L. E., Dabasinskas, C., & O'Connor, E. (2002). An information processing perspective on language impairment in children: Looking at both sides of the coin. *Topics in Language Disorders, 22*(3), 1–14.

Sohlberg, M. M., & Mateer, C. A. (2001). *Cognitive rehabilitation: An integrative neuropsychological approach.* Guilford.

Sohlberg, M. M., & Turkstra, L. S. (2011). *Optimizing cognitive rehabilitation: Effective instructional methods.* Guilford.

Soak Your Head. (n.d.) *Soak your brain.* http://www.soakyour head.com/Default.aspx

Soto, G., & Yu, B. (2014). Considerations for the provision of services to bilingual children who use augmentative and alternative communication. *Augmentative & Alternative Communication, 30*(1), 83–92. https://doi.org/10.3109/0 7434618.2013.878751

Soto, X., Seven, Y., McKenna, M., Madsen, K., Peters-Sanders, L., Kelley, E., & Goldstein, H. (2020). Iterative development of a home review program to promote preschoolers' vocabulary skills: Social validity and learning outcomes.

Language, Speech, and Hearing Services in Schools, 51(2), 371–389. https://doi.org/ 10.1044/2019_LSHSS-19-00011

Southwood, F., & Russell, A. F. (2004). Comparison of conversation, freeplay, and story generation as methods of language elicitation. *Journal of Speech, Language, and Hearing Research, 47*, 366–376.

Southwood, F., & van Hout, R. (2010). Production of tense morphology by Afrikaans-speaking children with and without specific language impairment. *Journal of Speech, Language, and Hearing Research, 53*, 394–413.

Spanoudis, G. S. (2016). Theory of mind and specific language impairment in school-age children. *Journal of Communication Disorders, 61*, 83–96. https://doi.org/10.1016/j.jcomdis.2016.04.003

Spanoudis, G. S., Papadopoulos, T. C., & Spyrou, S. (2019). Specific language impairment and reading disability: Categorical distinction or continuum? *Journal of Learning Disabilities, 52*, 3–14. https://doi.org/10.1177/00222 19418775111

Spaulding, T. J. (2010). Investigating mechanisms of suppression in preschool children with specific language impairment. *Journal of Speech, Language, and Hearing Research, 53*, 725–738.

Spaulding, T. J., Plante, E., & Farinella, K. A. (2006), Eligibility criteria for language impairment: Is the low end of normal always appropriate? *Language, Speech, and Hearing Services in Schools, 37*, 61–72.

Spencer, E. J., Goldstein, H., Sherman, A., Noe, S., Tabbah, R., Ziolkowski, R., & Schneider, N. (2012). Effects of an automated vocabulary and comprehension intervention: An early efficacy study. *Journal of Early Intervention, 34*, 195–221.

Spencer, E. J., Schuele, C. M., Guillot, K., & Lee, M. (2008). Phonological awareness skill of speech-language pathologists and other educators. *Language, Speech, and Hearing Services in Schools, 39*, 512–520.

Spencer, T. D., Kajian, M., Petersen, D. B., & Bilyk, N. (2013). Effects of an individualized narrative intervention on children's storytelling and comprehension skills. *Journal of Early Intervention, 35*, 243–269. https://doi.org/10.1177/1053815114540002

Spencer, T. D., & Petersen, D. B. (2018). Bridging oral and written language: An oral narrative language intervention study with writing outcomes. *Language, Speech, and Hearing Services in Schools, 49*, 569–581. https://doi.org/10.1044/2018_LSHSS-17-0030

Spencer, T. D., & Petersen, D. B. (2019). Narrative intervention: Principles to practice. *Language, Speech, and Hearing Services in Schools, 50*, 1081–1096. https://doi.org/10.1044/2020_LSHSS-20-00015

Spencer, T. D., Petersen, D. B., & Adams, J. L. (2015). Tier 2 language intervention for diverse preschoolers: An early-stage randomized control group study following an analysis of response to intervention. *American Journal of Speech-Language Pathology, 24*, 619–636. https://doi.org/10.1044/2015_AJSLP-14-0101

Spencer, T. D., Petersen, D. B., Slocum, T. A., & Allen, M. M. (2015). Large group narrative intervention in Head Start classrooms: Implications for response to intervention. *Journal of Early Childhood Research, 13*(2), 196–217. https://doi.org/10.1177/1476718X13515419

Spencer, T. D., & Slocum, T. A. (2010). The effect of a narrative intervention on story retelling and personal story generation skills of preschoolers with risk factors and narrative language delays. *Journal of Early Intervention, 32*(3), 178–199. https://doi.org/10.1177/1053815110379124

Spinelli, F., & Terrell, B. (1984). Remediation in context. *Topics in Language Disorders, 5*(1), 29–40.

Stables, A. (2003). Learning, identity and classroom dialogue. *Journal of Educational Enquiry, 4*(1), 1–18. http://scholar.google.com/scholar_lookup?hl=en&publication_year=2003&pages=1-18&issue=1&title=Learning%2C+identity+and+classroom+dialogue

Stahl, S. A., & Nagy, W. E. (2006). *Teaching word meanings*. Erlbaum.

Stanovich, K. E. (2000). *Progress in understanding reading: Scientific foundations and new frontiers*. Guilford.

Stanton-Chapman, T. L., Chapman, D. A., Kaiser, A. P., & Hancock, T. B. (2004). Cumulative risk and low-income children's language development. *Topics in Early Childhood Special Education, 24*, 227–238.

St Clair, M. C., Forrest, C. L., Kok Yew, S. G., & Gibson, J. L. (2019). Early risk factors and emotional difficulties in children at risk of developmental language disorder: A population cohort study. *Journal of Speech, Language, and Hearing Research, 62*, 2750–2771. https://doi.org/10.1044/2018_JSLHR-L-18-0061

St Clair, M. C., Pickles, A., Durkin, K., & Conti-Ramsden, G. (2011). A longitudinal study of behavioral, emotional and social difficulties in individuals with a history of specific language impairment (SLI). *Journal of Communication Disorders, 44*, 186–199. https://doi.org/10.1016/j.jcomdis.2010.09.004

St Clair-Thompson, H. L., & Gathercole, S. E. (2006). Executive functions and achievements in school: Shifting, updating, inhibition and working memory. *Quarterly Journal of Experimental Psychology, 59*, 745–759. https://doi.org/10.1080/17470210500162854 http://scholar.google.com/scholar_lookup?hl=en&publication_year=2006&pages=745-759&author=H.+L.+St+Clair-Thompson&author=S.+E.+Gathercole&title=Quarterly+Journal+of+Experimental+Psychology

Steel, G., Rose, M., & Eadie, P. (2016). The production of complement clauses in children with language impairment. *Journal of Speech, Language, and Hearing Research, 59*, 330–341. https://doi.org/10.1044/2015_JSLHR-L-15-0001

Steele, S. C., & Watkins, R. V. (2010). Learning word meanings during reading by children with language learning disability and typically-developing peers. *Clinical Linguistics & Phonetics, 24*(7), 520–539. https://doi.org/10.3109/02699200903532474

REFERENCES

Steffani, S. A. (2007, Spring). Identifying embedded and conjoined complex sentences: Making it simple. *Contemporary Issues in Communication Science and Disorders, 34*, 44–54.

Stein, N., & Glenn, C. (1979). An analysis of story comprehension in elementary school children. In R. Freedle (Ed.), *New directions in discourse processing* (Vol. 2, pp. 53–120). Ablex.

Stevens, C., Fanning, J., Coch, D., Sanders, L., & Neville, H. (2008). Neural mechanisms of selective auditory attention are enhanced by computerized training: Electrophysiological evidence from language-impaired and typically developing children. *Brain Research, 1205*, 55–69.

Stickler, K. R. (1987). *Guide to analysis of language transcripts.* Thinking Publications.

Stirman, S. W., Miller, C. J., Toder, K., & Calloway, A. (2013). Development of a framework and coding system for modifications and adaptations of evidence-based interventions. *Implementation Science, 8*(1), 65. https://doi.org/10.1186/1748-5908-8-65

Stockman, I. J. (2007). Social–political influences on research practices: Examining language acquisition by African American children. In B. Bailey & C. Lucas (Eds.), *Sociolinguistic variation: Theory, method, and applications* (pp. 297–317). Cambridge University Press.

Stockman, I. J. (2008). Toward validation of a minimal competence phonetic core for African American children. *Journal of Speech, Language, and Hearing Research, 51*, 1244–1262.

Stockman, I. J. (2010). A review of developmental and applied language research on African American children: From a deficit to difference perspective on dialect differences. *Language, Speech, and Hearing Services in Schools, 41*, 23–38.

Stockman, I. J., Karasinski, L., & Guillory, B. (2008). The use of conversational repairs by African American preschoolers. *Language, Speech, and Hearing Services in Schools, 39*, 461–474.

Stone, W. L., & Yoder, P. J. (2001). Predicting spoken language level in children with autism spectrum disorders. *Autism, 5*, 341–361.

Storkel, H. L. (2001). Learning new words: Phonotactic probability in language development. *Journal of Speech, Language, and Hearing Research, 44*, 1321–1337.

Storkel, H. L. (2004). The emerging lexicon of children with phonological delays: Phonotactic constraints and probability in acquisition. *Journal of Speech, Language, and Hearing Research, 47*, 1194–1212.

Storkel, H. L., & Adlof, S. M. (2009). The effect of semantic set size on word learning by preschool children. *Journal of Speech, Language, and Hearing Research, 52*, 306–320.

Storkel, H. L., Komesidou, R., Pezold, M. J., Pitt, A. R., Fleming, K. K., & Swinburne Romine, R. (2019). The impact of dose and dose frequency on word learning by kindergarten children with developmental language disorder during interactive book reading. *Language, Speech, and Hearing Services in Schools, 50*, 518–539. https://doi.org/10.1044/2019_LSHSS-VOIA-18-0131

Storkel, H. L., & Maekawa, J. (2005). A comparison of homonym and novel word learning: The role of phonotactic probability and word frequency. *Journal of Child Language, 32*, 827–853.

Storkel, H. L., & Morrisette, M. L. (2002). The lexicon and phonology: Interactions in language acquisition. *Language, Speech, and Hearing Services in Schools, 33*, 24–37.

Streissguth, A., & O'Malley, K. D. (2001). Neuropsychiatric implications and long-term consequences of fetal alcohol spectrum disorders. *Seminars in Clinical Neuropsychiatry, 5*, 177–190.

Stronach, S. T., & Wetherby, A. M. (2017). Observed and parent-report measures of social communication in toddlers with and without autism spectrum disorder across race/ethnicity. *American Journal of Speech-Language Pathology, 26*, 355–368. https://doi.org/10.1044/2016_AJSLP-15-0089

Sturm, J. M., & Nelson, N. W. (1997). Formal classroom lessons: New perspectives on a familiar discourse event. *Language, Speech, and Hearing Services in Schools, 28*, 255–273.

Sullivan, A., & Bal, A. (2013). Disproportionality in special education: Effects of individual and school variables on disability risk. *Exceptional Children, 79*(4), 475–494. https://doi.org/10.1177/001440291307900406

Sullivan, P. M., & Knutson, J. F. (2000). Maltreatment and disabilities: A population-based epidemiological study. *Child Abuse & Neglect, 24*, 1257–1275.

Sultana, N., Wong, L. L., & Purdy, S. C. (2019). Natural language input: Maternal education, socioeconomic deprivation, and language outcomes in typically developing children. *Language, Speech, and Hearing Services in Schools, 50*, 1049–1070. https://doi.org/10.1044/2020_LSHSS-19-00095

Sun, L., & Nippold, M. A. (2012). Narrative writing in children and adolescents: Examining the literate lexicon. *Language, Speech, and Hearing Services in Schools, 43*, 2–13.

Sundara, M., Demuth, K., & Kuhl, P. K. (2011). Sentence position effects on children's perception and production of English third person singular –s. *Journal of Speech, Language, and Hearing Research, 54*, 55–71.

Swanson, H. L. (2017). Verbal and visual–spatial working memory: What develops over a life span? *Developmental Psychology, 53*, 971–995.

Swanson, L. A., Fey, M. E., Mills, C. E., & Hood, L. S. (2005). Use of narrative-based language intervention with children who have specific language impairment. *American Journal of Speech-Language Pathology, 14*, 131–143.

Swineford, L. B., Thurm, A., Baird, G., Wetherby, A. M., & Swedo, S. (2014). Social (pragmatic) communication disorder: A research review of this new DSM-5 diagnostic category. *Journal of Neurodevelopmental Disorders, 6*, 41–49.

Tabors, P. O., Snow, C. E., & Dickinson, D. K. (2001). Homes and schools together: Supporting language and literacy development. In D. K. Dickinson & P. O. Tabors (Eds.), *Beginning literacy with language* (pp. 313–334). Brookes.

Tager-Flusberg, H. (2000). The challenge of studying language development in autism. In L. Menn & N. Bernstein Ratner (Eds.), *Methods for studying language production* (pp. 313–332). Erlbaum.

Tager-Flusberg, H. (2004). Do autism and specific language impairment represent overlapping language disorders? In M. L. Rice & S. F. Warren (Eds.), *Developmental language disorders: From phenotypes to etiologies* (pp. 31–52). Erlbaum.

Tager-Flusberg, H. (2016). Risk factors associated with language in autism spectrum disorder: Clues to underlying mechanisms. *Journal of Speech, Language, and Hearing Research, 59*, 143–154. https://doi.org/10.1044/2015_JSLHR-L-15-0146

Tager-Flusberg, H., & Kasari, C. (2013). Minimally verbal school-aged children with autism spectrum disorder: The neglected end of the spectrum. *Autism Research, 6*(6), 468–478. https://doi.org/10.1002/aur.1329

Tager-Flusberg, H., Paul, R., & Lord, C. E. (2005). Language and communication in autism. In F. Volkmar, R. Paul, A. Klin, & D. J. Cohen (Eds.), *Handbook of autism and pervasive developmental disorder* (3rd ed., Vol. 1, pp. 335–364). Wiley. https://doi.org/10.1002/9780470939345.ch12

Tamborella, A., & Singer, B. D. (2015, November). *Realistic ways to help students with LLD meet Common Core State Standards for syntax*. Paper presented at the annual convention of the American Speech-Language-Hearing Association, Denver, CO.

Tambyraja, S. R., Farquharson, K., Logan, J. A. R., & Justice, L. M. (2015). Decoding skills in children with language impairment: Contributions of phonological processing and classroom experiences. *American Journal of Speech-Language Pathology, 24*, 177–188. https://doi.org/10.1044/2015_AJSLP-14-0054

Tannenbaum, K. R., Torgesen, J. K., & Wagner, R. K. (2006). Relationships between word knowledge and reading comprehension in third-grade children. *Scientific Studies of Reading, 10*, 381–398. https://doi.org/10.1207/s1532799xssr1004_3

TechEd Marketing. (2022). *Inspiration-10*. https://www.inspiration-at.com

Tek, S., Mesite, L., Fein, D., & Naigles, L. (2014). Longitudinal analyses of expressive language development reveal two distinct language profiles among young children with autism spectrum disorders. *Journal of Autism and Developmental Disorders, 44*, 75–89.

Terrell, P., & Watson, M. (2018). Laying a firm foundation: Embedding evidence-based emergent literacy practices into early intervention and preschool environments. *Language, Speech, and Hearing Services in Schools, 49*, 148–164. https://doi.org/10.1044/2017_LSHSS-17-0053

Terry, N. P., Connor, C. M., Thomas-Tate, S., & Love, M. (2010). Examining relationships among dialect variation, literacy skills, and school context in first grade. *Journal of Speech, Language, and Hearing Research, 53*, 126–145.

Thal, D., Jackson-Maldonado, D., & Acosta, D. (2000). Validity of a parent-report measure of vocabulary and grammar for Spanish-speaking toddlers. *Journal of Speech, Language, and Hearing Research, 43*, 1087–1100.

Theakston, A., & Lieven, E. (2017). Multiunit sequences in first language acquisition. *Topics in Cognitive Science, 9*(3), 588–603. https://doi.org/10.1111/tops.12268

Theakston, A., Lieven, E., & Tomasello, M. (2003). The role of input in the acquisition of third person singular verbs in English. *Journal of Speech, Language, and Hearing Research, 46*, 863–877.

Theodore, R. M., Demuth, K., & Shattuck-Hufnagel, S. (2011). Acoustic evidence for positional and complexity effects on children's production of plural –s. *Journal of Speech, Language, and Hearing Research, 54*, 539–548.

Theodore, R. M., Demuth, K., & Shattuck-Hufnagel, S. (2015). Examination of the locus of positional effects on children's production of plural –s: Considerations from local and global speech planning. *Journal of Speech, Language, and Hearing Research, 58*, 946–953. https://doi.org/10.1044/2015_JSLHR-L-14-0208

Therrien, M. C. C., Light, J., & Pope, L. (2016). Systematic review of the effects of interventions to promote peer interactions for children who use aided AAC. *Augmentative and Alternative Communication, 32*, 81–93. https://doi.org/10.3109/07434618.2016.1146331

Thiemann, K. S., & Goldstein, H. (2004). Effects of peer training and written text cueing on social communication of school-age children with pervasive developmental disorder. *Journal of Speech, Language, and Hearing Research, 47*, 126–144. https://doi.org/10.1044/1092-4388(2004/012)

Thiemann-Bourque, K., Brady, N., McGuff, S., Stump, K., & Naylor, A. (2016). Picture exchange communication system and Pals: A peer-mediated augmentative and alternative communication intervention for minimally verbal preschoolers with autism. *Journal of Speech, Language, and Hearing Research, 59*, 1133–1145. https://doi.org/10.1044/2016_JSLHR-L-15-0313

Thiemann-Bourque, K., Feldmiller, S., Hoffman, L., & Johner, S. (2018). Incorporating a peer-mediated approach into speech-generating device intervention: Effects on communication of preschoolers with autism spectrum disorder. *Journal of Speech, Language, and Hearing Disorders, 61*, 2045–2061. https://doi.org/10.1044/2018_JSLHR-L-17-0424

Thiemann-Bourque, K. S., McGuff, S., & Goldstein, H. (2017). Training peer partners to use a speech-generating device with classmates with autism spectrum disorder: Exploring communication outcomes across preschool contexts. *Journal of Speech, Language, and Hearing Disorders, 60*, 2648–2662. https://doi.org/10.1044/2017_JSLHR-L-17-0049

Thiessen, E. D. (2017). What's statistical about learning? Insights from modelling statistical learning as a set of memory processes. *Philosophical Transactions of the Royal Society of London Series B: Biological Sciences, 372*20160056. https://doi.org/10.1098/Rstb.2016.0056

Thistle, J. J., & Wilkinson, K. (2009). The effects of color cues on typically developing preschoolers' speed of locating a target line drawing: Implications for augmentative and alternative communication display design. *American Journal of Speech-Language Pathology, 18,* 231–240.

Thomas-Tate, S., Washington, J., Craig, H., & Packard, M. (2006). Performance of African American preschool and kindergarten students on the Expressive Vocabulary Test. *Language, Speech, and Hearing Services in Schools, 37,* 143–149.

Thomas-Tate, S., Washington, J., & Edwards, J. (2004). Standardized assessment of phonological awareness skills in low-income African American first graders. *American Journal of Speech-Language Pathology, 13,* 182–190.

Thompson, P. A., Hulme, C., Nash, H. M., Gooch, D., Hayiou-Thomas, E., & Snowling, M. J. (2015). Developmental dyslexia: Predicting individual risk. *Journal of Child Psychology and Psychiatry, 56,* 976–987. https://doi.org/10.1111/jcpp.12412 http://scholar.google.com/scholar_lookup?hl=en&volume=56&publication_year=2015&pages=976-987&journal=The+Journal+of+Child+Psychology+and+Psychiatry&author=P.+A.+Thompson&author=C.+Hulme&author=H.+M.+Nash&author=D.+Gooch&author=E.+Hayiou-Thomas&author=M.+J.+Snowling&title=Developmental+dyslexia%3A+Predicting+individual+risk

Thordardottir, E. (2008). Language-specific effects of task demands on the manifestation of specific language impairment: A comparison of English and Icelandic. *Journal of Speech, Language, and Hearing Research, 51,* 922–937.

Thordardottir, E., & Brandeker, M. (2013). The effect of bilingual exposure versus language impairment on nonword repetition and sentence imitation scores. *Journal of Communication Disorders, 46,* 1–16.

Thordardottir, E., Kehayla, E., Mazer, B., Lessard, N., Majnemer, A., Sutton, A., . . . Chillingaryan, G. (2011). Sensitivity and specificity of French language and processing measures for the identification of primary language impairment. *Journal of Speech, Language, and Hearing Research, 54,* 580–597.

Thorell, L., Lindqvist, S., Nutley, S., Bohlin, G., & Klingberg, T. (2009). Training and transfer effects of executive functions in preschool children. *Developmental Science, 12,* 106–113.

Thorne, J. C. (2004). *The Semantic Elaboration Coding System.* Unpublished training manual, University of Washington, Seattle, WA.

Thorne, J. C. (2006). *Tallying reference errors in narratives.* https://johncthorne.wordpress.com

Thorne, J. C., & Coggins, T. E. (2016). Cohesive referencing errors during narrative production as clinical evidence of central nervous system abnormality in school-aged children with fetal alcohol spectrum disorders. *American Journal of Speech-Language Pathology, 25,* 532–546. https://doi.org/10.1044/2016_AJSLP-15-0124

Thorne, J. C., Coggins, T. E., Carmichael Olson, H., & Astley, S. J. (2007). Exploring the utility of narrative analysis is diagnostic decision making: Picture-bound reference, elaboration, and fetal alcohol spectrum disorders. *Journal of Speech, Language, and Hearing Research, 50,* 459–474.

Thothathiri, M., & Snedeker, J. (2008). Syntactic priming during language comprehension in three- and four-year-old children. *Journal of Memory and Language, 58,* 188–213.

Thoughtful Learning. (2017). *Write Away.* https://k12.thoughtfullearning.com/products/write-away

Threats, T. (2013). WHO's international classification of functioning, disability, and health: A framework for clinical and research outcomes. In L. C. Golper & C. M. Frattali (Eds.), *Outcomes in speech-language pathology* (2nd ed.). Thieme.

Throneburg, R. N., Calvert, L. K., Sturm, J. M., Paramboukas, A. M., & Paul, P. (2000). A comparison of service delivery models: Effects on curricular vocabulary skills in the school setting. *American Journal of Speech-Language Pathology, 9,* 10–20.

Thurm, A., Manwaring, S. S., Swineford, L., & Farmer, C. (2015). Longitudinal study of symptom severity and language in minimally verbal children with autism. *Journal of Child Psychology and Psychiatry, 56*(1), 97–104. https://doi.org/10.1111/jcpp.12285

Tilstra, J., & McMaster, K. (2007). Productivity, fluency, and grammaticality measures from narratives: Potential indicators of language proficiency? *Communication Disorders Quarterly, 29,* 43–53.

Timler, G. R. (2014). Use of the Children's Communication Checklist–2 for classification of language impairment risk in young school-age children with attention-deficit/hyperactivity disorder. *American Journal of Speech-Language Pathology, 23,* 73–83. https://doi.org/10.1044/1058-0360 (2013/12-0164)

Timler, G. R. (2018a, April 1). Similar . . . but very different: Determining when a child has social communication disorder versus autism spectrum disorder can be tricky. Here are some key considerations. *ASHA Leader, 23*(4). https://doi.org/10.1044/leader.FTR2.23042018.56

Timler, G. R. (2018b). Using language sample analysis to assess pragmatic skills in school-age children and adolescents. *Perspectives, 3*(1), 23–35. https://doi.org/10.1044/persp3.SIG1.23

Timler, G. R., Vogler-Elias, D., & McGill, K. F. (2007). Strategies for promoting generalization of social communication skills in preschoolers and school-aged children. *Topics in Language Disorders, 27,* 167–181.

Tomas, E., Demuth, K., & Petocz, P. (2017). The role of frequency in learning morphophonological alternations: Implications for children with specific language impairment. *Journal of Speech, Language, and Hearing Disorders, 60,* 1316–1329. https://doi.org/10.1044/2016_JSLHR-L-16-0138

Tomblin, J. B. (2014). Educational and psychosocial outcomes of language impairment in kindergarten. In J. B. Tomblin & M. A. Nippold (Eds.), *Understanding individual differences in language development across the school years* (pp. 166–203). Psychology Press.

Tomblin, J. B., Barker, B. A., Spencer, L. J., Zhang, X., & Gantz, B. J. (2005). The effect of age at cochlear implant initial stimulation on expressive language growth in infants and toddlers. *Journal of Speech, Language, and Hearing Research, 48*, 853–867.

Tomblin, J. B., Mainela-Arnold, E., & Zhang, X. (2007). Procedural learning in adolescents with and without specific language impairment. *Language Learning and Development, 3*(4), 269–293. https://doi.org/10.1080/15475440701377477

Tomblin, J. B., Records, N. L., Buckwalter, P., Zhang, X., Smith, E., & O'Brien, M. (1997). Prevalence of specific language impairment in kindergarten children. *Journal of Speech, Language, and Hearing Research, 40*(6), 1245–1260. https://doi.org/10.1044/jslhr.4006.1245

Tomblin, J. B., & Zhang, X. (2006). The dimensionality of language ability in school-age children. *Journal of Speech, Language, and Hearing Research, 49*, 1193–1208. https://doi.org/10.1044/1092-4388(2006/086)

Tönsing, K. M., Dada, S., & Alant, E. (2014). Teaching graphic symbol combinations to children with limited speech during shared story reading. *Augmentative and Alternative Communication, 30*, 279–297. https://doi.org/10.3109/07434618.2014.965846

Tönsing, K. M., & Tesner, H. (1999). Story grammar analysis of pre-schoolers' narratives: An investigation into the influence of task parameters. *South African Journal of Communication Disorders, 46*, 37–44.

Topál, J., Gergely, G., Miklósi, Á., Erdőhegyi, Á., & Csibra, G. (2008). Infants' perseverative search errors are induced by pragmatic misinterpretation. *Science, 321*(5897), 1831–1834.

Torgesen, J. K. (2004). Avoiding the devastating downward spiral: The evidence that early intervention prevents reading failure. *American Educator, 28*(3), 6–19. http://scholar.google.com/scholar_lookup?hl=en&volume=28&publication_year=2004&pages=6-19&journal=American+Educator&issue=3&author=J.+K.+Torgesen&title=Avoiding+the+devastating+downward+spiral%3A+The+evidence+that+early+intervention+prevents+reading+failure

Torgesen, J. K., & Bryant, B. R. (2013). *Test of Phonological Awareness, Second Edition (TOPA-2+)*. Pro-Ed.

Torgesen, J. K., Rashotte, C. A., & Alexander, A. W. (2001). Principles of fluency instruction in reading: Relationships with established empirical outcomes. In M. Wolf (Ed.), *Dyslexia, fluency and the brain* (pp. 332–355). York Press.

Torkildsen, J., Dailey, N., Aguilar, J., Gómez, R., & Plante, E. (2013). Exemplar variability facilitates rapid learning of an otherwise unlearnable grammar by individuals with language-based learning disability. *Journal of Speech, Language, and Hearing Research, 56*, 618–629.

Torppa, M., Lyytinen, P., Erskine, J., Eklund, K., & Lyytinen, H. (2010). Language development, literacy skills, and predictive connections to reading in Finnish children with and without familial risk for dyslexia. *Journal of Learning Disabilities, 43*, 308–321.

Tosh, R., Arnott, W., & Scarinci, N. (2017). Parent-implemented home therapy programmes for speech and language:

A systematic review. *International Journal of Language & Communication Disorders, 52*, 253–269. https://doi.org/10.1111/1460-6984.12280

Towey, M., Whitcomb, J., & Bray, C. (2004, November). *Print–sound–story–talk: A successful early reading first program.* Paper presented at the American Speech-Language-Hearing Association Annual Convention, Philadelphia, PA.

Townsend, D., Filippini, A., Collins, P., & Biancarosa, G. (2012). Evidence for the importance of academic word knowledge for the academic achievement of diverse middle school students. *Elementary School Journal, 112*(3), 497–518. https://doi.org/10.1086/663301

Treiman, R. (2017). Learning to spell: Phonology and beyond. *Cognitive Neuropsychology, 34*(3–4), 83–93. https://doi.org/10.1080/02643294.2017.1337630 http://scholar.google.com/scholar_lookup?hl=en&volume=34&publication_year=2017&pages=83-93&journal=Cognitive+Neuropsychology&issue=3%E2%80%934&author=R.+Treiman&title=Learning+to+spell%3A+Phonology+and+beyond

Trembath, D., Westerveld, M., & Shellshear, L. (2016). Assessing spoken language outcomes in children with ASD: A systematic review. *Current Developmental Disorders Reports, 3*, 33–45.

Troia, G. A. (2013). Writing instruction within a response-to-intervention framework. In S. Graham, C. A. MacArthur, & J. Fitzgerald (Eds.), *Best practices in writing instruction* (2nd ed., pp. 403–427). Guilford. http://scholar.google.com/scholar_lookup?hl=en&publication_year=2013&pages=403-427&author=G.+A.+Troia&title=Best+practices+in+writing+instruction

Tubul-Lavy, G., Jokel, A., Leon-Attia, O., & Gabis, L. V. (2020). Content words in child-directed speech of mothers toward children with autism spectrum disorder. *American Journal of Speech-Language Pathology, 29*, 1434–1447. https://doi.org/10.1044/2020_AJSLP-19-00170

Tucker, J., & McGuire, W. (2004). *Epidemiology of preterm birth.* BMJ.

Tunmer, W. E., & Chapman, J. W. (2012). Does set for variability mediate the influence of vocabulary knowledge on the development of word recognition skills? *Scientific Studies of Reading, 16*, 122–140. https://doi.org/10.1080/10888438.2010.542527 http://scholar.google.com/scholar_lookup?hl=en&volume=16&publication_year=2012&pages=122-140&journal=Scientific+Studies+of+Reading&author=W.+E.+Tunmer&author=J.+W.+Chapman&title=Does+set+for+variability+mediate+the+influence+of+vocabulary+knowledge+on+the+development+of+word+recognition+skills%3F

Tunmer, W. E., & Greaney, K. (2010). Defining dyslexia. *Journal of Learning Disabilities, 43*(3), 229–243.

Turkstra, L. S., Ciccia, A., & Seaton, C. (2003). Interactive behaviors in adolescent conversation dyads. *Language, Speech, and Hearing Services in Schools, 34*, 117–127.

Tyack, D., & Gottsleben, R. (1977). *Language sampling, analysis, and training: A handbook for teachers and clinicians.* Consulting Psychologists Press.

Tymms, P., Merrell, C., & Bailey, K. (2017). The long-term impact of effective teaching, *School Effectiveness and*

School Improvement: An International Journal of Research, Policy and Practice, 1–20. https://doi.org/10.1080/09243453.2017.1404478

Tymms, P., Merrell, C., & Bailey, K. (2018). The long-term impact of effective teaching. *School Effectiveness and School Improvement, 29*, 242–261. https://doi.org/10.1080/09243453.2017.1404478

Uccelli, P., Barr, C. D., Dobbs, C. L., Galloway, E. P., Meneses, A., & Sanchez, E. (2015). Core Academic Language Skills (CALS): An expanded operational construct and a novel instrument to chart school-relevant language proficiency in preadolescent and adolescent learners. *Applied Psycholinguistics, 36*(5), 1077–1109. https://doi.org/10.1017/S014271641400006X http://scholar.google.com/scholar_lookup?hl=en&publication_year=2014&title=Applied+Psycholinguistics

Uccelli, P., Galloway, E., Barr, C. D., Meneses, A., & Dobbs, C. L. (2015). Beyond vocabulary: Exploring cross-disciplinary academic-language proficiency and its association with reading comprehension. *Reading Research Quarterly, 50*(3), 337–356. https://doi.org/10.1002/rrq.104

Uccelli, P., & Páez, M. M. (2007). Narrative and vocabulary development of bilingual children from kindergarten to first grade: Developmental changes. *Language, Speech, and Hearing Services in Schools, 38*(3), 225–236.

Ukrainetz, T. A. (2006). *Contextualized language intervention: Scaffolding preK–12 literacy achievement.* Thinking Publications.

Ukrainetz, T. A. (2019). Sketch and speak: An expository intervention using note-taking and oral practice for children with language-related learning disabilities. *Journal of Speech, Language, and Hearing Services in Schools, 50*, 53–70. https://doi.org/10.1044/2018_LSHSS-18-0047

Ukrainetz, T. A., & Gillam, R. B. (2009). The expressive elaboration of imaginative narratives by children with specific language impairment. *Journal of Speech, Language, and Hearing Research, 52*, 883–898.

Ukrainetz, T. A., Justice, L. M., Kaderavek, J. N., Eisenberg, S. L., Gillam, R. B., & Harm, H. M. (2005). The development of expressive elaboration in fictional narratives. *Journal of Speech, Language, and Hearing Research, 48*, 1363–1377.

Ukrainetz, T. A., Ross, C., & Harm, H. (2009). An investigation of treatment scheduling for phonemic awareness with kindergartners who are at risk for reading difficulties. *Language, Speech, and Hearing Services in Schools, 40*, 86–100.

Ullman, M., & Pierpont, E. (2005). Specific language impairment is not specific to language: The procedural deficit hypothesis. *Cortex, 41*(3), 399–433. https://doi.org/10.1016/S0010-9452(08)70276-4

U.S. Bureau of the Census. (2011). *Census brief: Overview of race and Hispanic origin.* https://www.census.gov/content/dam/Census/library/publications/2011/dec/c2010br-02.pdf

U.S. Department of Education. (2016). *Our nations English learners.* https://www2.ed.gov/datastory/el-characteristics/index.html#one

U.S. Department of Education. (2018). *IDEA.* https://sites.ed.gov/idea/regs/b/a/300.8/c/10

U.S. Department of State. (2019). *FY 2018 annual report on intercountry adoption.* https://travel.state.gov/content/dam/NEWadoptionassets/pdfs/Tab%201%20Annual%20Report%20on%20Intercountry%20Adoptions.pdf

U.S. Housing and Urban Development. (2021). *2020 annual homeless assessment report Part* (HUD No. 21-041). https://www.hud.gov/press/press_releases_media_advisories/hud_no_21_041

U.S. National Institute of Mental Health. (2021, September) *Attention-deficit/hyperactive disorder.* https://www.nimh.nih.gov/health/topics/attention-deficit-hyperactivity-disorder-adhd

U.S. National Library of Medicine. (2010, December 15). *Mental retardation.* http://www.nlm.nih.gov/medlineplus/ency/article/001523.htm

van Berkel-van Hoof, L., Hermans, D., Knoors, H., & Verhoeven, L. (2019). Effects of signs on word learning by children with developmental language disorder. *Journal of Speech, Language, and Hearing Research, 62*, 1798–1812. https://doi.org/10.1044/2019_JSLHR-L-18-0275

VanDerHeyden, A., Snyder, P., Broussard, C., & Ramsdell, K. (2008). Measuring response to early literacy intervention with preschoolers at risk. *Topics in Early Childhood Special Education, 27*, 232–249. https://doi.org/10.1177/0271121407311240

VanDerHeyden, A., Witt, J., & Gilbertson, D. (2007). A multiyear evaluation of the effects of a response to intervention (RTI) model on identification of children for special education. *Journal of School Psychology, 45*, 225–256.

van Kleeck, A. (1995). Emphasizing form and meaning separately in prereading and early reading instruction. *Topics in Language Disorders, 16*(1), 27–49.

van Kleeck, A. (2003). Research on book sharing: Another critical look. In A. van Kleeck, S. A. Stahl, & E. Bauer (Eds.), *On reading to children: Parents and teachers* (pp. 271–320). Erlbaum.

van Kleeck, A. (2013). Guiding parents from diverse cultural backgrounds to promote language skills in preschoolers with language disorders: Two challenges and proposed solutions for them. *Perspectives on Language Learning and Education, 20*, 78–85. http://scholar.google.com/scholar_lookup?hl=en&publication_year=2013&pages=78-85&title=Guiding+parents+from+diverse+cultural+backgrounds+to+promote+language+skills+in+preschoolers+with+language+disorders%3A+Two+challenges+and+proposed+solutions+for+them

van Kleeck, A. (2014). Distinguishing between casual talk and academic talk beginning in the preschool years: An important consideration for speech-language pathologists. *American Journal of Speech-Language Pathology, 23*, 724–741. https://doi.org/10.1044/2014_AJSLP-14-0032

van Kleeck, A., & Schwarz, A. L. (2011). Making "academic talk" explicit: Research directions for fostering classroom discourse skills in children from nonmainstream cultures. *Revue Suisse des Sciences de l'Éducation, 33*, 1–18. http://scholar.google.com/scholar_lookup?hl=en&publication_year=2011&pages=1-18&title=Making+%E2%80%9Cacademic+talk%E2%80%9D+explicit%3A+Research+direc

tions+for+fostering+classroom+discourse+skills+in+children+from+nonmainstream+cultures

van Kleeck, A., Schwarz, A. L., Fey, M., Kaiser, A., Miller, J. & Weitsman, E. (2010). Should we use telegraphic or grammatical input in the early stages of language development with children who have language impairments? A meta-analysis of the research and expert opinion. *American Journal of Speech-Language Pathology*, *19*, 3–21. https://doi.org/10.1044/1058-0360(2009/08-0075)

van Kleeck, A., Vander Woude, J., & Hammett, L. (2006). Fostering literal and inferential language skills in Head Start preschoolers with language impairment using scripted-sharing discussions. *American Journal of Speech-Language Pathology*, *15*, 89–95.

Van Naarden Braun, K., Christensen, D., Doernberg, N., Schieve, L., Rice, C., Wiggins, L., . . . Yeargin-Allsopp, M. (2015). Trends in the prevalence of autism spectrum disorder, cerebral palsy, hearing loss, intellectual disability, and vision impairment, metropolitan Atlanta, 1991–2010. *PLoS One*, *10*, e0124120.

van Viersen, S., Kroesbergen, E. H., Slot, E. M., & de Bree, E. H. (2016). High reading skills mask dyslexia in gifted children. *Journal of Learning Disabilities*, *49*, 189–199. https://doi.org/10.1177/0022219414538517

Vaughn, S., Mathes, P., Linan-Thompson, S., Cirino, P., Carlson, C., Pollard-Durodola, S., . . . Francis, D. (2006). Effectiveness of an English intervention for first-grade English language learners at risk for reading problems. *Elementary School Journal*, *107*, 153–180.

Venker, C. E., Bolt, D. M., Meyer, A., Sindberg, H., Ellis Weismer, S., & Tager-Flusberg, H. (2015). Parent telegraphic speech use and spoken language in preschoolers with ASD. *Journal of Speech, Language, and Hearing Research*, *58*, 1733–1746. https://doi.org/10.1044/2015_JSLHR-L-14-0291

Verdon, S., McLeod, S., & Winsler, A. (2014). Language maintenance and loss in a population study of young Australian children. *Early Childhood Research Quarterly*, *29*, 168–181. https://doi.org/10.1016/j.ecresq.2013.12.003

Verhoeven, L., Aparici, M., Cahana-Amitay, D., van Hell, J. G., Kriz, S., & Viguié-Simon, A. (2002). Clause packaging in writing and speech: A cross-linguistic developmental analysis. *Written Language & Literacy*, *5*, 135–161. https://doi.org/10.1075/wll.5.2.02ver

Verly, M., Gerrits, R., Sleurs, C., Lagae, L., Sunaert, S., Zink, I., & Rommel, N. (2019). The mis-wired language network in children with developmental language disorder: Insights from DTI tractography. *Brain Imaging and Behavior*, *13*, 973–984.

Victorino, K. R., & Schwartz, R. G. (2015). Control of auditory attention in children with specific language impairment. *Journal of Speech, Language, and Hearing Research*, *58*, 1245–1257. https://doi.org/10.1044/2015_JSLHR-L-14-0181

Vigil, A., & van Kleeck, A. (1996). Clinical language teaching: Theories and principles to guide our responses when children miss our language targets. In M. Smith & J. Damico (Eds.), *Childhood language disorders* (pp. 64–96). Thieme.

Virtue, S., & Haberman, J., Clancy, Z., Parrish, T., & Beeman, M. (2006). Neural activity of inferences during story comprehension. *Brain Research*, *1084*, 104–114.

Virtue, S., & van den Broek, P. (2004). Hemispheric processing of anaphoric inferences: The activation of multiple antecedents. *Brain and Language*, *93*, 327–337.

Vogt, S. S., & Kauschke, C. (2017). With some help from others' hands: Iconic gesture helps semantic learning in children with specific language impairment. *Journal of Speech, Language, and Hearing Disorders*, *60*, 3213–3225. https://doi.org/10.1044/2017_JSLHR-L-17-0004

Volden, J. (2002). Features leading to judgments of inappropriacy in the language of speakers with autism: A preliminary study. *Journal of Speech-Language Pathology and Audiology*, *26*(3), 138–146.

Volden, J. (2004). Conversational repair in speakers with autism spectrum disorder. *International Journal of Language and Communication Disorders*, *39*, 171–189. http://scholar.google.com/scholar_lookup?hl=en&volume=57&publication_year=1986&pages=1454-1463&journal=Child+Development&author=M.+Tomasello&author=M.+J.+Farrar&title=Joint+attention+and+early+language

Volden, J., Coolican, J., Garon, N., White, J., & Bryson, S. (2009). Brief report: Pragmatic language in autism spectrum disorder: Relationships to measures of ability and disability. *Journal of Autism and Developmental Disorders*, *39*, 388–393.

Volden, J., Dodd, E., Engel, K., Smith, I. M., Szatmari, P., Fombonne, E., . . . Pathways in ASD Study Team. (2017). Beyond sentences: Using the Expression, Reception, and Recall of Narratives Instrument to assess communication in school-aged children with autism spectrum disorder. *Journal of Speech, Language, and Hearing Disorders*, *60*, 2228–2240. https://doi.org/10.1044/2017_JSLHR-L-16-0168

Volden, J., & Phillips, L. (2010). Measuring pragmatic language in speakers with autism spectrum disorders: Comparing the children's Communication Checklist–2 and the Test of Pragmatic Language. *American Journal of Speech-Language Pathology*, *19*, 204–212.

Vugs, B., Hendriks, M., Cuperus, J., Knoors, H., & Verhoeven, L. (2017). Developmental associations between working memory and language in children with specific language impairment: A longitudinal study. *Journal of Speech, Language, and Hearing Disorders*, *60*, 3284–3294. https://doi.org/10.1044/2017_JSLHR-L-17-0042

Vygotsky, L. (1978). *Mind in society: The development of higher psychological processes*. Harvard University Press.

Wada, R., Gillam, S. L., & Gillam, R. B. (2020). The use of structural priming and focused recasts to facilitate the production of subject- and object-focused relative clauses by school-age children with and without developmental language disorder. *American Journal of Speech-Language Pathology*, *29*, 1883–1895. https://doi.org/10.1044/2020_AJSLP-19-00090

Wadman, R., Durkin, K., & Conti-Ramsden, G. (2008). Self-esteem, shyness, and sociability in adolescents with specific language impairment (SLI). *Journal of Speech, Language, and Hearing Research, 51,* 938–952.

Wagner, R. E., Torgesen, J. K., & Rashotte, C. (1999). *Comprehensive Test of Phonological Processing (CTOPP).* Pro-Ed.

Wagner, R. K., Francis, D. J., & Morris, R. D. (2005). Identifying English language learners with learning disabilities: Key challenges and possible approaches. *Learning Disabilities Research & Practice, 20,* 6–15.

Wahlberg, T., & Magliano, J. P. (2004). The ability of high-functioning individuals with autism to comprehend written discourse. *Discourse Processes, 38*(1), 119–144.

Waite, M. C., Theodoros, D. G., Russell, T. G., & Cahill, L. M. (2010). Internet-based telehealth assessment of language using the CELF-4. *Language, Speech, and Hearing Services in Schools, 41,* 445–458.

Walters, C., Sevcik, R. A., & Romski, M. A. (2021). Spoken vocabulary outcomes of toddlers with developmental delay after parent-implemented augmented language intervention. *American Journal of Speech-Language Pathology, 3,* 1023–1037. https://doi.org/10.1044/2020_AJSLP-20-00093

Walton, K. M., & Ingersoll, B. R. (2014). The influence of maternal language responsiveness on the expressive speech production of children with autism spectrum disorders: A microanalysis of mother–child play interactions. *Autism, 19,* 421–432. https://doi.org/10.1177/1362361314523144

Wang, H. C., Nickels, L., Nation, K., & Castles, A. (2013). Predictors of orthographic learning of regular and irregular words. *Scientific Studies of Reading, 17,* 369–384. https://doi.org/10.1080/10888438.2012.749879

Wanzek, J., Gatlin, B., Al Otaiba, S., & Kim, Y. S. G. (2017). The impact of transcription writing interventions for first-grade students. *Reading & Writing Quarterly, 33*(5), 484–499. http://scholar.google.com/scholar_lookup?hl=en&volume=33&publication_year=2017&pages=484-499&journal=Reading+%26+Writing+Quarterly&issue=5&author=J.+Wanzek&author=B.+Gatlin&author=S.+Al+Otaiba&author=Y.+S.+G.+Kim&title=The+impact+of+transcription+writing+interventions+for+first-grade+students

Wanzek, J., & Vaughn, S. (2007). Research-based implications from extensive early reading interventions. *School Psychology Review, 36*(4), 541–561. http://scholar.google.com/scholar_lookup?hl=en&volume=36&publication_year=2007&pages=541-561&journal=School+Psychology+Review&issue=4&author=J.+Wanzek&author=S.+Vaughn&title=Research-based+implications+from+extensive+early+reading+interventions

Wanzek, J., Wexler, J., Vaughn, S., & Ciullo, S. (2010). Reading interventions for struggling readers in the upper elementary grades: A synthesis of 20 years of research. *Reading and Writing, 23*(8), 889–912. http://scholar.google.com/scholar_lookup?hl=en&volume=23&publication_year=2010&pages=889-912&journal=Reading+and+Writing&issue=8&author=J.+Wanzek&author=J.+Wexler&

author=S.+Vaughn&author=S.+Ciullo&title=Reading+interventions+for+struggling+readers+in+the+upper+elementary+grades%3A+A+synthesis+of+20+years+of+research

Ward-Lonergan, J. M. (2010). Expository discourse in school-age children and adolescents with language disorders: Nature of the problem. In M. A. Nippold & C. M. Scott (Eds.), *Expository discourse in children, adolescents, and adults: Development and disorders* (pp. 155–189). Taylor & Francis.

Warlaumont, A., & Jarmulowicz, L. (2012). Caregivers' suffix frequencies and suffix acquisition by language impaired, late talking, and typically developing children. *Journal of Child Language, 39,* 1017–1042.

Warner, G., Moss, J., Smith, P., & Howlin, P. (2014). Autism characteristics and behavioural disturbances in ~500 children with Down's syndrome in England and Wales. *Autism Research, 7,* 433–441. https://doi.org/10.1002/aur.1371

Washington, J. A., Branum-Martin, L., Sun, C., & Lee-James, R. (2018). The impact of dialect density on the growth of language and reading in African American children. *Language, Speech, and Hearing Services in Schools, 49,* 232–247. https://doi.org/10.1044/2018_LSHSS-17-0063

Washington, J. A., & Craig, H. K. (1994). Dialectal forms during discourse of urban, African American preschoolers living in poverty. *Journal of Speech and Hearing Research, 37,* 816–823.

Washington, K. N. (2007). Using the ICF within speech language-pathology: Application to developmental language impairment. *International Journal of Speech-Language Pathology, 9*(3), 242–255.

Washington, K. N., Fritz, K., Crowe, K., Shaw, B., & Wright, R. (2019). Bilingual preschoolers' spontaneous productions: Considering Jamaican Creole and English. *Language, Speech, and Hearing Services in Schools, 50,* 179–195. https://doi.org/10.1044/2018_LSHSS-18-0072

Wasik, B. A., Bond, M. A., & Hindman, A. (2006). The effects of a language and literacy intervention on Head Start children and teachers. *Journal of Educational Psychology, 98,* 63–74.

Watkins, C. L., & Slocum, T. A. (2004). The components of direct instruction. In N. E. Marchand-Martella, T. A. Slocum, & R. C. Martella (Eds.), *Introduction to direct instruction* (pp. 28–65). Allyn & Bacon.

Watson, L. R., & Ozonoff, S. (2000). Pervasive developmental disorders. In T. L. Layton, E. Crais, & L. R. Watson (Eds.), *Handbook of early language impairment in children: Nature* (pp. 109–161). Delmar.

Watt, N., Wetherby, A., & Shumway, S. (2006). Prelinguistic predictors of language outcome at 3 years of age. *Journal of Speech, Language, and Hearing Research, 49*(6), 1224–1237. https://doi.org/10.1044/1092-4388(2006/088)

Way, N., Reddy, R., & Rhodes, J. (2007). Students' perceptions of school climate during the middle school years: Associations with trajectories of psychological and behavioral adjustment. *American Journal of Community Psychology*, *40*(3–4), 194–213. https://https://doi.org/org/10.1007/s10464-007-9143-y

Wayman, K. I., Lynch, E. W., & Hanson, M. J. (1990). Home-based early childhood services: Cultural sensitivity in a family systems approach. *Topics in Early Childhood Special Education*, *10*(4), 56–75.

Webb, S. J., Jones, E. J. H., Kelly, J., & Dawson, G. (2014). The motivation for very early intervention for infants at high risk for autism spectrum disorders. *International Journal of Speech-Language Pathology*, *16*, 36–42. https://doi.org/10.3109/17549507.2013.861018

Weiner, F. (1988). *Parrot Easy Language Sample Analysis (PELSA)* [Computer program]. Parrot Software.

Weinreb, L. F., Buckner, J. C., Williams, V., & Nicholson, J. (2006). A comparison of the health and mental health status of homeless mothers in Worcester, Mass: 1993 and 2003. *American Journal of Public Health*, *96*, 1444–1448.

Weitzman, E., & Greenberg, J. (2002). *Learning language and loving it* (2nd ed.). Hanen Center.

Wells, G. (1985). *Language development in the pre-school years*. Cambridge University Press.

Welsh, M., Parke, R. D., Widaman, K., & O'Neil, R. (2001). Linkages between children's social and academic competence: A longitudinal analysis. *Journal of School Psychology*, *39*, 463–481.

Wentzel, M. (2000, November 29). UR first to identify autistic gene. *Democrat and Chronicle*, pp. 1A, 10A.

Werfel, K. L., Eisel Hendricks, A., & Schuele, C. M. (2017). The potential of past tense marking in oral reading as a clinical marker of specific language impairment in school-age children. *Journal of Speech, Language, and Hearing Disorders*, *60*, 3561–3572. https://doi.org/10.1044/2017_JSLHR-L-17-0115

Werfel, K. L., & Krimm, H. (2017). A preliminary comparison of reading subtypes in a clinical sample of children with specific language impairment. *Journal of Speech, Language, and Hearing Disorders*, *60*, 2680–2686. https://doi.org/10.1044/2017_JSLHR-L-17-0059

Westby, C. E. (1984). Development of narrative language abilities. In G. Wallach & K. Butler (Eds.), *Language learning disabilities in school-age children* (pp. 103–127). Williams & Wilkins.

Westby, C. E. (2005). Assessing and remediating text comprehension problems. In H. W. Catts & A. G. Kamhi (Eds.), *Language and reading disabilities* (2nd ed., pp. 157–232). Pearson.

Westby, C. E. (2007). Child maltreatment: A global issue. *Language, Speech, and Hearing Services in Schools*, *38*, 140–148.

Westby, C. E., & Clauser, P. S. (2005). The right stuff for writing: Assessing and facilitating written language. In H. W. Catts & A. G. Kamhi (Eds.), *Language and reading disabilities* (2nd ed., pp. 274–348). Pearson.

Westby, C. E., & Culatta, B. (2016). Telling tales: Personal event narratives and life stories. *Language, Speech, and Hearing Services in Schools*, *47*, 260–282. https://doi.org/10.1044/2016_LSHSS-15-0073

Westby, C. E., Culatta, B., Lawrence, B., & Hall-Kenyon, K. (2010). Summarizing expository texts. *Topics in Language Disorders*, *30*, 275–287. https://doi.org/10.1097/TLD.0b013e3181ff5a88

Westby, C. E., Van Dongen, R., & Maggart, Z. (1989). Assessing narrative competence. *Seminars in Speech and Language*, *10*, 63–76.

Westby, C., & Washington, K. N. (2017). Using the International Classification of Functioning, Disability and Health in assessment and intervention of school-aged children with language impairments. *Language, Speech, and Hearing Services in Schools*, *48*, 137–152. https://doi.org/10.1044/2017_LSHSS-16-0037

Wester Oxelgren, U., Myrelid, A., Annerén, G., Ekstam, B., Göransson, C., Holmbom, A., . . . Fernell, E. (2017). Prevalence of autism and attention-deficit-hyperactivity disorder in Down syndrome: A population-based study. *Developmental Medicine & Child Neurology*, *59*, 276–283. https://doi.org/10.1111/dmcn.13217

Westerveld, M. F., & Moran, C. A. (2011). Expository language skills of young school-age children. *Language, Speech, and Hearing Services in Schools*, *42*, 182–193.

Westerveld, M. F., Paynter, J., Brignell, A., & Reilly, S. (2020). Brief report: No differences in code-related emergent literacy skills in well-matched 4-year-old children with and without ASD. *Journal of Autism and Developmental Disorders*, *50*, 3060–3065. https://doi.org/10.1007/s10803-020-04407-5

Westerveld, M. F., Paynter, J., O'Leary, K., & Trembath, D. (2018). Preschool predictors of reading ability in the first year of schooling in children with ASD. *Autism Research*, *11*, 1332–1344. https://doi.org/10.1002/aur.1999

Westerveld, M. F., Paynter, J., Trembath, D., Webster, A. A., Hodge, A. M., & Roberts, J. (2017). The emergent literacy skills of preschool children with autism spectrum disorder. *Journal of Autism and Developmental Disorders*, *47*, 424–438. https://doi.org/10.1007/s10803-016-2964-5

Westerveld, M. F., Paynter, J., & Wicks, R. (2020). Shared book reading behaviors of parents and their verbal preschoolers on the autism spectrum. *Journal of Autism and Developmental Disorders*, *50*, 3005–3017. https://doi.org/10.1007/s10803-020-04406-6

Westerveld, M. F., & Roberts, J. M. A. (2017). The oral narrative comprehension and production abilities of verbal preschoolers on the autism spectrum. *Language, Speech, and Hearing Services in Schools*, *48*, 260–272. https://doi.org/10.1044/2017_LSHSS-17-0003

Westerveld, M. F., Trembath, D., Shellshear, L., & Paynter, J. (2016). A systematic review of the literature on emergent literacy skills of preschool children with autism spectrum disorder. *Journal of Special Education*, *50*(1), 37–48. https://doi.org/10.1177/0022466915613593

Wetherby, A. M., Guthrie, W., Hooker, J. L., Delehanty, A., Day, T. N., Woods, J., . . . (2021). The Early Screening for Autism and Communication Disorders: Field-testing an autism-specific screening tool for children 12 to 36 months of age. *Autism*, *25*, 2112–2123. https://doi.org/10.1177/13623613211012526

REFERENCES

Wetherby, A. M., Prizant, B. M., & Schuler, A. (2000). Understanding the nature of communication and language impairments. In A. Wetherby & B. Prizant (Eds.), *Autism spectrum disorders: A transactional developmental perspective* (pp. 109–141). Brookes.

Wetherby, A. M., & Woods, J. J. (2006). Early social interaction project for children with autism spectrum disorders beginning in the second year of life: A preliminary study. *Topics in Early Childhood Special Education, 26,* 67–82.

Wetherby, A., Woods, J., & Lord, C. (2007). *ESAC: Early Screening for Autism and Communication Disorders.* Unpublished manual, Florida State University, Tallahassee, FL.

Weyer, M. (2018, January 2). *Dual- and English-language learners.* National Council of State legislatures. https://www.ncsl.org/research/education/english-dual-language-learners.aspx

White, P. J., O'Reilly, M., Streusand, W., Levine, A., Sigafoos, J., Lancioni, G., . . . Aguilar, J. (2011). Best practices for teaching joint attention: A systematic review of the intervention literature. *Research in Autism Spectrum Disorders, 5*(4), 1283–1295. https://doi.org/10.1016/j.rasd.2011.02.003

Whitehouse, A. J. (2010). Is there a sex ratio difference in the familial aggregation of specific language impairment? A meta-analysis. *Journal of Speech, Language, and Hearing Research, 53,* 1015–1025.

Wiederholt, J. L., & Bryant, B. R. (2012). *Gray Oral Reading Test, Fifth Edition.* Pro-Ed.

Wiig, E. H. (1995). Teaching prosocial communication. In D. F. Tibbits (Ed.), *Language intervention: Beyond the primary grades. For clinicians by clinicians.* Pro-Ed.

Wiig, E. H., & Semel, E. M. (1984). *Language assessment and intervention for the learning disabled* (2nd ed.). Merrill/Macmillan.

Wiig, E. H., Semel, E., & Secord, W. A. (2013). *Clinical Evaluation of Language Fundamentals, Fifth Edition (CELF-5).* Pearson.

Wilcox, M. J., Bacon, C. K., & Greer, D. C. (2005). *Evidence-based early language intervention: Caregiver verbal responsivity training.* http://www.asu.edu/clas/icrp/research/presentations/p1/pdf2.pdf

Wilcox, M. J., & Woods, J. (2011). Participation as a basis for developing early intervention outcomes. *Language, Speech, and Hearing Services in Schools, 42,* 365–378.

Wilkinson, G. S. (1995). *Wide Range of Achievement Test–3.*

Wilkinson, G. S., & Robertson, G. J. (2017). *Wide Range Achievement Test, Fifth Edition (WRAT-5).* Pearson.

Willcutt, E. G. (2012). The prevalence of DSM-IV attention-deficit/hyperactivity disorder: A meta-analytic review. *Neurotherapeutics, 9,* 490–499.

Williams, G. J., Larkin, R. F., Rose, N. V., Whitaker, E., Roeser, J., & Wood, C. (2021). Orthographic knowledge and clue word facilitated spelling in children with developmental language disorder. *Journal of Speech, Language, and Hearing Research, 64,* 3909–3927. https://doi.org/10.1044/2021_JSLHR-20-00710

Williams, H., Hughes, N., Williams, W. H., Chitsabesan, P., Walesby, R. C., Mounce, L. T. A., & Clasby, B. (2015). The prevalence of traumatic brain injury among young offenders in custody: A systematic review. *Journal of Head Trauma Rehabilitation, 30,* 94–105. https://doi.org/10.1097/HTR.0000000000000124

Williams, K. J., Walker, M. A., Vaughn, S., & Wanzek, J. (2017). A synthesis of reading and spelling interventions and their effects on spelling outcomes for students with learning disabilities. *Journal of Learning Disabilities, 50*(3), 286–297. http://scholar.google.com/scholar_lookup?hl=en&volume=50&publication_year=2017&pages=286-297&journal=Journal+of+Learning+Disabilities&issue=3&author=K.+J.+Williams&author=M.+A.+Walker&author=S.+Vaughn&author=J.+Wanzek&title=A+synthesis+of+reading+and+spelling+interventions+and+their+effects+on+spelling+outcomes+for+students+with+learning+disabilities

Williams, K. T. (2018). *Expressive Vocabulary Test, Third Edition (EVT-3).* Pearson.

Williamson, P., Carnahan, C. R., Birri, N., & Swpboda, C. (2015). Improving comprehension of narrative using character event maps for high school students with autism spectrum disorder. *Journal of Special Education, 49,* 28–38. https://doi.org/10.1177/0022466914521301

Windsor, J., Scott, C. M., & Street, C. K. (2000). Verb and noun morphology in the spoken and written language of children with language learning disabilities. *Journal of Speech, Language, and Hearing Research, 43,* 1322–1336.

Wing, C., Kohnert, K., Pham, G., Cordero, K. N., Ebert, K. D., Kan, P. F., & Blaiser, K. (2007). Culturally consistent treatment for late talkers. *Communication Disorders Quarterly, 29*(1), 20–27.

Winner, M. G. (2013). *Why teach social thinking? Questioning our assumptions about what it means to learn social skills.* Think Social Publishing.

Winstanley, M., Webb, R. T., & Conti-Ramsden, G. (2018). More or less likely to offend? Young adults with a history of identified developmental language disorders. *International Journal of Language & Communication Disorders, 53,* 256–270. https://doi.org/10.1111/1460-6984.12339

Wittke, K., & Spaulding, T. J. (2018). Which preschool children with specific language impairment receive language intervention? *Language, Speech, and Hearing Services in Schools, 49,* 59–71. https://doi.org/10.1044/2017_LSHSS-17-0024

Wodka, E. L., Mathy, P., & Kalb, L. (2013). Predictors of phrase and fluent speech in children with autism and severe language delay. *Pediatrics, 131*(4), e1128–e1134. https://doi.org/10.1542/peds.2012-2221

Wolf, M. (2007). *Proust and the squid: The story and science of the reading brain.* HarperCollins.

Wolf, M., & Katzir-Cohen, T. (2001). Reading fluency and its intervention. *Scientific Studies of Reading, 5,* 211–239.

Wolfe, M. B. W. (2005). Memory for narrative and expository text: Independent influences of semantic associations and text organization. *Journal of Experimental Psychology, 31,* 359–364. https://doi.org/10.1037/0278-7393.31.2.359

Wolfram, W., & Schilling, N. (Eds.). (2016). *American English, dialects and variation.* Wiley.

Wolter, J. A., & Apel, K. (2010). Initial acquisition of mental graphemic representations in children with language impairment. *Journal of Speech, Language, and Hearing Research, 53*, 179–195.

Wolter, J. A., Gibson, F. E., & Slocum, T. A. (2020). A dynamic measure of morphological awareness and first-grade literacy skill. *Language, Speech, and Hearing Services in Schools, 51*, 617–639. https://doi.org/10.1044/2020_LSHSS-19-00047

Wolter, J. A., & Green, L. (2013). Morphological awareness intervention in school-age children with language and literacy deficits: A case study. *Topics in Language Disorders, 33*, 27–41. https://doi.org/10.1097/TLD.0b013e318280f5aa

Wolter, J. A., Wood, A., & D'Zatko, K. W. (2009). The influence of morphological awareness on the literacy development of first-grade children. *Language, Speech, and Hearing Services in Schools, 40*, 286–298.

Wong, B. Y. (2000). Writing strategies instruction for expository essays for adolescents with and without learning disabilities. *Topics in Language Disorders, 20*(4), 244.

Wong, B. Y., Butler, D. L., Ficzere, S. A., & Kuperis, S. (1996). Teaching low achievers and students with learning disabilities to plan, write, and revise opinion essays. *Journal of Learning Disabilities, 29*(2), 197–212.

Wood, C., Diehm, E. A., & Callender, M. F. (2016). An investigation of language environment analysis measures for Spanish–English bilingual preschoolers from migrant low-socioeconomic-status backgrounds. *Language, Speech, and Hearing Services in Schools, 47*, 123–134. https://doi.org/10.1044/2015_LSHSS-14-0115

Wood, C., Fitton, L., Petscher, Y., Rodriguez, E., Sunderman, G., & Lim, T. (2018). The effect of e-book vocabulary instruction on Spanish–English speaking children. *Journal of Speech, Language, and Hearing Disorders, 61*, 1945–1969. https://doi.org/10.1044/2018_JSLHR-L-17-0368

Wood, T. S., Pratt, A. S., Durant, K., McMillen, S., Peña, E., & Bedore, L. (2021). Contribution of nonverbal cognitive skills on bilingual children's grammatical performance: Influence of exposure, task type, and language of assessment. *Languages, 6*, 36. https://doi.org/10.3390/languages6010036

Woodcock, R. W. (2011). *Woodcock Reading Mastery Tests, Third Edition* (WRMT-III). Pearson.

Woodcock, R. W., McGrew, K. S., & Mather, N. (2001). *Woodcock–Johnson III Tests of Cognitive Abilities*. Riverside.

Woods, J. J., & Wetherby, A. M. (2003). Early identification of and intervention for infants and toddlers who are at risk for autism spectrum disorder. *Language, Speech, and Hearing Services in Schools, 34*, 180–193. https://doi.org/10.1044/0161-1461(2003/015)

Woods, J. J., Wilcox, M. J., Friedman, M., & Murch, T. (2011). Collaborative consultation in natural environments: Strategies to enhance family-centered supports and services. *Language, Speech, and Hearing Services in Schools, 42*, 379–392.

World Health Assembly. (2001). https://apps.who.int/iris/handle/10665/260183

World Health Organization. (2001, May 22). *International Classification of Functioning, Disability and Health (ICF).* Resolution WHA54.21. https://www.who.int/standards/classifications/international-classification-of-functioning-disability-and-health

World Health Organization. (2010). *Mental retardation: From knowledge to action.* http://www.searo.who.int/en/Section1174/Section1199/Section1567/Section1825_8090.htm

World Health Organization (2018, February 18). *Preterm Birth.* https://www.who.int/news-room/fact-sheets/detail/preterm-birth

Woynaroski, T., Watson, L., Gardner, E., Newsom, C. R., Keceli-Kaysili, B., & Yoder, P. J. (2016). Early predictors of growth in diversity of key consonants used in communication in initially preverbal children with autism spectrum disorder. *Journal of Autism and Developmental Disorders, 46*, 1013–1024.

Wray, C., Saunders, N., McGuire, R., Cousins, G., & Frazier Norbury, C. (2017). Gesture production in language impairment: It's quality, not quantity, that matters. *Journal of Speech, Language, and Hearing Disorders, 60*, 969–982. https://doi.org/10.1044/2016_JSLHR-L-16-0141

Wright, T. S., & Cervetti, G. N. (2017). A systematic review of the research on vocabulary instruction that impacts text comprehension. *Reading Research Quarterly, 52*, 203–226. https://doi.org/10.1002/rrq.163

Wright Karem, R., & Washington, K. N. (2021). The cultural and diagnostic appropriateness of standardized assessments for dual language learners: A focus on Jamaican preschoolers. *Language, Speech, and Hearing Services in Schools, 52*, 807–826. https://doi.org/10.1044/2021_LSHSS-20-00106

Wright Karem, R., Washington, K. N., Crowe, K., Jenkins, A., Leon, M., Kokotek, L., . . . Westby, C. (2019). Current methods of evaluating the language abilities of multilingual preschoolers: A scoping review using the International Classification of Functioning, Disability and Health–Children and Youth Version. *Language, Speech, and Hearing Services in Schools, 50*, 434–451. https://doi.org/10.1044/2019_LSHSS-18-0128

Wyatt, T. (2012). Assessment of multicultural and international clients with communication disorders. In D. E. Battle (Ed.), *Communication disorders in multicultural and international populations* (4th ed., pp. 243–278.). Elsevier.

Xin, J. F., & Leonard, D. A. (2015). Using iPads to teach communication skills of students with autism. *Journal of Autism and Developmental Disorders, 45*, 4154–4164.

Yang, H., & Gray, S. (2017). Executive function in preschoolers with primary language impairment. *Journal of Speech, Language, and Hearing Disorders, 60*, 379–392. https://doi.org/10.1044/2016_JSLHR-L-15-0267

Yee Mikami, A., Münch, L. P., &, Hudec, K. L. (2018). Associations between peer functioning and verbal ability among children with and without attention-deficit/hyperactivity disorder. *Journal of Emotional and Behavioral Disorders, 26*, 93–105.

Ylvisaker, M., & DeBonis, D. (2000). Executive function impairment in adolescence: TBI and ADHD. *Topics in Language Disorders, 20*(2), 29–57.

Yoder, P., Fey, M., & Warren, S. (2012). Studying the impact of intensity is important but complicated. *International Journal of Speech-Language Pathology, 14*, 410–413.

Yoder, P. J., & McDuffie, A. (2002). Treatment of primary language disorders in early childhood: Evidence of efficacy. In P. Accardo, B. Rogers, & A. Capute (Eds.), *Disorders of language development* (pp. 151–177). York Press.

Yoder, P. J., Molfese, D., & Gardner, E. (2011). Initial mean length of utterance predicts the relative efficacy of two grammatical treatments in preschoolers with specific language impairment. *Journal of Speech, Language, and Hearing Research, 54*, 1170–1181.

Yoder, P. J., & Stone, W. L. (2006). A randomized comparison of the effect of two prelinguistic communication interventions on the acquisition of spoken communication in preschoolers with ASD. *Journal of Speech, Language, and Hearing Research, 49*(4), 698–711. https://doi.org/10.1044/1092-4388(2006/051)

Yoder, P. J., & Warren, S. F. (2002). Effects of prelinguistic milieu reaching and parent responsivity education on dyads involving children with intellectual disabilities. *Journal of Speech, Language, and Hearing Research, 45*, 1158–1174.

Yoder, P. J., Watson, L., & Lambert, W. (2015). Value-added predictors of expressive and receptive language growth in initially nonverbal preschoolers with autism spectrum disorders. *Journal of Autism and Developmental Disorders, 45*(5), 1254–1270. https://doi.org/10.1007/s10803-014-2286-4

Young, E., Diehl, J., Morris, D., Hyman, S., & Bennetto, L. (2005). The use of two language tests to identify pragmatic language problems in children with autism spectrum disorders. *Language, Speech, and Hearing Services in Schools, 36*, 62–72.

Yu, B. (2013). Issues in bilingualism and heritage language maintenance: Perspectives of minority-language mothers of children with autism spectrum disorders. *American Journal of Speech-Language Pathology, 22*, 10–24. https://doi.org/10.1044/1058-0360(2012/10-0078)

Yuan, H., & Dollaghan, C. (2018). Measuring the diagnostic features of social (pragmatic) communication disorder: An exploratory study. *American Journal of Speech-Language Pathology, 27*, 647–656.

Zambrana, I. M., Pons, F., Eadie, P., & Ystrom, E. (2014). Trajectories of language delay from age 3 to 5: Persistence, recovery and late onset. *International Journal of Language & Communication Disorders, 49*, 304–316. https://doi.org/10.1111/1460-6984.12073

Zimmerman, E. (2018). Do infants born very premature and who have very low birth weight catch up with their full-term peers in their language abilities by early school age? *Journal of Speech, Language, and Hearing Disorders, 61*, 53–65. https://doi.org/10.1044/2017_JSLHR-L-16-0150

Zimmerman, I. L., Steiner, V. G., & Pond, R. E. (2011). *Preschool Language Scale, Fifth Edition*. Pearson.

Zipoli, R. P., & Kennedy, M. (2005). Evidence-based practice among speech-language pathologists: Attitudes, utilization, and barriers. *American Journal of Speech-Language Pathology, 14*, 208–220.

Zubrick, S. R., Taylor, C. L., Rice, M. L., & Slegers, D. W. (2007). Late language emergence at 24 months: An epidemiological study of prevalence, predictors, and covariates. *Journal of Speech, Language, and Hearing Research, 50*, 1562–1592. https://doi.org/10.1044/1092-4388(2007/106)

Zwaigenbaum, L., Bryson, S. E., Rogers, T., Roberts, W., Brian, J., & Szatmaxi, P. (2005). Behavioural manifestations of autism in the first year of life. *International Journal of Developmental Neuroscience, 23*, 143–152.

Zwitserlood, R., van Weerdenburg, M., Verhoeven, L., & Wijnen, F. (2015). Development of morphosyntactic accuracy and grammatical complexity in Dutch school-age children with SLI. *Journal of Speech, Language, and Hearing Research, 58*(3), 891–905. https://doi.org/10.1044/2015_JSLHR-L-14-00157

Index

Note: Page numbers in **bold** reference non-text material.

A

AAC (Augmentative and alternative communication), 123, 144, 146–148
  assessment, 146–148
  children with autism spectrum disorder and, 143
  communication
    partners, children with autism spectrum
     disorder and, 150
    training program, 148
  early communication intervention model and, 144–155
    types of, 145
  evidence-based practice, 145–146
  intervention, 148–154
  language system, building, 153–154
  role of environment, 152
  symbolic assessment, 123
  teaching to caregivers, 152–153
  vocabulary, 150–152
AAE (African American English)
  dialect, 314–315, 342
  dialectal scoring, 343
  Gullah/Geechee) dialect influenced, 344
  grammatical patterns, analysis techniques, 344
Abbreviated episodes, story grammar analysis, 291
Abuse, language disorders and, 91–94
Academic
  attainment, language disorders and, 26
  preparation, lack of, 308
  success, predictors of, 318
Action sequences, story grammar analysis, 291
Activities
  classroom structured, 525
  preliterate, 520
AD/HD (Attention-deficit/hyperactive disorder), 72–74
  fetal alcohol spectrum disorder and, 75
Adolescents
  classroom demands, 517
  functional intervention, linguistic awareness in classroom, 524–526
  morphological markers and, 42

  sampling, 203–206
    conversational partners, 205–206
    topics, 206
  with developmental language disorders, 38
Adoptions, international, 113
Adults
  teaching, 137
  verbal control of interactions, 372
Adverbial
  conjuncts/disjuncts, 255–256
  subordinate clauses, 340
African American children, with low socioeconomic status backgrounds, 350
African American English (AAE)
  dialect, 314–315, 342
  dialectal scoring, 343
  GG-influenced, 344
  grammatical patterns, analysis techniques, 344
  SLP and, 307
Alcohol, infant abuse and, 91
Alexithymia, 94
Alternative assessment approaches, 344–345
American Association on Intellectual and Developmental Disabilities, 77
American English
  learning as second language, 306
  speaking (MAE) children, 306
  standardized tests, 328
American Psychiatric Association, *Diagnostic and Statistical Manual of Mental Disorders*, 50, 56
American Speech-Language-Hearing Association (ASHA), 3, 18, 419
Area assessment, 119
Articles, 481
ASD (Autism spectrum disorder), 3, 25
  augmentative and alternative communication and, 143
  causal factors, 64–66
  characteristics of, 58–59
  communication partners and, 150
  development, 57–58
  early communication intervention, 140–144
    model and, 109–110

ASD (Autism spectrum disorder) *(continued)*
  intervention, 58
    techniques, 421–422
  language
    characteristics, 59–63
    disorders and, 56–66
  reading and, 572–573
  risk factors, 59
  severities of, **57**
  vocabulary, 150–152
ASHA (American Speech-Language-Hearing
    Association), 3, 18, 419
Asperger's syndrome, 57
Assessment
  alternative approaches, 344–345
  approaches, descriptive, 168–173
  area, 119
  challenge of accurate, 314
  children
    presymbolic, 122–123
    symbolic, 123–125
  children with language disorders and, 174–193
    descriptive assessment approaches, 168–173
    integrated functional assessment strategy,
      174–193
    normal measures, 161–168
  communication
    organizing early language, 128–130
    steps, 129–130
  described, 119
  dynamic, 132, 192
  early communication intervention model and,
    118–133
    family, 120
    formal, 128
    infants with diverse backgrounds, 133
    informed communication, 120–128
    organizing early language, 128–133
    transdisciplinary model of, 119–120
  ELLs (English language learners), overcoming bias
    in, 319
  fast-mapping, 344
  importance of accurate, 319
  informal measures of, 331–342
  of information-processing skills, 341–342
  language, location of, 326
  measures
    normal, 161–168
    psychological vs. descriptive approaches,
      160–173
  model, for English language learners, 322–342
  play based interactional, 132

of preschool and school age children, 157–193
  descriptive assessment approaches, 168–173
  normal measures, 161–168
psychometric vs. descriptive approaches,
  descriptive assessment approaches, 168–173
Assistance, request for, 423
Attempts, story grammar analysis, 289
Attention
  call for, 422–423
  controlled, 46
  difficulties, 68
  intellectual developmental disorder and, 84
  information processing and, 29–30
Attention-deficit/hyperactive disorder (ADHD),
  72–74
  fetal alcohol spectrum disorder (FASD) and, 75
Augmentative and alternative communication,
  assessment, 146–148
  children with autism spectrum disorder and, 143
  communication
    partners, children with autism spectrum
      disorder and, 150
    training program, 148
  early communication intervention model and,
    144–155
    types of, 145
  evidence-based practice, 145–146
  intervention, 148–154
  language system, building, 153–154
  symbolic assessment, 123
  teaching to caregivers, 152–153
Autism Diagnostic Observation Schedule, 199
Autism spectrum disorder (ASD), 3, 25
  augmentative and alternative communication
    and, 143
  causal factors, 64–66
  characteristics of, 58–59
  communication partners and, 150
  development, 57–58
  early communication intervention, 140–144
    model and, 109–110
  early intervention, 58
  intervention techniques, 421–422
  language
    characteristics, 59–63
    disorders and, 56–66
  reading and, 572–573
  risk factors, 59
  severities of, **57**
  vocabulary, 150–152
Automaticity, working memory and, 471–472
Automobiles, traumatic brain injury and, 86

INDEX

737

Auxiliary verbs, 478
Awareness
  intervention for, **470**
  metapragmatic, 525–526
  morphological, 446–447
  taxonomic, 330

B

Backgrounds, diverse
  difference or disorder, 306–307
  language assessment
    child who is ELL, 316–321
    ELLs assessment model, 322–342
    model of, 346–350
  state of service delivery, 307–316
    lack of academic preparation, 308
    lack of assessment tools, 315–316
    unfamiliarity with, 308–315
Behavior regulation, children with language
    disorders and, 26
Behavioral factors
  ASD, 59
  assessment
    presymbolic, 122–123
    symbolic, 123–125
BESA (Bilingual English Spanish Assessment), 316
BESOS (Bilingual English Spanish Oral Screener),
    316
Bias, negative, countering, 343
Bilingual English Spanish Assessment (BESA), 316
Bilingual English Spanish Oral Screener (BESOS),
    316
Bilingual English–Spanish Assessment, 329
Bilingual Language Assessment Battery: Preschool
    Teacher Report, 323
Biological factors
  intellectual developmental disorder, 82
  learning/disabilities and, 70–71
  maltreatment and, 93
  specific language impairment, 43–44
Birth,
  preterm
    causes/consequences of, 116–118
    early communication intervention model and,
      115–118
    incidence of, 116
  weight, fetal alcohol spectrum disorder and, 75
Blended intervention, 135
Blindness
  defined, 112
  light perception, 112

Book sharing, interactive, 450–451
Brain
  executive function of, 31
  language disorders and, 27
Brain Injury Association of America, 86
Breakdowns, 404
Broca's area, language disorders and, 27
Buildups, 404
Bullying, children with language disorders and, 26

C

Call for attention, 422–423
Caregivers
  child interactions with, 121–122
  conversation style, 372–375
  early communication intervention model and,
    105
  interview of, 131
  speech language pathologist and, 505
  teaching augmentative and alternative
    communication to, 152–153
Casual chains, story organization, 286
CATALISE, 3
Causal factors
  attention deficit/hyperactive disorder and, 73
  communication impairments, 108
  intellectual developmental disorder, 82, **83–84**
  of language disorders, 3
  learning/disabilities and, 70–71
  maltreatment and, 93–94
  neurocognitive disorders and, 90–91
CBLI (Curriculum-based intervention model),
    513–518
  barriers to, classroom demands, 515
  instructional approaches, 517–518
CCPs (Childhood care providers). *See* Caregivers
CCSS (Common core state standards), 497–498
CD (Clausal density), 295
CDC (Centers for Disease Control and Prevention),
    prevalence of ASD, 56
CEF (Central executive function), brain, 31
Centers for Disease Control and Prevention (CDC),
    prevalence of ASD, 56
Central executive function (CEF), brain, 31
Central nervous system, anatomy/function of,
    attention deficit/hyperactive disorder and, 74
Cerebral palsy
  characteristics/causes of, **111**
  early communication intervention model and,
    111–112
  intellectual developmental disorder and, 77

Cerebrovascular accident (CVA), 86, 90
Certification programs, Columbia University, 308
Channel availability, conversations, 252
Chemicals, prenatal/postnatal exposure to, 26
Childhood
   care providers (CCPs). *See* Caregivers
   schizophrenia, 96–97
Children
   actively involve, 362
   African American
     with low socioeconomic status backgrounds
      backgrounds,314, 350
   assessment of
     descriptive assessment approaches, 168–173
     normal measures, 161–168
   caregiver interactions with, 121–122
   classroom support of, 539–543
   communication deficits and, 102
   from culturally linguistically diverse backgrounds,
     375–378
   developmental trajectories, 24–25
   with developmental language disorders, 38, **39**
   developmental language disorders and
     morphology and, 42
     pragmatics, 40
     semantics, 40–42
     syntax and, 42
   early communication intervention model and,
     105, 108–118
     established risk, 108–113
     individualized, 106
     at risk, 113–118
   ELLs (English language learners), language
     disorders characteristics, **324**
   integrated functional assessment strategy
     dynamic assessment, 192
     formal language testing, 180–188
     related cognitive factors assessment, 188–192
     sampling, 192–193
   interview questions, with Culturally linguistically
     diverse backgrounds, **327–328**
   presymbolic behaviors, 122–123
   psychometric vs. descriptive approaches, 160–173
     descriptive assessment approaches, 168–173
     normal assessment measures, 161–168
   social communication disorder, language
     characteristics, 51
   spontaneous verbalizations, 374
   talking with, 537–539
   with ASD, language characteristics, **61**
   with language impairment, recognizing, **506**
   with late-emerging language, 24

   with learning disability, language characteristics,
     69
Children's literature, use of, 523–524
Children's Test of Nonword Repetition, 190
Choice making, 407
CINAHL, 18
Classification of Functioning, Disability and
     Health (WHO), international classification
     framework, 159–160
Classroom
   aids, speech language pathologist and, 505
   demands, 515–517
     adolescents, 517
     critical thinking, 515–516
     listening skills, 516
     oral language, supporting written, 516–517
   facilitation of language, 527–536
   functional intervention, 513
     see also Functional intervention
   instructional strategies, **519**
   linguistic awareness, 524–525
   structured activities, 525
   support of children, 539–543
Clausal density (CD), 295
Clauses, relative, 488
CLD (Culturally linguistically diverse) backgrounds
   children with, 488–491
     SLP (Speech language pathologist) errors and,
      307
     syntax/morphology and, 488–491
CLSA (computer-assisted language sample analysis),
     301–303
Cocaine, drug exposed infants and, 75
Code switching, linguistic, 332
Cogmed Working Memory Training, 471
Cognitive deficits
   described, 88
   factors, assessment of related, 180–188
Cognitive considerations
   intervention techniques, 418–420
     information processing, 419–420
Cohesion
   intervention techniques, 442–443
   types of, **340**
Cohesive devices
   conversations, 253–254
   microstructure devices, 296–300
   used in English, **254**
Collaborative teaching, 501–503
   training model for, **545**
Color, use of, 148
Columbia University, certification programs, 308

INDEX

739

Common core state standards (CCSS), 497–498
Communication
  ASD (Autism spectrum disorder) and, 60
  assessment
    organizing early language, 128–130
    steps, 129–130
  context dimensions of, 9–10
  described, 121
  event, described, 232–251
  first approach, 5
  forms/means of, 121
  impairments, causal factors, 108
  partners
    children with autism spectrum disorder
      and, augmentative and alternative
      communication), 150
    intervention team and, 371–372
  screening, 129
  social vs. nonsocial, 235–236
  success, 121
  training program, augmentative and alternative
    communication, 148
Communication and Symbolic Behavior Scales
    Behavior Sample (CSBS-BS), 128
Communication Disorders Quarterly, 316
Competing Language Processing Task, 191–192
Competing sources of input approach, exposure to
    grammatical targets, 389–390
Complete episodes, story grammar analysis, 291
Complex
  episodes, story grammar analysis, 291
  WM (Working memory), 191
Complexity, syntactic, 341
Comprehension
  attention and, 46–47
  children with developmental language disorders
    and, **39**
  deficits, reading and, 560–561
  intervention techniques, 443
Computer-aided analysis, SUGAR (Sampling
    Utterances and Grammatical Analysis
    Revised), 602
Concepts, culture and, 308
Conceptual scoring, 330
Congenital malformation, brain injury and, 86
Conjoined clauses, 485–488
Conjoining, 279, 282–283
Conjunctions, 459–461
  described, 255
Conjuncts, Adverbial, 255–256
Constructionism, 125
Constructionist patterns, **127**

Content
  communication context, 9
  generalization, 12
Context
  conversational, 382
  cues, 447–448
  elicitation, 201–202
  generalization, 12–13
Contextual support, continuum of, **207**
Contingency
  hierarchy of conversational, **410**
  pragmatic, 381
  requiring a response, 406
Contingent query, 408–409
Continuum of function, 33
Contrast teaching, 379
  described, 366
Contrastive stress, 256
Controlled attention, 191
Conversation, 201
  samples, language sampling and, 207–218
Conversational
  context, 382
  contingencies, hierarchy of, **410**
  milieu, 393–411
    focused stimulation, 397–398
    imitation, 398
    modeling, 393–397
    priming, 399
  narratives, 526
  partners, 205–206
    adolescent sampling, 205–206
    language sample analysis and, 256
  samples, 207–209
    evocative techniques, 209
    length of, 208–209
  techniques, evocative, 209
Conversational abilities
  intervention techniques, 427–435
    conversational repair, 433–435
    entering a conversation, 429–430
    presuppositions, 429–431
    referential skills, 431–433
    turn taking, 433
  repairs, 434–435
Conversations, 236–243
  breakdowns of, 247–249
  channel availability, 252
  cohesive devices, 253–254
    used in English, **254**
  entering, 428–430
  initiation, 236

Conversations *(continued)*
  maintenance, 236–237
  manipulating context, top-down teaching, 411–412
  reference, 254
  referential, 252–253
  repair of, 249–251
    strategy, 250–251
  termination, 237
  topics, 237–243
    analysis format, 237
    initiation, 237–240
    maintenance of, 241–242
    manner of, **240**
    termination of, 242–243
    types of, **239**
  turn taking, 244–247
    density, 245
    duration of, 246–247
    informativeness., 246
    overlap, 247
    sequencing, 246
    types of, **245**
Convulsive disorders, brain injury and, 86
Correction model/request, 406–407
Cortical anomalies, language disorders and, 27
Critical-thinking, 515
  classroom demands, 515–516
  tasks, 204
CSBS-BS (Communication and Symbolic Behavior Scales Behavior Sample), 128
CUBED Narrative Language Measures, 285
Cues
  nonlinguistic, 434
  teaching, 15
Cultural
  competence, defined, 309
  congruency, 312
  curriculum, 513
  humility, 310–311
  orientation continuum, 312
  variants, influence assessment of, **309**
Culturally diverse backgrounds
  difference or disorder, 306–307
  language assessment
    child who is ELL, 316–321
    ELLs assessment model, 322–342
    model of, 346–350
  reading and, 557–558
  state of service delivery, 307–316
    lack of academic preparation, 308
    lack of assessment tools, 315–316
    unfamiliarity with, 308–315

Culturally linguistically diverse (CLD) backgrounds, 488–491
  children with, 488–491
  SLP (Speech language pathologist) errors and, 307
Culturally responsive interaction, 138–139
Culture
  defined, 308
  early communication intervention model and, 104–105
  educating self on, 311–315
  infants with diverse backgrounds, 133
Cultures, 311–312
  unfamiliarity with diverse, 308–315
C-units, 268, **272**
Curricula, language-focused, 518
Curriculum, SLP (Speech language pathologist) and, 543
Curriculum-based intervention model (CBLI), 513–518
  barriers to, 515–517
  instructional approaches, 517–518
CVA (Cerebrovascular accident), 86, 90

D

DA (Dynamic assessment), 132, 337
  English language learners, 334–336
  of narrative ability, 341
Data
  analysis of, 132
    reading and, 568–569
  collection, reading assessment and, 564–568
  gathering, preplanning/preliminary, 130
DC (Direct consequences), story grammar analysis, 289
DD (Developmental disability), prevalence of, 101
De facto curriculum, 513
Deaf-blindness, early communication intervention model and, 112–113
Deafness, 97
  early communication intervention model and, 112–113
  prevalence of, 112
Decision
  of appropriateness, 235
  evidence-based practice, 17–19
  making/recommendations, 132–133
  points/paths, language assessment, **159**
Deductive teaching procedures, 367
Deictic skills, 211, 214–215
DELV-NR (Diagnostic Evaluation of Language Variation, Norm Referenced), 343

INDEX

DELV-ST (Diagnostic Evaluation of Language
    Variation–Screener Test), 346
Demographic factors, ASD, 59
Density, defined, 234–235
Department of Education, 306
Department of Housing and Urban Development,
    on homeless people, 314–315
Depression, language disorders and, 27
Descriptions, elicited, 201
Descriptive
    assessment approaches, psychological vs.
        descriptive approaches, 168–173
    story grammar analysis, 290
Development language disorders (DLD), 34–49
    causal factors, 43–45
        biological, 43–44
        processing, 44–45
        social-environmental, 44
    described, 36, 38
    dyslexia and, 563–564
    language characteristics, 38–42
        morphology and, 42
        pragmatics of, 40
        semantics, 40–42
        syntax and, 42
    linguistic context/functions and, 345
    predominance of, 44
    processing factors and, 44–49
    psychosocial adjustment, 37–38
    social-environmental factors and, 44
Developmental Disabilities Assistance and Bill of
    Rights Act, 101
Developmental
    disability (DD), prevalence of, 101
    outcomes, 24–26
    trajectories, children, 24–25
Developmental Reciprocity Treatment, **373**
Diagnostic and Statistical Manual of Mental Disorders,
    50, 56
Diagnostic categories
    language disorders, 3, 32–52
        broad groupings, 34
        continuum of function, 33
Diagnostic Evaluation of Language Variation
    Norm Referenced (DELV-NR), 343
    Screener Test (DELV-ST), 346
Dialects, 314
    seven forms of, 344–345
Diana v. State Board of Education, 315, 316
Direct
    access (DA), 337
        ELLs (English language learners), 334–336
    consequences (DC), story grammar analysis, 289

linguistic cues, 400–401
    mand model, 401
reference, 211
Directive
    intervention, 135
    styles, characteristics of, **373**
Discourse
    communication context, 9
    levels, of semantic complexity, **524**
    mode of, 9
    organization, 215
Discrimination
    intellectual developmental disorder and, 84–85
    information processing and, 30
    skills, working memory and, 71
Disjuncts, Adverbial, 255–256
Diverse backgrounds
    difference or disorder, 306–307
    language assessment
        child who is ELL, 316–321
        ELLs assessment model, 322–342
        model of, 346–350
    state of service delivery, 307–316
        lack of academic preparation, 308
        lack of assessment tools, 315–316
        unfamiliarity with, 308–315
DLD (Development language disorders), 34–49
    causal factors, 43–45
        biological, 43–44
        processing, 44–45
        social-environmental, 44
    described, 36, 38
    dyslexia and, 563–564
    language characteristics, 38–42
        morphology and, 42
        pragmatics of, 40
        semantics, 40–42
        syntax and, 42
    linguistic context/functions and, 345
    predominance of, 44
    processing factors and, 44–49
    psychosocial adjustment, 37–38
    social-environmental factors and, 44
DLL (Dual language learner), 306
DMMA (Dynamic Measure of Morphological
    Awareness), 192
Down syndrome (DS)
    intellectual developmental disorder and, 77, 79
    prevalence of ASD, 57
Drug exposed infants, 75–76, 91
DS (Down syndrome), 57
    intellectual developmental disorder and, 77, 79
    prevalence of ASD, 57

Dual language learner (DLL), 306
Duration, defined, 234
Dynamic assessment (DA), 132, 192
  English language learners, 334–336
  of narrative ability, 341
Dynamic Measure of Morphological Awareness
    (DMMA), 192
Dynamic procedures, 339
Dyslexia
  described, 67
  learning disorders and, 72
  reading and, 562–564
    assessment and, 570–572

E

Early
  language, semantic patterns, **126**
  syntax, 127–128
Early communication intervention (ECI), 128, 130
  augmentative and alternative communication
      assessment, 133, 146–148
      evidence-based practice, 145–146
      family, 120
      formal, 128
      infants with diverse backgrounds, 133
      informed communication, 120–128
      intervention, 148–154
      organizing early language, 128–133
      process, **130**
      transdisciplinary model of, 119–120
      vocabulary, 150–152
  augmentative/alternative, 144–155
  checklists, 133
  children served in, 108–118
    established risk, 108–113
    at risk, 113–118
  established risk, 108–113
  individualized
    for child, 106
    for family, 106
  intervention, 133–144
    children with ASD, 140–144
    culturally responsive, 138–139
    hybrid model, 139–140
    natural settings/partners, 135–137
    record keeping, 134
    strategies, 135
  legal basis for, 102–103
  model, 103–107
    cultural concerns, 104–105
    families and, 104

team approach, 104
  natural environment, 106–107
  optimal services, 135
  at risk children, 113–118
  SLPs role in, 107
  telehealth, 134
Early intervention (EI), 58, 102
  ASD, 58
  described, 102
  intervention, 573
EBP (Evidence-based practice), 17–19
  decision-making process, 17–18
  early communication intervention model and,
      145–146
Echolalia, 60
ECI (Early communication intervention) model,
      102, 145
  assessment, 118–133, 146–148
    families and, 104, 120
    formal, 128
    infants with diverse backgrounds, 133
    informed communication, 120–128
    organizing early language, 128–133
    process, **130**
    transdisciplinary model of, 119–120
  augmentative and alternative communication,
      144–155
    vocabulary, 150–152
  children served in, 108–118
    established risk, 108–113
  cultural concerns, 104–105
  established risk, 108–113
  evidence based practice and, 145–146
  individualized
    for child, 106
    for family, 106
  intervention, 133–144
    children with ASD, 140–144
    culturally responsive, 138–139
    evidence-based practice, 145–146
    hybrid model, 139–140
    natural settings/partners, 135–137
    record keeping, 134
    strategies, 135
    use of daily routines, 134
  legal basis for, 102–103
  model, 103–107
  natural environment, 106–107
  optimal services, 135
  at risk children, 113–118
  SLPs role in, 107
  team approach, 104

INDEX **743**

telehealth, 134
Educational changes, 497–503
    collaborative teaching, 501–503
    common core state standards, 497–498
    inclusion, 500–501
    response to invitation, 498–500
    outcomes, 24–26
EF (Executive function), 31
    described, 41
    working memory deficits, 41
Effective
    instruction, semantic, 448–452
    learners, 71
EI (Early intervention), 58, 102
    ASD, 58
    described, 102
Elaboration, 295, 462
    verb phrase 484
Elicitation
    Intentions, **212–214**
    of morphosyntactic features, **217**
Ellipsis, defined, 200, 255
ELLs (English language learners), 306
    academic success predictors of, 318
    dynamic assessment, 336
    identified, 317–319
    integrated assessment model, 322–342
        assessing, 326–342
        assessment preparation, 325–326
        pre-evaluation process, 323–325
    language
        assessment of, 316–319
        differences and, 3
        disorders and, characteristics of children with,
        324
    narrative analysis, 334–336
    test scores and, 307
ELOs (Embedded learning opportunities), 519–520
Embedded
    clauses, 485–488
        embedded/conjoined, 485–488
    learning opportunities, 519–520
Embedding, 279, 282–283
Emerging, language disorders, 25
Emotional
    awareness/expression, teaching, **426**
    difficulties, 68
Employment, language disorders and, 26
EMT (Enhanced milieu training), 137
    en Español, 137
Encephalopathy, brain injury and, 86
English-based tests, 315

English language learners (ELLs), 306
    dynamic assessment, 334–336
    identified, 317–319
    integrated assessment model, 322–342
        assessing, 326–342
        assessment preparation, 325–326
        pre-evaluation process, 323–325
    language
        assessment of, 316–319
        differences and, 3
    narrative analysis, 334–336
    screening tests, for English language learners,
        children and, 325
    test scores and, 307
English-language screening tests, English language
        learning child and, 325
English morphological errors, **334**
Enhanced milieu training (EMT), 137
Episode knowledge, narrative structure, 439–440
Episodes, story grammar analysis, 291
Equality, defined, 310
Equity, defined, 310
ERIC, 18
Error repetition/request, 408
Established risk
    early communication intervention, 108–113
    examples, **109**
Ethnographic analysis, **235**
Evaluation of Response to Intervention Practices for
        Elementary School Reading, 499
Evaluations, described, 119
Evidence-based practice (EBP), 17–19
    augmentative and alternative communication,
        145–146
    decision-making process, 17–18
Executive function, 31
    described, 41
    working memory deficits, 45–48
Expansion request, 409
Explicit instruction
    manipulating context and, 391–393
    semantic, 452
Expository discourse, 204
Expressive elaboration, 295
Expressive Vocabulary Test, 346
Extension, 403

F

Fables, 204
Facilitation, of language, classroom requirements,
        527–536

Facilitators, language, 14–15
Falls, traumatic brain injury and, 86
Familial risk factors, 26
Families
  culturally diverse, interaction guidelines, **376**
  events, scripts found in, 362
  from culturally linguistically diverse backgrounds, 375–378
  early communication intervention model and, 104, 106
FASD (Fetal alcohol spectrum disorder), 74–75
  early communication intervention model and, 114–115
  international adoptions and, 113
Fast ForWord Language, 471
Fast-mapping assessments, 344
Feedback, teaching adults, 137
Fetal alcohol spectrum disorder (FASD), 74–75
  early communication intervention model and, 114–115
  international adoptions and, 113
Figurative language, 267, 467–469
Figure-ground perception, 68
First phase syntax, 127
Five Intervention Principles for Verbal Working Memory, **541**
Fluharty Speech and Language Screening Test, 343
Fluid reasoning, 46, 191
Focused temporal chains, story organization, 286
Formal assessment, 128
Four-step teaching cycle, 340
Fragile X syndrome (FXS), 380
  gestures and, 122
  intellectual developmental disorder and, 77, 79
  morphology, 81–82
  pragmatics, 79–81
  semantics, 81
  syntax, 81–82
Fraternal twins, attention deficit/hyperactive disorder and, 74
Free-play sampling, 199, 201
Frequency data, defined, 234
Frog, Where Are You? 340
Functional intervention, 505
  approach, 5–6
  curriculum-based intervention model, 513–515
    barriers to, 515–517
    instructional approaches, 517–518
  classroom model elements, child at risk identification, 506–512
  curriculum-based, 513–518
  instituting classroom model, 543–547

language facilitation, 527–543
  classroom language requirements, 527–536
  classroom support for children, 539–543
  talking with children, 537–539
language intervention, language arts and, 505–506
linguistic awareness in classroom, 518–526
  adolescents, 524–526
  preschool, 518–524
  school-age, 524–526
recent educational changes, 497–503
  collaborative teaching, 501–503
  common core state standards, 497–498
  inclusion, 500–501
  response to invitation, 498–500
SLP's role, 503–505
Functional intervention model
generalized variables, 363–382
  contingencies, 380–381
  language teachers, 370–379
  location, 381–382
  teaching cues, 379–380
  teaching items, 365–367
  teaching method, 367–370
  teaching targets, 364–365
guidelines, 357–363
  actively involve child, 362
  be a reinforcer, 358–359
  closely approximate natural learning, 359
  first design a generalized plan, 363
  follow child's lead, 360–361
  follow developmental, 359–360
  influence of context on language, 362
  scripts use in family events, 362
Functional target selection, 13
Future tense, 478
FXS (Fragile X syndrome), 380
  gestures and, 122
  intellectual developmental disorder and, 77, 79
  morphology, 81–82
  pragmatics, 79–81
  semantics, 81
  syntax, 81–82

G

GEM model of working memory, 45–46
Generalization, 5
  content, 12
  context, 12–13
  factors affecting, 11
  in intervention, 10–17
    lack of, 10

INDEX

lack of, 364
optimum, 14
plan format, **363**
variables, 11–17, 364–382
  categories of, 12–13
Generalized variables
  functional intervention model, 363–382
    contingencies, 380–381
    language teachers, 370–379
    location, 381–382
    teaching cues, 379–380
    teaching method, 367–370
    teaching targets, 364–365
Genetics, attention deficit/hyperactive disorder
  and, 74
Gesture comprehension
  ASD, 60
  TDL, 60
GG (Gullah/Geechee) dialect, 344
Google, 18
Google Cloud Speech, 225
GOs (Graphic organizers), 542–543
GoTalk 4+, 150
Graduated prompting, 336
Grammatical targets
  exposure to, 389–391
    competing sources of input approach,
      389–390
    high variable approach, 390–391
    input informativeness approach, 389
  utterances, percent, 272
Graphic organizers (GOs), 542–543
Group sessions, peer, 371
Guidelines, narrative structure, 437–438
Gullah/Geechee (GG) dialect, 344

H

Head blows, traumatic brain injury and, 86
Heaps, story organization, 286
Hepatitis B & C, international adoptions and, 113
Heritage language, maintenance of, 324
Hidden curriculum, 513
Hierarchy, 410
  of conversational contingencies, **410**
High
  point analysis, 287–288
  variable approach, exposure to grammatical
    targets, 390–391
Home
  based intervention, 106
  review, enhanced, 446

Homeless, 314
  parents empowered by intervention, 375
Homework monitoring, 539
Hybrid model, early communication intervention,
  139–140
Hypotheses, formulating, 132

I

ICF (international classification framework),
  159–160
ICF-CY (International Classification of Functioning,
  Disability and Health–Children and Youth),
  317
IDD (Intellectual developmental disorder), 33, 109
  aspects of, 76
  biological factors, 64, 82
  causal factors, 82, **83–84**
  children with, 360
  differences in, 77
  established risk and, 108
  fetal alcohol spectrum disorder and, 75
  focus groups, 79
  language and, 79
    characteristics, 79–82
    disorders and, 76–86
  morphology and, 81–82
  mothers of children with, 82
  narrative samples and, 218
  processing factors, 65, 84–86
    attention and, 84
    discrimination and, 84–85
    memory and, 85
    organization and, 85
    transfer and, 86
  severity of, **78**
  social-environmental factors of, 82
  socioeconomic status and, 77
  syntax and, 81–82
  tests and, 188
IDEA (Individuals with Disabilities Education Act),
  66, 102
  guidelines, 325
  principles of intervention, 103
  response to intervention and, 498
Identification, teaching steps in, 435
IE (Initiating event), story grammar analysis, 289
IFSP (Individualized Family Service Plan), 106
Imaginative language, 520–521
Imitation, 403
  conversational milieu, 398
Incidental teaching, 135

Inclusion philosophy, 500–501
Indirect
  linguistic cues, 401–402
  reference, 211
Individualization, importance of, 13
Individualized Family Service Plan (IFSP), 106
Individuals with Disabilities Education Act (IDEA), 102
  guidelines, 325
  principles of intervention, 103
  RTI (Response to intervention) and, 498
Individuals with Disabilities Education Improvement Act, 500
Infants
  with diverse backgrounds, 133
  drug exposed, 75–76
  low-birth-weight, early communication intervention model and, 115–118
  preterm, early communication intervention model and, 115–118
Infection, brain injury and, 86
Inferencing, 552–553
  reading and, language disorders and, 561
Infinitives
  developmental language disorders and, 42
  top-down model of intervention, **486–487**
Inflections, morphological, 42
Informal assessment measures, 331–342, 348–350
Information
  processing, 29–31, 189
    assessment of skills of, 341–342
    cognitive considerations, intervention techniques, 419–420
  request for, 423–424
Initiation, conversations, 236
Initiating event (IE), story grammar analysis, 289
Input informativeness approach, exposure to grammatical targets, 389
Instituting classroom model, functional intervention, 543–547
Instruction
  effective, semantic, 448–452
  explicit, semantic, 452
  multimodality, 450
  teach-model-coach-review approach, 137
Instructional strategies, **519**
Integrated assessment model, 322–342
Integrated functional strategy, 174–193
  dynamic assessment, 192
  formal language testing, integrated functional assessment strategy, 180–188
  psychological vs. descriptive approaches, 174–193
    observation, 177–179

referral/screening/questionnaire/interview, 175–177
  related cognitive factors assessment, 188–192
  sampling, 192–193
Integrated Model for Assessment of ELLS, 322–342
  assessing, 326–342
    formal tests/measures, 325–331
    informal assessment measures, 331–342
  assessment preparation, 325–326
  pre-evaluation process, 323–325
Intellectual developmental disorder (IDD), 33, 109
  aspects of, 76
  biological factors, 64, 82
  causal factors, 82, **83–84**
  children with, 360
  differences in, 77
  established risk and, 108
  fetal alcohol spectrum disorder and, 75
  focus groups, 79
  language and, 79
    characteristics, 79–82
    disorders and, 76–86
  morphology and, 81–82
  mothers of children with, 82
  narrative samples and, 218
  pragmatics, 81, **420**
  progressing factors of, 65, 84–86
    attention and, 84
    discrimination and, 84–85
    memory and, 85
    organization and, 85
    transfer and, 86
  severity of, **78**
  social-environmental factors of, 82
  socioeconomic status and, 77
  syntax and, 81–82
  tests and, 188
Intentions
  elicitation, **212–214**
  intervention techniques, 422–427
    call for attention, 422–423
    pragmatics, 422–427
    request for assistance, 423
    request for information, 423–424
    request for objects, 424
    statements, 427
  language use, 258–261
    age of mastery, **260**
    of children, **259**
Interaction, culturally responsive, 138–139
Interactional observation, 131
Interactive
  book sharing, 450–451

episodes, story grammar analysis, 291
style, guide for, parents'/teachers,' **537**
Internal plan (IP), story grammar analysis, 289
Internal response (IR), story grammar analysis, 289
International adoptions, 113
International classification framework (ICF), 159–160
International Classification of Functioning, Disability and Health–Children and Youth (ICF-CY), 317
Internet, use of, 18
Interpreters, use of, 319–320
Intervention
  approaches
    communication-first, 5
    comparison of, **7**
    early, verbal, **124**
    functional, 5–6
    home-based, 106
    hybrid model, 139–140
    pragmatics role in, 6–8
    traditional, 4–5
  approximate natural learning, 359
  for awareness, **470**
  contexts of, 362
  early communication intervention model and, 133–144
    use of daily routines, 134
  enables SLP to, 357
  generalization in, 10–17
    lack of, 10
  language, 11
  natural settings/partners, 135–137
  parent
    assisted blended, 422
    implemented language, 375
  peer, 371
  principles, Individuals with Disabilities Education Act, 103
  purposes of, 355
  reading, language-based, 573–595
  semantic, 445
  stimulus-response-reinforcement of, 4
  strategies/techniques, synchrony of, 312
  for working memory, **470**
  for writing, 605–613
Intervention techniques
  cognitive considerations, 418–420
    information processing, 419–420
  conversational abilities, 427–435
    conversational repair, 433–435
    entering a conversation, 429–430
    presuppositions, 429–431
    referential skills, 431–433

    turn taking, 433
  microcomputer use and, 491–492
  morphology, 472–482
  narration, 436–443
    cohesion, 442–443
    structure, 436–442
  pragmatics, 421–443
    autism spectrum disorder, 421–422
    intentions, 422–427
    social skills, 421–422
  semantics, 444–453
    categories/relational webs, 454–461
    comprehension, 466–467
    contextual cues, 447–448
    effective instruction, 448–452
    explicit instruction, 452
    figurative language, 467–469
    morphological awareness, 446
    networks, 447
    verbal working memory, 469–472
    vocabulary, 444–453
    word meaning, 444–453
    word retrieval /categorization, 461–466
    word selection, 445–446
  syntax, 472–488
Interview
  integrated functional assessment strategy, 175–177
    format, **178–179**
  questions, children with culturally linguistic diverse backgrounds, **327–328**
Intestinal parasites, international adoptions and, 113
Iodine insufficiency, international adoptions and, 113
IP (Internal plan), story grammar analysis, 289
IR (Internal response), story grammar analysis, 289
Irregular verbs, **282**

J

Journal of Speech and Hearing Research, 3
Journal of Speech, Language, and Hearing Research, 3

K

"Konglish" (Korean–English), 329

L

Labels, discussed, 32–33
Language, 2–4
  autism spectrum disorder and, 60

748 LANGUAGE DISORDERS: A FUNCTIONAL APPROACH TO ASSESSMENT AND INTERVENTION IN CHILDREN

Language *(continued)*
  assessment
    aspects of, 180–187
    decision points/paths, **159**
    location of, 326
  characteristics of, 68–70
  comprehension, 41, 466–467
  dialects, 314
  early, semantic patterns, **126**
  educating self on, 311–315
  external, 540–541
  facilitation, 527–543
    classroom requirements, 527–536
    talking with children, 537–539
  facilitators, 14–15
  figurative, 267, 467–469
  heritage, maintenance of, 324
  imaginative function of, 520–521
  influence of context on, 362
  of language, talking with children, 537–539
  literacy play, 38
  literate, 295–296
  models
    peers as, 538–539
    of related aspects of, **8**
  oral, difficulties, 72
  organizing early, assessment, 128–130
  play, 38
  processing, 41
  quantitative measures of, **271**
  sampling, 331–332
    collecting guidelines, **332**
  setting contexts, 198–206
    conversational partners, 205–206
    settings and tasks, 199–205
  social tool of, 2, 14
  standardized assessment, scoring procedures,
    343
  as a visual mode
    intervention, 505–506
    language arts, 505–506
    reading, 551–564
    writing, 595–613
  verbal working memory and, 48–49
Language and Language Behavior Abstracts (LLBA),
  18
Language
  assessment, of NMAE (Non-mainstream American
    English), 341–342
  characteristics
    attention deficit/hyperactive disorder, 73
    ASD, 59–63

    drug exposed infants and, 76
    intellectual (and, 79–82
    maltreatment and, 92, **93**
    neurocognitive disorders and, 88–89
  development, preschool children, **280–281**
  difference, 3
  focused curricula, 518
  form, language samples and, 216–218
  functions, situations with potential to elicit a
    variety of, **210**
  impairment, recognizing children with, **506**
  intervention, 11
  knowledge in LTM, 195
  learning, dialects, 314
  skills, needed in first three grades, **509–510**
  teachers/teaching, 370–379
    strategy, effectiveness of, 6
    techniques, **394–396**
  testing, formal, integrated functional assessment
    strategy, 180–188
Language-based intervention
  reading and, 573–595
    early literacy, 573
    preschool children, 574–581
    school-age children, 581–595
  writing
    extended writing, 605–609
    sentence construction/composition, 612–613
    spelling, 609–612
Language disorders, 2–4, 306
  academic attainment and, 26
  ASD, 56–66
    characteristics of, 58–59
    development, 56–57
    language characteristics, 59–63
    risk factors, 59
  aspects of, 28–29
  casual
    categories of, 3
    factors of, 3
  categories of, **35**
  co-occurrence of, 2
  defined, 3
  diagnostic categories, 3, 32–52
    broad groupings, 34
    continuum of function, 33
  implications of, 98
  intellectual developmental disorder and, 76–86
  intervention approaches, traditional, 4–5
  language awareness, contribution to, 559–560
  learning/disability/specific learning disorder and,
    66–76

attention deficit/hyperactive disorder, 72–74
causal factors, 70–71
described, 66–68
drug/alcohol exposure, 74–76
dyslexia, 72
language characteristics, 68
LLE (late language emergence), 95–96
long-term effects of, 25
maltreatment, 91–94
neurocognitive disorders and, 86–91
neurology and, 27–28
outcomes, developmental/educational, 24–26
pragmatic, 73
prevalence of, 23–24
reading and, 558–564
comprehension deficits, 560–561
inferencing deficits, 561
risk factors, 26–29
Language Exposure Assessment Tool (LEAT), 323
Language facilitation
functional intervention, 527–543
classroom language requirements, 527–536
classroom support for children, 539–543
Language sample analysis (LSA)
described, 232
levels of, **233–234**
communication event, 232–251
methods, **257–258**
traditional, 232
within utterances, 256–284
conjunction, 265–266
content, 261–265
conversational partners and, 256
form, 268–284
language use, 256–261
lexical diversity, 262–264
lexical items, 261–262
negatives, 266–267
passive voice, 267
prepositions, 267
word finding, 267
word relationships, 264
Language sampling
child awareness, 198
collecting, 207–223
conversation samples, 207–218
narrative samples and, 218–223
collecting written samples, 224
extent of language of, 196
planning, 196–206
representativeness of, 196–197
sampling contexts, 198–206

recording samples, 224
transcribing samples, 224–228
utterances, 226–228
Language use, 256–261
disruptions, 256, 258
intentions, 258–261
age of mastery, **260**
of children, **259**
Languages
testing in both, 321
unfamiliarity with diverse, 308–315
Large samples, collecting, 207–218
Larry P. v. Riles, 315, 316
Late language emergence (LLE), 95–96, 108
early communication intervention model and,
114
Late
emerging language, 24
late talkers, 24
Latency, defined, 234
Latino/Latina communities, collectivist values of,
312
LD (Learning disability)
defined, 67
described, 67–68
Lead, exposure to, 26
Learners, effective, 71
Learning, generalization in, 11
Learning disability (LD), 66–67
defined, 67
described, 67–68
Least
LRE, 103, 134
prompts, system of, 379, 411
LEAT (Language Exposure Assessment Tool), 323
Lexical similarity, 446
Light perception, blindness, 112
Linguistic
awareness, classroom, 524–525
code switching, 332
cues
direct, 400–401
indirect, 401–402
devices, 253
forms, targeted, 14
systems, miniature, **483**
Linguistic contexts
manipulating context, 389–411
common ground, 391–393
exposure to grammatical targets, 389–391
Linguistically diverse background
difference or disorder, 306–307

Linguistically diverse background *(continued)*
　language assessment
　　child who is ELL, 316–321
　　ELLs assessment model, 322–342
　　model of, 346–350
　state of service delivery, 307–316
　　lack of assessment tools, 315–316
　　unfamiliarity with, 308–315
Listening skills, classroom demands, 516
Literate language, 295–296
Literature, children's, use of, 523–524
LLE (Late language emergence), 95–96, 108
Location, of teaching, 16
Long-term memory (LTM), 45
　language knowledge in, 195
Low-birth-weight infants, early communication
　　intervention model and, 115–118
Low socioeconomic status (SES)
　African American children and, 314
　communication disorders and, 24
LRE (Least restrictive environment), 103, 134
LSA (Language sample analysis)
　described, 232
　levels of, **233–234**
　　across utterances and partners, 251–256
　　communication event, 232–251
　　within utterances, 256–284
　narrative analysis, 284–301
　traditional, 232
　within utterances, 256–284
　　conjunction, 265–266
　　content, 261–265
　　conversational partners and, 256
　　form, 268–284
　　language use, 256–261
　　lexical diversity, 262–264
　　lexical items, 261–262
　　negatives, 266–267
　　passive voice, 267
　　prepositions, 267
　　word relationships, 264
LTM (Long-term memory), 45
　language knowledge in, 195

M

*MacArthur–Bates Communicative Development
　Inventory* (MCDI), 128
　checklists, 133
Macrostructure analysis, 285–292
　high-point, 287–288
　narrative-level, 286–287

story grammar, 288–292
MAE (American English-speaking) children, 306
Maintenance, conversations, 236–237
Maltreatment
　early communication intervention model and,
　　114–115
　language disorders and, 91–94
Mand model, direct linguistic cues, 401
Manipulating context
　conversations, top-down teaching, 411–412
　linguistic contexts, 389–411
　　common ground, 391–393
　　contingencies, 402–411
　　conversational milieu, 393–411
　　direct linguistic cues, 400–401
　　exposure to grammatical targets, 389–391
　　indirect linguistic cues, 401–402
　nonlinguistic contexts, 385–389
Mass learning, 356
Materials, use of, 203
Maternal sensitivity, language disorders and, 27
MCDI (*MacArthur– Bates Communicative Development
　　Inventory*), 128
　checklists, 133
Mean length of utterance (MLU), 268–270
　in morphemes (MLUM), 373
Mean syntactic length (MSL), 268, 270
Meaning, defined, 444
Mediated learning experience (MLE), 336–337
　example of, **338**
MEDLINE, 18
Memory
　described, 71
　difficulties, 68
　intellectual developmental disorder and, 85
　information processing and, 30
　phonological, 470
　procedural, 44
　storage, 462
　working capacity, 471
Mental retardation. *See* Intellectual developmental
　　disorder (IDD)
Mercury, exposure to, 26
Meta-analysis, 17
Metacognitive terms, **512**
Metalinguistic terms, **512**
Metapragmatics, 525–526
Microcomputer, intervention techniques and,
　　491–492
Microstructure analysis
　cohesive devices, 296–300
　expressive elaboration, 295

measures, **294**
  quantitative measures of, 293–295
  literate language, literate language, 295–296
  narrative analysis, 293–300
Minimally directive verbal feedback to children, **374**
MLE (Mediated learning experience), 336–337
  example of, **338**
MLU (Mean length of utterance), 268–270
MLU^M (Mean length of utterance in morphemes), 373
Modeling, 149
Monitoring, homework, 539
Morbidity, defined, 115
Morphological
  analysis, narrative analysis and, 273–274
  assessment, DMMA (Dynamic Measure of Morphological Awareness), 192
  awareness, 446–447
    reading and, 569–570
  errors, most frequent in English, **334**
Morphology
  autism spectrum disorder and, 62–63
  children with developmental language disorders and, **39**
  FXS (Fragile X syndrome), 81–82
  intervention techniques, 472–482
  language, 70
  maltreatment and, 93
  neurocognitive disorders and, 90
  syntax and, 472–482
  verbs, 473–476
    phonological variations of endings, 476
    tenses, 473–476
Morphosyntactic features, elicitation of, **217**
Morphosyntax subtest, 329
Motor
  difficulties, 67–68
  vehicles, traumatic brain injury and, 86
MSL (Mean syntactic length), 268, 270
Multimodality instruction, 450
Mutism, selective, 97

N

Narration
  intervention techniques, 436–443
    structure, 436–442
Narrative
  analysis
    CLSA (computer-assisted language sample analysis), 301–303
    ELLs (English language learners), 334–336

language sample analysis, 284–301
  macrostructure, 285–292
  microstructure, 293–300
  morphological analysis and, 273–274
  reliability of, 300–301
  syntactic analysis, 274–275
  validity of, 300–301
development, preschool, 523
frames, 218–219
level analysis, 286–287
retells, narrative structure, 440
samples, 216–218
  intellectual developmental disorder and, 218
  language sampling and, 218–223
  prompting hierarchy for, **222**
structure, 436–442
  episode knowledge, 439–440
  guidelines, 437–438
  narrative retells, 440
  reminiscing, 438–439
teaching, steps in, **441**
test, 187
Narrative Assessment Protocol, 285
Narrative Language Measure (NLM), CUBED, 285
Narratives
  collecting, 219–220
  conversational, 526
  personal, 200
  personal event, 221–223
  retelling, 220–221
  story organization, 286–287
  structural properties of, **292**
  types of, **340**
National Center for Education Statistics, 518
National Library of Medicine, PubMed, 18
Natural
  environments, 106
  learning
    approximate, 359
    models, 359
Navajo culture, speech/language diversity and, 308
Negative bias, countering, 343
Neglect
  children with language disorders and, 26
  early communication intervention model and, 114–115
  language disorders and, 91–94
Networks
  semantic, 445
  semantics, 447
Neurocognitive disorders, 86–91
  causal factors and, 90

Neurocognitive disorders *(continued)*
  language characteristics and, 88–89
  morphology and, 90
  pragmatics and, 89
  semantics and, 89
  syntax and, 90
  traumatic brain injury, 86–90
Neurodevelopmental disorder, alcohol-related, 74
Neuroimaging, language disorders and, 27–28
Neurological factors, ASD, 59
Neurology, language disorders and, 27–28
NLM (Narrative Language Measure), CUBED, 285
NMAE (Non-mainstream American English), 306
  language assessment of, 341–342
    model, 346–351
  language profiles of, 307
Nonlinguistic
  contexts
    described, 386
    language elicitation and, **387–388**
    manipulating context, 385–389
  cues, 434
Non-mainstream American English (NMAE), 306
  language profiles of, 307
Nonsocial speech, described, 235
Nonverbal deficits, 56
Nonword repetition (NWR) tasks, 190
Nonword Repetition Task (NRT), 191
Noun phrase (NP), 275
  elaboration, 484
  elements of, **276**
NP (Noun phrase), 275
  elaboration, 484
  elements of, **276**
NRT (Nonword Repetition Task), 191

O

Objects, request for, 424
Observation
  features to note, **180**
  integrated functional assessment strategy, 177–179
  interactional, 131
  reliability of, 179
Official curriculum, 513
Open-ended questions, **131**
  using target word, 449
Oral
  language
    classroom demands, supporting written, 516–517
    difficulties, 72

sample, transcribing samples, 224–228
Organization
  discourse, 215
  intellectual developmental disorder and, 85
  information processing and, 30
Otitis media, 97
Outcomes, developmental/educational, 24–26

P

Parallel sentence production, 399
Parasites, international adoptions and, 113
Parents
  assisted blended intervention, 422
  early communication intervention model and, 105
  implemented language interventions, 375
  SLP (Speech language pathologist) nd, 505
  teaching, 375
Parkinson's disease, 86
Participant characteristics, communication context, 9
Particles, verb, 479
PECS (Picture Exchange Communication System), 148
Peer
  group sessions, 371
  intervention, 371
  as language models, 538–539
  social groups, 371
  as training facilitators, **539**
Persisting, language disorders, 25
Personal narratives, 200, 221–223
Personality changes, PTSD (Post-traumatic stress disorder) and, 88
Phonological
  STM (Short-term memory), 470
  awareness, reading and, 569
Phonology, children with developmental language disorders and, **39**
Picture Exchange Communication System (PECS), 148
Play
  based interactional assessment, 132
  described, 119
  training format for, 522
Plural pronouns, 480–481
Polychlorinated biphenyls, exposure to, 26
Post-traumatic stress disorder (PTSD), 88
Pragmatic
  contingency, 381
  language disorders, 73

INDEX

Pragmatics
  autism spectrum disorder and, 61–62
  children with developmental language disorders
    and, **39**, 40
  fragile X syndrome, 79–81
  intervention approaches and, 6–8
  intervention techniques, 421–443
    autism spectrum disorder, 421–422
    intentions, 422–427
    social skills, 421–422
  language, 69
    samples and, 209–215
  neurocognitive disorders and, 89
Perceptual difficulties, 68
Predictability, defined, 199
Preliterate activities, 520
Prenatal
  drug/alcohol exposure, 74–76
  environment, attention deficit/hyperactive
    disorder and, 74
Prepositions, 482
Preschool
  preliterate activities, 520
  replica/role-play, 520–522
  teachers, 378–379
Preschool children
  assessment of, 157–193
    descriptive assessment approaches, 168–173
    integrated functional assessment strategy,
      174–193
  children with developmental language disorders
    and, pragmatics, 40
  executive function deficits and, 47
  functional intervention, linguistic awareness in
    classroom, 524–526
  integrated functional assessment strategy
    dynamic assessment, 192
    formal language testing, 180–188
    related cognitive factors assessment, 188–192
    sampling, 192–193
  intervention, emerging-literacy, 574–581
  language development, **280–281**
  late-emerging language, 24
  psychometric vs. descriptive approaches,
    160–173
    descriptive assessment approaches, 168–173
    normal assessment measures, 161–168
  sampling, 201–203
Preservation, 68
Presuppositional skills, 211, 214–215
Presuppositions, 430
Presymbolic behaviors, children, 122–123

Preterm birth, 115
  causes/consequences of, 116–118
  incidence of, 116
  infants, early communication intervention model
    and, 115–118
Preverbal intentions, early, intervention, **124**
Priming, conversational milieu, 399
Primitive temporal narratives, story organization,
  286
Probes, testing/structured, 132
Procedural memory, 44
Procedures, dynamic, 339
Processes, information processing and, 30–31
Processing factors
  development language disorders, 44–49
  intellectual developmental disorder, 84–86
  learning/disabilities and, 71
Prompting, graduated, 336
Prompts, system of least, 379, 411
Pronouns, 480
  development language disorders and, 42
  plural, 480–481
Psychometric vs. descriptive procedures, 160–173
  descriptive assessment approaches, 168–173
  normal assessment measures, 161–168
PsycINFO, 18
PTSD (Post-traumatic stress disorder), 88
PubMed, 18
Purpose, communication context, 9

Q

Qualitative terms, 457
Quantitative
  measures, 268
    of language, **271**
  terms, 456–457
Questionnaire, 131
  integrated functional assessment strategy, 175–177
    format, **178–179**
Questions
  interview questions, children with Culturally
    linguistically diverse backgrounds, **327–328**
  open-ended, **131**
    using target word, 449

R

Rate, WM (Working memory) and, 471–472
Ratings, teacher, using Bilingual Language
    Assessment Battery: Preschool Teacher Report,
    323

754 LANGUAGE DISORDERS: A FUNCTIONAL APPROACH TO ASSESSMENT AND INTERVENTION IN CHILDREN

Reaction
story grammar analysis, 289
teaching steps in, 435
Reading, 551–558, 573–595
assessment of, 564–573
children with autism spectrum disorder and, 572–573
comprehension, 570
data collection, 564–568
dyslexia, 570–572
phonological awareness and, 569
comprehension/inferencing, 552–553
data analysis, 568–569
dyslexia and, 72, 562–564
familial risk factors, 26
intervention, language-based, 573–595
language disorders and, 558–564
comprehension deficits, 560–561
culturally diverse backgrounds and, 557–558
inferencing deficits, 561
morphological awareness and, 569–570
problems, 553–557
Reasoning, fluid, 46
Recast sentences, 404
Reciprocity, deficits in, 56
Record keeping, 134
Reduction error repetition/request, 407–408
Reference, defined, 254
Referential, conversations, 252–253
Referral
of children, **507**
integrated functional assessment strategy, 175–177
Reformulation, 403
Reinforcement rate, importance of, 149
Relational words, 455–456
Relationships, deficits in, 56
Relative clauses, 488
Reliability, 296–300
of narrative analysis, 300–301
Reminiscing, narrative structure, 438–439
Repairs, requests for, teaching, 434–435
Repetition request, 409
Repetitive motor movements, autism spectrum disorder and, 56
Replica
play themes, **521**
preschool, 520–522
Replying, 425–426
conversational, as reinforcers, 380
Requests
age and comprehension of, **211**
for repair, teaching steps in, 434–435

responding to, 424–425
Resolving, language disorders, 24–25
Response
contingencies requiring a, 406
interaction, 135
to intervention (RTI), 325, 498–500
response to, **498**
verbal, 15
Restricted, repetitive patterns of interest, behavior, or activity (RRIBs), autism spectrum disorder and, 56
Retells, narrative structure, 440
Risk
at-risk children, early communication intervention model and, 113–118
established
early communication intervention model and, 108–113
examples, **109**
factors
abuse/neglect, 91
caregiver, 91
language disorders, 26–29
Role-play, 201
preschool, 520–522
Routines, use of daily, 134
RRIBs (Restricted, repetitive patterns of interest, behavior, or activity), autism spectrum disorder and, 56
RTI (Response to intervention), 325, 498–500
response to, **498**
Rule
learning, 360
teaching approach, 368

S

Samples
collecting
large, 207–218
narrative, 218–223
conversational, 207–209
recording, 224
transcribing samples, 218–223
Sampling, 132, 192–193
free-play, 199
integrated functional assessment strategy, children with word disorders, 192–193
language. *see* Language sampling
Sampling Utterances and Grammatical Analysis Revised (SUGAR), 170, 198, 202, 270, 273
computer-aided analysis, 602

INDEX

designed for computers, 302
website, 277, 284
SCD (Social communication disorder), 49–52
causal factors, 52
language characteristics, 51
Scenes, use of, 148
Schizophrenia, childhood, 96–97
School
administrators, SLP (Speech language pathologist) nd, 505
culture curriculum, 513
School-age children
assessment of, 157–193
descriptive assessment approaches, 168–173
integrated functional assessment strategy, 174–193
with developmental language disorders, 38
functional intervention, linguistic awareness in classroom, 524–526
integrated functional assessment strategy
dynamic assessment, 192
sampling, 192–193
intervention, language-based reading intervention and, 581–595
psychometric vs. descriptive approaches, 160–173
descriptive assessment approaches, 168–173
normal assessment measures, 161–168
sampling, 201–203
Scoring, conceptual, 330
Screening
communication, 129
English-language tests, for English language learners, child and, 325
integrated functional assessment strategy, 175–177
Scripts, 218–219
found in family events, 362
Second language learning, 312–313
Seizures, intellectual developmental disorder and, 77
Selective mutism, 97
Self-correction request, 408
Semantic
categories, 454–461
classes, 454
complexity, discourse levels of, **524**
intervention, 445
networks, 445, 447
similarity, 446
teaching, 445
classes, 454
testing, Spanish–English for English language learners children, 329

Semantics
autism spectrum disorder and, 62–63
categories of, **266**
children with
culturally linguistically diverse backgrounds, 488–491
developmental language disorders and, **39**
feature similarities, analyzing, **449**
fragile X syndrome, 81
intervention techniques
categories/relational webs, 454–461
comprehension, 466–467
effective instruction, 448–452
explicit instruction, 452
figurative language, 467–469
morphological awareness, 446–447
networks, 447
verbal working memory, 469–472
vocabulary, 444–453
word meaning, 444–453
word retrieval /categorization, 461–466
word selection, 445–446
language, 69
samples and, 215–216
maltreatment and, 93
neurocognitive disorders and, 89
patterns, early language, **126**
subtest, 329
Semantic–syntactic rules, 125
Sensory integration, 68
Sentence
initial overlaps of, 247
parallel production, 399
types, word order and, 482–488
types of, 279
Sequence, defined, 235
story organization, 286
SES (Low socioeconomic status)
African American children and, 314
communication disorders and, 24
considerations with children from, 453
early communication intervention model and, 113–114
health and, 77
intellectual developmental disorder and, 78
Setting, communication context, 9
Settings statement, story grammar analysis, 289
Shape Coding system, 391
Short-term memory (STM), 45
intellectual developmental disorder and, 85
phonological, 470
Side-by-side teaching, 325

SKILL 441–442
SLD (Specific learning disorder), 66. *see also* Dyslexia
SLI (Specific language impairment), 35
SLP (Speech language pathologist)
  classroom functional intervention and, 503–505
  curriculum and, 543
  early communication intervention model and, 107
  evaluation errors made by, 307
  language sampling and, 197
    contrivance, 198
  prevalence of bilingual clients, 307
  training model for, **545**
Small-group instruction, 325
Soak Your Brain, 471
Social
  communication, 50
  communication disorder, 49–52
    causal factors, 52
    language characteristics, 51
  disinhibition, defined, 88
  groups, peer, 371
  interaction, autism spectrum disorder and, 60
  knowledge, 430
  Security Administration, Supplemental Security Income Program, communication disorders and, 24
  skills, intervention techniques, 421–422
  speech, described, 235
Social Thinking, 422
Social vs. nonsocial communication, 235–236
  environmental factors
    developmental language disorders and, 44
    intellectual developmental disorder and, 82
    learning/disabilities and, 71
    maltreatment and, 93–94
Sociodramatic, script training, **522**
Socioeconomic status (SES)
  health and, 77
  intellectual developmental disorder and, 78
Socioemotional problems, language disorders and, 26
Southern White English (SWE), dialectal scoring, 343
"Spanglish" (Spanish–English), 329
Spanish–English for English language learners children, semantic testing, 329
Spatial terms, 457–459
  common, **459**
Specific
  language impairment (SLI), 35
  learning disorder (SLD), 66. *see also* Dyslexia
    dyslexia as, 67

Speech disorders, co-occurrence of, 2
Speech language pathologist (SLP)
  classroom functional intervention and, 503–505
    classroom aids, 505
    parents/caregivers, 505
    school administrators, 505
    teachers, 503–504
  curriculum and, 543
  early communication intervention model and, 107
  evaluation errors made by, 307
  language sampling and
    contrivance, 198
    control, 197
  prevalence of bilingual clients, 307
  training model for, **545**
Spelling, assessment of, 603–605
Spidergram, 450, **451**
Spontaneous verbalizations, children and, 374
Sports injury, traumatic brain injury and, 86
Standardized
  language assessment, scoring procedures, 343
  tests, 146, 189
    careful use of, 342–343
    formal tests/measures, 346–347
Statistical learning, defined, 38
Stay, Play, Talk model, 150
Stimulation
  focused, conversational milieu, 397–398
  only approaches, 367
Stimulus-response-reinforcement models of intervention, 4
STM (Short-term memory), 45
  intellectual developmental disorder and, 85
  phonological, 470
Story
  grammar analysis, 288–292, **293**
    elements of, 289
    examples, **290**
  language sample analysis, 292
  organization, stages of, 286–287
  retelling, 201, 220
Strategies, intervention, 134
Stress, contrastive, 256
Stroke, 86, 90
Structural priming, 399
Structure, defined, 199
Structured
  activities, classroom, 525
  probes, 132
  TEACCHing, 422
Style switching, 251

INDEX   **757**

Stylistic variations, 251
Subcortical anomalies, language disorders and, 27
Subjective teacher ratings, using Bilingual Language
       Assessment Battery: Preschool Teacher Report,
       323
Subordinate clauses, adverbial, 340
SUGAR (Sampling Utterances and Grammatical
       Analysis Revised), 170, 202, 270, 273
   computer-aided analysis, 602
   designed for computers, 302
   website, 277, 284
Supplemental Security Income Program,
       communication disorders and, 24
Supporting Knowledge in Language and Literacy
       (SKILL), 441–442
SWE (Southern White English), dialectal scoring,
       343
Symbolic assessment, 123–125
Syntactic analysis, narrative analysis, 274–275
Syntactic complexity, measures of, 341
Syntax
   children with developmental language disorders
      and, **39**
   early, 127–128
   first phase, 127
   fragile X syndrome, 81–82
   intervention techniques, 472–488
   language, 70
   maltreatment and, 93
   morphology and, 472–482
   neurocognitive disorders and, 90
System of least prompts, 379, 411
Systems model, 517

T

Target word, open-ended questions using, 449
Targets, selection of functional, 13
Taxonomic
   approaches, 462–464
   awareness, 330
TBI (Traumatic brain injury), 3, 86–90
   symptoms of, 87
TDL (Typically developing language), 24, 108
   gesture comprehension, 60
   language disorders and, 25
   social confidence and, 38
Teach–model–coach–review instructional approach,
      137
Teacher ratings, using Bilingual Language
      Assessment Battery: Preschool Teacher Report,
      323

Teachers
   preschool, 378–379
   referral of children, **507**
   SLP (Speech language pathologist) nd, 503–504
Teaching
   ACC to caregivers, 152–153
   adults, 137
   cues, 15, 379–380
   deductive procedure, 367
   identification, 435
   incidental, 135
   items, 13–14, 365–367
   location of, 16
   model, four-step cycle, 340
   reaction, 435
   requests for repairs, steps in, 434–435
   semantic, 445
      classes, 454
   targets, 13, 364–365
Telehealth, 134
Temporal terms, 457–459
   common, **459**
Termination, conversations, 237
Test
   formal/measures, 326, 328–331
   modification, 187–188
   narrative, 187
Testing
   language, formal, 180–188
   probes, 132
Test-teach-retest, 336
Test–teach–test format, 132
Theory of mind (ToM), defined, 40
Top-down teaching, 411–412
Topics
   conversations, 237–243
      analysis format, 237
      initiation, 237–240
   initiation, 239
      manner of, **240**
      types of, **239**
   maintenance of, 241–242
   termination of, 242–243
Tourette syndrome, 34
Toys, use of, 203
Traditional intervention approaches, 4–5
Training model, for collaborating teachers/SLPs, **545**
Transcriber, 225
Transdisciplinary mode of assessment, 119–120
Transfer, intellectual developmental disorder and, 86
Traumatic brain injury (TBI), 3, 86–90
   symptoms of, 87

Trisomy 21. *See* Down syndrome (DS)
Tuberculosis, international adoptions and, 113
Tumors, brain injury and, 86
T-units, 268, 270, **272**
Turn taking
conversational abilities, 433–434
conversations, 244–247
density, 245
duration of, 246–247
latency, 246
overlap, 247
sequencing, 246
types of, **245**
topic rating format, **248**
Turnabouts, 409
variety of, **433**
Twins
attention deficit/hyperactive disorder and, 74
language disorders of, 44
Typically developing language (TDL), 24, 108
with developmental language disorders, 38
gesture comprehension, 60
language disorders and, 25
social confidence and, 38

U

Unfocused temporal chains, story organization, 286
University of Iowa, studies by, 2
U.S. majority culture, speech/language diversity and, 308
Utterance
boundaries, **226**
pairs, definitions/examples of, **243**
Utterances
defined, 207
grammatical percent, 272
sample, new structures likely in, **284**
transcribing, 226–228

V

Validity, of narrative analysis, 300–301
Variables
affecting generalization, 11–17
contingencies/consequences, 15–16
language facilitators, 14–15
location, 16
teaching clues, 15–16
teaching items, 13–14
teaching method, 14
teaching targets, 13

Vehicular accidents, traumatic brain injury and, 86
Verbal
intentions, early, preverbal, **124**
responses, 15
Verbal working memory (VWM), 45, 48, 341
assessment, 190–191
intellectual developmental disorder and, 85
language and, 48–49
Verbs
auxiliary, 478
BE, special cases for, 476–478
development language disorders and, 42
irregular, **282**
particles, 479
phrase (VP), 277–279
elaboration, 484
elements of, **278**
Vietnamese culture, speech/language diversity and, 308
Visual
stimuli, working memory resources and, 471
supports, working memory, 542
Vocabulary
augmentative and alternative communication, 150–152
acquisition, 444
Vocabulary Acquisition and Usage for Late Talkers methodology, 450
VP (Verb phrase), 277–279
elaboration, 484
elements of, **278**
VWM (Verbal working memory), 45, 48, 341
assessment, 190–191
intellectual developmental disorder and and, 85
language and, 48–49

W

Wernicke's area, 71
language disorders and, 27
WHO (World Health Organization), 103
ICF (international classification framework), 159–160
WM (Working memory), 31, 45, 189–190
capacity, 471
complex, 191
deficits, 45–48
discrimination skills and, 71
GEM model of, 45–46
intervention for, **470**
mechanisms, 47
visual supports, 542

INDEX **759**

Word
  finding, difficulties, 461
  knowledge, 444
  meaning, acquired by, 444
  order, sentence types and, 482–488
  pairs, comparative, **458**
  retrieval, 451, 464–466
    categorization, 461–462
Words
  culture and, 308
  finding, 267
  relational, 455–456
  short, developmental language disorders and, 42
Working memory (WM), 31, 45, 189–190
  capacity, 471
  complex, 191
  deficits, 45–48
  discrimination skills and, 71
  GEM model of, 45–46
  intervention for, **470**
  mechanisms, 47
  visual supports, 542
World Health Organization (WHO), 103

Writing, 595–605
  assessment of, 598–605
    data analysis, 600–602
    data collection, 598–600
    spelling, 603–605
  dyslexia and, 72
  familial risk factors, 26
  language-based intervention, 605–613
    extended writing, 605–609
    spelling, 609–612
Written language
  collecting samples for, 224
  supporting oral, 516–517

U

U.S. Department of Education, 306
U.S. Department of Housing and Urban
    Development, on homeless people, 314–315

Y

Young adults, social confidence of, 38